AF843681

To Dr Betty

With kindest regards
from Jayesh Mehta

Myeloma

Edited by

JAYESH MEHTA, MD
Professor of Medicine
Director, Hematopoietic Stem Cell Transplant Program
Division of Hematology/Oncology, Northwestern University Medical School
The Robert H Lurie Comprehensive Cancer Center of Northwestern University
Chicago, IL, USA

SEEMA SINGHAL, MD
Professor of Medicine
Director, Multiple Myeloma Program
Division of Hematology/Oncology, Northwestern University Medical School
The Robert H Lurie Comprehensive Cancer Center of Northwestern University
Chicago, IL, USA

MARTIN DUNITZ

First published in the United Kingdom in 2002
by Martin Dunitz Ltd, The Livery House, 7–9 Pratt Street, London NW1 0AE

Tel.: +44(0) 20 74822202
Fax.: +44(0) 20 72670159
E-mail: info@dunitz.co.uk
Website: http://www.dunitz.co.uk

A CIP record for this book is available from the British Library.

ISBN 1–901865–50–9

Distributed in the USA by:
Fulfilment Center
Taylor & Francis
7625 Empire Drive
Florence, KY 41042, USA
Toll Free Tel.: +1 800 634 7064
E-mail: cserve@routledge_ny.com

Distributed in Canada by:
Taylor & Francis
74 Rolark Drive
Scarborough, Ontario M1R 4G2, Canada
Toll Free Tel.: +1 877 226 2237
E-mail: tal_fran@istar.ca

Distributed in the rest of the world by
ITPS Limited
Cheriton House
North Way
Andover, Hampshire SP10 5BE, UK
Tel.: +44 (0)1264 332424
E-mail: reception@itps.co.uk

Composition by J&L Composition Ltd, Filey, North Yorkshire
Printed and bound in Spain by Tallers Grafics Soler, SA

Contents

Foreword

It is a great pleasure to introduce and preview this comprehensive new text on myeloma and related diseases. Three decades ago, when President Richard Nixon declared War On Cancer, the biology and treatment of myeloma could be covered in a few pages of an internal medicine textbook. In the 1970s and 1980s knowledge and interest increased, and longer chapters appeared in both medicine and hematology/oncology texts. Subsequently, several textbooks devoted entirely to myeloma have been published. However, the multi-author text co-edited by Jayesh Mehta and Seema Singhal is a very welcome addition. As they emphasize in their Preface, physicians, scientists and patients can greatly benefit from the detailed focus spanning 29 chapters. The international authorship is especially helpful in broadening the perspective and introducing nuances of opinion both about the understanding of the various disease entities as well as the treatment thereof.

For those interested in biology, the concise summary of molecular biology in Chapter 2 is especially useful. Likewise, the very comprehensive analysis of the potential involvement (or not) of Kaposi's sarcoma herpes virus (herpes virus 8) in the pathogenesis of myeloma illustrates the complexity of evaluating such associations. A whole chapter (Chapter 8) devoted to angiogenesis is valuable in considering new treatment modalities, even though the mechanisms underlying the clinical activity of thalidomide remain to be fully elucidated.

The basics of epidemiology, clinical features and prognostic factors are presented well. Chapters 12, 13 and 14 dealing respectively with neurological, renal and infectious complications of myeloma are extremely valuable. Written by experts in these subspecialty areas, they add substantially to the comprehensive value of the text. The role of imaging is a constant source of questions; thus a chapter devoted to that aspect is appreciated.

The six chapters (18–23) devoted to therapy cover current approaches to management extremely well, especially in the areas of high dose therapy and transplantation. For example, the discussion of one versus two transplants helps evaluate this ongoing controversy. With so many new treatments currently in clinical trials (e.g. PS (LDP) 341 and IMiDs), I can foresee one or two new chapters in future editions.

The final chapters (24–29) are a welcome aspect of this new volume, highlighting in some detail areas not frequently touched upon. Separate discussions of multicentric Castleman's and light chain deposition disease serve as important resources for those faced with these less common entities.

Overall, it is very reassuring to have a state of the art text to guide basic understanding and decision-making. I am sure that this will become a frequently consulted book, which can lead to better outcomes for patients living with myeloma and related diseases.

Brian G M Durie
Chairman, International Myeloma Foundation
Cedars-Sinai Comprehensive Cancer Center
Los Angeles, USA

Preface

New developments in molecular biology, immunology, cytogenetics, and imaging studies have changed our understanding of plasma cell disorders considerably over the last few years. With this has come much refinement of the clinical approach to patients with myeloma. From high-dose melphalan to thalidomide, to newer agents such as CC5013 and PS-341, the number of active treatment options available is increasing steadily. The availability of cytokines such as erythropoietin, and powerful bisphosphonates such as pamidronate and zoledronate, has contributed significantly to improved symptom control by ameliorating major complications of myeloma.

Despite all this, it appears that myeloma is probably not curable by any available therapy except an allogeneic hematopoietic stem cell transplant. Yet, with skilled, sequential use of various treatment steps, it is possible to obtain extended disease control with good quality of life.

We have attempted to deal with all aspects of myeloma and related diseases in this book to complement clinical practice as well as laboratory research. We hope that this volume will be useful to practicing physicians and scientists working in this field, and also to patients who desire deeper information about their disease.

We are very grateful to the distinguished international panel of experts who have contributed their knowledge and experience to this work. We hope that their insight will provide comprehensive information and stimulate further research in this disease.

Jayesh Mehta
Seema Singhal

Contributors

Julia Almeida, MD
Departmento de Medicina
Centro de Investigación del Cáncer
Universidad de Salamanca
Hospital Universitario de Salamanca
P. de San Vicente n° 58-182
Salamanca 37007
Spain

Kenneth C Anderson, MD
Dana Farber Cancer Institute
44 Binney Street
Boston, MA 02115-6084
USA

Edgardo JC Angtuaco, MD
Department of Radiology
University of Arkansas for Medical Sciences
4301 West Markham Street
Little Rock, AR 72205
USA

Ramesh Avva, MD
Department of Radiology
University of Arkansas for Medical Sciences
4301 West Markham Street
Little Rock, AR 72205
USA

Reiner Bartl, MD
Department of Internal Medicine III
Klinikum Grosshaden
University of Munich
Marchioninistrasse 15
81377 Munich
Germany

James R Berenson, MD
Department of Medicine
Hematology/Oncology
Cedars-Sinai Medical Center
8700 Beverly Blvd BM-1 Room 100
Los Angeles, CA 90048
USA

Amy Chadburn, MD
Department of Pathology
Cornell University
School of Medical Sciences
New York, NY 10021
USA

Helen Chapel, MB Bchir, MD, FRCP, FRCPath
Department of Clinical Immunology
Level 7
John Radcliffe Hospital
Headley Way
Headington
Oxford OX3 9DU
UK

William S Dalton, PhD, MD
Interdisciplinary Oncology
H Lee Moffitt Cancer Center
12902 Magnolia Drive
Tampa, FL 33612
USA

Franco Dammacco, MD
Department of Biomedical Sciences and Human Oncology
Section of Internal Medicine and Clinical Oncology
Policlinico
Piazza Giulio Cesare 11
I-70124 Bari
Italy

Meletios A Dimopoulos, MD
Department of Clinical Therapeutics
Alexandra Hospital
80 Vas. Sofias
Athens 11528
Greece

Angela Dispenzieri, MD
Division of Hematology and Internal Medicine
Mayo Clinic
200 First Street SW
Rochester, MN 55905
USA

Bertha Frisch, MD
Departments of Hematology and Pathology
Ichilov Hospital and Sackler School of Medicine
University of Tel Aviv 69978
Israel

Elke Fritz, MD
Department of Medicine and Oncology
Wilhelminenspital
Montleartstrasse
A-1171 Vienna
Austria

Glauco Frizzera, MD
Hematopathology Laboratory
NYU Presbyterian Hospital
East 68th Street, Room Starr 715
New York, NY 10021
USA

John Gibson, FRACP, FRCPA
Institute of Hematology
Royal Prince Alfred Hospital
Missenden Road
Camperdown, NSW 2050
Australia

Kenneth C Gorson, MD
Division of Neurology
St Elizabeth Hospital
736 Cambridge Street
Boston, MA 02135
USA

Phillip R Greipp, MD
Division of Hematology and Internal Medicine
Mayo Clinic Rochester
200 First Street SW
Rochester, MN 55905
USA

Morie A Gertz, MD
Division of Hematology and Internal Medicine
Mayo Clinic
200 First Street SW
Rochester, MN 55905
USA

Jean-Luc Harousseau, MD
Hematology Department
Hotel Dieu
Place Alexis Ricordeau
44035 Nantes
France

Guillermo A Herrera, MD
Department of Pathology
School of Medicine in Shreveport
LSU Medical Center
1501 Kings Highway
Shreveport, LA 71130-3932
USA

Theo Hronas, MD
Baptist Medical Center
Little Rock, AR 72205
USA

Sundar Jagannath, MD
Multiple Myeloma Service
St Vincent's Comprehensive Cancer Center
325 W 15th Street
New York, NY 10011
USA

Douglas E Joshua, FRACP, FRCPA
Institute of Hematology
Royal Prince Alfred Hospital
Missenden Road
Camperdown, NSW 2050
Australia

Peter Kelleher MB BS, PhD, MRCP, MRCPath
Department of Clinical Immunology
Level 7
John Radcliffe Hospital
Headley Way
Headington
Oxford OX3 9DU
UK

Bernard Klein, PhD
INSERM U475
99 Rue Puech Villa
34197 Montpellier, Cedex 5
France

Robert A Kyle, MD
Department of Laboratory Medicine and Pathology
Hilton 920
Mayo Clinic Rochester
200 First Street SW
Rochester, MN 55905
USA

Martha Q Lacy, MD
Division of Hematology and Internal Medicine
Mayo Clinic
200 First Street SW
Rochester, MN 55905
USA

Terry H Landowski, MD
Interdisciplinary Oncology
H Lee Moffitt Cancer Center
12902 Magnolia Drive
Tampa, FL 33612
USA

Henk M Lokhorst, MD, PhD
University Medical Center Utrecht
Department of Haematology
Heidelberglaan 100
3584 CX Utrecht
The Netherlands

Heinz Ludwig, MD
Department of Medicine and Oncology
Wilhelminenspital
Montleartstrasse
A-1171 Vienna
Austria

Jayesh Mehta, MD
Hematopoietic Stem Cell Transplant Program
Divsion of Hematology/Oncology
Northwestern University Medical School
Robert H Lurie Comprehensive Cancer Center
of Northwestern University
Chicago, IL 60611-4492
USA

Philippe Moreau, MD
Hematology Department
Hotel Dieu
Place Alexis Ricordeau
44035 Nantes
France

Angela Moulopoulos, MD
4 Ivis Street Ekali
Athens 14565
Greece

Alberto Orfao, MD
Servicio de Citometría
Departamento de Medicina
Centro de Investigación del Cáncer
Universidad de Salamanca
Hospital Universitario de Salamanca
P. de San Vicente n° 58-182
Salamanca 37007
Spain

Ray Powles, MD, FRCP, FRCPath
Leukaemia and Myeloma Units
Royal Marsden Hospital
Downs Road
Sutton
Surrey SM2 5PT
UK

Noopur Raje, MD
Dana Farber Cancer Institute
44 Binney Street
Boston, MA 02115-6084
USA

S Vincent Rajkumar, MD
Division of Hematology and Internal Medicine
Mayo Cancer Center
200 First Street SW
Rochester, MN 55905
USA

Domenico Ribatti, MD
Department of Human Anatomy and Histology
Policlinico
Piazza Giulio Cesare 11
I-70124 Bari
Italy

Allan H Ropper, MD
Division of Neurology
St Elizabeth Hospital
736 Cambridge Street
Boston, MA 02135
USA

Jesus F San Miguel, MD
Servicio de Hematología
Centro de Investigación del Cáncer
Hospital Universitario de Salamanca
P. de San Vicente n° 58-182
Salamanca 37007
Spain

Jeffrey R Sawyer, PhD
Cytogenetics Laboratory
Arkansas Children's Hospital
800 Marshall Street
Little Rock, AR 72202
USA

Seema Singhal, MD
Multiple Myeloma Program
Divsion of Hematology/Oncology
Northwestern University Medical School
Robert H Lurie Comprehensive Cancer Center
of Northwestern University
Chicago, IL 60611-4492
USA

Sudhir V Shah, MD
Division of Nephrology
University of Arkansas for Medical Sciences
4301 West Markham Street
Little Rock, AR 72205
USA

Mary Jo Shaver-Lewis, MD
Division of Nephrology
University of Arkansas for Medical Sciences
4301 West Markham Street
Little Rock, AR 772205
USA

Dennis C Shrieve, MD, PhD
Radiation Oncology
University of Utah School of Medicine
50 North Medical Drive
Salt Lake City, UT 84132-1801
USA

Bhawna Sirohi, MBBS, DCH
Leukaemia and Myeloma Units
Royal Marsden Hospital
Downs Road
Sutton
Surrey SM2 5PT
UK

Alan Solomon, MD
Human Immunology and Cancer Program
University of Tennessee
Graduate School of Medicine
1924 Alcoa Highway
Knoxville, TN 37920-6999
USA

Karin Tarte, PhD
INSERM U475
99 Rue Puech Villa
34197 Montpellier Cedex 5
France

Jennifer Treleaven, MD, FRCP, FRCPath
Leukaemia and Myeloma Units
Royal Marsden Hospital
Downs Road
Sutton
Surrey SM2 5PT
UK

Angelo Vacca, MD
Department of Biomedical Sciences and Human Oncology
Section of Internal Medicine and Clinical Oncology
Policlinico
Piazza Giulio Cesare 11
I-70124 Bari
Italy

Deborah T Weiss, BS
Human Immunology and Cancer Program
University of Tennessee
Graduate School of Medicine
1924 Alcoa Highway
Knoxville, TN 37920-6999
USA

Qing Yi, MD, PhD
Myeloma and Transplantation Research Center
University of Arkansas for Medical Sciences
4301 West Markham Street
Little Rock, AR 72205
USA

Athanasios Zomas, MD
Department of Clinical Hematology
"G Gennimatas" General Hospital of Athens
154 Mesogeion Avenue, Holargos
Athens
Greece

Part 1

Biology

1

Plasma cells and immunoglobulins

S Vincent Rajkumar, Phillip R Greipp

CONTENTS • **Introduction** • **Plasma cells** • **Immunoglobulins**

INTRODUCTION

To understand myeloma and its biology, it is important to study the nature of plasma cells and the immunoglobulins secreted by them. The first section of this chapter is devoted to plasma cells: their structure, function, and proliferation. The second half of the chapter focuses on immunoglobulins, and includes a detailed description of the various classes and their structure. Of critical importance are the genetic events that lead to immunoglobulin synthesis; these events are also discussed.

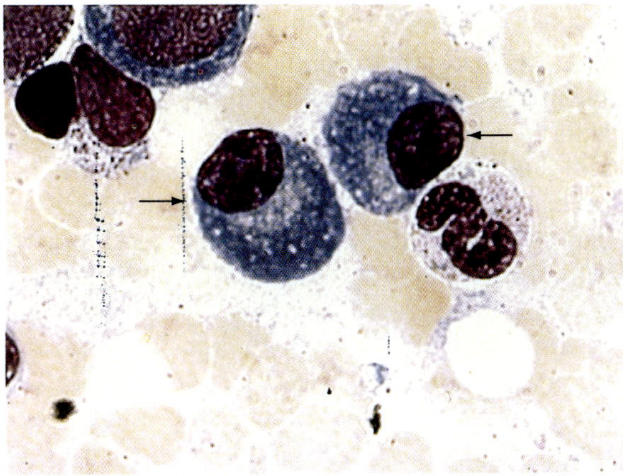

Figure 1.1 Normal mature plasma cell (arrows). Note the clumped chromatin, eccentric nucleus, and perinuclear hof.

PLASMA CELLS

Structure and morphology of plasma cells

Light microscopy

A normal mature plasma cell is easily recognized by its oval shape, eccentrically placed nucleus, and abundant basophilic cytoplasm (Figure 1.1). Its size ranges from 9 to 20 μm in diameter (with a mean cell diameter of about 14 μm).[1] A perinuclear clearing, or hof region, is the site of the Golgi apparatus. This well-developed Golgi apparatus accounts for the eccentric location of the nucleus. The nuclear chromatin is condensed, and nucleoli are not seen.

In myeloma, plasma cell morphology is more variable. In some patients, most cells are typical small mature cells. In others, more immature and atypical forms are found: the cells may be larger, bi- or multinuclear, with scanty cytoplasm, or with a fine nuclear chromatin pattern. Abnormal inclusions may be present. Sometimes the morphology is more lymphoid or lymphoplasmacytic. In many instances, it is not possible to differentiate a neoplastic plasma cell from a non-neoplastic cell by morphological features alone.

Most patients with myeloma have more than 10% plasma cells in the bone marrow; the average is 30–40%. Often, the cells are present in sheets, aggregates, or 'clones'. In monoclonal gammopathy of undetermined significance (MGUS), the plasma cell is often less atypical than in myeloma, but the morphology may be conspicuously immature. Characteristically in MGUS, plasma cells account for fewer than 10% of bone marrow cells.[2]

Normally, plasma cells are present in the medullary cords and germinal centers of lymph nodes, in the bone marrow, and in the white pulp and periarteriolar sheaths of the spleen. They can also be found in the lamina propria of the intestine and the thymus.

Electron microscopy

The electron-microscopic appearance of a plasma cell is illustrated in Figure 1.2.[1] The characteristic perinuclear hof region contains the Golgi apparatus, in which immunoglobulins are processed before secretion. Electron microscopy shows a highly developed rough endoplasmic reticulum with numerous ribosomes, essential for immunoglobulin synthesis. The blue cytoplasmic staining in light-microscopic preparations is due to abundant RNA. Mitochondria are present between the strands of endoplasmic reticulum.

Sometimes in myeloma, excess cytoplasmic immunoglobulin causes plasma cells to balloon, giving them the appearance of cells seen in Gaucher's disease. Accumulation of excess immunoglobulin can also lead to acidophilic, round cytoplasmic inclusions called 'Russell bodies'. However, none of these features is pathognomonic of myeloma.

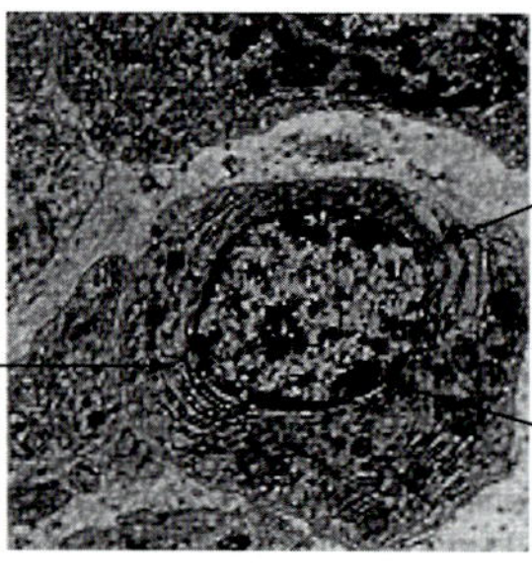

Figure 1.2 Electron micrograph of normal plasma cell showing abundant endoplasmic reticulum (ER), Golgi apparatus (GA), and mitochondria (M).

Establishing clonality of plasma cells in myeloma and other plasma cell disorders

Clonality in plasma cell disorders is typically inferred by identifying a monoclonal immunoglobulin component in the serum or urine. Immunohistochemical staining for the light chains, κ and λ, is not always necessary. The normal ratio of κ-staining to λ-staining plasma cells in the bone marrow is 2 : 1. A κ/λ ratio greater than 4 : 1 implies the presence of a monoclonal population of κ light-chain-restricted plasma cells. Similarly, a ratio of 1 : 2 or less infers a λ light-chain-restricted clone. Flow cytometry may also be used to determine light-chain restriction on bone marrow aspirates as well as in peripheral blood samples.

Immunophenotypic features

Plasma cells express various surface molecules (Table 1.1).[3–5] The immunophenotypic features of plasma cells may be studied by immunohistochemistry or flow cytometry. Plasma cells characteristically express the CD38 antigen and show negative or dim staining for CD45.[6] CD38 is expressed by several cells in the hematopoietic system, and is not specific for plasma cells. However, CD38 is expressed to a higher intensity in plasma cells than in most other cells. The combination of CD38 positivity and dim or negative staining for CD45 is the immunophenotypic hallmark of plasma cells.

Plasma cells also typically express plasma cell antigen 1 (PCA-1),[7] CD28, CD31, CD54 (ICAM-1), CD24, CD40, and CD44 (HCAM)[4,8] In addition, they express cytoplasmic immunoglobulin, but unlike blood B lymphocytes, they typically lack surface immunoglobulin. Plasma cells may sometimes show reactivity to a small extent to other non-lineage-restricted markers such as myeloid and stem cell markers. In myeloma, plasma cells also express receptors for growth factors such as interleukin (IL)-6, IL-1, estrogens, and glucocorticoids.

Table 1.1 Immunophenotypic features of normal and malignant plasma cells

Plasma cells	CD38	CD45	CD54 (ICAM-1)	CD44 (HCAM)	CD24	CD56 (NCAM)	CD58 (LFA-3)
Normal and MGUS[a]	+	−/dim	+	+	+	−	−
Myeloma	+	−/dim	+	+	+	+	+

[a] Monoclonal gammopathy of undetermined significance.

Unlike B lymphocytes, plasma cells are in most cases typically negative for CD20 and CD21 and class II HLA antigens and positive for CD28 and PCA-1. They are also $CD2^-$. However, in 20–30% of cases, myeloma cells may express CD20.

There may be differences in immunophenotypic features between normal/MGUS and myeloma plasma cells (Table 1.1).[9] Previous studies have suggested that loss of plasma cell CD56 (NCAM) expression in multiple myeloma defines a unique subset of patients and that CD56 expression reliably discriminates between MGUS and multiple myeloma.[10, 11] In a study of 55 patients with myeloma and 23 with MGUS, 78% of patients with myeloma had strong expression of CD56; all patients with MGUS were $CD56^-$.[12] However, contradictory results have been reported. We conducted a study of 68 untreated patients with myeloma from a single institution to define the clinicopathologic correlates of CD56 expression. We found CD56 expression in 55% of patients with myeloma.[13] The lack of CD56 expression did not define a unique clinicopathologic or prognostic entity in myeloma. Strong CD56 expression was also found in some patients with MGUS. One explanation for the CD56 negativity observed in many patients with MGUS may be contamination of the scant number of monoclonal MGUS plasma cells with normal plasma cells. The expression of CD56 on myeloma cells is unexpected. CD56 myeloma cells do not have the functional activity of natural killer cells, and the expression appears to be aberrant.[12] CD58 (leukemia-function-associated antigen 3, LFA-3) is also usually expressed on myelomatous plasma cells but not on normal or MGUS plasma cells.[4,6,12,14,15] In addition, the $CD19^-CD56^+$ phenotype has been proposed as a specific feature of myeloma cells. Normal plasma cells are typically $CD19^+CD56^-$.[5,7] However, none of these differences is sensitive and specific enough to allow MGUS and myeloma to be distinguished in clinical practice.

Certain immunophenotypic features have been suggested to have prognostic value. $CD20^+$ plasma cells in myeloma have been associated with a more aggressive course of disease.[16] The presence or coexpression of CD10 or surface immunoglobulin may also represent a poor prognostic feature. However, the prognostic value of CD10 in myeloma is unclear, because conflicting results have been reported.[16–18] Furthermore, usually only 15% of myeloma cells are positive for CD10. The presence of surface immunoglobulin may also be indicative of a more immature plasma cell clone. It does not appear that any of these immunophenotypic characteristics of plasma cells have independent prognostic value in myeloma.

Certain surface adhesion molecules described above may be important in the homing ability of plasma cells for bone marrow.[7] CD56 and other adhesion molecules on the myeloma cell surface may be important in the pathogenesis of bone lesions in myeloma.

Plasma cells also express syndecan-1 (CD138), a low-affinity receptor for basic fibroblast growth factor (bFGF). It has been shown with flow cytometry that plasma cells in almost all patients with myeloma and MGUS express syndecan-1 on their surface, a factor that is useful in the detection of malignant plasma cells in the peripheral blood and bone marrow.[19] In contrast, B cells from patients with chronic lymphocytic leukemia do not express syndecan-1. Studies have shown that syndecan-1 induces apoptosis, inhibits the growth of myeloma cells, and mediates decreased osteoclast and increased osteoblast differentiation.[20] The role of syndecan-1 in the pathogenesis of myeloma is being actively investigated. The relationship of syndecan-1 and bound bFGF to angiogenesis also remains to be studied.

Variations in plasma cell morphology in myeloma and their significance

On the basis of morphologic features, it is possible to identify a subset of myeloma characterized by immature plasmablasts. To limit interobserver variation, a strict definition of plasmablastic morphology is required.[21] Accordingly, plasmablasts are defined as follows (Figure 1.3):

- a fine reticular nuclear chromatin pattern with minimal or no chromatin clumping;
- large nuclear size (estimated to be > 10 μm) or a large nucleolus (estimated to be > 2 μm);
- cytoplasm with very little or no hof region;
- less abundant cytoplasm (less than one-half the nuclear area).

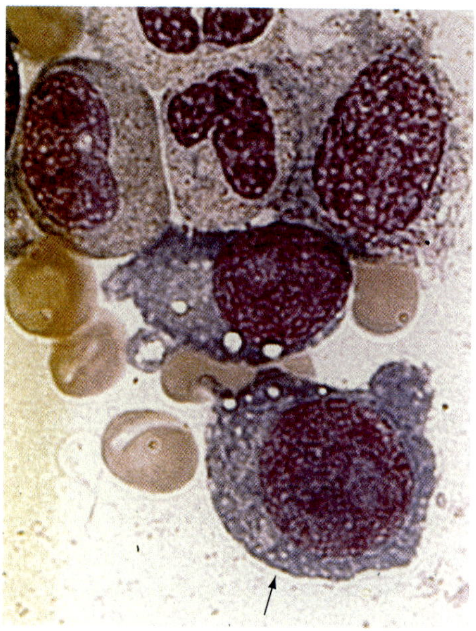

Figure 1.3 Plasmablast (arrow). Note the fine chromatin, large nucleus, scanty cytoplasm, and absence of perinuclear hof.

All four of these criteria must be fulfilled for a plasma cell to be defined as a plasmablast. A well-spread area of the slide is chosen, about 500 plasma cells are identified, and the percentage of plasmablasts is estimated. Plasmablastic morphology is considered to be present (plasmablastic myeloma) when 2% or more of the plasma cells in the bone marrow are plasmablasts.

With the above criteria, a large study by the Eastern Cooperative Oncology Group (ECOG) of 453 patients with newly diagnosed myeloma demonstrated that plasmablastic morphology is a powerful independent adverse prognostic factor for survival.[21] In this study, the median overall survival was 1.9 years for patients with plasmablastic myeloma and 3.7 years for those with non-plasmablastic morphology. A similar difference was also noted in progression-free survival. In another study, performed at the Mayo Clinic, plasmablastic morphology was an important predictor of poor survival following autologous transplantation for relapsed or refractory myeloma.[22] In this study, overall survival following transplantation was significantly worse for patients with plasmablastic morphology than for those without (median survival 5 months and 24 months, respectively). Also, progression-free survival was shortened (median time 4 months and 12 months, respectively). Other groups have also confirmed the prognostic value of plasmablastic morphology in myeloma.

Plasmablastic morphology is associated with an increased incidence of cytogenetic abnormalities.[22] There is also a correlation with other prognostic and biologic factors, such as plasma cell labeling index (PCLI), serum level of calcium, and incidence of *ras* mutations.[21] However, the precise reason why plasmablastic morphology leads to poor survival is unknown.

In some cases, plasma cells appear to be immature because of their nuclear characteristics, but do not meet the criteria for a plasmablast because of an abundance of cytoplasm. These cells are defined as 'immature plasma cells' (Figure 1.4). The prognostic significance of immature plasma cells in the absence of plasmablastic morphology has not been clearly defined.[23]

Detection of circulating plasma cells

Plasma cells are not frequently seen in the circulation. In myeloma, an increased number of circulating plasma cells may be detected with a slide-based immunofluorescence technique,[24] similar to the technique described below for determining the PCLI. Circulating plasma cells may also be detected by flow cytometry.[25] An increased number of circulating plasma cells in myeloma and amyloidosis is an indicator of poor prognosis.[24,26]

Summary

- Normal mature plasma cells are characterized by an oval shape, eccentric nucleus, and abundant basophilic cytoplasm.

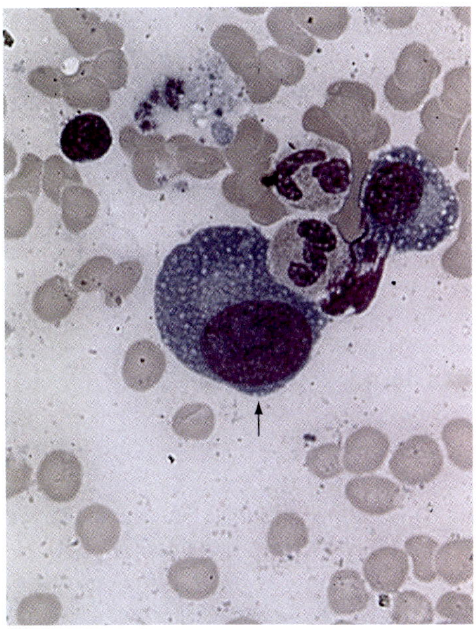

Figure 1.4 Immature plasma cell (arrow). Note the resemblance of the nucleus to those of plasmablasts, but immature plasma cells have abundant cytoplasm.

- The characteristic perinuclear hof region on light microscopy contains the Golgi apparatus.
- More variable plasma cell morphology is seen in patients with myeloma than in normal subjects.
- Clonality in plasma cell neoplasms may be assessed by κ/λ restriction.
- Combination of CD38 positivity and dim /negative staining for CD45 is the identifying immunophenotypic hallmark of plasma cells.
- Plasma cells express syndecan-1, a low-affinity receptor for bFGF.
- CD56 and CD58 are present on myelomatous plasma cells but not on normal plasma cells.
- Plasmablastic morphology is a powerful independent predictor of poor survival in myeloma.

Development of plasma cells

Most circulating B lymphocytes are naive (virgin) cells that have not been exposed to an activating antigen. Their lifespan is about one week in the absence of antigenic activation. Plasma cells are derived from B lymphocytes that have been activated by antigenic stimuli (Figure 1.5).

When an antigen enters the body, it usually reaches the regional lymph nodes (or other organs of the reticuloendothelial system) and is captured.[27] The site of antigen processing is determined by the route of entry into the body. For instance, intra-abdominal or subcutaneous entry of the antigen usually results in antigen processing in the regional lymph nodes. An intravenous route of entry leads to antibody production in the spleen or bone marrow. Antigens that enter through the gastrointestinal tract or respiratory mucosa are processed in subepithelial lymphoid tissues.[27]

In lymph nodes, antigens are captured in the medulla mainly by macrophages, and in the cortical regions by dendritic cells. Some antigen escapes the lymph nodes and is processed by the spleen or liver.

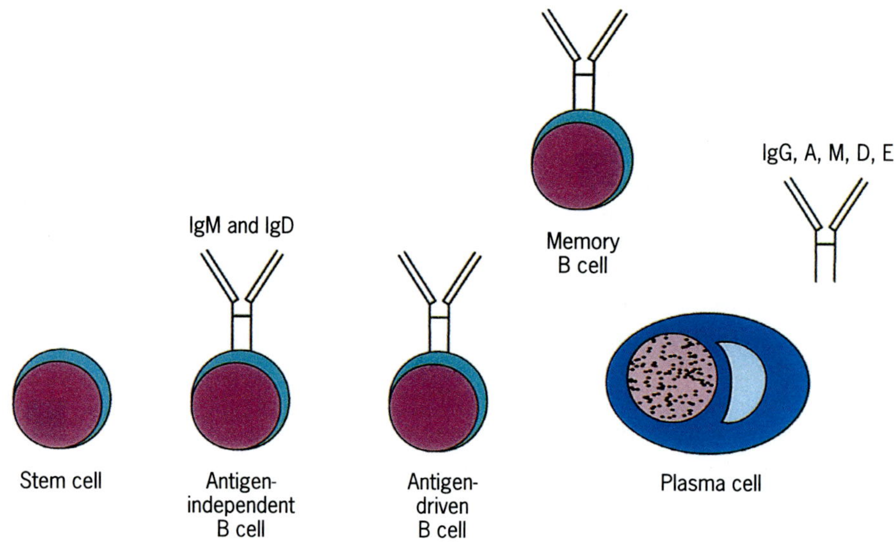

Figure 1.5
Maturation of B cell to plasma cell and memory cell by antigenic stimulation.

The primary follicles of lymph nodes contain mainly B lymphocytes as well as the helper subset of T cells. When stimulated by antigens, B lymphocytes transform into blasts that divide and give rise to germinal centers. At this point, the primary follicle is known as a 'secondary follicle'. Antigenic binding occurs on the IgM molecule on the cell surface of B lymphocytes. This initiates a process by which B cells transform into immunoglobulin-secreting plasma cells and move into the medullary cords.[28,29] Antigenic stimulation leads to activation of signaling pathways that results in cell division, increased expression of immunoglobulin mRNAs, and the development of a large endoplasmic reticulum and Golgi region.[1,27–30] The cytoplasm of the B lymphocyte also enlarges. These changes result in the progressive differentiation of B lymphocytes into plasmablasts, immature plasma cells, and, finally, mature plasma cells. The result is a clone of plasma cells that synthesizes and secretes immunoglobulins (antibodies).

The initial antibodies secreted by B lymphocytes are predominantly IgM (primary immune response). Subsequently, a 'class switch' occurs that leads to a shift from IgM secretion to IgG secretion. This is a result of a switch in the heavy-chain type from μ to γ or α or ε. These genetic events are discussed below in the section on immunoglobulins. The initial IgM antibody is produced for about one week. IgG antibody is the principal antibody secreted after the class switch, in 4–7 days. This class switch can happen during the primary response if antigenic stimulation is sustained. Subsequent exposure to the same antigen leads to stimulation of memory B cells and consists of a more rapid and larger response, known as the 'secondary immune response'. The secondary immune response is usually IgG or, in some instances, IgA or IgE, depending on the type of antigenic stimulation.

Some B lymphocytes are also converted to memory B cells that are able to mount a quicker plasma cell response when challenged with the same antigen at a later date (immunologic memory).[31] These memory cells circulate for years. Recent studies have suggested that CD40–CD40 ligand, OX–OX40 ligand, and other cytokines and intracellular transcriptional factors contribute to B-lymphocyte differentiation control along either the plasma cell pathway or the memory B-cell pathway.[32] In addition, B lymphocytes also process and degrade protein antigens to peptides and express them on their cell surface in association with major histocompatibility complex (MHC) class II molecules and act as antigen-presenting cells (APC).

Antigen activation of B lymphocytes also involves interactions with the helper T cells that have been activated by the same antigen. Several T-cell cytokines are involved in the maturation of B lymphocytes, including IL-3, IL-4, IL-5, transforming growth factor (TGF)-β, and interferon-γ. These cytokines also have an important role in class switching. Certain antigens are capable of activating B cells independently of T cells. These generally are bacterial cell wall lipopolysaccharides. In general, protein antigens require T-cell interaction for B-cell activation.[5]

The primary function of plasma cells is the production and release of immunoglobulin antibodies as effectors of the humoral immune response. Plasma cells are terminally differentiated cells and have a low rate of DNA synthesis. This is consistent with the normal PCLI being less than 0.2% – in fact, it is usually 0.0% (see below). This also explains why it is difficult to detect plasma cell metaphases during conventional cytogenetic analysis.

Summary

- Antigenic binding to surface IgM on B lymphocytes activates signaling pathways that result in cell division, increased expression of immunoglobulin mRNAs, development of a large endoplasmic reticulum and Golgi region, and eventual transformation into plasma cells.
- Antigen-activated B lymphocytes can differentiate along the plasma cell pathway or the memory B-cell pathway.
- Initial antibody response is typically IgM, followed by a 'class switch' leading to IgG (or, less frequently, IgA/IgE) antibody production.
- Bacterial cell wall lipopolysaccharide antigens activate B cells in a T-cell independent fashion, in contrast to protein antigens, which require T-helper interaction.

Plasma cell proliferation in myeloma and its significance

Cytokines produced by plasma cells

Plasma cells produce various cytokines, including IL-6, which is a major proliferative cytokine for malignant plasma cells. They also secrete vascular endothelial growth factor (VEGF), which is one of the most important cytokines for angiogenesis. In addition, myeloma cells express IL-1β and tumor necrosis factor (TNF)-α, which are potent osteoclast-activating factors. The role of the major cytokines and other factors in the proliferation of normal and malignant plasma cells is summarized below and discussed in depth in Chapter 4.

Role of IL-6 in normal and malignant plasma cells

IL-6 is an important growth factor in the differentiation of normal B lymphocytes into plasma cells.[33,34] However, IL-6 does not generally induce proliferation of normal B lymphocytes or plasma cells.[7] In contrast, IL-6 may induce a significant proliferative response in myeloma cells.[33] Transgenic mice (C57BL/6) carrying the human IL-6 gene fused to a human immunoglobulin heavy-chain enhancer develop massive lethal (polyclonal) plasmacytosis.[35,36] The addition of exogenous IL-6 may enhance the growth of myeloma cells in vitro. This growth is inhibited by the introduction of anti-IL-6 antibody.[37] There is a correlation between the IL-6 responsiveness of myeloma cells and the PCLI.[38] The proliferative response of myeloma cells to IL-6 is a major factor that distinguishes malignant proliferating plasma cells from normal non-proliferating plasma cells, and is important in the pathogenesis of myeloma.[7] In addition, IL-6 may inhibit apoptosis, thus contributing to myeloma tumor burden.

IL-6 appears to play both an autocrine and a paracrine role in the growth and proliferation of myeloma cells.[33,39] Several studies have documented that IL-6 is an autocrine growth factor for human myeloma cells. Freshly isolated myeloma cells produce IL-6 and express its receptor. Monoclonal plasma cells from most myeloma patients with a high PCLI express IL-6 mRNA. In addition, it is also likely that paracrine sources of IL-6 production (bone marrow stromal cells) play a role in the pathogenesis of myeloma.[40]

Serum levels of IL-6 are increased in about one-third of patients with myeloma, and are increased more frequently in plasma cell leukemia. In contrast, IL-6 levels are rarely increased in MGUS.[38] The C-reactive protein level may serve as a surrogate marker for IL-6 levels.

Role of soluble IL-6 receptors (sIL-6R) in myeloma

The activity of IL-6 in myeloma appears to be modulated by the expression of soluble IL-6 receptors (sIL-6R).[7] In the presence of IL-6, sIL-6R associates with gp130 and leads to signal transduction and augmentation of the IL-6 proliferation effect.[41] An increased level of sIL-6R has independent, poor prognostic value in myeloma.[42,43]

Role of IL-1β

Normal plasma cells and plasma cells from patients with MGUS do not produce IL-1β. In contrast, plasma cells from almost all myeloma patients produce IL-1β.

IL-1β can induce the expression of genes for IL-6, colony-stimulating factors, and various adhesion molecules. Furthermore, it has been shown that myeloma cells can induce IL-6 production in marrow stromal cells. This appears to be mediated through endogenously released IL-1β, and antibodies to IL-1β completely suppress IL-6 production.[44]

Aberrant expression of IL-1β may also induce the expression of adhesion molecules such as CD49d (VLA-4), CD44, CD54, and CD56, and other surface molecules on myeloma cells.[7]

Aberrant IL-1β production may be a critical factor that contributes to the progression of MGUS to myeloma.[45] IL-1β has potent osteoclast-activating factor (OAF) activity, and may be the predominant factor responsible for the development of osteolytic lesions in myeloma.[7,46]

PCLI

The PCLI is a measure of the proliferative rate of plasma cells.[47] The assay can be performed on both bone marrow and peripheral blood [48]. It is based on the detection of bromo-2-deoxyuridine incorporation into DNA, which occurs in proliferating cells. The normal PCLI is 0.2% or less. A PCLI of 1% or greater is classified as 'high'.

The PCLI is performed using a slide-based immunofluorescence method.[47,49] Briefly, bone-marrow mononuclear cells are isolated on Ficoll–Hypaque, and 1×10^6 cells are incubated for 1 hour at 37°C in RPMI-1640 containing 10 μmol/l bromo-2-deoxyuridine, 1 μmol/l fluorodeoxyuridine, 10% fetal calf serum, and antibiotics. After the cells are washed with phosphate-buffered saline, cytospin slides are made and fixed in 95% ethanol. Next, 20 μg of BU-1 monoclonal antibody (antibody to bromo-2-deoxyuridine; Amersham Corporation, Arlington Heights, IL) is added, and the cells are incubated for 30 minutes at room temperature and washed once again. After washing, 8 μg of goat anti-mouse IgG labeled with rhodamine isothiocyanate is added to detect the BU-1 antibody. Subsequently, monospecific anti-κ or anti-λ, labeled with fluorescein isothiocyanate to identify the plasma cells, is added. At least 500 cells staining positive for the same cytoplasmic light-chain isotype as the patient's M protein are counted, and the PCLI is the percentage of these cells that show positive nuclear fluorescence for BU-1 antibody (Figure 1.6).

The PCLI has major clinical significance because of the consistent association between poor survival and high PCLI values.[43,49] By using the same immunofluorescence methods described above, it is also possible to quantitate circulating peripheral blood plasma cells and determine a peripheral blood labeling index.[48] Such estimations have prognostic value in both myeloma and amyloidosis.[24,26]

Other factors that influence plasma cell proliferation in myeloma

Various biologic variables appear to enhance the proliferation of plasma cells in myeloma. As discussed above, IL-6 is a major cytokine that influences plasma cell proliferation. Increased levels of sIL-6R are also seen in myeloma, and this leads to an enhanced proliferative response

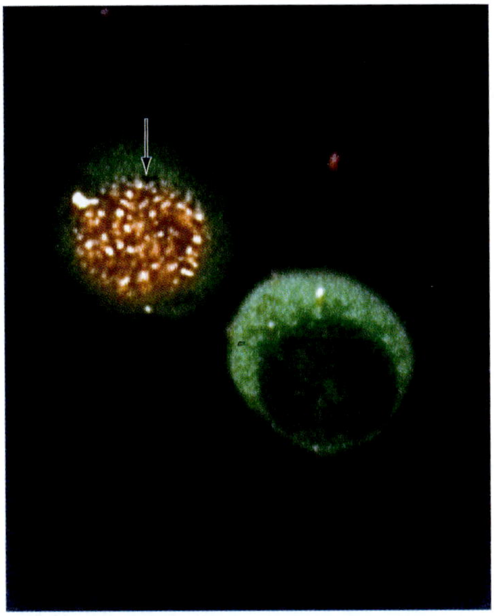

Figure 1.6 Plasma cell labeling index (PCLI). Immunofluorescence photomicrograph showing two plasma cells that stain positive for cytoplasmic immunoglobulin and one plasma cell with a nucleus that stains positive (labeled) for bromodeoxyuridine (arrow).

of plasma cells to IL-6 and a poor outcome clinically.

The cell surface Ku autoantigen may mediate adhesion of tumor cells to each other and to bone marrow stromal cells and to human fibronectin.[50] The Ku antigen may also play a role in both autocrine and paracrine IL-6-mediated myeloma cell proliferation.

Cytogenetic abnormalities are often present in myeloma, especially at the time of relapse.[51] These abnormalities can be detected using conventional karyotypic analysis or other techniques such as fluorescence in situ hybridization (FISH) or fiber FISH.[52,53] The presence of cytogenetic abnormalities has an adverse effect on outcome following stem cell transplantation for myeloma.[54] The correlation between the presence of cytogenetic abnormalities and a high PCLI is good. Studies have shown that, compared with patients with a normal karyotype, patients with an abnormal clone on cytogenetic analysis have a higher PCLI (median 0.2 and 1.4, respectively).[55] In addition, as the percentage of abnormal metaphases increases, the PCLI and bone marrow plasma cell percentage increase significantly.[56] Although this relationship may be the result of cytogenetic abnormalities becoming more apparent with a high PCLI and with bone marrow involvement with myeloma, the strong correlation of these factors with the percentage of abnormal metaphases suggests a growth advantage offered by chromosomal abnormalities to the neoplastic plasma cell.

It has been suggested that conventional karyotypic analyses underestimate the frequency of 14q32 translocations in myeloma.[57] Translocations of 14q32 appear to be a nearly universal phenomenon when a combination of FISH techniques, Southern blot assay (to identify illegitimate switch recombination fragments containing sequences from only one heavy chain class switch region), and cytogenetic analysis is applied.[58] These translocations most frequently include 11q13 (the site of the cyclin D1 gene) and 4p16 (the site of the fibroblast growth factor receptor 3 gene) as partner loci. Several other regions, such as 1p13, 8q24, 12q24, 16q23, and 21q22, can also serve as promiscuous partner loci for the 14q32 translocations. In many cases, partner chromosomes have not been identified.

Plasma cells also express VEGF, a potent angiogenic cytokine.[59] This expression is also increased by IL-6 stimulation. There is early evidence that bone marrow angiogenesis is increased in myeloma and is of prognostic value.[60–63] Higher levels of bone marrow angiogenesis are correlated positively with the PCLI, suggesting that increased angiogenesis is associated with accelerated plasma cell proliferation.[64] Thus, there is potential for the use of antiangiogenic agents in the treatment of myeloma.

Summary

- IL-6 is an important cytokine for the differentiation of B lymphocytes into plasma cells.
- IL-6 does not induce proliferation of normal B lymphocytes or plasma cells, but it has a significant proliferative and antiapoptotic effect on myeloma cells.
- IL-6 likely has both an autocrine and a paracrine role in myeloma cell proliferation.

- IL-6 activity in myeloma is modulated by the expression of soluble IL-6 receptors.
- IL-1β may mediate the release of IL-6 by marrow stromal cells.
- Aberrant IL-1β production appears to be a critical factor in the progression of MGUS to myeloma.
- Proliferative activity of plasma cells is quantified by the PCLI, which has independent prognostic value in myeloma.
- Cytogenetic abnormalities and increased levels of bone marrow angiogenesis may increase the proliferative rate and decrease the apoptotic rate of malignant plasma cells.

IMMUNOGLOBULINS

Immunoglobulins (antibodies) constitute the humoral immune response to a foreign antigen. They are secretory products of plasma cells. The genetic events that are involved in immunoglobulin synthesis and structure and the various classes of immunoglobulins are reviewed below.

Genetics of immunoglobulin synthesis

Each immunoglobulin molecule has two heavy and two light chains (Figure 1.7). The five types of heavy chains are denoted by the Greek letters μ, δ, γ, α, and ε. The type of heavy chain present determines the class of the immunoglobulin: IgM, IgD, IgG, IgA, and IgE, respectively. The two types of light chain are denoted by the Greek letters κ and λ. Each immunoglobulin molecule has either a κ or a λ subtype of light chain in association with one of the types of heavy chain.

The immunoglobulin molecule is formed by the fusion of various genetic regions through a unique series of recombinations detailed below.[65–68] The heavy-chain locus is located on chromosome 14, the κ light-chain locus on chromosome 2, and the λ light-chain locus on chromosome 22 (Figure 1.8).

Each heavy chain and light chain is formed by the rearrangement and fusion of several noncontiguous genes. The variable portion of each heavy chain is formed by fusion of three genes: V_H (variable), D_H (diversity), and J_H (joining). There are more than 100–150 different V_H genes

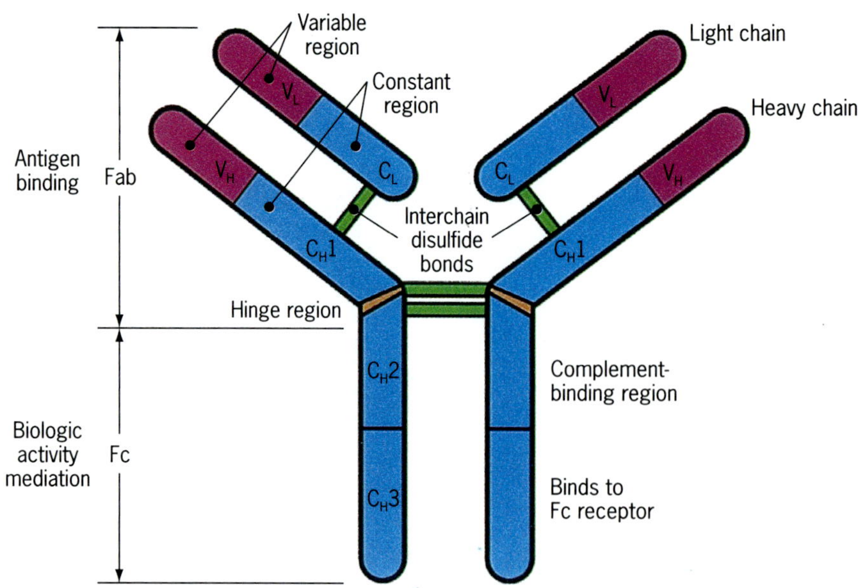

Figure 1.7 Diagram of immunoglobulin molecule structure. (From Kyle and Lust.[79] By permission of Churchill Livingstone.)

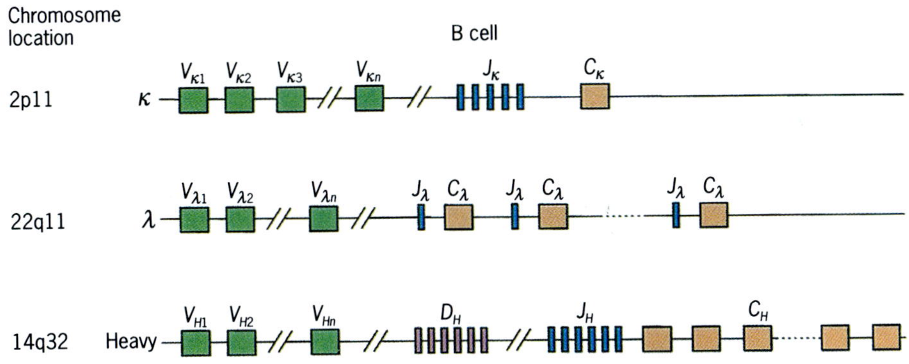

Figure 1.8 Diagram of immunoglobulin heavy- and light-chain loci. *C*, constant; *D*, diversity; *J*, joining; *V*, variable. (From Kyle and Lust.[79] By permission of Churchill Livingstone.)

(of which 60–70 are functional and available for recombination), 30 different D_H genes, and 6 functional J_H genes on chromosome 14.[69] By a process of DNA rearrangement, one V_H gene, one D_H gene, and one J_H gene are brought into proximity to form a $V_HD_HJ_H$ gene (Figure 1.9). The D_HJ_H rearrangement occurs first, and then the $V_HD_HJ_H$ recombination takes place. This unique $V_HD_HJ_H$ recombination codes for the variable region of the heavy chain and is transcribed as a single unit into RNA.[69] Subsequently, this RNA is spliced together with one of several constant region RNAs that code for the constant regions of the five types of heavy chains (μ, γ, α, ε, or δ) to determine the class of immunoglobulin that is formed (Figure 1.9). Successful recombination, as described above in one allele, inhibits such rearrangements from occurring in the other allele

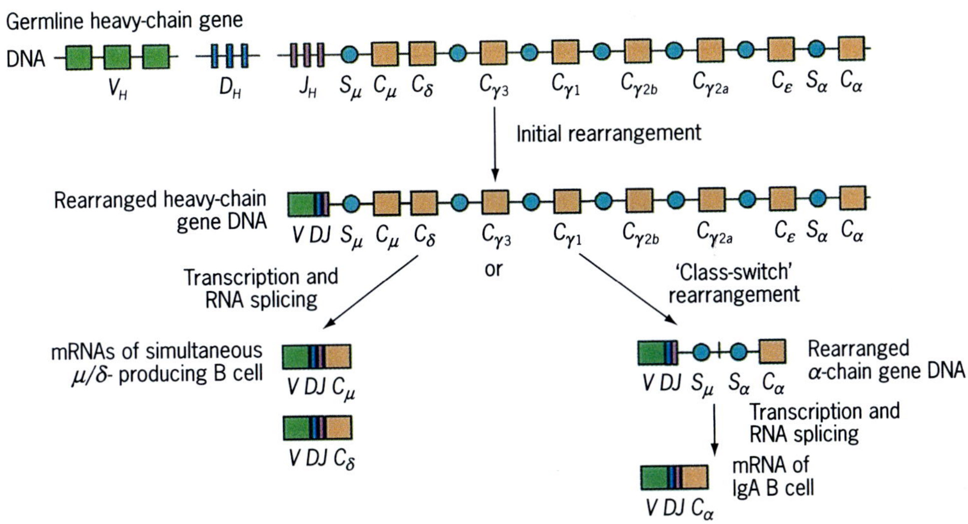

Figure 1.9 Diagram of the *VDJ* heavy-chain gene recombination and initial mRNA splicing to form μ- or δ-chain mRNA. Also shown is the 'class switch' rearrangement and α-chain mRNA formation. *C*, constant; *D*, diversity; *J*, joining; *V*, variable. The 'class-switch' rearrangement occurs at switch regions (S). (From Kyle and Lust.[79] By permission of Churchill Livingstone.)

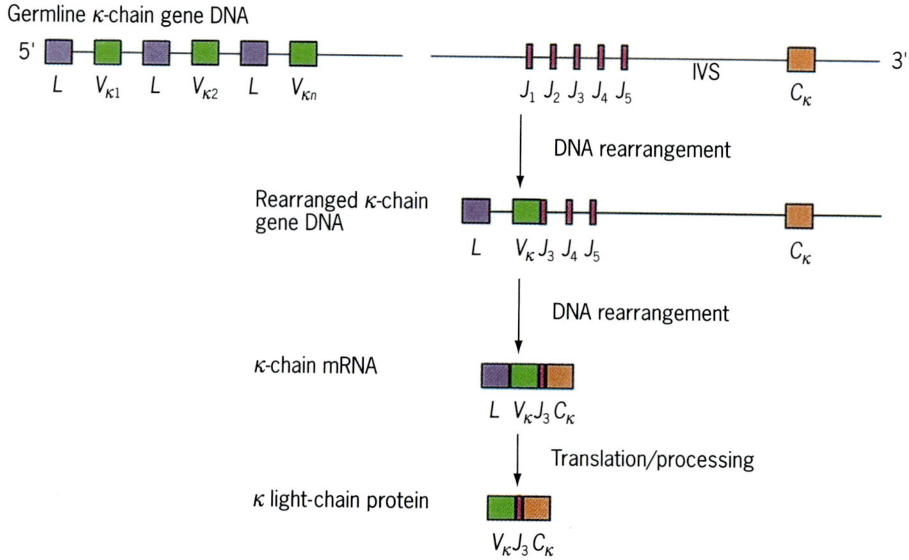

Figure 1.10 Diagram of κ-chain gene recombination. *L*, leader sequence; *D*, diversity; *J*, joining; *V*, variable; IVS, intervening sequence. The leader sequence accompanies each *V* gene. (From Kyle and Lust.[79] By permission of Churchill Livingstone.)

(allelic exclusion). Heavy-chain recombination and expression of a fully assembled heavy-chain molecule occur in the pre-B-cell stage of B-lineage differentiation.

Similarly, the variable portion of light-chain is formed by the recombination of one V_L gene with one J_L gene (V_LJ_L gene) (Figure 1.10). There are no D_L genes for the light chains. Light-chain rearrangement is enhanced by successful heavy-chain rearrangement. Similar to heavy chains, there are numerous V_L genes (76 different V_κ genes and 10 different families of V_λ genes) and several J_L genes (5 J_κ and 7 J_λ genes), leading to diversity in the structure of each light chain. Recombination of the V_L and J_L segments on chromosome 2 leads to a κ light chain, and recombination on chromosome 22 leads to a λ light chain. After recombination has taken place on chromosome 2 and a κ light-chain rearrangement takes place, λ light-chain rearrangement does not proceed. If κ light chains are not rearranged, then λ rearrangement takes place. After successful recombination, transcription to RNA occurs. RNA splicing with the RNAs coding for the constant regions of the κ or λ light chains results in mRNA that codes for complete κ and λ light chains, respectively.

$V_HD_HJ_H$ and V_LJ_L recombinations are catalyzed by protein products coded by the *RAG-1* and *RAG-2* genes on chromosome 11q13.[69,70] These gene products appear to activate a unique recombinase that is critical for both heavy- and light-chain recombination events.[71] The same recombinase also appears to be critical for T-cell-receptor rearrangements. It appears that transcriptional activation of the V_H, D_H, J_H and V_L, J_L segments is important for recombinase to act, and may involve hypomethylation of the gene segments.[69]

The diversity of the *V*, *D*, and *J* segments in the human genome leads to the diverse repertoire of antibodies that can be generated. In addition, insertion of extra nucleotides in the junctional region and somatic mutational events in the variable regions lead to vast and unlimited antibody diversity.

Generally, in naive B cells, the RNA coded for by the rearranged heavy-chain regions ($V_HD_HJ_H$) fuses with RNA coding for the μ and δ constant genes to produce IgM and IgD immunoglobulins, respectively. During the class switch that occurs with subsequent antigen stimulation, the rearranged $V_H D_H J_H$ genes are brought next to a different constant-region class. For example, if the $V_H D_H J_H$ region is brought into proximity with the $\gamma 1$ region, a class switch occurs from IgM to IgG1.

Summary

- The variable portion of each heavy chain is formed by rearrangement and fusion of one V_H (variable) gene with one D_H (diversity) and one J_H (joining) gene.
- Intact heavy-chain mRNA is formed by RNA splicing of the products of the fused $V_H D_H J_H$ gene and one of the constant-chain genes.
- A similar process takes place in the synthesis of light chains, initiated by the fusion of a V_L gene with a J_L gene.
- $V_H D_H J_H$ and $V_L J_L$ recombinations are catalyzed by protein products coded by the *RAG-1* and *RAG-2* genes on chromosome 11q13 that activate a unique recombinase enzyme.
- The diversity of the *V*, *D*, and *J* segments available for recombination is partly responsible for the diverse repertoire of antibodies that can be generated.

Structure of the immunoglobulins

Heavy- and light-chain structure

The immunoglobulin molecule is composed of two heavy chains and two light chains (Figure 1.7).[72,73] Each heavy chain has approximately 440–450 amino acid residues, and each light chain has about 214. The amino acids are numbered in increasing order from the amino terminal of the immunoglobulin molecule.

Because myeloma is a neoplastic, clonal process, the malignant cells and the secreted immunoglobulin are either κ- or λ-restricted, which readily enables determination of clonality. Certain plasma cell disorders are characterized by the predominance of one light-chain subtype over the other. For instance, in amyloidosis, λ light chain is predominant. In contrast, the light chains are usually the κ subtype in Fanconi syndrome.

Each heavy chain and light chain has a heterogeneous variable region in the amino end of the molecule. In addition, each light chain also has one constant region (C_L), and each heavy chain has three (or four) constant regions. In the case of IgG, which has three heavy-chain constant regions, these segments are called $C_\gamma 1$, $C_\gamma 2$, and $C_\gamma 3$ (Figure 1.7). The constant region of the immunoglobulin molecule binds to the Fc receptor and complement. The constant regions of the heavy and light chains share significant homology in amino acid sequence with members of the same heavy/light-chain class.

The light chains and heavy chains are bound together by disulfide bridges, and the heavy chains are bound to each other by two disulfide bridges. In addition, both heavy chains and light chains contain intrachain disulfide bonds.

Variable regions, complementarity-determining regions, and antibody diversity

Both heavy chains and light chains have a variable region in their amino ends. It is this variable region that confers specificity to the antibody, enabling it to target a defined antigen. Both heavy chains and light chains contain within the variable region short stretches of amino acid sequences that are hypervariable. These hypervariable regions are in direct contact with the antigen, and permit the formation of many sites where the antibody interacts with the antigen in a specific and intimate manner. These amino acid segments responsible for antigen recognition and binding are also called 'complementary-determining regions' (CDRs).[74] Portions of the variable region that do not come in direct contact with the antigen are called 'framework areas' (FRs), and they provide a stable domain structure to the immunoglobulin molecule. Each variable region of each heavy chain and light chain contains three CDRs and four FRs. Together, the six CDRs form the antigen-binding site.[69]

The three regions of hypervariability in the light chains have been identified in amino acid positions 24–34, 50–56, and 89–97, and are denoted as light-chain CDRs 1, 2, and 3, respectively.[75,76] Similar hypervariable regions in the heavy chains are in positions 30–37, 51–68, and 101–110, and are denoted as heavy-chain CDRs 1, 2, and 3, respectively.[77–79] Another hypervariable region in the heavy chain between CDR2 and CDR3 at amino acid positions 84–88 is not involved in antigen binding.

Heavy-chain CDR3 regions, in particular, are extremely heterogeneous, and are one of the main factors responsible for the magnitude of antibody diversity that is achieved. They form the most variable segment of the immunoglobulin molecule. The primary reason for the extreme variability of the heavy-chain CDR3 region is that this region encompasses the portion of the rearranged gene where the three heavy-chain gene segments V_H, D_H, and J_H are joined.[69,80] It is coded for by the 3′ end of V_H, all of D_H, and the 5′end of J_H. In addition, several other factors contribute to the diversity of the CDR3 region. First, the segment of DNA coding for this region often contains 'N-region' nucleotides that are randomly inserted at the V_HD_H and D_HJ_H junctions by terminal deoxytransferase (Tdt). Second, the terminal nucleotides of the V_H, D_H, and J_H regions may also be randomly deleted by nucleases. Third, the orientation of the D_H gene may be switched and the gene rearranged with the 3′ end in proximity with the 3′ end of the V_H gene. These events greatly increase the diversity of the amino acid sequence coded for by the CDR3 region. Also, somatic mutations described below account for the incredible diversity of antibodies.

Hinge region

A hinge region is located between the first and second constant fragments, C_H1 and C_H2, of the immunoglobulin molecule. It consists mainly of cysteine and proline residues.[27] The cysteine residues form the heavy-chain disulfide bridges. This region does not fold well because of its unique amino acid sequence, and is susceptible to enzymatic cleavage.

Enzymatic fragmentation

Treatment of the immunoglobulin molecule with papain leads to two Fab fragments and one Fc fragment. The Fc fragment is composed of the constant regions of the immunoglobulin molecule. Digestion with pepsin cleaves the immunoglobulin molecule to a single fused Fab(2) fragment and one Fc fragment.

Somatic mutations of immunoglobulins

Somatic mutations occur in germinal centers and greatly increase the repertoire of antibodies available. The mutations are confined to the coding regions of the rearranged immunoglobulin genes. They occur only in antigen-activated cells of advanced differentiation. These mutations may serve to increase the binding affinity to a given antigen. Somatic mutations have been described in myeloma cells.[81] This indicates that the target cell of malignant transformation in multiple myeloma may be a B-lineage cell that already has undergone antigenic selection.[82] Monoclonal cells of B lineage with a CDR3 sequence identical to that of the myeloma clone can be detected in the peripheral blood of patients with myeloma, representing different stages of B-cell differentiation, such as $CD34^+$, $CD20^+CD10^+$, $CD20^+CD21^+$, and $CD20^+CD19^-$ cells.[82–85]

Summary

- Each heavy chain and light chain has a heterogeneous variable region in the amino end of the molecule.
- Each light chain also has one constant region (C_L), and each heavy chain has three or four constant regions.
- Both heavy chains and light chains contain within the variable region short stretches of amino acid sequences that are hypervariable, called 'complementary-determining regions' (CDRs).
- CDRs are in direct contact with the antigen in a specific and intimate manner.
- Heavy-chain CDR3 is the most variable of the CDRs, and is one of the principal reasons for the magnitude of antibody diversity that can be achieved.
- Somatic mutations in the rearranged immunoglobulin genes occur in antigen-activated

cells of advanced differentiation, and serve to increase the binding affinity to a given antigen and further increase the antibody repertoire.

Immunoglobulin subtypes

The five types of immunoglobulins and their major properties are summarized in Table 1.2. The discussion below focuses on the unique features of each type of immunoglobulin.

Immunoglobulin G (IgG)

Most of the antibodies produced by activation of memory cells (the secondary immune response) are of the IgG class. The variable region of the IgG heavy chains and light chains contain approximately 110 amino acid residues, and the constant region for the IgG heavy chain contains more than 300 amino acids.[79] The three constant regions of the IgG heavy molecule, $C_{\gamma 1}$, $C_{\gamma 2}$, and $C_{\gamma 3}$, share homology within the IgG class. Each of the heavy-chain constant regions is approximately 110 amino acid residues long. Each light chain consists of 210 amino acid residues. The variable portion of the light chain consisting of about 107 amino acid residues is responsible for the unique heat-soluble properties of Bence Jones protein.

The four subclasses of IgG are IgG1, IgG2, IgG3, and IgG4 (Table 1.3). The half-lives of IgG1, IgG2, and IgG4 are approximately three weeks, while that of IgG3 is much shorter, 7–8 days. This appears to be a result of a much longer hinge region that is easily digested by proteolytic enzymes.

Each subclass of the IgG family has different functional properties. Only IgG1 and IgG3 fix complement through the classic pathway. IgG1 is directed against isoagglutinins, viruses, Rh antigen, and diphtheria toxoid. IgG4 is the class of antibody directed against factor VIII and factor IX. IgG2 antibodies are directed against lipopolysaccharides and polysaccharide antigens. IgG3 is also directed against viruses and Rh antigen. All four IgG subtypes cross the placenta.

There is no difference between patients with myeloma and those with MGUS in the distribution of the IgG subclass. The subclasses do not

Table 1.2 Properties of human immunoglobulins

Feature	IgG	IgA	IgM	IgD	IgE
Subclasses	IgG1, IgG2, IgG3, IgG4	IgA1, IgA2	None	None	None
Molecular weight (kDa)	150	160–400	900	180	200
Serum concentration (mg/dl)	700–1500	60–400	60–300	0–14	0.05
Half-life (days)	23 (IgG1, IgG2, IgG4); 7 (IgG3)	5.8	5.1	2.8	2.3
Synthetic rate per day (mg/kg)	33	24	6.7	0.4	0.02
Molecular form	Monomer	Monomer, dimer	Pentamer	Monomer	Monomer
Sedimentation constant *S*	6.6	7, 11	19	7	8
Complement activation	Classic pathway (IgG1, IgG3); alternate pathway (IgG4)	Alternate pathway	Classic pathway	Alternate pathway	None
Placental transfer	Yes	No	No	No	No

Table 1.3 Properties of IgG subclasses

Property	IgG1	IgG2	IgG3	IgG4
Percentage of serum IgG	70	20	6	4
Examples of antigens targeted	Staphylococcal protein A, isoagglutinins, Rh antigen	Staphylococcal protein A, tetanus toxoid, lipopolysaccharides, polysaccharides	Viruses	Anti-factor VIII and IX antibodies
Fix complement	Yes	No	Yes	No
Tendency to aggregate	No	No	Yes	No
React with anti-Ig antibodies	Yes	Yes	No	Yes

bear any unique clinical characteristics in myeloma and have no prognostic value. Myeloma in which the monoclonal protein is of the IgG2 subclass is associated with a greater tendency to suppress residual IgG.[86]

Immunoglobulin A (IgA)

IgA has the tendency to form dimers. Increased IgA concentrations may lead to increased concentration of polymers and result in increased serum viscosity. Hence, hyperviscosity syndromes are seen in patients with high IgA levels.

The two subtypes of IgA are IgA1 and IgA2. Most IgA (90%) is of the IgA1 subclass. IgA2 molecules do not have disulfide bonds linking the light and heavy chains; instead, they are bound non-covalently. IgA has a much shorter half-life (5.8 days) than IgG. Consequently, the daily production of IgA is equal to that of IgG despite a serum concentration that is 10 times less. IgA fixes complement through the alternative pathway.

The ratio of IgA1 to IgA2 in myeloma is identical to what is seen in the normal healthy population. IgA2 is associated with IgA nephropathy and Henoch–Schönlein purpura. In contrast, IgA1 is associated with lupus nephritis.

IgA is a class of antibody secreted by glands lining the gastrointestinal and respiratory tracts. It is also found in tears, urine, and colostrum. The secretory form of IgA consists of two IgA molecules linked together through disulfide bonds to a glycoprotein (Figure 1.11). This glycoprotein is called the 'secretory component' of IgA. It is this secretory component (molecular weight 60–80 kDa) that is responsible for the resistance of secretory IgA molecules to digestion by trypsin and pepsin. IgA dimers and polymers are linked to each other by a joining (J) chain, which has a molecular weight of 15 kDa and binds to the Fc portion by disulfide bonds. The molecular weight of secretory IgA is 380 kDa, including the IgA molecule, the J chain, and the secretory component.

The secretory IgA molecule has both antibacterial and antiviral activity, which is of significance especially in upper respiratory tract infections. It protects the host from invasion of the epithelial surfaces by various microorganisms. Secretory IgA is also a helpful mediator of the degranulation of eosinophils.

Immunoglobulin M (IgM)

IgM consists of five subunits that are linked together by disulfide bonds (Figure 1.12). The pentameric nature of IgM leads to a high molecular weight of approximately 900 kDa. Each subunit has a structure similar to that of IgG, with two heavy chains and two light chains. The μ chain consists of four constant regions, unlike the IgG γ chain, which has three constant regions. In contrast to IgG, the IgM molecule does not have a hinge region. The five subunits of IgM are also held together by J

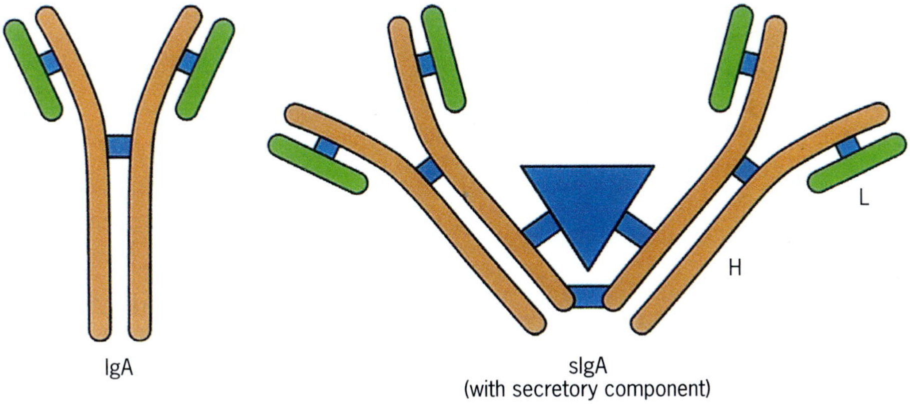

Figure 1.11 Diagram of IgA and secretory IgA (sIgA) molecules. H, heavy chain; L, light chain. (From Kyle RA, Berger RC, Gleich GJ. Diagnosis of syndromes associated with hyperglobulinemia. *Med Clin North Am* 1970; **54**: 917–38. By permission of WB Saunders Company.)

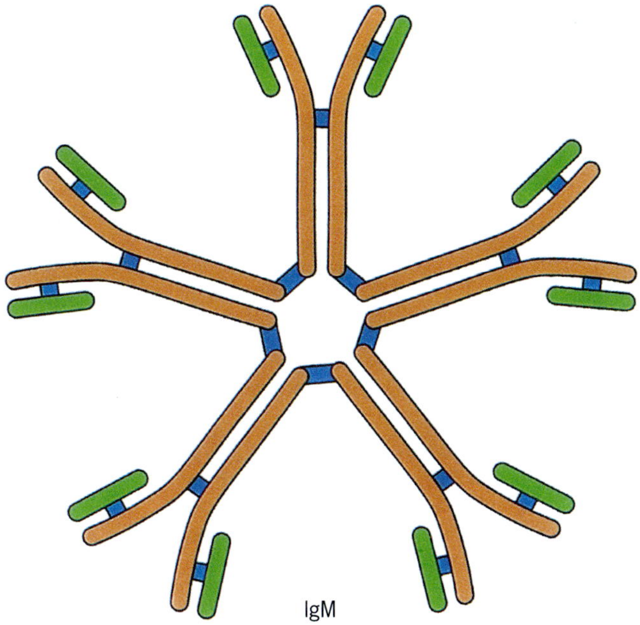

Figure 1.12 Diagram of IgM pentameric structure. (From Kyle RA, Berger RC, Gleich GJ. Diagnosis of syndromes associated with hyperglobulinemia. *Med Clin North Am* 1970; **54**: 917–38. By permission of WB Saunders Company.)

chains identical to those of IgA. Examples of IgM antibodies are cold agglutinins, rheumatoid factor, and isoagglutinins.

The initial antibodies secreted by B lymphocytes are of the IgM subtype. IgM antibodies activate complement by the classic pathway. In addition, all antigen-naive B lymphocytes express a monomeric IgM on the surface, which acts as an antigen-recognizing receptor. The membrane IgM molecule is anchored at the carboxy terminal to the cytoplasmic membrane through a hydrophobic segment.

The high concentrations of IgM seen in Waldenström's macroglobulinemia lead to hyperviscosity symptoms. Most (80%) molecular IgM proteins are the κ subtype.

Immunoglobulin D (IgD)

Normally, IgD is present on the surface of most B lymphocytes. A very small amount is also present in the serum. Most IgD molecules have the λ light-chain isotype. IgD has a very short half-life (2.8 days). There is a unique trimodal distribution of IgD at concentrations of approximately 0.25, 5, and 35 IU/ml. This may suggest a genetic inheritance pattern in normal persons. IgD is extremely sensitive to heat and proteases. Each δ heavy chain has three constant regions. The functional role of IgD is unknown. Most patients with IgD monoclonal protein have either multiple myeloma or primary amyloidosis; IgD MGUS is rare.

Immunoglobulin E (IgE)

IgE is an important mediator of allergy. It is present on the surface of both basophils and mast cells. Antigen–antibody interaction involving the IgE molecule results in release of histamine, which leads to an anaphylactic/allergic type of reaction.

IgE, similar to IgD, has a short half-life (2.3 days). Similar to the IgM molecule, the heavy chain of IgE has four constant domains and lacks a hinge region. Serum levels of IgE are increased in patients with atopic conditions such as asthma. The physiologic role of IgE is not known.

Summary

- IgG accounts for more than 75% of serum immunoglobulins.
- IgG has four subclasses – IgG1, IgG2, IgG3, and IgG4 – that have unique chemical and functional properties.
- IgA has a tendency to form dimers, and similar to IgM, increased IgA levels may lead to a hyperviscosity syndrome.
- IgA also exists in a secretory form that has antibacterial and antiviral activity and protects the host epithelial surfaces from invasion by various microorganisms.
- IgM exists as a pentamer, with a high molecular weight of 900 kDa.
- The initial antibody response in activated B cells is of the IgM class.
- Normally, IgD is present on the surface of most B lymphocytes, and a very small amount is present in the serum as circulating immunoglobulin.
- IgE is an important mediator of allergy and is present on the surface of both basophils and mast cells.

REFERENCES

1. Kay NE, Douglas SD. Morphology of lymphocytes and plasma cells. In: *Williams Hematology*, 5th edn (Beutler E, Lichtman MA, Coller BS et al, eds). New York: McGraw-Hill, 1995: 907–15.
2. Kyle RA. 'Benign' monoclonal gammopathy – after 20 to 35 years of follow-up. *Mayo Clin Proc* 1993; **68**: 26–36.
3. Ruiz-Arguelles GJ, San Miguel JF. Cell surface markers in multiple myeloma, *Mayo Clin Proc* 1994; **69**: 684–90.
4. San Miguel JF, Garcia-Sanz R, Gonzalez M et al. Immunophenotype and DNA cell content in multiple myeloma. *Baillière's Clin Haematol* 1995; **8**: 735–59.
5. Maclennan IC, Hardie DL, Ball J et al. Antibody-secreting cells and their origins. In: *Myeloma. Biology and Management* (Malpas JS, Bergsagel DE, Kyle RA, eds). Oxford: Oxford University Press, 1995: 30–49.
6. Leo R, Boeker M, Peest D et al. Multiparameter analyses of normal and malignant human plasma cells: $Cd38^{++}$, $Cd56^{+}$, $Cd54^{+}$, Cig^{+} is the common phenotype of myeloma cells. *Ann Hematol* 1992; **64**: 132–9.
7. Lust JA, Donovan KA. Biology and transition of monoclonal gammopathy of undetermined significance (MGUS) to multiple myeloma. *Cancer Control* 1998; **5**: 209–17.
8. Hamilton MS, Ball J, Bromidge E et al. Surface antigen expression of human neoplastic plasma cells includes molecules associated with lymphocyte recirculation and adhesion. *Br J Haematol* 1991; **78**: 60–5.
9. Helfrich MH, Livingston E, Franklin IM et al. Expression of adhesion molecules in malignant plasma cells in multiple myeloma: comparison with normal plasma cells and functional significance. *Blood Rev* 1997; **11**: 28–38.
10. Kaiser U, Auerbach B, Oldenburg M. The neural cell adhesion molecule NCAM in multiple myeloma. *Leuk Lymphoma* 1996; **20**: 389–95.
11. Van Riet I, De Waele M, Remels L et al. Expression of cytoadhesion molecules (Cd56, Cd54, Cd18 and Cd29) by myeloma plasma cells. *Br J Haematol* 1991; **79**: 421–7.
12. Van Camp B, Durie BG, Spier C et al. Plasma cells in multiple myeloma express a natural killer cell-associated antigen: Cd56 (Nkh-1; Leu-19). *Blood* 1990; **76**: 377–82.

13. Mathew P, Ahmann GJ, Witzig TE et al. Clinicopathological correlates of CD56 expression in multiple myeloma: a unique entity? *Br J Haematol* 1995; **90**: 459–61.
14. Sonneveld P, Durie BG, Lokhorst HM et al. Analysis of multidrug-resistance (MDR-1) glycoprotein and CD56 expression to separate monoclonal gammopathy from multiple myeloma. *Br J Haematol* 1993; **83**: 63–7.
15. Barker HF, Ball J, Drew M et al. The role of adhesion molecules in multiple myeloma. *Leuk Lymphoma* 1992; **8**: 189–196.
16. San Miguel JF, Gonzalez M, Gascon A et al. Immunophenotypic heterogeneity of multiple myeloma: influence on the biology and clinical course of the disease. Castellano-Leones (Spain) Cooperative Group for the Study of Monoclonal Gammopathies. *Br J Haematol* 1991; **77**: 185–90.
17. Durie BG, Grogan TM. CALLA-positive myeloma: an aggressive subtype with poor survival. *Blood* 1985; **66**: 229–32.
18. Epstein J, Xiao HQ, He XY. Markers of multiple hematopoietic-cell lineages in multiple myeloma. *N Engl J Med* 1990; **322**: 664–8.
19. Witzig TE, Kimlinger T, Stenson M et al. Syndecan-1 expression on malignant cells from the blood and marrow of patients with plasma cell proliferative disorders and B-cell chronic lymphocytic leukemia. *Leuk Lymphoma* 1998; **31**: 167–75.
20. Dhodapkar MV, Abe E, Theus A et al. Syndecan-1 is a multifunctional regulator of myeloma pathobiology: control of tumor cell survival, growth, and bone cell differentiation. *Blood* 1998; **91**: 2679–88.
21. Greipp PR, Leong T, Bennett JM et al. Plasmablastic morphology – an independent prognostic factor with clinical and laboratory correlates: Eastern Cooperative Oncology Group (ECOG) myeloma trial E9486 report by the ECOG Myeloma Laboratory Group. *Blood* 1998; **91**: 2501–7.
22. Rajkumar SV, Fonseca R, Lacy MQ et al. Plasmablastic morphology is an independent predictor of poor survival following autologous stem-cell transplantation for multiple myeloma. *J Clin Oncol* 1999; **17**: 1551–7.
23. Murakami H, Nemoto K, Sawamura M et al. Prognostic relevance of morphological classification in multiple myeloma. *Acta Haematol* 1992; **87**: 113–17.
24. Witzig TE, Gertz MA, Lust JA et al. Peripheral blood monoclonal plasma cells as a predictor of survival in patients with multiple myeloma. *Blood* 1996; **88**: 1780–7.
25. Witzig TE, Gertz MA, Pineda AA et al. Detection of monoclonal plasma cells in the peripheral blood stem cell harvests of patients with multiple myeloma. *Br J Haematol* 1995; **89**: 640–2.
26. Rajkumar SV, McElroy EA Jr, Ansell SM et al. Circulating peripheral blood plasma cells have prognostic significance in primary systemic amyloidosis. *Blood* 1998; **92**(Suppl 1): 261a.
27. Paraskevas F. Cell interactions in the immune response. In: *Wintrobe's Clinical Hematology,* 10th edn. Vol 1 (Lee GR, Foerster J, Lukens J et al, eds). Baltimore: Williams & Wilkins, 1999: 570–614.
28. Gold MR, DeFranco AL. Biochemistry of B lymphocyte activation. *Adv Immunol* 1994; **55**: 221–95.
29. Hentges F. B lymphocyte ontogeny and immunoglobulin production. *Clin Exp Immunol* 1994; **1**: 3–9.
30. Lodish H, Berk A, Ziparsky SL et al. *Molecular Cell Biology*, 4th edn. New York: WH Freeman, 2000: 168–79.
31. Ahmed R, Gray D. Immunological memory and protective immunity: understanding their relation. *Science* 1996; **272**: 54–60.
32. Liu YJ, Banchereau J. Regulation of B-cell commitment to plasma cells or to memory B cells. *Semin Immunol* 1997; **9**: 235–40.
33. Kishimoto T. The biology of interleukin-6. *Blood* 1989; **74**: 1–10.
34. Klein B, Zhang XG, Lu ZY et al. Interleukin-6 in human multiple myeloma. *Blood* 1995; **85**: 863–72.
35. Potter M, Mushinski JF, Mushinski EB et al. Avian v-myc replaces chromosomal translocation in murine plasmacytomagenesis. *Science* 1987; **235**: 787–9.
36. Clynes R, Wax J, Stanton LW et al. Rapid induction of IgM-secreting murine plasmacytomas by pristane and an immunoglobulin heavy-chain promoter/enhancer-driven c-myc/v-Ha-ras retrovirus. *Proc Natl Acad Sci USA* 1988; **85**: 6067–71.
37. Kawano M, Hirano T, Matsuda T et al. Autocrine generation and requirement of BSF-2/IL-6 for human multiple myelomas. *Nature* 1988; **332**: 83–5.
38. Zhang XG, Klein B, Bataille R. Interleukin-6 is a potent myeloma-cell growth factor in patients with aggressive multiple myeloma. *Blood* 1989; **74**: 11–13.

39. Donovan KA, Lacy MQ, Kline MP et al. Contrast in cytokine expression between patients with monoclonal gammopathy of undetermined significance or multiple myeloma. *Leukemia* 1998; **12**: 593–600.
40. Klein B, Zhang XG, Jourdan M et al. Paracrine rather than autocrine regulation of myeloma-cell growth and differentiation by interleukin-6. *Blood* 1989; **73**: 517–26.
41. Lust JA, Donovan KA, Kline MP et al. Isolation of an mRNA encoding a soluble form of the human interleukin-6 receptor. *Cytokine* 1992; **4**: 96–100.
42. Greipp PR, Gaillard JP, Kalish LA et al. Independent prognostic value for serum soluble interleukin-6 receptor (sIL-6R) in Eastern Cooperative Oncology Group (ECOG) Myeloma Trial E9487. *Proc Am Soc Clin Oncol* 1993; **12**: 404.
43. Greipp PR. Prognosis in myeloma. *Mayo Clin Proc* 1994; **69**: 895–902.
44. Carter A, Merchav S, Silvian-Draxler I et al. The role of interleukin-1 and tumour necrosis factor-alpha in human multiple myeloma. *Br J Haematol* 1990; **74**: 424–31.
45. Greipp PR, Lust JA. Pathogenetic relation between monoclonal gammopathies of undetermined significance and multiple myeloma. *Stem Cells* 1995; **2**: 10–21.
46. Torcia M, Lucibello M, Vannier E et al. Modulation of osteoclast-activating factor activity of multiple myeloma bone marrow cells by different interleukin-1 inhibitors. *Exp Hematol* 1996; **24**: 868–74.
47. Greipp PR, Witzig TE, Gonchoroff NJ. Immunofluorescent plasma cell labeling indices (Li) using a monoclonal antibody (Bu-1). *Am J Hematol* 1985; **20**: 289–92.
48. Witzig TE, Gonchoroff NJ, Katzmann JA et al. Peripheral blood B cell labeling indices are a measure of disease activity in patients with monoclonal gammopathies. *J Clin Oncol* 1988; **6**: 1041–6.
49. Greipp PR, Lust JA, O'Fallon WM et al. Plasma cell labeling index and beta 2–microglobulin predict survival independent of thymidine kinase and C-reactive protein in multiple myeloma. *Blood* 1993; **81**: 3382–7.
50. Teoh G, Urashima M, Greenfield EA et al. The 86-kD subunit of Ku autoantigen mediates homotypic and heterotypic adhesion of multiple myeloma cells. *J Clin Invest* 1998; **101**: 1379–88.
51. Dewald GW, Kyle RA, Hicks GA et al. The clinical significance of cytogenetic studies in 100 patients with multiple myeloma, plasma cell leukemia, or amyloidosis. *Blood* 1985; **66**: 380–90.
52. Fonseca R, Ahmann GJ, Juneau AL et al. Cytogenetic abnormalities in multiple myeloma and related plasma cell disorders: a comparison of conventional cytogenetic analysis to fluorescent in situ hybridization with simultaneous cytoplasmic immunoglobulin staining. *Blood* 1997; **90**(Suppl 1): 349a.
53. Nishida K, Tamura A, Nakazawa N et al. The Ig heavy chain gene is frequently involved in chromosomal translocations in multiple myeloma and plasma cell leukemia as detected by in situ hybridization. *Blood* 1997; **90**: 526–34.
54. Tricot G, Sawyer JR, Jagannath S et al. Unique role of cytogenetics in the prognosis of patients with myeloma receiving high-dose therapy and autotransplants. *J Clin Oncol* 1997; **15**: 2659–66.
55. Rajkumar SV, Fonseca R, Lacy MQ et al. Abnormal cytogenetics predict for poor survival after peripheral blood stem cell transplantation in relapsed multiple myeloma. *Blood* 1997; **90**(Suppl 1): 527a.
56. Rajkumar SV, Fonseca R, Dewald GW et al. Cytogenetic abnormalities correlate with the plasma cell labeling index and extent of bone marrow involvement in myeloma. *Cancer Genet Cytogenet* 1999; **113**: 73–7.
57. Bergsagel PL, Nardini E, Brents L et al. IgH translocations in multiple myeloma: a nearly universal event that rarely involves c-myc. *Curr Top Microbiol Immunol* 1997; **224**: 283–7.
58. Bergsagel PL, Chesi M, Nardini E et al. Promiscuous translocations into immunoglobulin heavy chain switch regions in multiple myeloma. *Proc Natl Acad Sci USA* 1996; **93**: 13931–6.
59. Dankbar B, Padro T, Mesters RM et al. VEGF is expressed by myeloma cells and stimulates IL-6 secretion by microvascular endothelial and marrow stromal cells. *Blood* 1998; **92**(Suppl 1): 681a.
60. Rajkumar SV, Fonseca R, Witzig TE et al. Bone marrow angiogenesis in complete responders after stem cell transplantation for multiple myeloma. *Leukemia* 1999; **13**: 469–72.
61. Rajkumar SV, Leong T, Roche PC. Prognostic value bone marrow angiogenesis in multiple myeloma. *Clin Cancer Res* 2000; **6**: 3111–16.

62. Vacca A, Ribatti D, Roncali L et al. Bone marrow angiogenesis and progression in multiple myeloma. *Br J Haematol* 1994; **87**: 503–8.
63. Munshi N, Wilson CS, Penn J et al. Angiogenesis in newly diagnosed multiple myeloma: poor prognosis with increased microvessel density (MVD) in bone marrow biopsies. *Blood* 1998; **92**(Suppl 1): 98a.
64. Vacca A, Di Loreto M, Ribatti D et al. Bone marrow of patients with active multiple myeloma: angiogenesis and plasma cell adhesion molecules LFA-1, VLA-4, LAM-1, and CD44. *Am J Hematol* 1995; **50**: 9–14.
65. Lieber MR, Chang CP, Gallo M et al. The mechanism of V(D)J recombination: Site-specificity, reaction fidelity and immunologic diversity. *Semin Immunol* 1994; **6**: 143–53.
66. Alt FW, Oltz EM, Young F et al. VDJ recombination. *Immunol Today* 1992; **13**: 306–14.
67. Schatz DG, Oettinger MA, Schlissel MS. V(D)J recombination: molecular biology and regulation. *Annu Rev Immunol* 1992; **10**: 359–83.
68. Seidman JG, Leder P. The arrangement and rearrangement of antibody genes. *Nature* 1978; **276**: 790–5.
69. Stewart AK, Schwartz RS. Immunoglobulin V regions and the B cell. *Blood* 1994; **83**: 1717–30.
70. Oettinger MA, Schatz DG, Gorka C et al. RAG-1 and RAG-2, adjacent genes that synergistically activate V(D)J recombination. *Science* 1990; **248**: 1517–23.
71. Yancopoulos GD, Blackwell TK, Suh H et al. Introduced T cell receptor variable region gene segments recombine in pre-B cells: evidence that B and T cells use a common recombinase. *Cell* 1986; **44**: 251–9.
72. Virella G, Wang AC. Immunoglobulin structure. *Immunol Ser* 1993; **58**: 75–90.
73. Buck CA. Immunoglobulin superfamily: structure, function and relationship to other receptor molecules. *Semin Cell Biol* 1992; **3**: 179–88.
74. Kirkham PM, Schroeder HW Jr. Antibody structure and the evolution of immunoglobulin V gene segments. *Semin Immunol* 1994; **6**: 347–60.
75. Wu TT, Kabat EA. An analysis of the sequences of the variable regions of Bence Jones proteins and myeloma light chains and their implications for antibody complementarity. *J Exp Med* 1970; **132**: 211–50.
76. Capra JD, Kehoe JM, Williams RC Jr et al. Light chain sequences of human IgM cold agglutinins (variable-region subgroups/amino-acid sequence/kappa light chain/N-terminal). *Proc Natl Acad Sci USA* 1972; **69**: 40–3.
77. Pascual V, Capra JD. Human immunoglobulin heavy-chain variable region genes: organization, polymorphism, and expression. *Adv Immunol* 1991; **49**: 1–74.
78. Capra JD, Kehoe JM. Hypervariable regions, idiotypy, and the antibody-combining site. *Adv Immunol* 1975; **20**: 1–40.
79. Kyle RA, Lust JA. Immunoglobulins and laboratory recognition of monoclonal proteins. In: *Neoplastic Diseases of the Blood*, 3rd edn (Wiernik PH, Canellos GP, Dutcher JP, Kyle RA, eds). New York: Churchill Livingstone, 1996: 453–75.
80. VanDyk L, Meek K. Assembly of IgH CDR3: mechanism, regulation, and influence on antibody diversity. *Int Rev Immunol* 1992; **8**: 123–33.
81. Bakkus MH, Heirman C, Van Riet I et al. Evidence that multiple myeloma Ig heavy chain VDJ genes contain somatic mutations but show no intraclonal variation. *Blood* 1992; **80**: 2326–35.
82. Takishita M, Kosaka M. Multiple myeloma: new evidence and insights from the immunoglobulin heavy chain gene and phenotypes. *Leuk Lymphoma* 1995; **19**: 395–400.
83. Van Riet I, Bakkus M, De Greef C et al. Homing mechanisms in the etiopathogenesis of multiple myeloma. *Stem Cells* 1995; **2**: 22–7.
84. Bergsagel PL, Masellis Smith A, Belch AR et al. The blood B-cells and bone marrow plasma cells in patients with multiple myeloma share identical IgH rearrangements. *Curr Top Microbiol Immunol* 1995; **194**: 17–24.
85. Bergsagel PL, Smith AM, Szczepek A et al. In multiple myeloma, clonotypic B lymphocytes are detectable among $CD19^+$ peripheral blood cells expressing CD38, CD56, and monotypic Ig light chain. *Blood* 1995; **85**: 436–47.
86. Kyle RA, Gleich GJ. IgG subclasses in monoclonal gammopathy of undetermined significance. *J Lab Clin Med* 1982; **100**: 806–14.

2

Molecular biology of plasma cell disorders

Terry H Landowski, William S Dalton

CONTENTS • **Introduction** • **Anti-aptoptotic oncogenes** • **Pro-apoptotic genes** • **Growth-promoting oncogenes** • ***ras* mutations in myeloma** • **Tumor progression through additional mutations**

INTRODUCTION

Oncogenes activated in human tumors can be classified into two general categories: those promoting cell proliferation and those preventing cell death. The development and progression of cancer depends upon an imbalance between the two categories of genes. Because the disease course of myeloma is characterized by the latent accumulation of well-differentiated plasma cells that typically display low proliferative activity, it is reasonable to consider mechanisms that dysregulate the process of cell death as an initial step in the transformation process.

Aberrant expression of anti-apoptotic oncogenes has been identified in many tumor types, including myeloma. However, overexpression alone of the proteins encoded by these oncogenes may not be sufficient for full oncogenic transformation. As a normally quiescent cell, the plasma cell is likely to require a mitogenic signal to promote malignancy. The extension of the lifespan of myeloma tumor cells due to dysregulated expression of the antiapoptotic genes may facilitate disease progression by allowing the accumulation of additional oncogenic mutations.[1]

In contrast to certain hematologic malignancies such as chronic myeloid leukemia, no single genetic anomaly has been implicated in the pathogenesis of myeloma. Cytogenetic analysis of myeloma cells frequently demonstrates multiple mutations and chromosomal aberrations. As in many B-lymphocyte neoplasms, one of the most predominant aberrations identified in myeloma involves the dysregulation of proto-oncogenes by rearrangement with the immunoglobulin heavy-chain (IgH) locus (14q32) of the plasma cell.[2,3] Several lines of evidence indicate that although the original genetic insult occurs in the pre-B- or early B-cell population, lymphocyte development occurs along normal lines prior to antigenic stimulation.[4,5]

Plasma cell development originates in the bone marrow, and progresses through a number of sequential stages defined primarily by the status of immunoglobulin gene rearrangements.[6] The initial rearrangement of the heavy-chain locus in naive pro-B cells occurs within the bone marrow, and this is followed by negative selection for self-reactive antigens. Newly generated B cells that express self-reactive Ig are deleted by induction of programmed cell death through the ligation of cell surface death receptors and co-stimulatory molecules. Cells surviving the initial selection migrate out of the bone marrow to the spleen and lymph node germinal centers, where they undergo hypermutation of the *IgH* and *IgL* genes in response to foreign antigens. Following a secondary antigen challenge, plasmablasts selected for expression of high-affinity Ig receptors typically home to the bone marrow, where they differentiate into long-lived plasma cells.

The clonality of the IgH rearrangement seen in myeloma cells and the non-specific nature of the secreted immunoglobulin suggest that malignant cells in myeloma originate outside of the bone marrow; perhaps during a secondary gene recombination event.

Specific mutations occurring at either the pro-B-cell or plasmablast stage likely provide a survival advantage to the long-lived plasma cells, allowing the development of further mutations in and transformation to the malignant phenotype. Karyotype abnormalities and myeloma development are discussed in Chapter 5; see also the reviews in references 7–9. This chapter will focus on the potential mechanisms by which commonly dysregulated oncogenes may contribute to the pathogenesis and progression of myeloma.

ANTI-APOPTOTIC ONCOGENES

bcl-2

The *bcl-2* gene was one of the first to be identified as a proto-oncogene with anti-apoptotic activity.[10,11] Originally isolated from follicular B-cell lymphoma, the *bcl-2* gene is translocated into the *IgH* locus in over 80% of follicular B-cell malignancies, resulting in high constitutive expression of the protein product Bcl-2. This is a 25 kDa protein that has been shown to localize to the mitochondrial membrane, where it functions as an inhibitor of the apoptotic cascade.[12]

The frequency of *bcl-2* translocations t(14;18) is much lower in myeloma than in other B-cell malignancies. However, overexpression of Bcl-2 protein has been demonstrated in the majority of myeloma patient specimens and cell lines examined.[13–16]

Apoptosis, induced either by physiological or pharmaceutical means, is characterized by the activation of a proteolytic enzyme cascade that ultimately results in DNA fragmentation and cell death. One level of amplification and control in the apoptotic cascade involves a permeability transition of the mitochondria and the release of cytochrome *c* into the cytoplasmic space to form a quaternary complex for the activation of downstream effectors.[12,17–21] It has been proposed that Bcl-2 functions as an ion gate in the mitochondrial membrane, where it is believed to control the flow of ions such as calcium, prevent mitochondrial swelling, and inhibit the opening of membrane pores.

Overexpression of Bcl-2 allows the protein to form stable homodimers in the mitochondrial membrane, thereby preventing the release of cytochrome *c* and inhibiting the terminal steps of the apoptotic cascade. In addition, high levels of Bcl-2 protein leads to the formation of heterodimers with pro-apoptotic members of the Bcl family, including Bad and Bax, thereby blocking their pro-apoptotic function. Bcl-2 has been shown to efficiently inhibit programmed cell death by physiological mediators, such as cytokine deprivation,[22] tumor necrosis factor α (TNF-α), and Fas,[23] as well as the cytotoxicity of chemotherapeutic drugs.[20]

bcl-2 translocations have been identified in only 5–15% of myeloma cells. However, 80–100% of patients have been reported to express high levels of the Bcl-2 protein. The mechanism of *bcl-2* overexpression in myeloma tumors that do not contain the t(14;18) translocation is currently unknown. Recent studies have implicated *c-myb*, the cellular homologue of the transforming gene of the avian myeloblastosis virus, as a *bcl-2* transactivating factor.[24]

In addition to its role as an anti-apoptotic protein, Bcl-2 has recently been implicated as a regulatory molecule in cell cycle progression.[25,26] Overexpression of Bcl-2 has been shown to result in a 30–60% increase in the length of G_1 phase in a variety of cell types. There is an inverse relationship between Bcl-2 expression and the proliferative index of normal and malignant plasma cells.[27] In this study, myeloma cells from 49 patients with various stages of disease were examined for expression of Bcl-2 in relation to the location of the tumor. The lowest expression of Bcl-2 was identified in malignant plasma cells from extramedullary sites and reactive plasmacytosis, which displayed a high labeling index. In contrast, high levels of Bcl-2 protein were detected in plasma cells derived from bone marrows of normal individuals as well as myeloma patients. Bcl-2-positive cells proliferated minimally or not at all. These observations support the hypothesis that cell cycle kinetics may be intimately related to the regulation of programmed cell death, although the nature of this association is not well defined.

bcl-x$_L$

A second member of the Bcl-2 family with anti-apoptotic function is Bcl-x_L, which is constitutively expressed in a large number of patients with myeloma and myeloma cell lines; particularly those displaying resistance to chemotherapeutic drugs.[28] In contrast to the constitutive overexpression of Bcl-2, Bcl-x_L expression appears to be primarily controlled by cytokine-inducible promoters in hematopoietic cells. Interleukin (IL)-6 is considered to be the major growth factor in myeloma, and several established myeloma cell lines require IL-6 for survival. Signal transduction through the IL-6 receptor has been shown to induce the expression of Bcl-x_L.[29]

The myeloma cell line U266 is an IL-6-dependent cell line that produces high levels of IL-6 establishing an autocrine loop for its own survival. Recent studies have demonstrated that *bcl-x$_L$* expression is induced in the U266 cell line by a pathway involving the non-receptor tyrosine kinase Jak2, and the transcription factor STAT3.[30] Abrogation of the IL-6–Jak/STAT pathway by a Jak2 inhibitor or a dominant-negative STAT3 expression vector resulted in downregulation of the anti-apoptotic gene *bcl-x$_L$*, thereby reversing the inherent resistance of these cells to Fas-mediated apoptosis. STAT3 was found to be activated in the bone marrows of all 24 myeloma patient examined, suggesting that STAT3-mediated expression of Bcl-x_L may be a common mechanism of tumor cell survival in myeloma (Figure 2.1).

FGFR3

In addition to the high frequency of STAT3 activation in myeloma, STAT1 is also constitutively activated in some patients. The signal transduction pathways leading to STAT1 activation in myeloma tumor cells are not known at present. Recent studies have shown that STAT1 and STAT5 are activated by overexpression of mutant fibroblast growth factor receptor 3 (FGFR3).[31]

This may be particularly relevant to the pathogenesis of myeloma, since *FGFR3* is dysregulated by translocation to the *IgH* locus in approximately 25% of myeloma cell lines and patients, resulting in high constitutive expression of the receptor.[2,32] Additionally, myeloma cells with the *FGFR3* translocation t(4;14) frequently display additional mutations within the receptor, resulting in constitutive FGFR3 signaling in the absence of ligand stimulus.

FGFR3 is normally expressed in the lung, kidney, and the chondrocytes at the ends of growing bones where it is believed to regulate endochondral bone growth. In animal models, overexpression of mutant FGFR3 causes constitutive activation of STAT1, STAT5a, and STAT5b.[31,33] The specific role of FGFR3 signaling in myeloma is yet to be defined.

STAT1 and STAT5 activation have both been linked to cytokine-inducible survival signals in other hematopoietic cells. STAT1 was originally identified as a ligand-induced transcription factor in interferon-treated cells.[34,35] Subsequent studies have demonstrated STAT activation by interferons -α, -β, and -γ,[36] IL-2 …, -7, -9, -10 …, -13, and -15,[37–40] erythropoietin,[41] growth hormone, and other polypeptides.[42] For example, experiments have demonstrated that the stable expression of a dominant-negative form of STAT5 in the murine IL-3-dependent cell line Ba/F3 renders the cells more sensitive to

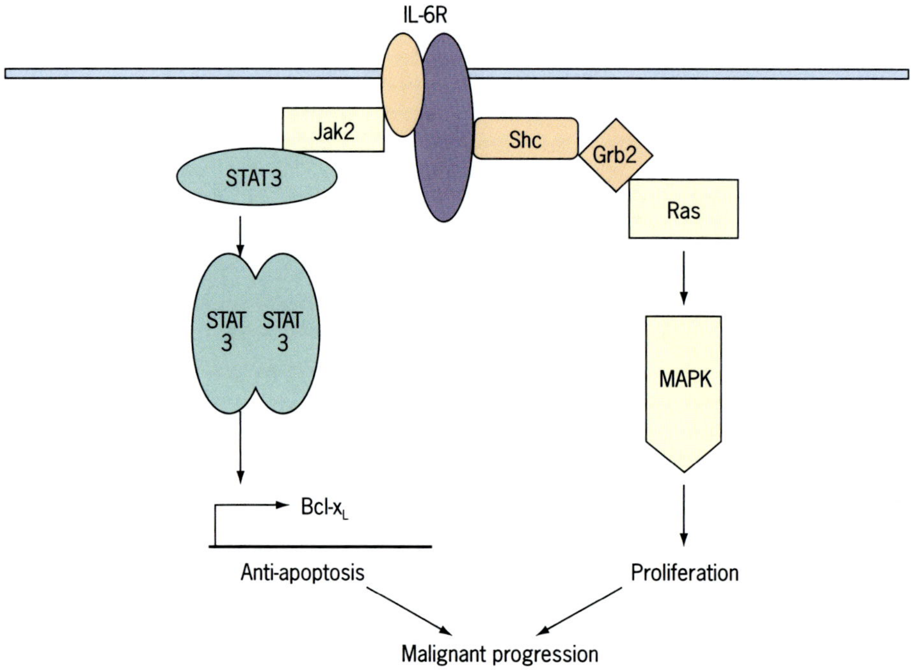

Figure 2.1 Cytokine receptor signal transduction pathways contribute to myeloma tumor progression. IL-6, the major plasma cell growth factor, activates the Jak/STAT signal transduction pathway, leading to phosphorylation and dimerization of STAT3 subunits. Activated STAT homo- or heterodimers translocate to the nucleus, where they bind DNA and initiate specific gene transcription. One of the genes transcriptionally regulated by the IL-6–Jak2/STAT3 signal transduction pathway is the anti-apoptotic gene *bcl-x*$_L$. Constitutive expression of anti-apoptotic factors by alterations in the cytokine receptor signal transduction pathways provides for extended survival of myeloma cells, and allows accumulation of additional transforming mutations.

apoptosis due to IL-3 withdrawal.[43] Similarly, transfection of the same cell line with a constitutively activated STAT5 mutant conferred growth-factor independence through overexpression of Bcl-x$_L$ and the serine/threonine kinase Pim-1.[37] With these studies and more, it is becoming increasingly clear that genes regulated by the STAT family of transcriptional activators are highly cell-type-specific, and different cells are likely to respond to death (or growth) stimuli in different manners.

PRO-APOPTOTIC GENES

Just as overexpression of anti-apoptotic genes may contribute to the pathogenesis of myeloma, underexpression or inactivating mutations in pro-apoptotic genes could have a similar effect. The Fas/Fas-ligand (CD95/CD95L) system of apoptosis plays a central role in the regulation of hemostasis by elimination of self-reactive lymphocytes during ontogeny, and of activated lymphocytes following an immune response (for reviews, see references 44–46). Aberrant expression or function of the Fas antigen has been associated with both human and animal disease characterized by lymphadenopathy, hypergammaglobulinemia, and autoimmunity.[47–50]

Several recent reports have identified Fas antigen expression on primary myeloma cells as well as cultured myeloma cell lines.[51–53] However, not all myeloma cells are capable of undergoing apoptosis in response to cross-linkage with anti-Fas antibody.[54,55] Examination of the Fas antigen cDNA in bone marrow samples obtained from 54 patients with myeloma identified mutations in the signal-transducing region of the Fas antigen that may account for the functional deficiencies identified in those studies.[56] Thus, Fas antigen mutations may contribute to the pathogenesis and progression of some hematological malignancies (Figure 2.2).

GROWTH-PROMOTING ONCOGENES

One of the more frequently identified translocations in myeloma is t(11;14), which results in constitutive overexpression of the cell cycle regulator cyclin D1.[3,57] In normal cells, D-type cyclins function as growth factor sensors and provide the required signal between mitogenic cues and the cell cycle machinery. Constitutive activation of the D-type cyclin pathway by mutations or overexpression of cyclin D1 may provide a mechanism for myeloma tumor cells to escape from growth factor dependence and promote tumorigenesis.

When quiescent cells enter the cell cycle, genes encoding D-type cyclins are induced in response to mitogenic signals. As cells progress through G_1 phase, the cyclins assemble with their catalytic partners, the cyclin-dependent kinases Cdk4 and Cdk6.[58] Assembled cyclin D–Cdk complexes then enter the cell nucleus, where they must be phosphorylated by a Cdk-activating kinase (CAK) for subsequent phosphorylation of protein substrates, most notably the tumor suppressor gene, *Rb*. Phosphorylation of the Rb protein is initiated by the D-type cyclins at the onset of G_1, and is maintained throughout the cell cycle by the E-type cyclins.

In its hypophosphorylated form, Rb associates with the transcription factor E2F, preventing E2F-dependent transcription of genes required for mitosis. Phosphorylation of Rb, initially by cyclin D and subsequently by cyclin

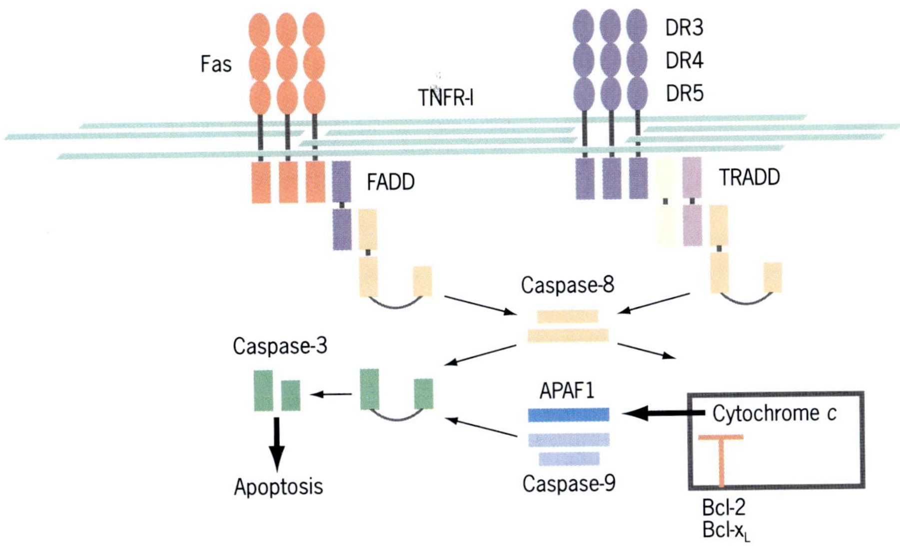

Figure 2.2 Apoptotic signal transduction by death receptors of the tumor necrosis factor receptor (TNFR) family. Ligand binding of the death receptors Fas (CD95) or DR3, DR4, DR5 leads to oligomerization of the receptor and recruitment of signaling molecules to a death-inducing signal complex (DISC). This complex includes the adapter proteins FADD (Fas-associated death domain) and/or TRADD (TNFR-associated death domain), and a cysteine protease, caspase-8. Cleavage and activation of caspase-8 initiates a proteolytic cascade ultimately resulting in the death of the cell. Alterations affecting the signal domain of the Fas death receptor prevent DISC formation, and inhibit the apoptotic signal pathway, allowing myeloma tumor cells to escape immune surveillance.

E, disrupts the Rb–E2F interaction, allowing E2F transcriptional activity.

In untransformed cells, the induction of cyclin D expression and its association with CDKs are independently regulated by mitogen-induced kinases, providing a two-signal check on cyclin D activity. Myeloma cells with translocation and overexpression of cyclin D1 have lost one of the checks on cyclin D1 function. An additional mutation in a growth factor receptor or signal transduction pathway under the circumstances can circumvent the second required mitogenic signal, resulting in a transformed phenotype. One of the most frequently identified mutations in all human cancer, including myeloma, is that of the signal transduction protein, Ras.[59,60]

ras MUTATIONS IN MYELOMA

The proto-oncogene *ras* was the first gene to be implicated in human cancer.[61–63] Initially identified as transforming oncogenes of the Harvey (H-*ras*) and Kirsten (K-*ras*) murine sarcoma viruses, the eukaryotic genome contains three non-transforming homologues of the *ras* gene located on different chromosomes. The three functional genes, H-*ras*, N-*ras*, and K-*ras*, have a very similar structure and function, but vary in intron size and structure, ranging in size from 3 kb to 35 kb.

The protein product of each of these genes is approximately 21 kDa in size, and encodes a signal transduction molecule that cycles between the active guanosine diphosphate (GDP)-bound and the inactive guanosine triphosphate (GTP)-bound state. Cell surface receptors activate the p21 protein through intrinsic tyrosine kinase activity or through phosphorylation by associated non-receptor tyrosine kinase messengers, resulting in the exchange of GDP for GTP. This activation initiates a sequence of events known as the MAP kinase (mitogen-activated protein kinase) cascade, and results in the transcriptional activation of various genes, including cyclin D1.[64] Activated p21 is returned to the inactive state by recruitment and association with a GTPase-activating protein (Ras-GAP), which hydrolyzes the bound GTP to GDP. Activating mutations in the *ras* proto-oncogene typically involve a single base change, impairing the GTPase activity of the Ras-GAP molecule, and resulting in constitutive activation of the Ras-MAP kinase cascade.

One of the cell surface receptors known to activate the Ras–MAP kinase pathway is the IL-6 receptor. In addition to the IL-6/Jak/STAT signal transduction pathway leading to the expression of anti-apoptotic factors, IL-6 has been shown to induce myeloma cell proliferation via the Ras–MAP kinase pathway.[65,66]

Two independent studies have demonstrated that IL-6 treatment of myeloma cell lines induces phosphorylation of the signaling intermediates Shc and Grb2, followed by ras translocation and MAP kinase activation. Ogata et al[66] demonstrated that this activity occurred only in myeloma cell lines capable of proliferation in response to IL-6, suggesting that IL-6 signaling through the Ras–MAP kinase pathway is an important event in promoting the growth of myeloma cells. Oncogenic *ras* mutations in myeloma cells result in constitutive activation of the MAP kinase pathway, and allow IL-6-independent proliferation; presumably through overexpression of cyclin D1 or other mitogen-responsive genes.

Examination of myeloma cells for oncogenic *ras* mutations has revealed activating K- or N-*ras* mutations in 30–47% of patients.[67–69] More importantly, the incidence of *ras* mutations correlated with a number of critical clinical parameters.[69] The median survival of patients with K-*ras* mutations was approximately 2.0 years, compared with 3.7 years for patients without K-*ras* mutations. These data suggest that *ras* mutations may be associated with disease progression, and may be useful as prognostic indicators in myeloma patients.

TUMOR PROGRESSION THROUGH ADDITIONAL MUTATIONS

Translocations resulting in dysregulation of anti-apoptotic genes or cell cycle regulatory genes have been demonstrated in approximately 50% of myeloma patients. Both of these events then allow the accumulation of additional oncogenic mutations that may contribute to disease progression and poor response to therapy. In addition to the correlation identified between *ras* mutations and advanced disease, mutations in the tumor suppressor gene *p53* have also been associated with resistance to chemotherapeutic drugs and a poor prognosis in myeloma.[70,71]

The tumor suppressor gene *p53* encodes for DNA-binding protein p53 with a diverse range of biological activities.[72,73] High-level expression of wild-type p53 has two outcomes: cell cycle arrest or apoptosis. The *p53* gene is proposed to be responsible for maintaining stability of the genome, and both cell cycle arrest and apoptosis can be considered mechanisms by which this may be accomplished. In the presence of DNA damage, cells with fully functional p53 will undergo cell cycle arrest to allow DNA repair. In the case of extensive damage, or insufficient DNA repair, the cell can be committed to p53-dependent cell death. In either situation, the propagation of potentially deleterious mutations can thus be averted.

The exact mechanism used by the cell to determine whether it will arrest or die is currently unknown; however, p53 has been shown to play a central role in both processes, and is proposed to be the pivotal molecule. Tumors that have aberrant p53 function through point mutations or gene deletion are frequently unable to arrest in G_1, or demonstrate a resistance to apoptosis mediated by DNA-damaging agents.

DNA strand breaks induced by cytotoxic agents or ionizing radiation lead to rapid accumulation of p53 protein.[74] This induction of *p53* expression is not a transcriptional event since levels of *p53* mRNA do not significantly change following DNA damage. Rather, the elevated levels of p53 protein are primarily attributed to enhanced protein stability and reduced degradation mediated by association with the Mdm2 protein. Additional post-translational modifications, including phosphorylation and acetylation, further activate the p53 protein and modulate its interactions with DNA and other regulatory proteins.

Analysis of a broad spectrum of human malignancies has identified 'hot spots' within the *p53* coding region that display a large number of point mutations. The vast majority of *p53* mutations have been localized to highly conserved regions in the sequence-specific DNA-binding domain.

One of the best-characterized functions of p53 is the initiation of cell cycle arrest either at G_1 or G_2/M following genotoxic stress. Cell cycle arrest depends on the transactivation of target genes by wild-type p53, primarily the cyclin-dependent kinase inhibitor $p21^{Cip1}$. Up-regulation of p21 expression by p53 has been shown to inhibit cyclin E/Cdk2 and cyclinA/Cdk2 activities, thereby preventing the phosphorylation of Rb and blocking cell cycle transit.

When the DNA damage incurred by a cell exceeds the capacity of the cell to repair the damage, the cell will undergo p53–dependent apoptosis. p53 transactivation of the pro-apoptotic protein Bax has been identified as one potential mechanism of p53-dependent cell death. Bax, a member of the Bcl-2 family, has been shown to be transcriptionally activated by p53, and is thought to be the primary means by which p53 induces cell death.[75,76] Just as the anti-apoptotic members of the Bcl-2 family form homo- and heterodimers to inhibit mitochondrial permeability transition, the pro-apoptotic family members promote mitochondrial pore formation and cytochrome *c* release.[77–79]

The incidence of *p53* mutations in myeloma is relatively low; ranging from 13% to 24%,[71,80,81] but a strong correlation has been identified between altered *p53* expression and resistance to chemotherapy.[82] This suggests that *p53* mutations may not play a major role in the initial pathogenesis of myeloma but may contribute to disease progression and the development of multidrug resistance, which is frequently seen in relapsed disease.[70,83]

Additional genetic lesions have been identified in myeloma cells, but their function is poorly understood. These include the genes encoding for the transcription factors c-Myc and c-Maf.[1,9,81] Although c-*myc* is frequently identified as an IgH translocation in murine myeloma, the frequency of c-*myc* translocations in human myeloma is less than 20%.[2,84] However, immunocytochemical examination of c-Myc expression has demonstrated high levels of protein in up to 53% of myeloma patients.[81,85] c-Myc is a transcription factor that was discovered as the cellular homologue of the transforming oncogene of several chicken retroviruses.[86,87] As with many proto-oncogenes, dysregulation of *myc* alone is not generally sufficient for oncogenic transformation, and a second oncogenic signal is required as well. Myc proteins are transcription factors of the helix–loop/leucine zipper family that activate transcription as obligate heterodimers with a partner protein, Max. The activity of the heterodimeric complex is primarily regulated by Myc : Max ratios. In normal cells, c-*myc* expression is strictly regulated in a growth-factor-dependent manner. In non-hematologic malignancies, dysregulation of c-*myc* expression is most commonly seen as a result of mutations in signaling pathways that regulate c-*myc* expression, suggesting that *myc* activation is a late event in tumor progression. Recently, mutations in the 5′ untranslated region of the c-*myc* gene have been identified in myeloma. These mutations contribute to the stability and accumulation of the protein.[88] Myc overexpression is associated with a rapid induction of cyclin E–Cdk2 kinase activity, hyperphosphorylation of Rb, and cell cycle progression in the absence of mitogenic signaling, thus fulfilling the requirements for a proliferative stimulus to the quiescent plasma cell. However, the exact role of c-*myc* activation in the pathogenesis of myeloma requires further investigation.

A second member of the helix–loop/leucine zipper family of transcription factors recently found to be frequently translocated in myeloma is that encoded by the proto-oncogene c-*maf*.[89] c-Maf is a highly tissue-specific transcription factor responsible for the expression of IL-4 in a subset of T helper cells.[90] Ectopic expression of c-Maf in non-IL-4-expressing B cells is sufficient to induce expression of the endogenous IL-4 gene, suggesting that dysregulation of the c-*maf* gene in B-cell malignancies, including myeloma, could contribute to the tumorigenic phenotype. The mechanism of c-Maf/IL-4 transformation in myeloma cells is highly speculative at present; however, IL-4 has been shown to induce resistance to physiological mediators of cell death in B cells.[91] This may very possibly be mediated by STAT activation and transcription of anti-apoptotic genes of the *bcl-2* family, such as *mcl-1*.[92,93] Plasma cells with the t(16;22) translocation would be protected from elimination by the immune system, allowing extended survival, and the accumulation of additional mutations.

The broad spectrum of karyotypic alterations seen in myeloma cells supports the hypothesis that the pathogenesis of myeloma is a multistep process (Figure 2.3). A recurring theme in the molecular anomalies is the initial survival advantage gained by chromosomal translocations, most likely during V(D)J recombination. This event gives rise to a pre-neoplastic plasma cell that is resistant to physiological mechanisms of elimination. The long-lived plasma cell remains dormant, possibly for a very long time, until a second signal promotes proliferation and immortality. An extended lifespan allows the accumulation of later additional mutations, resulting in the selection of a single clone expressing the malignant phenotype.

Because of the dormant nature of the untransformed plasma cell, the prospects for early detection and intervention in myeloma are minimal at best. However, later mutations, such as *p53* and *ras*, are more closely correlated with disease progression, and may represent molecular targets for rational drug design. Strategies to target these later molecular events may require long-term maintenance therapy. This may be reasonable, because agents directed against fundamental molecular mechanisms provide greater biological specificity, and increase the likelihood that the drug effect will be confined to the tumor cells.

Many of the molecular targets in signal transduction pathways represent common mechanisms used to regulate multiple cellular

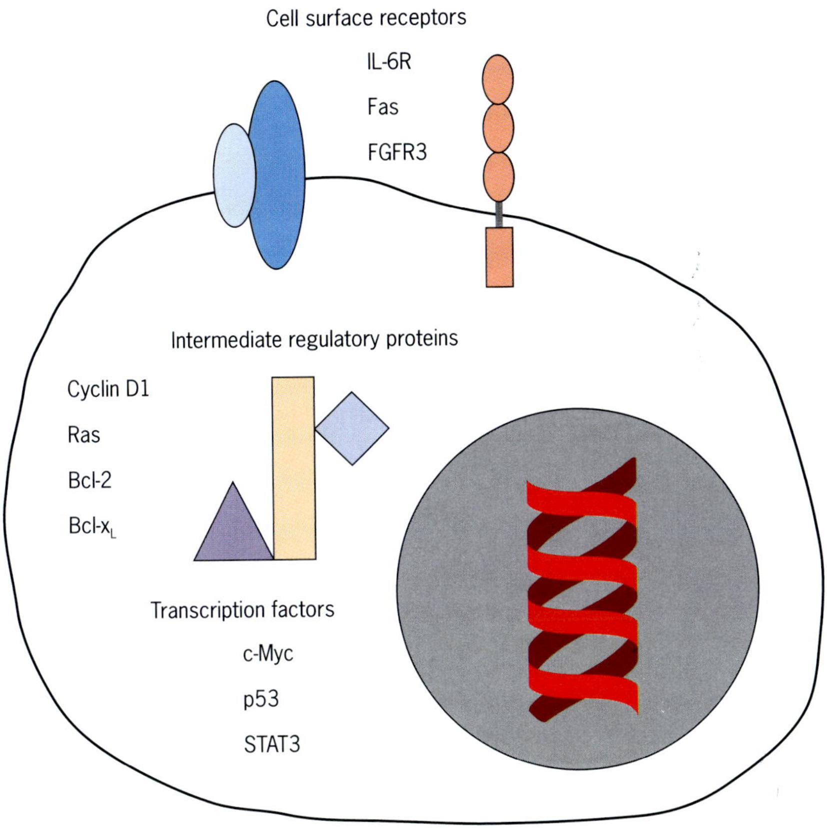

Figure 2.3 Commonly dysregulated oncogenes in myeloma. Normal signal transduction pathways include molecules that contribute to both cell proliferation and cell death. Aberrant regulation of either of these pathways may contribute to the pathogenesis and progression of human tumors. The figure shows just some of the proteins encoded by genes that have been implicated in the molecular pathogenesis of myeloma.

functions, thus exemplifying the complexity of rational drug design. Further understanding of the transformation process and the pathways involved in malignant progression is essential to the development of effective therapeutic agents.

REFERENCES

1. Pope B, Brown R, Luo XF, et al. Disease progression in patients with multiple myeloma is associated with a concurrent alteration in the expression of both oncogenes and tumor suppressor genes and can be monitored by the oncoprotein phenotype. *Leuk Lymphoma* 1997; **25**: 545–54.
2. Avet-Loiseau H, Li JY, Facon T, et al. High incidence of translocation t(11;14)(q13;q32) and t(4;14)(p16;q32) in patients with plasma cell malignancies. *Cancer Res* 1999; **58**: 5640–5.
3. Bergsagel PL, Chesi M, Nardini E, et al. Promiscuous translocations into immunoglobulin heavy chain switch regions in multiple myeloma. *Proc Natl Acad Sci USA* 1996; **93**: 13931–6.
4. Barlogie B, Epstein J, Selvanayagam P, Alexanian R. Plasma cell myeloma – new biological insights and advances in therapy. *Blood* 1989; **73**: 865–79.
5. Niesvizky R, Siegel D, Michaeli J. Biology and treatment of multiple myeloma. *Blood Rev* 1993; **7**: 24–33.
6. Rudin CM, Thompson CB. B-cell development and maturation. *Semin Oncol* 1998; **25**: 435–46.

7. Berenson JR, Vescio RA, Said J. Multiple myeloma: the cells of origin – a two way street. *Leukemia* 1998; **12**: 121–7.
8. Komada Y, Zhou YW, Zhang XL et al. Fas receptor (CD95)-mediated apoptosis is induced in leukemic cells entering G1B compartment of the cell cycle. *Blood* 1995; **86**: 3848–60.
9. Hallek M, Bergsagel PL, Anderson KC. Multiple myeloma: increasing evidence for a multistep transformation process. *Blood* 1998; **91**: 3–21.
10. Hockenbery DM. bcl-2, a novel regulator of cell death. *BioEssays* 1995; **17**: 631–8.
11. Strasser A, Huang DCS, Vaux DL. The role of the bcl-2/ced-9 gene family in cancer and general implications of defects in cell death control for tumorigenesis and resistance to chemotherapy. *Biochim Biophys Acta* 1997; **1333**: F151–78.
12. Reed JC. Double identity for proteins of the Bcl-2 family. *Nature* 1997; **19**: 773–6.
13. Pettersson M, Jernberg-Wiklund H, Larsson LG et al. Expression of the bcl-2 gene in human multiple myeloma cell lines and normal plasma cells. *Blood* 1992; **79**: 495–502.
14. Harada H, Hata H, Yoshida M et al. Expression of Bcl-2 family of proteins in fresh myeloma cells. *Leukemia* 1998; **12**: 1817–20.
15. Hamilton MS, Barker HF, Ball J et al. Normal and neoplastic human plasma cells express bcl-2 antigen. *Leukemia* 1991; **5**: 768–71.
16. Nishida K, Taniwaki M, Misawa S, Abe T. Nonrandom rearrangement of chromosome 14 at band q32.33 in human lymphoid malignancies with mature B-cell phenotype. *Cancer Res* 1989; **49**: 1275–81.
17. Schlessinger PH, Gross A, Yin XM et al. Comparison of the ion channel characteristics of proapoptotic Bax and antiapoptotic Bcl-2. *Proc Natl Acad Sci USA* 1997; **94**: 11357–62.
18. Yang J, Liu X, Bhalla K et al. Prevention of apoptosis by Bcl-2: release of cytochrome c from mitochondria blocked. *Science* 1997; **275**: 1129–32.
19. Sattler M, Liang H, Nettesheim D et al. Structure of Bcl-x_L–Bak peptide complex: recognition between regulators of apoptosis. *Science* 1997; **275**: 983–6.
20. Decaudin D, Geley S, Hirsch T et al. Bcl-2 and Bcl-X_L antagonize the mitochondrial dysfunction preceding nuclear apoptosis induced by chemotherapeutic agents. *Cancer Res* 1997; **57**: 62–7.
21. Kluck RM, Bossy-Wetzel E, Green DR, Newmeyer DD. The release of cytochrome c from mitochondria: a primary site for Bcl-2 regulation of apoptosis. *Science* 1997; **275**: 1132–6.
22. Johnson BW, Boise LH. Bcl-2 and caspase inhibition cooperate to inhibit tumor necrosis factor-alpha-induced cell death in a Bcl-2 cleavage-independent fashion. *J Biol Chem* 1999; **274**: 18552–8.
23. Weller M, Malipiero U, Aguzzi A et al. Protooncogene bcl-2 gene transfer abrogates Fas/APO-1 antibody-mediated apoptosis of human malignant glioma cells and confers resistance to chemotherapeutic drugs and therapeutic irradiation. *J Clin Invest* 1995; **95**: 2633–43.
24. Salomoni P, Perrotti D, Martinez R et al. Resistance to apoptosis in CTLL-2 cells constitutively expressing c-Myb is associated with induction of Bcl-2 expression and Myb-dependent regulation of bcl-2 promoter activity. *Proc Natl Acad Sci USA* 1997; **94**: 3296–301.
25. Mazel S, Burtrum D, Petrie HT. Regulation of cell division cycle progression by bcl-2 expression: a potential mechanism for inhibition of programmed cell death. *J Exp Med* 1996; **183**: 2219–26.
26. Vairo G, Innes KM, Adams JM. Bcl-2 has a cell cycle inhibitory function separable from its enhancement of cell survival. *Oncogene* 1996; **13**: 1511–19.
27. Puthier D, Pellat-Deceunynck C, Barille S et al. Differential expression of Bcl-2 in human plasma cell disorders according to proliferation status and malignancy. *Leukemia* 1999; **12**: 289–94.
28. Tu Y, Renner S, Xu F et al. Bcl-X expression in multiple myeloma: possible indicator of chemoresistance. *Cancer Res* 1998; **58**: 256–62.
29. Schwarze MMK, Hawley RG. Prevention of myeloma cell apoptosis by ectopic bcl-2 expression or interleukin 6-mediated up-regulation of bcl-x_L. *Cancer Res* 1995; **55**: 2262–65.
30. Catlett-Falcone R, Landowski TH, Oshiro MM et al. Constitutive activation of Stat3 signaling confers resistance to apoptosis in human U266 myeloma cells. *Immunity* 1999; **10**: 105–15.
31. Li C, Chen L, Iwata T et al. A Lys644Glu substitution in fibroblast growth factor receptor 3 (FGFR3) causes dwarfism in mice by activation of STATs and ink4 cell cycle inhibitors. *Hum Mol Genet* 1999; **8**: 35–44.
32. Chesi M, Nardini E, Brents LA et al. Frequent translocation t(4;14)(p16.3;q32.3) in multiple myeloma is associated with increased expression and activating mutations of fibroblast growth factor receptor 3. *Nature Genet* 1997; **16**: 260–4.

33. Su WCS, Kitagawa M, Xue N et al. Activation of Stat1 by mutant fibroblast growth-factor receptor in thanatophoric dysplasia type II dwarfism. *Nature* 1997; **386**: 288–92.
34. Darnell JE Jr, Kerr IM, Stark GR. Jak–STAT pathways and transcriptional activation in response to IFNs and other extracellular signaling proteins. *Science* 1994; **264**: 1415–21.
35. Darnell JE Jr. STATs and gene regulation. *Science* 1997; **277**: 1630–5.
36. Bromberg JF, Horvath CM, Wen Z et al. Transcriptionally active Stat1 is required for the antiproliferative effects of both interferon α and interferon γ. *Proc Natl Acad Sci USA* 1996; **93**: 7673–8.
37. Nosaka T, Kawashima T, Misawa K et al. STAT5 as a molecular regulator of proliferation, differentiation and apoptosis in hematopoietic cells. *EMBO J* 1999; **17**: 4754–65.
38. Demoulin JB, Van Roost E, Stevens M et al. Distinct roles for STAT1, STAT3, and STAT5 in differentiation gene induction and apoptosis inhibition by interleukin-9. *J Biol Chem* 1999; **274**: 25855–61.
39. Moriggl R, Sexl V, Piekorz R et al. Stat5 activation is uniquely associated with cytokine signaling in peripheral T cells. *Immunity* 1999; **11**: 225–30.
40. Socolvsky M, Fallon AE, Wang S et al. Fetal anemia and apoptosis of red cell progenitors in Stat5a$^{-/-}$Stat5b$^{-/-}$ mice: a direct role for Stat5 in Bcl-X_L induction. *Cell* 1999; **98**: 181–91.
41. Silva M, Benito A, Sanz C et al. Erythropoietin can induce the expression of bcl-x_L through Stat5 in erythropoietin-dependent progenitor cell lines. *J Biol Chem* 1999; **274**: 22165–9.
42. Leaman DW, Leung S, Li X, Stark GR. Regulation of STAT-dependent pathways by growth factors and cytokines. *FASEB J* 1996; **10**: 1578–88.
43. Dumon S, Santos SC, Debierre-Grockiego F et al. IL-3 dependent regulation of Bcl-x_L gene expression by STAT5 in a bone marrow derived cell line. *Oncogene* 1999; **18**: 4191–9.
44. van Parijs L, Abbas AK. Role of Fas-mediated cell death in the regulation of immune responses. *Curr Opin Immunol* 1996; **8**: 355–61.
45. Lynch DH, Ramsdell F, Alderson MR. Fas and FasL in the homeostatic regulation of immune responses. *Immunol Today* 1995; **16**: 569–74.
46. Nagata S, Golstein P. The Fas death factor. *Science* 1995; **267**: 1449–56.
47. Rieux-Laucat F, Le Deist F, Hivroz C et al. Mutations in Fas associated with human lymphoproliferative syndrome and autoimmunity. *Science* 1995; **268**: 1347–9.
48. Fisher GH, Rosenberg FJ, Straus SE et al. Dominant interfering Fas gene mutations impair apoptosis in a human autoimmune lymphoproliferative syndrome. *Cell* 1995; **81**: 935–46.
49. Takahashi T, Tanaka M, Brannan CI et al. Generalized lymphoproliferative disease in mice, caused by a point mutation in the Fas ligand. *Cell* 1994; **76**: 969–76.
50. Watanabe-Fukunaga R, Brannan CI, Copeland NG et al. Lymphoproliferation disorder in mice explained by defects in Fas antigen that mediates apoptosis. *Nature* 1992; **356**: 314–17.
51. Mandik L, Nguyen KAT, Erikson J. Fas receptor expression on B-lineage cells. *Eur J Immunol* 1995; **25**: 3148–54.
52. Dirks W, Schone S, Uphoff C et al. Expression and function of CD95 (Fas/APO-1) in leukaemia-lymphoma tumor lines. *Br J Haematol* 1997; **96**: 584–93.
53. Wang J, Taniuchi I, Maekawa Y et al. Expression and function of Fas antigen on activated murine B cells. *Eur J Immunol* 1996; **26**: 92–6.
54. Westendorf JJ, Lammert JM, Jelinek DF. Expression and function of Fas (APO-1/CD95) in patient myeloma cells and myeloma cell lines. *Blood* 1995; **85**: 3566–76.
55. Shima Y, Nishimoto N, Ogata A et al. Myeloma cells express Fas antigen/APO-1 (CD95) but only some are sensitive to anti-Fas antibody resulting in apoptosis. *Blood* 1995; **85**: 757–64.
56. Landowski TH, Qu N, Buyuksal I et al. Mutations in the Fas antigen of multiple myeloma patients. *Blood* 1997; **90**: 4266–70.
57. Gabrea A, Bergsagel PL, Chesi M et al. Insertion of excised IgH switch sequences causes overexpression of cyclin D1 in a myeloma tumor cell. *Mol Cell* 1999; **3**: 119–23.
58. Scherr CJ. Cancer cell cycles. *Science* 1996; **274**: 1672–7.
59. Marshall MS. Ras target proteins in eukaryotic cells. *FASEB J* 1995; **9**: 1311–18.
60. Filmus J, Robles AI, Shi W et al. Induction of cyclin D1 overexpression by activated ras. *Oncogene* 1994; **9**: 3627–33.
61. Harvey JJ. An unidentified virus which causes the rapid production of tumors in mice. *Nature* 1964; **204**: 1104–5.
62. Der CJ, Krontiris TG, Cooper GM. Transforming genes of human bladder and lung carcinoma cell

lines are homologous to the ras genes of Harvey and Kirsten sarcoma viruses. *Proc Natl Acad Sci USA* 1982; **79**: 3637–40.
63. Barbacid M. Ras genes. *Annu Rev Biochem* 1987; **56**: 779–827.
64. Winston JT, Coats SR, Wang YZ, Pledger W. Regulation of the cell cycle machinery by oncogenic *ras*. *Oncogene* 1996; **12**: 127–34.
65. Neumann C, Zehentmaier G, Danhauser-Riedl S et al. Interleukin-6 induces tyrosine phosphorylation of the Ras activating protein Shc, and its complex formation with Grb2 in the human multiple myeloma cell line LP-1. *Eur J Immunol* 1996; **26**: 379–84.
66. Ogata A, Chauhan D, Teoh G et al. IL-6 triggers cell growth via the ras-dependent mitogen-activated protein kinase cascade. *J Immunol* 1997; **159**: 2212–21.
67. Portier M, Moles JP, Mazars GR et al. p53 and RAS gene mutations in multiple myeloma. *Oncogene* 1992; **7**: 2539–43.
68. Corradini P, Ladetto M, Inghirami G et al. N- and K-Ras oncogenes in plasma cell dyscrasias. *Leuk Lymphoma* 1994; **15**: 17–20.
69. Liu P, Leong T, Quam L et al. Activating mutations of N- and K-ras in multiple myeloma show different clinical associations: analysis of the Eastern Cooperative Oncology Group phase III trial. *Blood* 1996; **88**: 2699–706.
70. Lowe SW, Ruley HE, Jacks T, Housman DE. p53–dependent apoptosis modulates the cytotoxicity of anticancer agents. *Cell* 1993; **74**: 957–67.
71. Neri A, Baldini L, Trecca D et al. p53 gene mutations in multiple myeloma are associated with advanced forms of malignancy. *Blood* 1993; **81**: 128–35.
72. Ko LJ, Prives C. p53: puzzle and paradigm. *Genes Dev* 1996; **10**: 1054–72.
73. Giacca AJ, Kastan MB. The complexity of p53 modulation: emerging patterns from divergent signals. *Genes Dev* 1998; **12**: 2973–83.
74. Nelson WG, Kastan MB. DNA strand breaks: the DNA template alterations that trigger p53–dependent DNA damage response pathways. *Mol Cell Biol* 1994; **14**: 1815–23.
75. Miyashita T, Reed JC. Tumor suppressor p53 is a direct transcriptional activator of the human bax gene. *Cell* 1995; **80**: 293–9.
76. McCurrach ME, Connor TMF, Knudson CM et al. bax-deficiency promotes drug resistance and oncogenic transformation by attenuating - p53-dependent apoptosis. *Proc Natl Acad Sci USA* 1997; **94**: 2345–9.
77. Zamzami N, Brenner C, Marzo I et al. Subcellular and submitochondrial mode of action of Bcl-2-like oncoproteins. *Oncogene* 1998; **16**: 2265–82.
78. Tsujimoto Y. Role of Bcl-2 family proteins in apoptosis: apoptosomes or mitochondria? *Genes Cells* 1998; **3**: 697–707.
79. Ding HF, Fisher DE. Mechanisms of p53–mediated apoptosis. *Crit Rev Oncol* 1998; **9**: 83–98.
80. Preudhomme C, Facon T, Zandecki M et al. Rare occurrence of p53 gene mutations in multiple myeloma. *Br J Haematol* 1992; **81**: 440–3.
81. Brown RD, Pope B, Luo XF et al. The oncoprotein phenotype of plasma cells from patients with multiple myeloma. *Leuk Lymphoma* 1994; **16**: 147–56.
82. Egle A, Villunger A, Marshitz I et al. Expression of Apo-1/Fas (CD95), Bcl-2, Bax and Bcl-x in myeloma cell lines: relationship between responsiveness to anti-Fas mab and p53 functional status. *Br J Haematol* 1997; **97**: 418–28.
83. Wattel E, Preudhomme C, Hecquet B et al. p53 mutations are associated with resistance to chemotherapy and short survival in hematologic malignancies. *Blood* 1994; **84**: 3148–57.
84. Rao PH, Cigudosa JC, Ning Y et al. Multicolor spectral karyotyping identifies new recurring breakpoints and translocations in multiple myeloma. *Blood* 1999; **92**: 1743–8.
85. Kuehl WM, Brents LA, Chesi M et al. Dysregulation of c-myc in multiple myeloma. *Curr Top Microbiol Immunol* 1997; **224**: 277–82.
86. Nesbit CE, Tersak JM, Prochownik EV. MYC oncogenes and human neoplastic disease. *Oncogene* 1999; **18**: 3004–16.
87. Bouchard C, Staller P, Eilers M. Control of cell proliferation by Myc. *Trends Cell Biol* 1998; **8**: 202–6.
88. Paulin FE, West MJ, Sullivan NF et al. Aberrant translational control of the c-myc gene in multiple myeloma. *Oncogene* 1996; **13**: 505–13.
89. Chesi M, Bergsagel PL, Shonukan OO et al. Frequent dysregulation of the c-maf proto-oncogene at 16q23 by translocation to an Ig locus in multiple myeloma. *Blood* 1998; **91**: 4457–63.
90. Ho IC, Hodge MR, Rooney JW, Glimcher LH. The proto-oncogene c-maf is responsible for tissue-specific expression of interleukin-4. *Cell* 1996; **88**: 973–83.
91. Foote LC, Howard RG, Marshak-Rothstein A, Rothstein TL. IL-4 induces Fas resistance in B cells. *J Immunol* 1996; **157:** 2749–53.

92. Zhou P, Qian L, Bieszczad CK et al. Mcl-1 in transgenic mice promotes survival in a spectrum of hematopoietic cell types and immortalization in the myeloid lineage. *Blood* 1998; **92**: 3226–39.

93. Lomo J, Smeland EB, Krajewski S et al. Expression of the Bcl-2 homologue Mcl-1 correlates with survival of peripheral blood B lymphocytes. *Cancer Res* 1996; **56**: 40–3.

3

The role of viruses in the pathogenesis of plasma cell disorders

Karin Tarte, Bernard Klein

CONTENTS • **Introduction** • **Biology of KSHV** • **KSHV and Castleman's disease** • **KSHV and myeloma** • **KSHV and Waldenström's macroglobulinaemia** • **KSHV and primary amyloidosis** • **Other viruses in plasma cell disorders**

INTRODUCTION

The causal role of viruses in the pathogenesis of some B-cell lymphoproliferative disorders was clearly established several years ago with the recognition of Epstein–Barr virus (EBV)-induced neoplasia. EBV is a human γ-herpesvirus which can immortalize B cells in vitro, and is involved in some forms of malignant lymphoma (Burkitt's lymphoma, AIDS-related lymphoma, post-transplantation lymphoproliferative disorders, and Hodgkin's disease).[1] A number of EBV genes, including viral homologues of interleukin (IL)-10 and *bcl-2*, participate in its transforming potential.

Plasma cell disorders include several heterogeneous neoplastic and non-neoplastic diseases with a wide range of clinical and biological manifestations. Until recently, no etiologic relationship could be demonstrated between a virus and any one of these diseases. However, the recent identification of Kaposi sarcoma-associated herpesvirus (KSHV), also called human herpesvirus-8 (HHV-8), a new γ-herpesvirus, has shed new light on the role of viruses in B-cell neoplasia.[2]

Detection of KSHV DNA by polymerase-chain reaction (PCR), epidemiological studies, and serologic assays support the causal role of KSHV in all forms of Kaposi sarcoma conclusively.[3–7] Although KSHV is not widely present in the general population, its prevalence is higher in Uganda and Sardinia in association with a higher rate of classical Kaposi sarcoma.[6,8–11] KSHV has also been linked with B-cell primary effusion lymphoma (PEL), and KSHV-infected PEL cell lines have provided a convenient tool to study KSHV-related tumorigenesis.[12,13]

In this chapter, we shall review in detail the evidence supporting an association of KSHV with a subset of Castleman's disease, and attempt to clarify the challenging question of the association of KSHV with myeloma, Waldenström's macroglobulinaemia, and primary amyloidosis.

BIOLOGY OF KSHV

The KSHV genome is approximatively 165 kb in length, and codes for at least 81 genes.[14] It contains numerous open reading frames (ORFs) numbered from ORF 4 to ORF 75 according to their homology with corresponding genes of herpesvirus saimiri (HVS), the prototypical member of the rhadinovirus genus. Several KSHV genes that are not found in HVS are designed ORF K1 to ORF K15.

Eleven KSHV ORFs have been identified as encoding for oncogenic or angiogenic factors, and have been thought to be involved in KSHV pathogenicity (Table 3.1).[15,16] Strikingly, the majority of them show homology with known cellular genes that code for secreted cytokines or for proteins involved in cell cycle regulation, cell death, and cell signalling.

Four ORFs (ORF 74, ORF K1, ORF K9, and ORF K12) have been shown to induce cellular transformation in vitro when transfected into rodent fibroblasts and to promote tumour formation in vivo. ORF 74 encodes for a viral G-protein-coupled receptor (vGPCR) constitutively activated and expressed in Kaposi sarcoma lesions and in PEL cell lines.[17,18] vGPCR stimulates signalling pathways linked to cell proliferation, and induces cell transformation in vitro and tumorigenicity in nude mice.[19] ORF K1 and ORF K12 are

Table 3.1 KSHV genes involved in cellular transformation and angiogenesis

Viral oncogenic or angiogenic factor	Transforming ORF[a]	Cellular expression[b]	Role in pathogenicity
ORF 16: vBcl-2		KS, PEL	Anti-apoptotic
ORF 72: vCyc		KS, PEL	Phosphorylation of Rb; transition G_1/S
ORF 73: LANA		KS, PEL	Inhibition of p53-mediated apoptosis
ORF 74: vGPCR	+	KS, PEL	Cell proliferation; constitutive activation of MAPK and PKC pathways; angiogenic (induction of VEGF)
ORF K1	+	KS, PEL	Constitutive signalling
ORF K2: vIL-6		PEL, CD, (KS)	Activation of gp130 pathway; proliferation of IL-6 dependent-cells
ORF K4: vMIP-II		KS, PEL	Angiogenic
ORF K6: vMIP-I		KS, PEL	Angiogenic
ORF K9: vIRF	+	PEL	Inhibition of IFN-α/β signaling
ORF K12: Kaposin	+	PEL, KS	?
ORF K13: vFLIP		?	Dominant-negative inhibition of CD95–induced apoptosis

[a] ORFs that are transforming after transfection are indicated as positive (+).
[b] KS, Kaposi sarcoma; PEL, primary effusion lymphoma.

transforming genes capable of inducing lymphoma in marmosets (K1)[20] and sarcoma in nude mice (K12).[21] The function of ORF K12 is unknown, but ORF K1 encodes a constitutively activated transmembrane signalling molecule.[22] KSHV ORF K9 has a conserved region derived from the interferon regulatory factor (IRF) family of proteins, and this viral IRF (vIRF) antagonizes class I interferon signalling.[23,24] In particular, it blocks the induction of $p21^{Waf1/Cip1}$ by interferon-β, an induction that correlates with cell cycle arrest. Additionally, interferons are potent inducers of major histocompatibility complex (MHC) class I expression, and the inhibition of interferon transduction by KSHV v-IRF could be a convenient way to escape the immune system. vIRF expression has been detected only in PEL cells and not in Kaposi sarcoma.[15,23] Unlike HVS, KSHV encodes for a D-type cyclin (ORF 72) that can phosphorylate the retinoblastoma protein Rb through interaction with Cdk6.[17,25,26] This phosphorylation leads to the release of active E2F factor in association with progression through the S phase of the cell cycle. Thus, KSHV encodes for at least two proteins, vCyc and vIRF, that could deregulate the G_1/S checkpoint.

KSHV also has pirated cellular genes involved in the control of cell death. Human Bcl-2 is known to block apoptosis induced by withdrawal of serum or growth factors, γ irradiation or cytotoxic drugs. KSHV carries a viral Bcl-2 with functional anti-apoptotic activities.[27,28] KSHV also encodes for a potential FLICE (caspase-8)-inhibitory protein, which contains two death-effector domains and is called vFLIP.[29] HVS vFLIP inhibits apoptosis induced by Fas (CD95). The function of KSHV vFLIP has not yet been studied, but it is possible that it could contribute to protecting infected host cells from apoptosis. In addition, the latent associated nuclear antigen (LANA) encoded by ORF 73 could contribute to K5 oncogenesis through inhibition of p53-mediated apoptosis.[30]

Finally, KSHV encodes for cytokines that could play autocrine and paracrine roles in infected tissues. Among them is viral IL-6 (vIL-6), which can bind to the gp130 IL-6 transducer chain and activate the Jak/STAT pathway.[23,31–33] vIL-6 shares several biological activities with human IL-6 (huIL-6). For example, it promotes growth and survival of the B9 murine IL-6-dependent cell line. vIL-6 is expressed in haematopoietic tissues but not in Kaposi sarcoma lesions, and is likely to contribute to the development of Castleman's disease. Two KSHV sequences show homology with macrophage inflammatory protein (MIP)-1: vMIP-I and vMIP-II.[23,32] These viral chemokines are biologically active, and may be involved in the pathogenesis of KSHV-related diseases by inducing angiogenesis.[34] vGPCR and vIL-6 are also angiogenic factors through induction of vascular endothelial growth factor (VEGF) secretion by infected cells.[19,35]

Unlike EBV, KSHV seems to have string tropism for both haematopoietic and non-haematopoietic cells. In Kaposi sarcoma lesions, KSHV has been shown by in situ hybridization to infect spindle cells, microvascular endothelial cells,[36,37] and monocytes.[38] KSHV DNA has been found in PEL B cells. In Kaposi sarcoma patients, the virus has been detected in peripheral blood mononuclear cells (PBMC), especially B cells[39,40] and monocytes,[38] and, in some cases, in T lymphocytes.[40,41] The tropism of KSHV for B cells has been confirmed by in vitro infection of human peripheral blood B lymphocytes.[42]

Surprisingly, despite having such strong tropism and all conceivable tools to trigger a malignancy, nobody has been able to transform any type of cell in vitro with KSHV infectious particles until recently. In the first report of the transformation of primary human endothelial cells by KSHV, the virus was present in only a subset of cultured cells, and paracrine mecanisms were responsible for the long-term proliferation and survival of uninfected cells.[43]

KSHV AND CASTLEMAN'S DISEASE

KSHV DNA can be reproducibly detected by PCR in multicentric plasma cell type or mixed-type Castleman's disease, but is only rarely found in localized forms of this lymphoproliferative disorder.[44–48] Nearly all HIV-seropositive patients and approximately 40% of HIV-seronegative patients with multicentric Castleman's disease (MCD) are infected with KSHV. This high rate of KSHV infection in HIV-infected MCD patients might explain why 75% of them develop Kaposi sarcoma, whereas Kaposi sarcoma occurs in only 11–13% of HIV-negative patients before or during the course of MCD (Table 3.2). In KSHV-infected patients with MCD, KSHV is found in involved lymph nodes as well as in PBMC, especially B lymphocytes.

Two studies strengthen the relationship between KSHV and MCD and suggest a causal role for KSHV in the pathogenesis of at least one subset of Castleman's disease. In the first report, three HIV-infected patients with MCD were studied.[49] In two of them, there was a strong correlation between clinical, biological, and virological events with concordance of fever, C-reactive protein levels, and KSHV DNA load in PBMC. The third patient was asymptomatic throughout the duration of the study, with a low level of KSHV DNA. In the second study, Parravicini et al[48] searched for the presence of KSHV DNA in the lymph nodes of 14 HIV-negative patients with confirmed Castleman's disease, including 11 patients with the plasma cell or mixed type and 3 patients with the hyaline vascular variant. None of the 3 hyaline vascular and 6 of the 11 plasma cell or mixed variant tissues were KSHV-positive by PCR. KSHV-infected patients had progressive MCD with systemic symptoms, and 5 of 6 died within 1–6 months of diagnosis. Conversely, the 5 patients with KSHV-negative plasma cell MCD were all free of disease after treatment.

The pathophysiological mechanisms underlying the induction of Castleman's disease by KSHV are unclear, but may in part be mediated by vIL-6. huIL-6 overexpression within the lesions is a classical feature of MCD,[50,51] and injection of a monoclonal anti-IL-6 antibody has been shown to be beneficial in patients with MCD.[52] In addition, retroviral transduction of IL-6 in mouse bone marrow leads to clinical and biological manifestations mimicking human Castleman's disease.[53] KSHV-encoded vIL-6 was detected by immunohistochemistry in all of six KSHV-infected plasma cell type MCD tissues.[48] In these cases, it is likely that vIL-6, in association with huIL-6, participates in the B-cell/plasma cell expansion by preventing cell apoptosis, stimulating cell proliferation, and eventually promoting plasma cell differentiation. vIL-6 should act essentially in a paracrine manner, since vIL-6-positive cells in the MCD lesions do not express CD20 B-cell antigen or CD138 plasma cell marker.[48]

Other KSHV genes could play a role in MCD pathogenesis. In particular, marked angiogenesis is central in this disease, which is characterized by a marked capillary proliferation with endothelial hyperplasia (Chapter 28). As described above, at least three KSHV ORFs

Table 3.2 Detection of KSHV by PCR from lymph nodes in patients with Castleman's disease

HIV serology	KSHV DNA positivity	Associated Kaposi sarcoma	Ref
Seropositive	14 of 14	9 of 14	44
	3 of 4	3 of 4	45
Total	**17 of 18 (94%)**	**11 of 18 (61%)**	
Seronegative	7 of 17	1 of 17	44
	1 of 6	0 of 6	45
	6 of 14	3 of 14	46,48
Total	**14 of 37 (38%)**	**4 of 37 (11%)**	

encode for proteins potentially involved in angiogenesis: vGPCR, vMIP-I and vMIP-II. Interestingly, vGPCR induces a secretion of VEGF by infected cells, and it has been shown that VEGF is expressed in Castleman's disease germinal centres but not in normal germinal centres.[54] In multicentric Castleman's disease, KSHV is essentially present in mantle zone large immunoblastic B cells.[55]

In conclusion, the association of KSHV and plasma cell type MCD seems indisputable on the basis of consistent PCR results and the relationship between Kaposi sarcoma and MCD. No large serological studies are available, probably because MCD is an uncommon disease. KSHV, by encoding for vIL-6 and for several angiogenic proteins, plays a paracrine role in MCD. Castleman's disease is a heterogeneous entity, and KSHV has not been clearly implicated in all forms of the disease. Nevertheless, it is necessary to design new therapeutic approaches for plasma cell type MCD with the aim of controlling the underlying KSHV infection.

KSHV AND MYELOMA

The general consensus is that huIL-6 produced by the bone marrow (BM) microenvironment is the major growth and survival factor for myeloma cells.[56,57] vIL-6 promotes the proliferation of myeloma cell lines.[58] The initial report from the University of California Los Angeles (UCLA) group,[59] showing the presence of KSHV DNA and vIL-6 transcripts in BM stromal dendritic cells of myeloma patients, provided an interesting and original model for myeloma pathogenesis. In addition, Rettig et al[59] suggested that the presence of KSHV in cultured BM stromal dendritic cells from two of eight patients with monoclonal gammopathy of undetermined significance (MGUS) could be used to explain the transformation of 25% of MGUS to myeloma.[59] However, this attractive hypothesis has not been confirmed by most of the groups studying it. Among the 23 studies published to date by independent laboratories, only 4 are consistent with a causal role for KSHV in myeloma[60–62] (Table 3.3). In an attempt to clarify the question of whether or not KSHV is associated with myeloma, we shall summarize these reports, with special reference to the type and the sensitivity of the methods used by the different investigators.

In their first report, the UCLA group detected KSHV by single PCR against ORF 26 (KS330 sequence) and by reverse-transcriptase (RT)-PCR against ORF K2 (vIL-6) in long-term cultured BM stromal dendritic cells from 15 of 15 patients with myeloma, but not in stromal cells from healthy individuals.[59] A French group also reported detecting KSHV ORF 26 in two of three long-term BM cultures from myeloma patients.[61] The UCLA group did not indicate the sensitivity of their PCR assays, but nearly all cultured cells were supposed to contain at least one virus copy, since they were labelled with an ORF 26 probe by in situ hybridization.[59] Such a high rate of infection should allow the detection of KSHV DNA by Southern blot, even without PCR amplification.

It is therefore hard to explain why four independent studies performed on 42 long-term BM stromal cell cultures using single or nested ORF 26 PCR failed to confirm these results.[63–66] The only positive case out of the 42 samples tested was only weakly positive using an unnested KS330 (ORF 26) PCR assay, and was negative by PCR for ORF 25 and on immunostaining for vIL-6 (ORF K2).[64]

A partial explanation for these discrepancies was proposed in a study by Tisdale et al,[67] who obtained BM stromal cells from 30 myeloma patients and assayed them for KSHV infection. They used nested PCR for two KSHV ORFs (ORF 26 and ORF 75), with a sensitivity of less than 3 genome copies per 200 000 cells, and a one-stage PCR for ORF 72, with a sensitivity of 30 genome copies per reaction. KSHV ORF 26 was detected at least once in 60% of the myeloma samples, 44% of human controls, and 85% of rhesus macaque samples. KSHV ORF 75 and KSHV ORF 72 were never detected, despite repeated testing. Only 2 of 15 myeloma samples gave a reproducible positive signal when the KS330 (ORF 26) nested PCR was repeated,

Table 3.3 Detection of KSHV in patients with myeloma

Sample	Technique	Samples analysed	Number of positive samples	Positive studies[a] (total number of studies)
Bone marrow dendritic cells	PCR ORF 26	90	36 (40%)	
	Other ORFs	42	3 (7%)	2 (7)
Bone marrow mononuclear cells	PCR ORF 26	141	1 (0.7%)	
	Other ORFs	8	0 (0%)	0 (8)
Bone marrow biopsies	PCR ORF 26	57	30 (53%)	
	Other ORFs	38	17 (45%)	3 (6)
Apheresis cells	PCR ORF 26	100	15 (15%)	1 (4)
$CD34^+$ cells	PCR ORF 26	42	3 (7%)	1 (3)
Monocyte-derived dendritic cells	PCR ORF 26	28	1 (3.5%)	0 (3)
$CD34^+$-derived dendritic cells	PCR ORF 26	10	0 (0%)	0 (3)
Sera	Serology	501	42 (8%)	1 (17)
Total				4 (23)

[a] Positive studies are those that concluded that KSHV is associated with myeloma.

suggesting that either the PCR was contaminated or that the amplified sequence was just at the limit of PCR detection. The authors concluded that a herpesvirus related to KSHV containing a sequence homologous to KSHV ORF 26, but not KSHV itself, was present at a low level in BM stromal cells in the general population.

In all the published studies, including that of Rettig et al,[59] KSHV was undetectable in fresh BM aspirates.[59,63–66,68–70] This could not be explained simply by an inhibition of Taq polymerase by heparin, as suggested by the UCLA group, since at least 22 negative samples had been treated with EDTA as an anticoagulant.[65]

In accordance with the assumption that KSHV-infected stromal cells are strongly adherent to bone in vivo, several groups have looked for KSHV in core BM biopsies. Berenson's group[71] has shown by ORF 72 in situ hybridization that 2–10% of cells in these BM biopsies were infected. However, despite such a high apparent rate of infection, only two of five studies were able to detect KSHV ORF 26 in a majority of paraffin-embedded BM biopsies from patients with myeloma.[60,61,64,66,72] In these two studies, the detection of KSHV required extensive PCR amplification with either 2 × 30 cycles[60] or 45 cycles.[61] No attempt was made to quantify genome copies in these two studies, and other KSHV ORFs were not assayed. Thus, other than the UCLA group, no report has confirmed that KSHV infects a high proportion of BM stromal cells in myeloma patients, such that enough vIL-6 could be produced locally to drive tumour cell proliferation.

Epidemiological studies also argue against an association between KSHV and myeloma. The prevalence of antibodies to KSHV is higher in southern Italy than in the USA or UK.[6] This is associated with a higher incidence of classic Kaposi sarcoma, but not of myeloma.[73] Similarly, the incidences of Kaposi sarcoma and myeloma worldwide do not correlate.[74]

Another major argument against an association between KSHV and myeloma is the lack of detection of antibodies against latent and lytic KSHV antigens in myeloma patients in 16 studies (20 patients KSHV-seropositive out of 474 tested; seroprevalence 4.2%; KSHV seroprevalence in the control group in the same studies 6.9%)[61,63–70,72,75–80] (Table 3.3). Only Gao et al[62] found an increased seroprevalence for KSHV (81%). However, this study raised several questions because of the very low antibody titres detected in myeloma patients and the higher frequency of anti-KSHV antibodies in sera from patients with other cancers (22%) than in the general population (6%); a finding that has not been reported elsewhere.

The low KSHV seroprevalence in myeloma patients does not support an association between myeloma and KSHV, because antibodies to KSHV are detected in 80–90% of Kaposi sarcoma patients at an early stage of the disease – even before clinical manifestations.[6,9,10,81] Several hypotheses have been proposed to explain these conflicting results.

The first is that myeloma patients are immunocompromised and have panhypogammaglobulinaemia, which would prevent the formation of antibodies to KSHV. However, in 7 of 17 studies, the humoral response of myeloma patients against two other herpesviruses (EBV and cytomegalovirus (CMV)) was checked, and was found to be similar to that of healthy individuals.[63,64,68,70,76–78] Also, the seroprevalence for KSHV in patients with MGUS, who have normal serum immunoglobulin levels, is low (4.5%, 4 patients seropositive out of 89).[64,69,70,75–77]

The second hypothesis is that myeloma patients are infected with a variant of KSHV that encodes for mutated antigens not recognized by the available serologic assays. The UCLA group in particular reports that KSHV ORF 65 is hypermutated in myeloma, and ORF 65-based seroassays could give false-negative results. However, a number of serologic studies employing LANA (ORF 73) detection have also yielded negative results. Hyjek et al[82] recently obtained the first KSHV-infected cell line from a myeloma patient with a malignant pleural effusion. They then tested sera from 59 patients with myeloma or MGUS in an immunofluorescence assay using this cell line instead of the PEL cell line as a source of KSHV antigens. The aim was to determine if myeloma patients were infected with a KSHV strain that did not cross-react with the KSHV strain implicated in PEL. Only 1 of 59 sera showed a positive reaction. This argues against the presence of a myeloma-specific KSHV strain in the majority of myeloma patients. The authors suggested that KSHV could be associated with an effusion phenotype that is found in PEL and occasional myeloma patients (myeloma with malignant effusion).

The third explanation is that KSHV has a particular tropism for dendritic cells in myeloma. Since dendritic cells are the only cells able to initiate an immune response, this could lead to an impaired viral antigen presentation, resulting in a poor anti-KSHV immune response.

The debate then shifts to the cells that are infected with KSHV in myeloma patients. Rettig et al[59] initially suggested that the infected stromal cells had some phenotypic characteristics of dendritic cells. Monocytes are the reservoir of the virus in patients with Kaposi sarcoma.[38] In the presence of appropriate cytokines, monocytes differentiate in vitro into immature dendritic cells, and vice versa.[83] However, dendritic cells are defined by a set of phenotypic, morphologic, and functional criteria, and there is no evidence to date that the putative KSHV-infected cells in myeloma patients are of dendritic cell origin. On the contrary, we and others have demonstrated that true, functional dendritic cells obtained from myeloma patients using adherent monocytes or $CD34^+$ progenitors are not infected with KSHV (1 of 28 and 0 of 10 positive samples, respectively).[69,80,84–86] The absence of PCR inhibitors in negative samples was checked in one study.[69] The only report that mentioned that apheresis cells collected during mobilization with chemotherapy and haematopoietic growth factor (a convenient source of adherent monocytes) or purified $CD34^+$ cells could be infected with KSHV was published by the UCLA group,[87] in contrast with data from three other groups.[84,86,88]

Given the lack of anti-KSHV antibodies in myeloma patients and the inconsistent PCR results, we have used another strategy to determine if these patients are infected with KSHV. KSHV must be under strict immune control in myeloma patients to explain the inability of the majority of laboratories to detect viral DNA using very sensitive methods. If this is the case, then, whatever the explanation for the negative serologic studies, other T-cell-mediated mechanisms must be involved in the maintenance of KSHV-infected cells at a low level. In patients with AIDS-associated Kaposi sarcoma, KSHV detection increases with a decrease in the $CD4^+$ cell count. Post-transplant Kaposi sarcoma is known to be essentially due to immunosuppression-dependent KSHV reactivation.

We hypothesized that if KSHV were present in myeloma patients, it should reactivate under conditions of severe and prolonged immunosuppression, when it could become detectable by PCR in BM aspirates.[89] We looked for KSHV DNA in BM aspirates from 10 myeloma patients treated by double high-dose chemotherapy and autotransplantation with $CD34^+$-selected cells. The grafts contained a mean of only $(0.11 \pm 0.08) \times 10^6$ $CD3^+$ cells/kg. Eight of ten patients remained $CD4^+$ lymphopenic ($<0.2 \times 10^9$/l) for up to a year and experienced multiple herpesvirus infections (two varicella, one herpes simplex, one herpes zoster, and six patients with antigen-positivity for CMV).

However, despite the use of a KS330 PCR assay allowing the detection of less than 5 genome copies in 150 000 cells and the lack of KSHV PCR inhibitors in negative samples, KSHV DNA was not detected in any of the BM samples collected 90, 180, and 360 days after the second high-dose chemotherapy. Thus, either the intensive therapy, which ablated immunity to several herpesviruses, did not effact anti-KSHV immunity, or KSHV was not present in our patients at all. Four of the ten patients relapsed during the one-year follow-up period. We were thus unable to confirm that there is a correlation between the presence of KSHV in BM of myeloma patients and their clinical outcome, as has been suggested by the UCLA group.[71]

Taken as a whole, epidemiological studies, serologic data, and PCR assays emphasize that KSHV does not seem to be implicated in the pathogenesis of myeloma, depsite the numerous hypotheses that have been proposed to explain the lack of consistent results. The possible relationship between KSHV and an effusion phenotype in lymphoma and myeloma is interesting, but further work is needed to elucidate this point.

KSHV AND WALDENSTRÖM'S MACROGLOBULINAEMIA

Waldenström's macroglobulinaemia shares some pathophysiological characteristics with myeloma, especially plasma cell differentiation (Chapter 27). A paracrine model, similar to that postulated for myeloma, was proposed for the pathogenesis of Waldenström's macroglobulinaemia, and the UCLA group reported the detection of KSHV DNA in the circulating dendritic cells of all four patients studied.[90]

These data have not been confirmed by other groups that have studied BM biopsies from patients with Waldenström's macroglobulinaemia.[61,66,91] Of the two groups that did detect KSHV DNA in myeloma patients, only Agbalika et al[61] were able to amplify KSHV DNA in 6 of 10 Waldenström patients using 45 cycles of KS330 PCR. The other group, which had found KSHV ORF 26 in 90% of myeloma BM biopsies, found only 1 positive sample among 20 Waldenström patients using the same PCR assay.[91] This single KSHV-positive patient was also infected with HIV, which confounded the results. Another study reported the lack of KSHV DNA and anti-KSHV antibodies in two Waldenström patients.[66]

In conclusion, based on the limited amount of published data, there is no evidence that KSHV is involved in the pathogenesis of Waldenström's macroglobulinaemia.

KSHV AND PRIMARY AMYLOIDOSIS

The UCLA group has also found KSHV by in situ hybridization in 3–7% of BM cells in 10 of 11 patients with primary amyloidosis.[90] The data currently available are insufficient[66] to conclude that there is an association between KSHV and primary (AL) amyloidosis.

OTHER VIRUSES IN PLASMA CELL DISORDERS

Hepatitis C virus and Waldenström's macroglobulinaemia

Santini et al[92] detected hepatitis C virus (HCV) RNA in the serum of all of six Waldenström patients studied. HCV was supposed to drive an activation of the immune system resulting in an expansion of B-cell clones that could eventually undergo malignant transformation. However, HCV has been found to be reproducibly associated only with Waldenström's disease that manifests cryoglobulinaemic activity; especially type II cryoglobulinaemia.[93–95] In monoclonal gammopathy without cryoglobulins, HCV prevalence is comparable to that in the appropriate matched control population.[95]

EBV and plasma cell disorders

EBV has not been causally involved in any plasma cell disorder. It has been detected in some cases of Castleman's disease,[96] without evidence of any role in the development of the disease.[49,97] In contrast to PEL, there is no evidence of EBV and KSHV co-localization in the same cells in Castleman's disease lesions.[48]

Human immunodeficiency virus and Castleman's disease

Castleman's disease occurs more frequently among HIV-seropositive persons.[97,98] AIDS-induced immunodeficiency as well as synergy between HIV proteins and cytokines[99] could explain the role of HIV as a cofactor in the emergence of the disease. The interaction between HIV and KSHV may also be important, since 100% of HIV-seropositive patients with Castleman's disease are also infected with KSHV.[44,45] For example, HIV-1 Tat is able to enhance the KSHV viral load,[100] whereas both MIP-I and MIP-II partially inhibit HIV infection of peripheral blood mononuclear cells.[22,24] Moreover, cytokines produced by HIV-1-infected cells can induce KSHV lytic replication.

REFERENCES

1. Rickinson AB, Kieff E. Epstein–Barr virus. In: *Fields Virology*, 3rd edn (Fields BN, Knipe DM, Howley PM, eds). Philadelphia: Lippincott-Raven, 1996: 2397–446.
2. Chang Y, Cesarman E, Pessin MS et al. Identification of herpesvirus-like DNA sequences in AIDS-associated Kaposi sarcoma. *Science* 1994; **266**: 1865–9.
3. Moore PS, Chang Y. Detection of herpesvirus-like DNA sequences in Kaposi sarcoma in patients with and without HIV infection. *N Engl J Med* 1995; **332**: 1181–5.
4. Huang YQ, Li JJ, Kaplan MH et al. Human herpesvirus-like nucleic acid in various forms of Kaposi sarcoma. *Lancet* 1995; **345**: 759–61.
5. Dupin N, Grandadam M, Calvez V et al. Herpesvirus-like DNA sequences in patients with Mediterranean Kaposi sarcoma. *Lancet* 1995; **345**: 761–2.
6. Gao SJ, Kingsley L, Li M et al. KSHV antibodies among Americans, Italians and Ugandans with and without Kaposi sarcoma. *Nature Med* 1996; **2**: 925–8.
7. Cesarman E, Chang Y, Moore PS et al. Kaposi sarcoma-associated herpesvirus-like DNA sequences in AIDS-related body-cavity-based lymphomas. *N Engl J Med* 1995; **332**: 1186–91.
8. Davis DA, Humphrey RW, Newcomb FM et al. Detection of serum antibodies to a Kaposi sarcoma-associated herpesvirus-specific peptide. *J Infect Dis* 1997; **175**: 1071–9.
9. Simpson GR, Schulz TF, Whitby D et al. Prevalence of Kaposi sarcoma associated herpesvirus infection measured by antibodies to recombinant capsid protein and latent

immunofluorescence antigen. *Lancet* 1996; **348**: 1133–8.
10. Lennette ET, Blackbourn DJ, Levy JA. Antibodies to human herpesvirus type 8 in the general population and in Kaposi sarcoma patients. *Lancet* 1996; **348**: 858–61.
11. Chatlynne LG, Lapps W, Handy M et al. Detection and titration of human herpesvirus-8–specific antibodies in sera from blood donors, acquired immunodeficiency syndrome patients, and Kaposi sarcoma patients using a whole virus enzyme-linked immunosorbent assay. *Blood* 1998; **92**: 53–8.
12. Renne R, Zhong W, Herndier B et al. Lytic growth of Kaposi sarcoma-associated herpesvirus (human herpesvirus 8) in culture. *Nature Med* 1996; **2**: 342–6.
13. Cesarman E, Moore PS, Rao PH et al. In vitro establishment and characterization of two acquired immunodeficiency syndrome-related lymphoma cell lines (BC-1 and BC-2) containing Kaposi sarcoma-associated herpesvirus-like (KSHV) DNA sequences. *Blood* 1995; **86**: 2708–14.
14. Renne R, Lagunoff M, Zhong W, Ganem D. The size and conformation of Kaposi sarcoma-associated herpesvirus (human herpesvirus 8) DNA in infected cells and virions. *J Virol* 1996; **70**: 8151–4.
15. Moore PS, Chang Y. Kaposi sarcoma-associated herpesvirus-encoded oncogenes and oncogenesis. *J Natl Cancer Inst Monogr* 1998; **23**: 65–71.
16. Neipel F, Albrecht JC, Fleckenstein B. Cell-homologous genes in the Kaposi sarcoma-associated rhadinovirus human herpesvirus 8: determinants of its pathogenicity? *J Virol* 1997; **71**: 4187–92.
17. Cesarman E, Nador RG, Bai F et al. Kaposi sarcoma-associated herpesvirus contains G protein-coupled receptor and cyclin D homologs which are expressed in Kaposi sarcoma and malignant lymphoma. *J Virol* 1996; **70**: 8218–23.
18. Arvanitakis L, Geras-Raaka E, Varma A et al. Human herpesvirus KSHV encodes a constitutively active G-protein-coupled receptor linked to cell proliferation. *Nature* 1997; **385**: 347–50.
19. Bais C, Santomasso B, Coso O et al. G-protein-coupled receptor of Kaposi sarcoma-associated herpesvirus is a viral oncogene and angiogenesis activator. *Nature* 1998; **391**: 86–9.
20. Lee H, Veazey R, Williams K et al. Deregulation of cell growth by the K1 gene of Kaposi sarcoma-associated herpesvirus. *Nature Med* 1998; **4**: 435–40.
21. Muralidhar S, Pumfery AM, Hassani M et al. Identification of kaposin (open reading frame K12) as a human herpesvirus 8 (Kaposi sarcoma-associated herpesvirus) transforming gene. *J Virol* 1998; **72**: 4980–8.
22. Lagunoff M, Majeti R, Weiss A, Ganem D. Deregulated signal transduction by the K1 gene product of Kaposi's sarcoma-associated herpesvirus. *Proc Natl Acad Sci USA* 1999; **96**: 5704–9.
23. Moore PS, Boshoff C, Weiss RA, Chang Y. Molecular mimicry of human cytokine and cytokine response pathway genes by KSHV. *Science* 1996; **274**: 1739–44.
24. Gao SJ, Boshoff C, Jayachandra S et al. KSHV ORF K9 (vIRF) is an oncogene which inhibits the interferon signaling pathway. *Oncogene* 1997; **15**: 1979–85.
25. Chang Y, Moore PS, Talbot SJ et al. Cyclin encoded by KS herpesvirus. *Nature* 1996; **382**: 410.
26. Godden-Kent D, Talbot SJ, Boshoff C et al. The cyclin encoded by Kaposi sarcoma-associated herpesvirus stimulates cdk6 to phosphorylate the retinoblastoma protein and histone H1. *J Virol* 1997; **71**: 4193–8.
27. Cheng EHY, Nicholas J, Bellows DS et al. A Bcl-2 homolog encoded by Kaposi sarcoma-associated virus, human herpesvirus 8, inhibits apoptosis but does not heterodimerize with Bax or Bak. *Proc Natl Acad Sci USA* 1997; **94**: 690–4.
28. Sarid R, Sato T, Bohenzky RA et al. Kaposi sarcoma-associated herpesvirus encodes a functional Bcl-2 homologue. *Nature Med* 1997; **3**: 293–8.
29. Thome M, Schneider P, Hofmann K et al. Viral FLICE-inhibitory proteins (FLIPs) prevent apoptosis induced by death receptors. *Nature* 1997; **386**: 517–21.
30. Friborg J Jr, Kong W-P, Hottiger MO, Nabel GJ. p53 inhibition by the LANA protein of KSHV protects against cell death. *Nature* 1999; **402**: 889–94.
31. Neipel F, Albrecht JC, Ensser A et al. Human herpesvirus 8 encodes a homolog of interleukin-6. *J Virol* 1997; **71**: 839–42.
32. Nicholas J, Ruvolo VR, Burns WH et al. Kaposi sarcoma-associated human herpesvirus-8 encodes homologues of macrophage inflammatory protein-1 and interleukin-6. *Nature Med* 1997; **3**: 287–92.
33. Molden J, Chang Y, You Y et al. A Kaposi sarcoma-associated herpesvirus-encoded cytokine homolog (vIL- 6) activates signaling through

the shared gp130 receptor subunit. *J Biol Chem* 1997; **272**: 19625–31.

34. Boshoff C, Endo Y, Collins PD et al. Angiogenic and HIV-inhibitory functions of KSHV-encoded chemokines. *Science* 1997; **278**: 290–4.
35. Aoki Y, Jaffe ES, Chang Y et al. Angiogenesis and hematopoiesis induced by Kaposi's sarcoma-associated herpesvirus-encoded interleukin-6. *Blood* 1999; **93**: 4034–43.
36. Boshoff C, Schulz TF, Kennedy MM et al. Kaposi sarcoma-associated herpesvirus infects endothelial and spindle cells. *Nature Med* 1995; **1**: 1274–8.
37. Staskus KA, Zhong W, Gebhard K et al. Kaposi sarcoma-associated herpesvirus gene expression in endothelial (spindle) tumor cells. *J Virol* 1997; **71**: 715–19.
38. Blasig C, Zietz C, Haar B et al. Monocytes in Kaposi sarcoma lesions are productively infected by human herpesvirus 8. *J Virol* 1997; **71**: 7963–8.
39. Ambroziak JA, Blackbourn DJ, Herndier BG et al. Herpes-like sequences in HIV-infected and uninfected Kaposi sarcoma patients. *Science* 1995; **268**: 582–3.
40. Harrington W Jr, Bagasra O, Sosa CE et al. Human herpesvirus type 8 DNA sequences in cell-free plasma and mononuclear cells of Kaposi sarcoma patients. *J Infect Dis* 1996; **174**: 1101–5.
41. Kikuta H, Itakura O, Taneichi K, Kohno M. Tropism of human herpesvirus 8 for peripheral blood lymphocytes in patients with Castleman's disease. *Br J Haematol* 1997; **99**: 790–3.
42. Mesri EA, Cesarman E, Arvanitakis L et al. Human herpesvirus-8/Kaposi sarcoma-associated herpesvirus is a new transmissible virus that infects B cells. *J Exp Med* 1996; **183**: 2385–90.
43. Flore O, Rafii S, Ely S et al. Transformation of primary human endothelial cells by Kaposi sarcoma- associated herpesvirus. *Nature* 1998; **394**: 588–92.
44. Soulier J, Grollet L, Oksenhendler E et al. Kaposi sarcoma-associated herpesvirus-like DNA sequences in multicentric Castleman's disease. *Blood* 1995; **86**: 1276–80.
45. Gessain A, Sudaka A, Briere J et al. Kaposi sarcoma-associated herpes-like virus (human herpesvirus type 8) DNA sequences in multicentric Castleman's disease: is there any relevant association in non-human immunodeficiency virus-infected patients? *Blood* 1996; **87**: 414–16.
46. Corbellino M, Poirel L, Aubin JT et al. The role of human herpesvirus 8 and Epstein–Barr virus in the pathogenesis of giant lymph node hyperplasia (Castleman's disease). *Clin Infect Dis* 1996; **22**: 1120–1.
47. Dupin N, Gorin I, Deleuze J et al. Herpes-like DNA sequences, AIDS-related tumors, and Castleman's disease. *N Engl J Med* 1995; **333**: 798.
48. Parravicini C, Corbellino M, Paulli M et al. Expression of a virus-derived cytokine, KSHV vIL-6, in HIV-seronegative Castleman's disease. *Am J Pathol* 1997; **151**: 1517–22.
49. Grandadam M, Dupin N, Calvez V et al. Exacerbations of clinical symptoms in human immunodeficiency virus type 1-infected patients with multicentric Castleman's disease are associated with a high increase in Kaposi sarcoma herpesvirus DNA load in peripheral blood mononuclear cells. *J Infect Dis* 1997; **175**: 1198–201.
50. Yoshizaki K, Matsuda T, Nishimoto N et al. Pathogenic significance of interleukin-6 (IL-6/BSF-2) in Castleman's disease. *Blood* 1989; **74**: 1360–7.
51. Leger-Ravet MB, Peuchmaur M, Devergne O et al. Interleukin-6 gene expression in Castleman's disease. *Blood* 1991; **78**: 2923–30.
52. Beck JT, Hsu SM, Wijdenes J et al. Alleviation of systemic manifestations of Castleman's disease by monoclonal anti-interleukin-6 antibody. *N Engl J Med* 1994; **330**: 602–5.
53. Brandt SJ, Bodine DM, Dunbar CE, Nienhuis AW. Dysregulated interleukin 6 expression produces a syndrome resembling Castleman's disease in mice. *J Clin Invest* 1990; **86**: 592–9.
54. Foss HD, Araujo I, Demel G et al. Expression of vascular endothelial growth factor in lymphomas and Castleman's disease. *J Pathol* 1997; **183**: 44–50.
55. Dupin N, Fisher C, Kellam P et al. Distribution of human herpesvirus-8 latently infected cells in Kaposi's sarcoma, multicentric Castleman's disease, and primary effusion lymphoma. *Proc Natl Acad Sci USA* 1999; **96**: 4546–51.
56. Klein B, Zhang XG, Lu ZY, Bataille R. Interleukin-6 in human multiple myeloma. *Blood* 1995; **85**: 863–72.
57. Klein B, Zhang XG, Jourdan M et al. Paracrine rather than autocrine regulation of myeloma-cell growth and differentiation by interleukin-6. *Blood* 1989; **73**: 517–26.
58. Burger R, Neipel F, Fleckenstein B et al. Human herpesvirus type 8 interleukin-6 homologue is functionally active on human myeloma cells. *Blood* 1998; **91**: 1858–63.
59. Rettig MB, Ma HJ, Vescio RA et al. Kaposi sarcoma-associated herpesvirus infection of bone

marrow dendritic cells from multiple myeloma patients. *Science* 1997; **276**: 1851–4.
60. Brousset P, Meggetto F, Attal M, Delsol G. Kaposi sarcoma-associated herpesvirus infection and multiple myeloma. *Science* 1997; **278**: 1972.
61. Agbalika F, Mariette X, Marolleau JP et al. Detection of human herpesvirus-8 DNA in bone marrow biopsies from patients with multiple myeloma and Waldenström's macroglobulinaemia. *Blood* 1998; **91**: 4393–4.
62. Gao SJ, Alsina M, Deng JH et al. Antibodies to Kaposi sarcoma-associated herpesvirus (human herpesvirus 8) in patients with multiple myeloma. *J Infect Dis* 1998; **178**: 846–9.
63. Masood R, Zheng T, Tupule A et al. Kaposi sarcoma-associated herpesvirus infection and multiple myeloma. *Science* 1997; **278**: 1970–1.
64. Olsen SJ, Tarte K, Sherman W et al. Evidence against KSHV infection in the pathogenesis of multiple myeloma. *Virus Res* 1998; **57**: 197–202.
65. Perna AM, Viviano E et al. No association between human herpesvirus type 8 infection and multiple myeloma. *J Natl Cancer Inst* 1998; **90**: 1013–14.
66. Bouscary D, Dupin N, Fichelson S et al. Lack of evidence of an association between HHV-8 and multiple myeloma. *Leukemia* 1998; **12**: 1840–1.
67. Tisdale JF, Stewart AK, Dickstein B et al. Molecular and serological examination of the relationship of human herpesvirus 8 to multiple myeloma: orf 26 sequences in bone marrow stroma are not restricted to myeloma patients and other regions of the genome are not detected. *Blood* 1998; **92**: 2681–7.
68. Parravicini C, Lauri E, Baldini L et al. Kaposi sarcoma-associated herpesvirus infection and multiple myeloma. *Science* 1997; **278**: 1969–70.
69. Yi Q, Ekman M, Anton D et al. Blood dendritic cells from myeloma patients are not infected with Kaposi sarcoma-associated herpesvirus (KSHV/HHV-8). *Blood* 1998; **92**: 402–4.
70. Schonrich G, Raftery M, Schnitzler P et al. Absence of a correlation between Kaposi sarcoma-associated herpesvirus (KSHV/HHV-8) and multiple myeloma. *Blood* 1998; **92**: 3474–5.
71. Said JW, Rettig MR, Heppner K et al. Localization of Kaposi sarcoma-associated herpesvirus in bone marrow biopsy samples from patients with multiple myeloma. *Blood* 1997; **90**: 4278–82.
72. Cathomas G, Stalder A, Kurrer MO et al. Multiple myeloma and HHV-8 infection. *Blood* 1998; **91**: 4391–3.
73. Masala G, Di Lollo S, Picoco C et al. Incidence rates of leukemias, lymphomas and myelomas in Italy: geographic distribution and NHL histotypes. *Int J Cancer* 1996; **68**: 156–9.
74. Hjalgrim H, Frisch M, Melbye M. Incidence rates of classical Kaposi sarcoma and multiple myeloma do not correlate. *Br J Cancer* 1998; **78**: 419–20.
75. Whitby D, Boshoff C, Luppi M, Torelli G. Kaposi sarcoma-associated herpesvirus infection and multiple myeloma. *Science* 1997; **278**: 1971–2.
76. Santarelli R, Angeloni A, Farina A et al. Lack of serologic association between human herpesvirus-8 infection and multiple myeloma and monoclonal gammopathies of undetermined significance. *J Natl Cancer Inst* 1998; **90**: 781–2.
77. Marcelin AG, Dupin N, Bouscary D et al. HHV-8 and multiple myeloma in France. *Lancet* 1997; **350**: 1144.
78. MacKenzie J, Sheldon J, Morgan G et al. HHV-8 and multiple myeloma in the UK. *Lancet* 1997; **350**: 1144–5.
79. Jaccard A, Touati M, Sol C et al. Human herpesvirus-8 and relatives of patients with plasmocytic diseases. *Blood* 1998; **92**: 3488.
80. Mitterer M, Mair W, Gatti D et al. Dendritic cells derived from bone marrow and CD34+ selected blood progenitor cells of myeloma patients, cultured in serum-free media, do not contain the Kaposi sarcoma herpesvirus genome. *Br J Haematol* 1998; **102**: 1338–40.
81. Gao SJ, Kingsley L, Hoover DR et al. Seroconversion to antibodies against Kaposi sarcoma-associated herpesvirus-related latent nuclear antigens before the development of Kaposi sarcoma. *N Engl J Med* 1996; **335**: 233–41.
82. Hyjek E, Rafii S, Flore O et al. KSHV/HHV-8 in myelomatous effusions: development of a cell line useful for serologic analysis and viral propagation. *Blood* 1998; **92** (Suppl 1): 96a.
83. Hart DN. Dendritic cells: unique leukocyte populations which control the primary immune response. *Blood* 1997; **90**: 3245–87.
84. Tarte K, Olsen SJ, Lu ZY et al. Clinical grade functional dendritic cells from patients with multiple myeloma are not infected with Kaposi sarcoma-associated herpesvirus. *Blood* 1998; **91**: 1852–7.
85. Cull GM, Timms JM, Haynes AP et al. Dendritic cells cultured from mononuclear cells and CD34 cells in myeloma do not harbour human herpesvirus 8. *Br J Haematol* 1998; **100**: 793–6.

86. De Greef C, Bakkus M, Heirman C et al. The absence of Kaposi sarcoma-associated herpesvirus (KSHV) DNA sequences in leukapheresis products and ex vivo expanded CD34+ cells in multiple myeloma (MM) patients. *Blood* 1997; **90**: 86a.
87. Vescio RA, Wu C, Rettig MB et al. The detection of KSHV is increased by mobilization chemotherapy and reduced in autografts by CD34-selection. *Blood* 1997; **90**: 565a.
88. Bellos F, Cremer FW, Ehrbrecht E et al. Leukapheresis cells of patients with multiple myeloma collected after mobilization with chemotherapy and G-CSF do not bear Kaposi sarcoma associated herpesvirus DNA. *Br J Haematol* 1998; **103**: 1192–7.
89. Tarte K, Olsen SJ, Rossi JF et al. Kaposi sarcoma-associated herpesvirus is not detected with immunosuppression in multiple myeloma. *Blood* 1998; **92**: 2186–8.
90. Rettig MB, Vescio R, Ma H et al. Detection of Kaposi sarcoma-associated herpesvirus in the dendritic cells of Waldenstrom's macroglobulinemia and primary amyloidosis patients. *Blood* 1997; **90**: 86a.
91. Brousset P, Theriault C, Roda D et al. Kaposi sarcoma-associated herpesvirus (KSHV) in bone marrow biopsies of patients with Waldenström's macroglobulinaemia. *Br J Haematol* 1998; **102**: 795–7.
92. Santini GF, Crovatto M, Modolo ML et al. Waldenström macroglobulinaemia: a role of HCV infection? *Blood* 1993; **82**: 2932.
93. Silvestri F, Barillari G, Fanin R et al. Risk of hepatitis C virus infection, Waldenström's macroglobulinaemia, and monoclonal gammopathies. *Blood* 1996; **88**: 1125–6.
94. Mussini C, Ghini M, Mascia MT et al. Monoclonal gammopathies and hepatitis C virus infection. *Blood* 1995; **85**: 1144–5.
95. Mangia A, Clemente R, Musto P et al. Hepatitis C virus infection and monoclonal gammopathies not associated with cryoglobulinemia. *Leukemia* 1996; **10**: 1209–13.
96. Hanson CA, Frizzera G, Patton DF et al. Clonal rearrangement for immunoglobulin and T-cell receptor genes in systemic Castleman's disease. Association with Epstein–Barr virus. *Am J Pathol* 1988; **131**: 84–91.
97. Oksenhendler E, Duarte M, Soulier J et al. Multicentric Castleman's disease in HIV infection: a clinical and pathological study of 20 patients. *AIDS* 1996; **10**: 61–7.
98. Peterson BA, Frizzera G. Multicentric Castleman's disease. *Semin Oncol* 1993; **20**: 636–47.
99. Ensoli B, Gendelman R, Markham P et al. Synergy between basic fibroblast growth factor and HIV-1 Tat protein in induction of Kaposi sarcoma. *Nature* 1994; **371**: 674–80.
100. Harrington W Jr, Sieczkowski L, Sosa C et al. Activation of HHV-8 by HIV-1 tat. *Lancet* 1997; **349**: 774–5.
101. Mercader M, Taddeo B, Panella JR et al. Induction of HHV-8 lytic cycle replication by inflammatory cytokines produced by HIV-1-infected T cells. *Am J Pathol* 2000; **156**: 1961–71.

4

Cytokine abnormalities in plasma cell disorders

Noopur Raje, Kenneth C Anderson

CONTENTS • Introduction • IL-6 as a growth factor for myeloma • IL-6 as a survival factor for myeloma • IL-6 as a morbidity factor in myeloma • Signaling of IL-6 in myeloma cells • IL-6 and cell cycle regulation • Role of viral IL-6 • IL-6 as a prognostic marker • In vivo role of IL-6 in plasma cell dyscrasias • Anti-IL-6-directed therapy for myeloma and other plasma cell dyscrasias • Cytokine abnormalities associated with bone disease • Interferons in plasma cell dyscrasias • Other cytokines in plasma cell dyscrasias • Summary and conclusions

INTRODUCTION

The cytokine milieu has a profound impact on the disease biology of plasma cell dyscrasias. The characterization of normal cellular physiology and pathophysiology, and the ability to produce purified proteins that regulate cellular function, have been pivotal in elucidating the role of cytokines in these disorders.

Cytokines are extracellular signaling molecules that activate a cascade of intracellular pathways, and regulate growth and differentiation. These growth factors bind to specific cell surface receptors and thereby establish a communication between malignant precursors and their microenvironment.

The malignant plasma cells are localized to the bone marrow (BM) in myeloma and other plasma cell dyscrasias, in close proximity with the BM stroma. They are long-lived cells with a low labeling index. These cells have a rearranged immunoglobulin (Ig) gene that is extensively somatically hypermutated.[1] These plasma cells, together with the BM stromal cells (BMSC), secrete cytokines that interact with their receptors and further support the growth and survival of the malignant clone.

Interleukin (IL)-6 is probably the most extensively studied cytokine in the pathogenesis of plasma cell dyscrasias, and serves as a model for studying cytokine interactions in these disorders. The role of IL-6 in disease pathogenesis stems from the fact that both immunoreactive as well as bioreactive IL-6 serum levels are elevated in myeloma patients and their levels correlate with tumor burden and serve as prognostic markers. More importantly, anti-IL-6 monoclonal antibody therapy can transiently reverse disease manifestations in myeloma.

IL-6 AS A GROWTH FACTOR FOR MYELOMA

IL-6 is a cytokine that has pleiotropic effects on hematopoietic and non-hematopoietic cells.[2–4] It induces purified B cells to differentiate into Ig-secreting plasma cells. It therefore mediates the expansion of plasmablastic cells as well as their malignant counterparts. The role of IL-6 as a key growth factor in myeloma was explored by

Kawano et al,[5] who showed that freshly isolated human myeloma cells secreted IL-6 as well as expressing the IL-6 receptor (gp80). Their studies demonstrated induction of DNA synthesis with exogenous IL-6, and its inhibition by the addition of anti-IL-6 antibodies. These observations are further supported by work undertaken in our laboratory and by others.[6–9] More recently, triggering of myeloma cells via cell surface CD40 has been shown to induce IL-6-mediated autocrine myeloma cell growth.[10–11]

Although controversy surrounds the exact source of IL-6 in myeloma, there is evidence to suggest both autocrine and paracrine production. IL-6-mediated paracrine myeloma cell growth is supported by observations that BMSC are the major source of IL-6 in myeloma,[12–14] that freshly isolated myeloma cells cultured without exogenous IL-6 rapidly stop proliferating,[7] and that adhesion of myeloma cells to BMSC upregulates IL-6 secretion by BMSC.[15–17]

In addition, adhesion of osteoblasts to myeloma cells appears sufficient to trigger IL-6 transcription and secretion by BMSC. This interaction likely involves adhesion molecules present on myeloma cells that bind to their respective receptors on BMSC. Adhesion molecules on tumor cells may in turn be regulated by the cytokine profile, besides directly influencing it. For example, the presence of certain adhesion molecules increases contact between myeloma cells and BMSC, and causes the release of IL-6 directly or by augmenting the release of other cytokines such as transforming growth factor β (TGF-β), which further augments IL-6 release. The presence of circulating cytokines may also alter adhesion molecule profile on tumor cells, for example downregulating of syndecan on myeloma cells and its influence on disease progression.

Cytokines such as IL-1β, tumor necrosis factor α, and TGF-β[18–20] secreted by tumor cells may also mediate paracrine production of IL-6. Several transactivating transcription factors, including NF-κB, NF-IL-6, and the AP-1 proteins c-Jun and c-Fos, also appear to mediate IL-6 induction.[21–23]

IL-6 AS A SURVIVAL FACTOR FOR MYELOMA

IL-6 supports the survival and/or expansion of myeloma cells not only by stimulating cell division, but also by preventing apoptosis induced by serum starvation,[24] or by treatment with compounds such as vitamin D_3 or its derivative EB 1089,[25] dexamethasone,[26] and anti-Fas antibodies.[27] Retinoic acid (RA) induces programmed cell death in myeloma cell lines by downregulating the IL-6 receptor (IL-6R) expression.[28] Similarly IL-6R antagonists, which block the activation of myeloma cells by IL-6, act as pro-apoptotic factors for myeloma cells.[29] Recent work undertaken in our laboratory has focused on the protective effects of IL-6 on myeloma cells from programmed cell death. We and others have attempted to delineate the signaling cascades involved in myeloma apoptosis and the protective role played by IL-6.[24,26,27,30,31]

IL-6 AS A MORBIDITY FACTOR IN MYELOMA

Besides playing a seminal role in the growth and survival of myeloma cells, IL-6 may directly contribute to the morbidity associated with myeloma. Its role as a potent osteoclast-activating factor accounts, at least in part, for the bony disease and hypercalcemia noted in myeloma.[32–34] IL-6 may also play a role in anemia seen in myeloma.[35] Finally, it may play a role in mediating the renal failure associated with myeloma, because IL-6 transgenic mice develop histopathologic changes characteristic of myeloma kidney.[36]

SIGNALING OF IL-6 IN MYELOMA CELLS

Stimulation of cells by IL-6 requires binding to IL-6R, which is composed of at least two subunits with molecular weights of 80 and 130 kDa, the α and β chains, also referred to as IL-6Rα (gp80) and IL-6Rβ (gp130).[3] Binding of IL-6 to gp80 induces tyrosine phosphorylation and association with gp130, the signal-transducing subunit of IL-6R, and the subsequent formation of gp130 homodimers.

The downstream signaling cascades have been extensively studied in the case of human IL-6. The homodimerization of gp130 results in activation of the Janus kinase (Jak) family of tyrosine kinases, Jak1, Jak2, and/or Tyk2.[37–39] The activated Jak family kinase members phosphorylate gp130. Following activation of these tyrosine kinases, three downstream pathways have been reported.[40–41]

First, the phosphorylated gp130 binds to the signal transducer and activator of transcription (STAT)3, which is phosphorylated by Jak family kinases; homodimers of phosphorylated STAT3 rapidly migrate to the nucleus and bind to IL-6 response elements on the promoter of IL-6-induced genes. Second, IL-6 phosphorylates STAT1, and the heterodimer of tyrosine-phosphorylated STAT1 and STAT3 binds the nuclear DNA sequence termed interferon-γ activated sequence (GAS) or Sis-inducible element (SIE). Finally IL-6 can also activate the Ras-dependent mitogen-activated protein kinase (MAPK) cascade with sequential activation of Shc (Src homology 2/α-collagen related), Grb2, son of sevenless 1 (Sos1), Ras, Raf, MEK, and MAPK; this cascade ultimately leads to activation of the transcription factors NF-IL-6 or AP-1 complex (Jun/Fos).

Characterization of the signaling cascades activated in myeloma cells with respect to IL-6-mediated growth has been studied in our laboratory.[42,43] Specifically, IL-6 proliferation of myeloma cells occurs via activation of the MAPK signaling cascade, evidenced by phosphorylation of Shc, co-immunoprecipitation of phosphorylated Shc with Sos1, and phosphorylation of Erk2 in patient and myeloma cell lines that are IL-6 responsive. More importantly MAPK antisense, but not sense, oligonucleotides (ODNs) inhibit IL-6-induced proliferation of myeloma patient cells and cell lines. The signaling cascades activated by IL-6 are summarized in Figure 4.1.

The signaling cascades mediating the anti-apoptotic effects of IL-6 appear to be different to those that mediate growth. For example, activation of various serine/threonine kinases, in particular stress-activated protein kinase (SAPK) and p38 kinase, are noted during apoptosis of myeloma cells induced by anti-FAS antibody or γ irradiation, but not by dexamethasone. The protective role of IL-6 in anti-FAS-induced apoptosis via inhibition of the Jnk/SAPK pathway has recently been shown.[27,30] IL-6 does not inhibit radiation-induced apoptosis in myeloma cells. In contrast, dexamethasone-induced apoptosis is associated with a significant decrease in the activities of MAPK and $p70^{RSK}$.[26] Importantly, IL-6 inhibits dexamethasone-induced apoptosis and down-regulates MAPK.

More recently, we have delineated the role of related adhesion focal tyrosine kinase (RAFTK), also known as proline-rich tyrosine kinase 2 (PYK2), during dexamethasone-induced apoptosis in myeloma cells.[31] Dexamethasone-induced apoptosis is associated with PYK2 tyrosine phosphorylation and kinase activity, as evidenced by phosphorylation of its substrate protein GST-HEF. IL-6 blocks dexamethasone-induced PYK2 tyrosine phosphorylation and apoptosis, and activates Src homology protein tyrosine phosphatase (SHPTP2), which modulates PYK2 tyrosine kinase activity.

These studies suggest that at least two signal cascades exist for apoptosis in myeloma – one is associated with cytochrome *c* (γ irradiation) and not influenced by IL-6, while the other is independent of cytochrome *c*, with IL-6 having a protective effect.[44] Delineation of these pathways will allow the use of novel treatment strategies that either trigger death or inhibit survival signals of tumor cells. A myeloma apoptosis model is depicted in Figure 4.2 with relation to IL-6.

Besides IL-6, the gp130 protein serves as a transducer for other cytokines such as ciliary neurotropic factor (CNTF), oncostatin M (OSM), leukemia-inhibitory factor (LIF), IL-11, and cardiotrophin-1.[2] These cytokines therefore share some biologic properties with IL-6, and might act on myeloma cells, although they have not been studied in great detail.

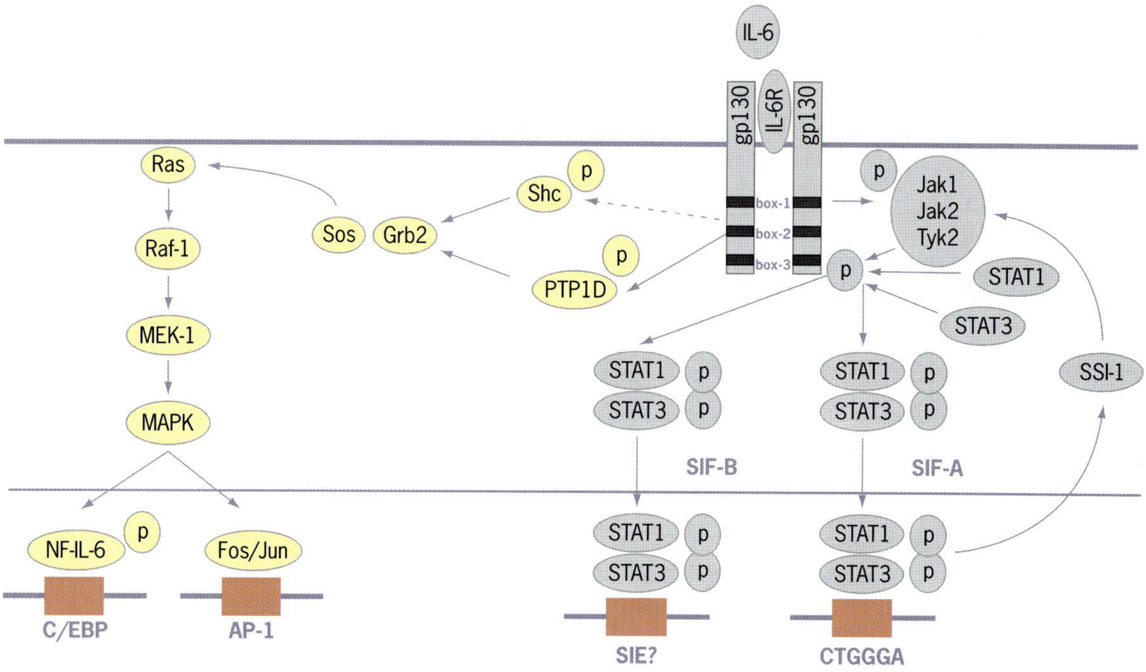

Figure 4.1 IL-6 signal transduction pathways. Binding of IL-6 to gp80 induces tyrosine phosphorylation and association with gp130, the signal-transducing subunit of IL6R, and the subsequent formation of gp130 homodimers. The homodimerization of gp130 results in activation of the Janus kinase (Jak) family of tyrosine kinases, Jak1, Jak2, and/or Tyk2. The activated Jak family kinase members phosphorylate gp130. Following activation of these tyrosine kinases, three downstream pathways are activated. First, the phosphorylated gp130 binds to STAT3, which is phosphorylated by Jak family kinases; homodimers of phosphorylated STAT3 rapidly migrate to the nucleus and bind to IL-6 response elements on the promoter of IL-6-induced genes. Second, IL-6 phosphorylates STAT1, and the heterodimer of tyrosine-phosphorylated STAT1 and STAT3 binds the nuclear DNA sequence termed interferon-γ activated sequence (GAS) or Sis-inducible element (SIE). Finally, IL-6 can also activate the Ras-dependent mitogen-activated protein kinase (MAPK) cascade, with sequential activation of Shc (Src homology 2/α-collagen related), Grb2, son of sevenless 1 (Sos1), Ras, Raf, MEK, and MAPK; this cascade ultimately leads to activation of the transcription factors NF-IL-6 or AP-1 complex (Jun/Fos). (Adapted from Treon SP, Anderson KC, Interleukin-6 in multiple myeloma and related plasma cell dyscrasias. *Curr Opin Hematol* 1998; **5**: 42–8.)

IL-6 AND CELL CYCLE REGULATION

Abnormalities of the retinoblastoma protein Rb and mutations of the *Rb* gene have been reported in up to 70% of myeloma patients and about 80% of myeloma cell lines.[45] Activated Rb blocks transition from G_1 to S phase of the cell cycle, whereas phosphorylated Rb releases this growth arrest. Exogenous IL-6 downregulates dephosphorylated Rb and decreases dephosphorylated Rb–E2F complexes, promoting myeloma cell growth by releasing growth arrest. Rb also upregulates autocrine release of IL-6 by myeloma cells, again promoting growth.

In addition, p21, another cell cycle regulatory protein, is constitutively expressed in the majority of myeloma cells, independently of the p53 status.[46] Its expression is upregulated by dexamethasone and downregulated by IL-6. Moreover, IL-6 inhibits the increase in p21 triggered by dexamethasone. Dexamethasone induces G_1 growth arrest in myeloma cells, whereas IL-6 counters this effect and facilitates G_1-to-S phase transition. Therefore IL-6, by its actions on Rb and p21, influences cell cycle kinetics and supports myeloma cell proliferation.

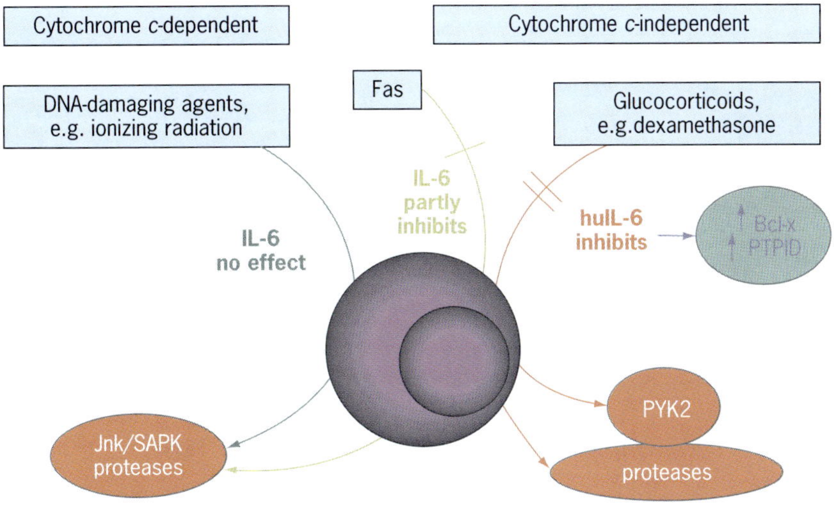

Figure 4.2 Role of IL-6 in myeloma apoptosis model. The signaling cascades mediating the anti-apoptotic effects of IL-6 are different from those that mediate growth. Anti-Fas antibody- or γ-irradiation-induced apoptosis of myeloma cells results in activation of stress-activated protein kinase (SAPK). Although IL-6 does not seem to rescue myeloma cells from radiation-induced apoptosis, it acts as a survival factor in anti-Fas-induced apoptosis via inhibition of the Jnk/SAPK pathway. In contrast, dexamethasone-induced apoptosis is associated with a significant decrease in the activities of MAPK and $p70^{RSK}$. IL-6 inhibits dexamethasone-induced apoptosis and downregulates MAPK. Importantly, dexamethasone-induced apoptosis is associated with protein-rich tyrosine kinase 2 (PYK2) tyrosine phosphorylation and kinase activity; conversely IL-6 blocks dexamethasone-induced PYK2 tyrosine phosphorylation and apoptosis and activates Src homology protein tyrosine phosphatase (SHPTP2), which modulates PYK2 tyrosine kinase activity. This model therefore suggests at least two signaling cascades for apoptosis in myeloma – one is associated with cytochrome *c* release from mitochondria (γ irradiation) and is not influenced by IL-6, while the other is independent of cytochrome *c*, with IL-6 having a protective effect.

ROLE OF VIRAL IL-6 (see also Chapter 3)

The recent detection of the Kaposi sarcoma-associated herpesvirus (KSHV; also known as human herpesvirus-8, HHV-8) in myeloma[47–50] and primary (AL) amyloidosis BMSC,[51] specifically dendritic cells (DC), is yet again an example of paracrine IL-6 production, because the KSHV genome encodes a homologue of the human IL-6 gene (huIL-6). Viral IL-6 (vIL-6) has been shown to support the growth of both human and murine myeloma cell lines,[52,53] as demonstrated by increased DNA synthesis in tritiated thymidine uptake studies. More importantly, vIL-6 has been able to rescue myeloma cell lines from serum-starvation-induced apoptosis, thereby suggesting its role as a survival factor. v-IL6 has also been transcribed in myeloma BM DC more often than in monoclonal gammopathy of unknown significance (MGUS), further suggesting its possible role in potentiating myeloma pathogenesis and progression.[47]

Distinct signal cascades are activated with huIL-6 versus vIL-6. Both cytokines activate gp130, Jak1, MAPK, and STAT3, but only huIL-6 induces phosphorylation of Tyk2, Jak2, STAT1, Shc and PTP1D. This therefore suggests that viral IL-6 might trigger a dual cascade – MAPK as well as Jak1/STAT3. Our studies also suggest that vIL-6 can inhibit dexamethasone-induced myeloma cell apoptosis. Therefore the role of vIL-6 as a proliferation and survival factor in myeloma and other plasma cell dyscrasias may complement that of human IL-6, and is the subject of ongoing studies.

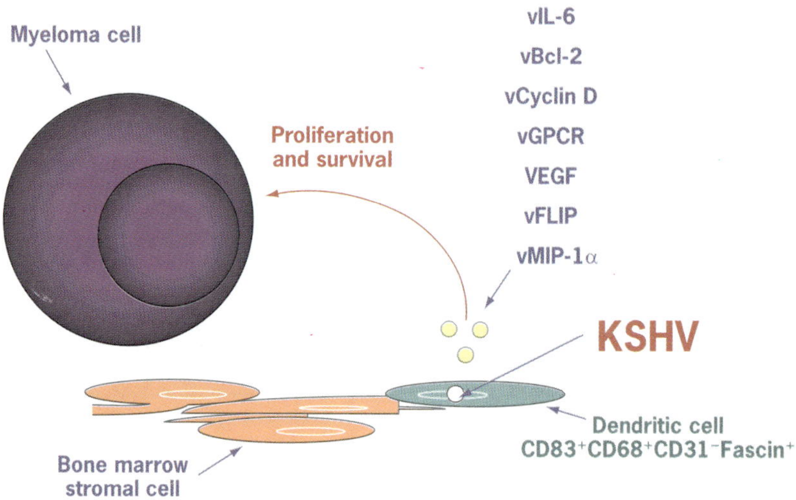

Figure 4.3 A hypothetical model for the role of KSHV in myeloma pathogenesis. The detection of KSHV in bone marrow stromal cells supports the theory of a paracrine role of IL-6 in myeloma pathogenesis. The KSHV genome encodes for vIL-6, which has been shown to support the growth and proliferation of myeloma cell lines. Besides vIL-6, KSHV encodes for other cellular genes and chemokines with homology to human proteins. Among these are the G-protein-coupled receptor (GPCR) or the IL-8R homologue, viral cyclin D, Bcl-2, viral FLICE inhibitory protein (vFLIP), macrophage inflammatory protein 1α (MIP-1α), and viral interferon regulatory factor (vIRF). These may play a significant role mediated either by anti-apoptotic signals or by increased tumor proliferation due to their oncogenic potential.

KSHV encodes for other cellular genes and chemokines with homology to the human proteins[54] (see Figure 4.3). Among these are the G-protein-coupled receptor (GPCR) or the IL-8R homologue and viral cyclin D. These two molecules have oncogenic potential, in that injection of GPCR-transfected NIH3T3 mouse cells into nude mice has resulted in production of tumors by induction of vascular endothelial growth factor (VEGF).[55] Viral cyclin D has a proliferative function via its capacity to phosphorylate Rb.[56] Others, such as vBcl-2, viral FLICE-inhibitory protein (vFLIP), macrophage inflammatory protein 1α (MIP-1α), and viral interferon regulatory factor (vIRF) may play a significant role mediated either by anti-apoptotic signals or by increased tumor proliferation. However, the presence of viral gene products in myeloma is controversial, and the role of KSHV in myeloma pathogenesis remains to be determined.

IL-6 AS A PROGNOSTIC MARKER

Multiple studies have shown that elevated levels of IL-6 in myeloma patients correlate with tumor burden and prognosis: high serum levels of IL-6 predict a poor prognosis and reflect active disease.[57,58] Several studies have also used soluble IL-6Rα levels as markers for disease progression.[59,60] These circulating soluble IL-6Rαs provide another potential mechanism making myeloma cells IL-6 sensitive and contributing to growth and expansion of myeloma cells. They are generated by receptor shedding from the cell membrane or by alternative RNA splicing.[61,62] Decreases in both serum IL-6 and IL-6Rα have been reported to accompany response to treatment.

IN VIVO ROLE OF IL-6 IN PLASMA CELL DYSCRASIAS

Besides strong evidence provided by soluble levels of IL-6 and IL-6Rα, and their correlation with disease status, the administration of murine monoclonal antibodies against huIL-6 to myeloma patients has been effective in inhibiting the growth of myeloma cells in vivo.[32]

Further in vivo evidence comes from studies demonstrating that huIL-6 transgenic mice develop plasmacytomas and plasmacytosis.[36,63] The role of IL-6 is further substantiated by studies in IL-6 gene knockout mice, which fail to develop pristane-induced plasmacytomas in the absence of IL-6.[64] In our studies with severe combined immunodeficient mice implanted with bilateral human bone grafts (SCID–hu mice), injected human myeloma cell lines grow only in xenografted human fetal bone implants, but not in murine BM. Moreover huIL-6, but not murine IL-6, is detected in the serum of these animals.[65]

More recently, a gp130 IL-6 transducer-dependent SCID model of human myeloma has been developed.[66] Agonist monoclonal antibodies to human gp130 transducer have been used, which support the growth of IL-6-dependent myeloma cell lines and short-term proliferation of primary myeloma cells. This model circumvents the problems associated with human IL-6 – specifically, its short half-life, toxicity, and lack of specificity. This and the SCID–hu mouse model will be particularly useful in studying disease biology and new therapeutic strategies in an in vivo setting.

ANTI-IL-6-DIRECTED THERAPY FOR MYELOMA AND OTHER PLASMA CELL DYSCRASIAS

Based on strong in vitro and in vivo evidence of the role of IL-6 in myeloma pathogenesis and progression, investigators have used cytokine-targeted antibody therapy. Klein et al[67] treated myeloma and plasma cell leukemia patients with murine anti-hu IL-6 antibodies. Although some responses were noted (decline in M component, serum calcium, and acute-phase reactants), no durable responses were seen.

The lack of sustained response could partially be attributed to the limitations of using murine antibodies: (a) the antibody levels achieved are inadequate to suppress circulating IL-6, (b) IL-6 and IL-6 antibody complexes form that retain some activity, (c) human antibodies develop to murine idiotypic determinants, and (d) IL-6R is upregulated in IL-6-deprived myeloma cells, enhancing their sensitivity to lower circulating IL-6 levels.[32,68] To overcome these pitfalls, investigators are using anti-IL-6 chimeric antibodies and anti-IL-6R antibodies.[69–71] More recently, investigators have developed IL-6 superantagonists that downregulate the growth of IL-6-dependent myeloma cell lines in vitro.[72–74] These agents bind to IL-6R and contain mutations that subsequently interfere with signaling of IL-6 and IL-6R complex via gp130.

Several cytokines, hormones, and drugs have been used that might act directly on IL-6, its receptor, or the complex formed with gp130. These include interferon (IFN)-α, IFN-γ, IL-4, all-*trans*-retinoic acid, bisphosphonates, glucocorticoids, vitamin D_3 derivatives, sex steroid hormones, and anti-estrogens.[25,75–78] IL-6 has also been fused with *Pseudomonas* exotoxin or diphtheria toxin, and has been shown to kill myeloma cells ex vivo in attempts to purge autologous BM prior to transplantation.[79,80]

CYTOKINE ABNORMALITIES ASSOCIATED WITH BONE DISEASE

Lytic lesions are the hallmark of myeloma, and are caused by increased recruitment of osteoclasts. Besides the profound role played by IL-6 and other members of the gp130 cytokine family (mainly LIF, IL-11, and OSM) in the development of bone lesions in myeloma patients,[34] Mundy et al.[81,82] detected bone-resorbing activity or osteoclast-stimulating factors (OSFs) in the supernatants of both myeloma cell lines and fresh patient cells. Cytokines such as IL-1β, tumor necrosis factor α (TNF-α), and TNF-β play an important role in bone resorption by inducing prostaglandin E_2 (PGE_2) and IL-6. Hematopoietic growth factors such as macrophage colony-stimulating factor (M-CSF) and TGF-β could also play a role. MIP-1α, known to induce osteoclast formation, has recently been detected in myeloma patients, and may also be an important OSF.[83]

INTERFERONS IN PLASMA CELL DYSCRASIAS

IFN-α has been used in the therapy of myeloma, with responses that have been variable[84] – at least partly because of the dual role played by this cytokine growth inhibition as well as proliferation. Although the rationale for the use of IFN-α in myeloma was its anti-proliferative action, it causes proliferation of fresh myeloma cells as well as stimulating the growth of IL-6-dependent myeloma cell lines.[85,86] Recent studies involving cell cycle regulatory genes and the differential induction of cyclin D2 and $p19^{INK4D}$ may be one of the key mechanisms underlying this heterogeneity.[87] IFN-α has been shown to cause growth arrest of hematopoietic cells by inhibition of Rb. IFN-α has been noted to upregulate cyclin D2 protein expression in myeloma cell lines that are growth responsive to IFN-α, but not in a cell line that is inhibited by IFN-α. It also stimulates an increase in Cdk4 and Cdk2 activity in growth-responsive cell lines, which correlated with G_1-to-S phase progression. Induction of p19 is noted in myeloma cell lines showing growth arrest, but not in those that are growth-responsive.

IFN-γ, on the other hand, has been reported to inhibit IL-6-dependent proliferation of fresh myeloma cells.[88] It did not affect endogenous IL-6 production, but seemed to act directly on myeloma cells. Interestingly, it also inhibits cytokine-mediated bone resorption. IFN-β has been shown to inhibit the proliferation of the myeloma cell line U266.[89] These effects are mediated, at least in part, by downmodulation of IL-6R. As a consequence, IFN-β reduces the IL-6-dependent tyrosine phosphorylation and activation of several signaling proteins, including Ras.

OTHER CYTOKINES IN PLASMA CELL DYSCRASIAS

Granulocyte colony-stimulating factor (G-CSF) is a hematopoietic growth factor with structural homology to IL-6. The G-CSF receptor also shares some homology with gp130. Both G-CSF and IL-6 induce activation of NF-IL-6, a transcription factor involved in the synthesis of IL-6. G-CSF is a potent growth factor for freshly explanted myeloma cells and cell lines.[90,91] The exact mechanism of this effect is unknown, as is its clinical significance because of the widespread use of G-CSF in mobilization schedules for autologous stem cell transplantation.

IL-10 is also a growth factor for myeloma cells, enhancing the proliferation of freshly explanted myeloma cells in short-term BM cultures.[92] It also supports the growth of myeloma cell lines. Because IL-10 has inhibitory effects on the production of IL-6, its effects are probably not mediated by IL-6. More likely, IL-10 enhances the responsiveness of myeloma cells by regulating the expression of other cytokines and cytokine receptors. IL-10 might increase the responsiveness of some myeloma cells to IL-11 by upregulating the expression of IL-11 receptors.[93] Moreover, IL-10 induces an autocrine OSM loop in human myeloma cells, probably by increasing the expression of LIF receptor, which, with gp130, forms a receptor for OSM.

Granulocyte–macrophage colony-stimulating factor (GM-CSF), IL-3, stem cell factor (SCF), TNF-α, hepatocyte growth factor (HGF), insulin-like growth factor 1 and 2 (IGF-1 and -2), and vascular endothelial growth factor (VEGF), are also potential myeloma growth factors, because they have been shown to stimulate growth and/or specific intracellular signaling events of myeloma cells or cell lines in vitro, often in a synergistic manner with IL-6.[94–96]

We have recently explored the biologic effects of TNF-α and VEGF in myeloma in order to identify new therapeutic targets via direct inhibition of these cytokines or by the use of drugs blocking NF-κB-mediated sequelae of TNF-α.[97,98]

SUMMARY AND CONCLUSIONS

In summary, IL-6 appears to be one of the key cytokines mediating tumor growth and survival in plasma cell dyscrasias. Besides its growth potential, it is responsible for much of the morbidity associated with these diseases. Other important cytokines include the IFNs and the OSFs. The association of KSHV with plasma cell dyscrasias also opens up a whole range of intriguing possibilities, since this viral genome encodes for various gene products with homology to human proteins known to have oncogenic and anti-apoptotic potential. Improved understanding of the complex cytokine interactions between tumor cells and their microenvironment will provide the rationale for novel treatment approaches that target signaling to either inhibit growth of tumor cells or enhance their apoptosis.

REFERENCES

1. Hallek M, Bergsagel PL, Anderson KC. Multiple myeloma: increasing evidence for a multistep transformation process. *Blood* 1998; **91**: 3–21.
2. Taga T, Kishimoto T. Cytokine receptors and signal transduction. *FASEB J* 1992; **6**: 3387–96.
3. Akira S, Taga T, Kishimoto T. Interleukin-6 in biology and medicine. *Adv Immunol* 1993; **54**: 1–78.
4. Hirano T, Akira S, Taga T, Kishimoto T. Biological and clinical aspects of interleukin-6. *Immunol Today* 1990; **11**: 443–9.
5. Kawano MM, Hirano T, Matsuda T et al. Autocrine generation and requirement of BSF-2/IL-6 for human multiple myeloma. *Nature* 1988; **332**: 83–5.
6. Anderson KC, Jones RC, Morimoto C et al. Response of purified myeloma cells to hematopoietic growth factors. *Blood* 1989; **73**: 1915–24.
7. Zhang XG, Klein B, Bataille R. Interleukin 6 is a potent myeloma cell growth factor in patients with aggressive multiple myeloma. *Blood* 1989; **74**: 11–13.
8. Barut BA, Zon LI, Cochran MK et al. Role of interleukin-6 in the growth of myeloma derived cell lines. *Leuk Res* 1992; **16**: 951–9.
9. Westendorf JJ, Ahmann GJ, Greipp PR et al. Establishment and characterization of three myeloma cell lines that demonstrate variable cytokine responses and abilities to produce autocrine interleukin-6. *Leukemia* 1996; **10**: 866–76.
10. Westendorf J, Ahmann G, Armitage R et al. CD40 expression in malignant plasma cells: role in stimulation of autocrine IL-6 secretion by a human myeloma cell line. *J Immunol* 1994; **152**: 117–28.
11. Urashima M, Chauhan D, Uchiyama H et al. CD40 ligand triggered interleukin-6 secretion in multiple myeloma. *Blood* 995; **85**: 1903–12.
12. Klein B, Zhang XG, Lu XY et al. Interleukin-6 in human multiple myeloma. *Blood* 1995; **85**: 863–72.
13. Lichtenstein A, Berenson D, Norman MP et al. Production of cytokines by bone marrow cells obtained from patients with multiple myeloma. *Blood* 1989; **74**: 1266–73.
14. Caligaris-Cappio F, Bergui L, Gregoretti M et al. Role of bone marrow stromal cells in growth of human multiple myeloma. *Blood* 1991; **77**: 2688–93.
15. Uchiyama H, Barut BA, Mohrbacher AF et al. Adhesion of human myeloma-derived cell lines to bone marrow stromal cells stimulates IL-6 secretion. *Blood* 993; **82**: 3712–20.
16. Chauhan D, Uchiyama H, Akbarali Y et al. Multiple myeloma cell adhesion-induced interleukin-6 expression in bone marrow stromal cells involves activation of NF-κB. *Blood* 1996; **87**: 1104–12.
17. Teoh G, Anderson KC. Interaction of tumor and host cells with adhesion and extracellular matrix molecules in the development of multiple myeloma. *Hematol Oncol Clin North Am* 1997; **11**: 27–42.
18. Carter A, Merchav S, Silvan-Draxler I, Tatarsky I. The role of interleukin-1 and tumor necrosis factor alpha in human multiple myeloma. *Br J Haematol* 1990; **74**: 424–31.
19. Lu ZY, Bataille R, Poubelle P et al. An interleukin 1 receptor antagonist blocks the IL-1 induced IL-6 paracrine production through a prostaglandin E2–related mechanism in multiple myeloma. *Stem Cells* 1995; **113**(Suppl): 28–34.
20. Urashima M, Ogata A, Chauhan D et al. Transforming growth factor β1: differential effects on multiple myeloma versus normal B cells. *Blood* 1996; **87**: 1928–38.
21. Isshiki H, Akira S, Tanabe O et al. Constitutive and IL-1 inducible factors interact with the IL-6 responsive element in the IL-6 gene. *Mol Cell Biol* 1990; **10**: 2757–62.
22. Muegge K, Vila M, Gusella GL et al. Interleukin 1 induction of the c-jun promoter. *Proc Natl Acad Sci USA* 1993; **90**: 7054–8.

23. Akira S, Isshiki H, Sugita T et al. A nuclear factor for IL-6 expression (NF-IL-6) is a member of the C/EBP family. *EMBO J* 1990; **9**: 1897–906.
24. Lichtenstein A, Tu Y, Fady C et al. Interleukin-6 inhibits apoptosis of malignant plasma cells. *Cell Immunol* 1995; **162**: 248–55.
25. Puthier D, Bataille R, Barille S et al. Myeloma cell growth arrest, apoptosis, and interleukin 6 receptor modulation induced by EB1089, a vitamin D3 derivative, alone or in association with dexamethasone. *Blood* 1996; **88**: 4659–66.
26. Chauhan D, Pandey P, Ogata A et al. Dexamethasone induces apoptosis of multiple myeloma cells in a JNK/SAP kinase independent mechanism. *Oncogene* 1997; **15**: 837–43.
27. Chauhan D, Kharbanda S, Ogata A et al. Interleukin-6 inhibits Fas-induced apoptosis and stress-activated protein kinase activation in multiple myeloma cells. *Blood* 1997; **89**: 227–34.
28. Levy Y, Labaume S, Colombel M, Brouet JC. Retinoic acid modulates the in vivo and in vitro growth of IL-6 autocrine human myeloma cell lines via induction of apoptosis. *Clin Exp Immunol* 1996; **104**: 167–72.
29. Demartis A, Bernassola F, Savino R et al. Interleukin-6 receptor superantagonists are potent inducers of human multiple myeloma cell death. *Cancer Res* 1996; **56**: 4213–18.
30. Xu F, Sharma S, Gardner S et al. Interleukin-6 induced inhibition of multiple myeloma cell apoptosis. support for the hypothesis that protection is mediated via inhibition of the JNK/SAPK pathway. *Blood* 1998; **92**: 241–51.
31. Chauhan D, Hideshima T, Pandey P et al. RAFTK/PYK2-dependent and independent apoptosis in multiple myeloma cells. *Oncogene* 1999; **18:** 6733–40.
32. Bataille R, Barlogie B, Yang Z et al. Biologic effects of anti-interleukin-6 murine monoclonal antibody in advanced multiple myeloma. *Blood* 1995; **86**: 685–91.
33. Ishimi Y, Miyaura C, Jin CH et al. IL-6 is produced by osteoblasts and induces bone resorption. *J Immunol* 1990; **145**: 3297–303.
34. Bataille R, Manolagas SC, Berenson JR. Pathogenesis and management of bone lesions in multiple myeloma. *Hematol Oncol Clin North Am* 1997; **11**: 349–61.
35. Nieken J, Mulder NH, Buter J et al. Recombinant human IL-6 induces a rapid and reversible anemia in cancer patients. *Blood* 1995; **86**: 900–5.
36. Fattori E, Della Rocca C, Costa P et al. Development of progressive kidney damage and myeloma kidney in interleukin-6 transgenic mice. *Blood* 1994; **83**: 2570–9.
37. Narazaki M, Witthuhn BA, Yoshida K et al. Activation of JAK2 kinase mediated by the interleukin 6 signal transducer gp130. *Proc Natl Acad Sci USA* 1994; **91**: 2285–9.
38. Stahl N, Boulton TG, Farruggella T et al. Association and activation of Jak–Tyk kinases by CNTF–LIF–OSM–IL-6 β receptor components. *Science* 1994; **263**: 92–5.
39. Matsuda T, Yamasaki Y, Hirano T. Interleukin-6–induced tyrosine phosphorylation of multiple proteins in murine hematopoietic lineage cells. *Biochem Biophys Res Commun* 1994; **200**: 821–8.
40. Kishimoto T, Taga T, Akira S. Cytokine signal transduction. *Cell* 1994; **76**: 253–62.
41. Kishimoto T, Akira S, Narazaki M, Taga T. Interleukin-6 family of cytokines and gp130. *Blood* 1995; **86**: 1243–54.
42. Ogata A, Chauhan D, Teoh G et al. Interleukin-6 triggers cell growth via the *ras*-dependent mitogen-activated protein kinase cascade. *J Immunol* 1997; **159**: 2212–21.
43. Ogata A, Chauhan D, Urashima M et al. Blockade of mitogen-activated protein kinase cascade signaling in interleukin-6 independent multiple myeloma cells. *Clin Cancer Res* 1997; **3**: 1017–22.
44. Chauhan D, Pandey P, Ogata A et al. Cytochrome-*c* dependent and independent induction of apoptosis in multiple myeloma cells. *J Biol Chem* 1997; **272**: 29 995–7.
45. Urashima M, Ogata A, Chauhan D et al. Interleukin-6 promotes multiple myeloma cell growth via phosphorylation of retinoblastoma protein. *Blood* 1996; **88**: 2219–27.
46. Urashima M, Teoh G, Chauhan D et al. Interleukin-6 overcomes $p21^{WAF1}$ upregulation and G1 growth arrest induced by dexamethasone and interferon-γ in multiple myeloma cells. *Blood* 1997; **90**: 279–89.
47. Rettig MB, Ma HJ, Vescio RA et al. Kaposi's sarcoma-associated herpesvirus infection of bone marrow dendritic cells from multiple myeloma patients. *Science* 1997; **276**: 1851–4.
48. Said JW, Rettig MR, Heppner K et al. Localization of Kaposi's sarcoma-associated herpesvirus in bone marrow biopsy samples from patients with multiple myeloma. *Blood* 1997; **90**: 4278–82.

49. Chauhan D, Bharti A, Raje N et al. Detection of Kaposi's sarcoma herpesvirus-8 DNA sequences in multiple myeloma bone marrow stromal cells. *Blood* 1999; **93**: 1482–6.
50. Raje N, Gong J, Chauhan D et al. Bone marrow and peripheral blood dendritic cells from patients with multiple myeloma are phenotypically and functionally normal. *Blood* 1999; **93**: 1487–95.
51. Raje N, Kica G, Chauhan D et al. Kaposi's sarcoma-associated herpesvirus gene sequences are detectable at low copy number in primary amyloidosis. *Amyloid* 2000; **7**: 126–32.
52. Hideshima T, Chauhan D, Teoh G et al. Signaling by Kaposi's sarcoma-associated herpesvirus encoded viral interleukin-6 in human interleukin-6 dependent cell lines. *Blood* 1998; **92**: 95a.
53. Burger R, Neipel F, Fleckenstein B et al. Human herpesvirus type 8 interleukin-6 homologue is functionally active on human myeloma cells. *Blood* 1998; **91**: 1858–63.
54. Whitby D, Boshoff C. Kaposi's sarcoma herpesvirus as a new paradigm for virus-induced oncogenesis. *Curr Opin Oncol* 1998; **10**: 405–12.
55. Bias C, Santomasso B, Coco O et al. G-protein-coupled receptor of Kaposi's sarcoma-associated herpesvirus is a viral oncogene and angiogenesis activator. *Nature* 1998; **391**: 86–9.
56. Cesarman E, Nador RG, Bai F et al. Kaposi's sarcoma-associated herpesvirus contains G protein-coupled receptor and cyclin D homologs which are expressed in Kaposi's sarcoma and malignant lymphoma. *J Virol* 1996; **70**: 8212–23.
57. Bataille R, Jourdan M, Zhang XG et al. Serum levels of interleukin-6, a potent myeloma cell growth factor, as a reflection of disease severity in plasma cell dyscrasias. *J Clin Invest* 1989; **84**: 2008–11.
58. Gaillard JP, Bataille R, Brailly H et al. Increased and highly stable levels of functional soluble interleukin-6 receptor in sera of patients with monoclonal gammopathy. *Eur J Immunol* 1993; **23**: 820–4.
59. Kyrtsonis MC, Dedoussis G, Zervas C et al. Soluble interleukin-6 receptor (sIL-6R), a new prognostic factor in multiple myeloma. *Br J Haematol* 1996; **93**: 398–400.
60. Pulkki K, Pelliniemi TT, Rajamaki A et al. Soluble interleukin-6 receptor as a prognostic factor in multiple myeloma. *Br J Haematol* 1996; **92**: 370–4.
61. Lust JA, Donovan KA, Kline MP et al. Isolation of an mRNA encoding a soluble form of the human interleukin-6 receptor. *Cytokine* 1992; **4**: 96–100.
62. Mullberg J, Dittrich E, Graeve L et al. Differential shedding of the two subunits of the interleukin-6 receptor. *FEBS Lett* 1992; **332**: 174–8.
63. Suematsu S, Matsukaka T, Matsuda T et al. Generation of plasmacytomas with the chromosomal translocation t(12;15) in interleukin-6 transgenic mice. *Proc Natl Acad Sci USA* 1994; **89**: 232–9.
64. Hilbert DM, Kopf M, Mock BA et al. Interleukin-6 is essential for the in vivo development of B lineage neoplasms. *J Exp Med* 1995; **182**: 243–8.
65. Urashima M, Chen BP, Chen S et al. The development of a model for the homing of multiple myeloma cells to human bone marrow. *Blood* 1997; **90**: 754–65.
66. Rebouissou C, Wijdenes J, Autissier P et al. A gp130 interleukin-6 transducer-dependent SCID model of human multiple myeloma. *Blood* 1998; **91**: 4727–37.
67. Klein B, Lu Y, Gaillard JP et al. Inhibiting IL-6 in human multiple myeloma. *Curr Top Microbiol Immunol* 1992; **182**: 236–44.
68. Mihara M, Koishihara Y, Fukui H et al. Murine antihuman IL-6 monoclonal antibody prolongs the half life in circulating blood and thus prolongs the bioactivity of human IL-6 in mice. *Immunology* 1991; **74**: 55–9.
69. van Zaanen HCT, Koopmans RP, Aarden LA et al. Endogenous interleukin 6 production in multiple myeloma patients treated with chimeric monoclonal anti-IL6 antibodies indicates the existence of a positive feed-back loop. *J Clin Invest* 1996; **98**: 1441–8.
70. Tsunernari T, Akamatsu KI, Kaiho SI et al. Therapeutic potential of humanized anti-interleukin 6 receptor antibody. antitumor activity in xenograft model of multiple myeloma. *Anticancer Res* 1996; **16**: 2537–44.
71. Suzuki H, Yasukawa K, Saito T et al. Anti-human interleukin 6 receptor antibody inhibits human myeloma growth in vivo. *Eur J Immunol* 1992; **22**: 1989–93.
72. Savino R, Ciapponi L, Lahm A et al, Rational design of a receptor super-antagonist of human interleukin-6. *EMBO J* 1994; **13**: 5863–70.
73. Ehlers M, de Hon FD, Klasse Bos H et al. Combining two mutations of human interleukin-6 that affect gp130 activation results in a potent interleukin-6 receptor antagonist on human myeloma cells. *J Biol Chem* 1995; **270**: 8158–63.
74. Sporeno E, Savino R, Ciapponi L et al. Human interleukin-6 receptor super antagonists with

high potency and wide spectrum on multiple myeloma cells. *Blood* 1996; **87**: 4510–19.
75. Lasfar A, Wietzerbin J, Billard C. Differential regulation of interleukin 6 receptors by interleukin 6 and interferons in multiple myeloma cell lines. *Eur J Immunol* 1994; **24**: 124–30.
76. Hermann F, Andreff M, Gruss HJ et al. Interleukin 4 inhibits growth of multiple myeloma by suppressing interleukin 6 expression. *Blood* 1991; **78**: 2070–8.
77. Ogata A, Nishimoto N, Shima Y, Yoshizaki K, Kishimoto T. Inhibitory effect of all-*trans* retinoic acid on the growth of freshly isolated myeloma cells via interference with interleukin-6 signal transduction. *Blood* 1994; **84**: 3040–6.
78. Ishikawa H, Tanaka H, Iwato K et al. Effect of glucocorticoids on the biologic activities of myeloma cells: inhibition of interleukin beta osteoclast activating factor induced bone resorption. *Blood* 1990; **75**: 715–20.
79. Kreitman R, Siegall CB, Fitzgerald DJP et al. Interleukin-6 fused to mutant form of pseudomonas exotoxin kills malignant cells form patients with multiple myeloma. *Blood* 1992; **79**: 1775–80.
80. Chadwick D, Jamal N, Messner HA et al. Differential sensitivity of human myeloma cell lines and bone marrow colony forming cells to a recombinant diphtheria toxin-interleukin-6 fusion protein. *Br J Haematol* 1993; **85**: 25–36.
81. Mundy GR, Raisz LG, Cooper RA et al. Evidence for the secretion of an osteoclast stimulating factor in myeloma. *N Engl J Med* 1974; **291**: 1041–6.
82. Mundy GR, Luben RA, Raisz LG et al. Bone resorbing activity in supernatants from lymphoid cell lines. *N Engl J Med* 1974; **290**: 867–71.
83. Alsina M, Choi SJ, Cruz JC et al. Overexpression of the osteoclast stimulatory factor (OSF), macrophage inflammatory protein 1-alpha (MIP1α) in multiple myeloma (MM). *Blood* 1998; **92**(Suppl): 680a.
84. Ludwig H, Cohen AM, Polliack A et al. Interferon-alpha for induction and maintenance in multiple myeloma: results of two multicenter randomized trials and summary of other studies. *Ann Oncol* 1995; **6**: 467–76.
85. Ludwig CU, Durie BG, Salmon SE, Moon TE. Tumor growth stimulation in vitro by interferons. *Eur J Cancer Clin Oncol* 1983; **19**: 1625–32.
86. Jourdan M, Zhang X-G, Portier M et al. IFN-alpha induced autocrine production of IL-6 in myeloma cell lines. *J Immunol* 1991; **147**: 4402–7.
87. Arora T, Jelinek DF. Differential myeloma cell responsiveness to interferon-α correlates with differential induction of p19 INK4d and cyclin D2 expression. *J Biol Chem* 1998; **273**: 11799–805.
88. Portier M, Zhang XG, Caron E et al. Gamma-interferon in multiple myeloma. inhibition of interleukin 6 dependent myeloma cell growth and downregulation of IL-6 receptor expression in vitro. *Blood* 1993; **81**: 3076–82.
89. Schwab M, Brini AT, Bosco MC et al. Disruption by interferon-α of an autocrine interleukin-6 growth loop in IL-6–dependent U266 myeloma cells by homologous and heterologous down-regulation of IL-6 receptor α- and β-chains. *J Clin Invest* 1994; **94**: 2317–25.
90. Klein B. Cytokines, cytokine receptors, transduction signals, and oncogenes in human multiple myeloma. *Semin Hematol* 1995; **32**: 4–19.
91. Chen-Kiang S, Hsu W, Natkunam Y, Zhang X. Nuclear signaling by interleukin-6. *Curr Opin Immunol* 1993; **5**: 124–8.
92. Lu ZY, Zhang XG, Rodriguez C et al. Interleukin-10 is a proliferation factor but not a differentiation factor for human myeloma cells. *Blood* 1995; **85**: 2521–7.
93. Lu ZY, Gu ZJ, Zhang XG et al. Interleukin-10 induces interleukin-11 responsiveness in human myeloma cell lines. *FEBS Lett* 1995; **377**: 515–18.
94. Zhang XG, Bataille R, Jourdan M et al. Granulocyte–macrophage colony-stimulating factor synergizes with interleukin-6 in supporting the proliferation of human myeloma cells. *Blood* 1990; **76**: 2599–605.
95. Freund GG, Kulas DT, Mooney RA. Insulin and IGF-1 increase mitogenesis and glucose metabolism in the multiple myeloma cell line, RPMI 8226. *J Immunol* 1993; **151**: 1811–20.
96. Borset M, Waage A, Brekke OL, Helseth E. TNF and IL-6 are potent growth factors for OH-2, a novel human myeloma cell line. *Eur J Haematol* 1994; **53**: 31–7.
97. Hideshima T, Chauhan D, Schlossman R et al. The role of tumor necrosis factor alpha in the pathophysiology of human multiple myeloma: therapeutic application. *Oncogene* 2001; **20**: 4519–27.
98. Podar K, Tai YT, Davies FE et al. Vascular endothelial growth factor triggers signaling cascades mediating multiple myeloma cell growth and migration. *Blood* 2001; **98**: 428–35.

5

Cytogenetics in plasma cell disorders

Jeffrey R Sawyer, Seema Singhal

INTRODUCTION

Myeloma is a clonal bone marrow disease characterized by the neoplastic transformation of differentiated B cells, in which over 90% of patients show a monoclonal protein production.[1] In contrast to normal plasma cells, myeloma cells are not terminally differentiated, and still have proliferative activity.[2]

Cytogenetic aberrations found in myeloma and other plasma cell disorders are not as well characterized as those seen in most other hematologic malignancies. In acute leukemias, the proliferative rate of the malignant cells is higher than that of the normal hematopoietic cells, and therefore abnormal cells predominate. However, in myeloma, the abnormal clone has a low proliferative activity in most patients, and therefore most analyzable metaphase spreads are derived from normal hematopoiesis.

Myeloma proceeds through a series of phases during malignant transformation, including a non-proliferative phase, an active phase with a small percentage of proliferating cells, and a fulminant phase with an increase in plasmablastic cells.[3] The sequential evolution of phenotypically distinct populations of myeloma plasma cells, in conjunction with morphological changes, suggests that myeloma plasma cells are the product of this continuous process of differentiation of an earlier progenitor cell.

Unfortunately, by the time that cytogenetic analysis is performed, it appears that in most patients the karyotype has already also evolved. The reported frequency of abnormal karyotypes in plasma cell dyscrasias varies considerably.[4–18] However, the most recent report from a large collaborative study found abnormal karyotypes in 15% of patients with Waldenström's macroglobulinemia (WM), 25% in monoclonal gammopathy of unknown significance (MGUS), 33% in myeloma, and 50% in plasma cell leukemia (PCL).[16]

CHROMOSOME ABNORMALITIES IN PLASMA CELL DISORDERS ARE NON-RANDOM

The overriding finding in modern cancer cytogenetics is that chromosome aberrations in cancer are non-random. It is important to distinguish between the two types of chromosome aberrations that occur in most cancers.[4] Primary chromosome aberrations are frequently found as sole aberrations and are often associated with a particular oncogene or tumor suppressor gene rearrangement. Secondary aberrations occur in addition to the primary aberrations and frequently dominate the karyotype during disease progression. These aberrations also occur in a non-random manner, and are probably associated with specific gene rearrangements.

No primary chromosome aberrations have yet been identified in plasma cell disorders, since no single aberration is seen in most patients. Secondary chromosome aberrations tend to dominate the karyotype by the time that myeloma is diagnosed, and therefore the chromosome abnormalities are usually quite complex. In many ways, the complex karyotypes found in myeloma are similar to those found in solid tumors.

Throughout this chapter, references are made to specific gene loci, and chromosome breakpoints found the plasma cell disorders. Figure 5.1 is a chromosome ideogram map showing the positions of these genes.

CHROMOSOME ABNORMALITIES IDENTIFIED BY GIESMA BANDING

Numerical aberrations

Myeloma is characterized at the Giesma banding level by complex karyotypes with frequent numerical and structural aberrations. The heterogeneous nature of myeloma karyotypes is

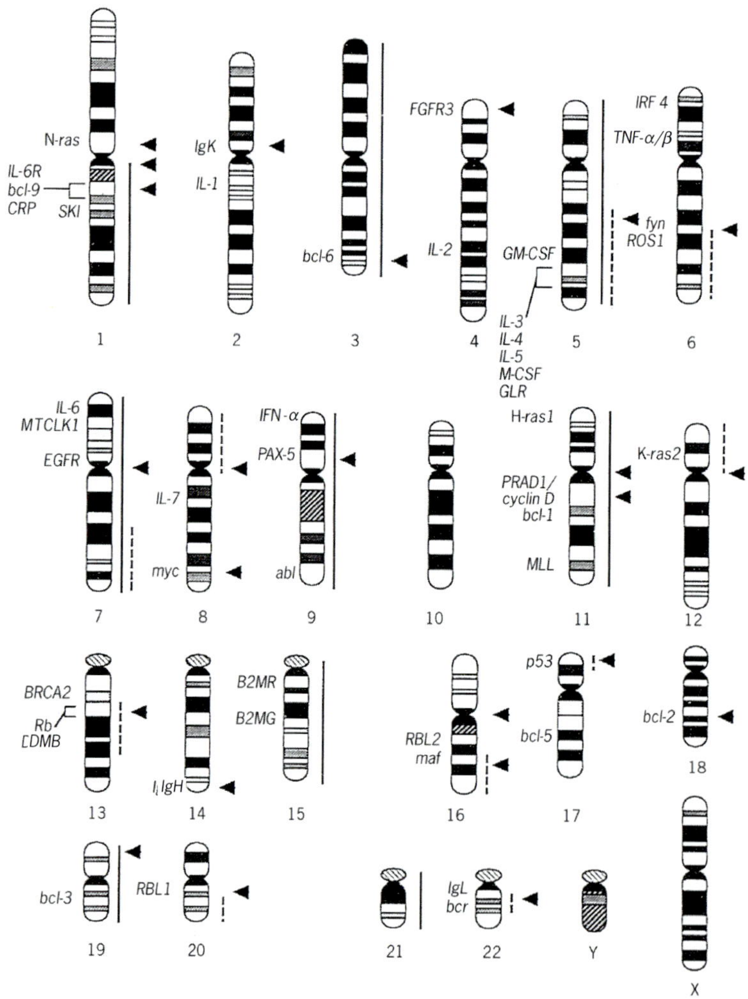

Figure 5.1 Chromosome ideogram showing the location of proto-oncogenes, tumor suppressor genes, and growth factors thought to be important in plasma cell disorders. Gene symbols are given to the left of each chromosome at the approximate chromosome band location. Breakpoints of recurring chromosome translocations are indicated by an arrowhead to the right of each chromosome. The solid vertical lines to the right indicate regions frequently present in triplicate, while the dashed vertical lines indicate regions that are frequently deleted.

consistent with the well-known clinical heterogeneity of the disease. High tumor burden and aggressive disease has been associated with high modal chromosome number and complex structural rearrangements.

The number of abnormal karyotypes reported in myeloma varies from 20% to 60%, but is about 40% in most published series.[5–18]

The most common numerical aberrations reported in myeloma are trisomies of chromosomes 3, 7, 9, 11, and 15, and monosomy of chromosome 13. The striking co-segregation of trisomies for these chromosomes suggests a consistent pattern of cytogenetic progression in myeloma (Figure 5.2). As the disease progresses, it seems likely that trisomies of chromosomes 9, 11, and 15 occur first, and the rest accumulate as intermediate steps prior to further karyotypic expansion and progression. The most striking chromosome losses are monosomy or deletion of chromosome 13 and, to a lesser extent, chromosome 16. Studies of the centrosome, a cell organelle involved with chromosome segregation, suggest that deregulated duplication and distribution of these structures may be implicated in numerical chromosome aberrations in many malignancies.[19–21]

Structural aberrations

The most consistent structural aberration in myeloma has been the presence of 14q+ chromosomal aberrations similar to those seen in other B-cell disorders. The reciprocal translocation t(11;14)(q13;q32) is the most frequent translocation detected by G-banding (Table 5.1).

In contrast to mantle cell lymphoma, where the breakpoint in the t(11;14) is clustered in the major translocation cluster (MTC) region, the breakpoint in myeloma is apparently different. Chesi et al[22] have demonstrated that in myeloma cell lines overexpressing cyclin D1, part of chromosome 11 is translocated into the gamma switch region, suggesting an error in switch recombination, while t(11;14) in mantle cell lymphoma invariably takes place into or near the *JH* segment, suggesting an error in *VDJ* recombination. These results are consistent with the fact that myeloma cells already have undergone *IgH* switch recombination, whereas mantle cell lymphomas generally have not.

Recently, several new recurring translocations have been identified in myeloma cell lines,

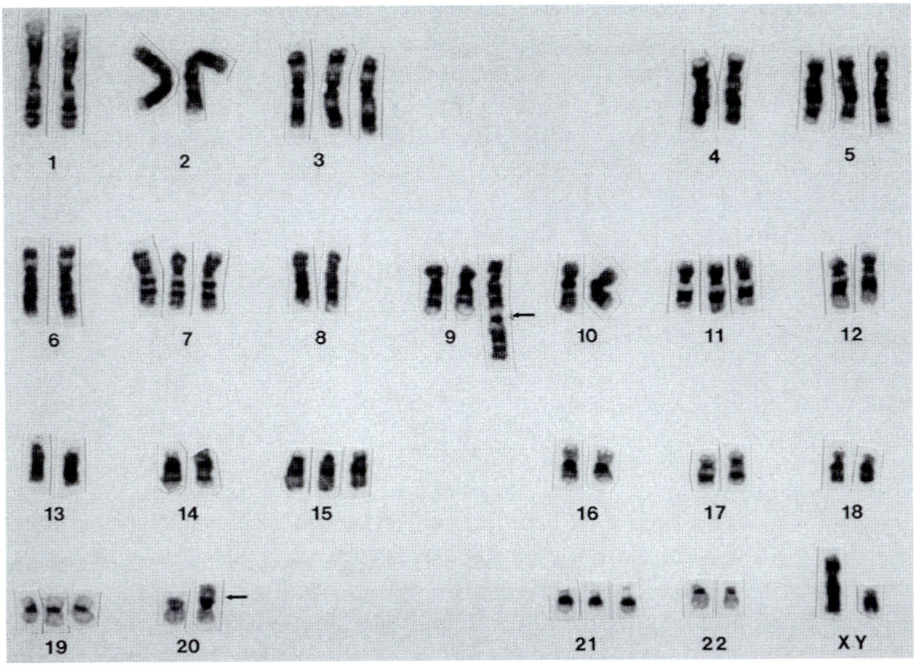

Figure 5.2 Giemsa band karyotype of a hyperdiploid cell in myeloma. Note the 'typical' numerical aberrations, including trisomies of chromosomes 3, 5, 7, 9, 11, 15, 19, and 21, all of which are common in myeloma. Structural aberrations include a whole-arm translocation of 1q to 9qter (arrow) and a derivative chromosome 20p (arrow).

Table 5.1 Common recurring structural chromosome aberrations in plasma cell disorders

Translocations	Frequency (%)	Involved genes	
t(11;14)(q13;q32)	25–30	*cyclin D1*	*IgH*
t(4;14)(p16.3;q32)	20–25	*FGFR3*	*IgH*
t(14;16)(q32;q22–23)	20–25	*IgH*	*MAF*
t(6;14)(p25;q32)	<5	*IRF4*	*IgH*
t(8;22)(q24;q32)	<5	*myc*	*IgL*
t(8;14)(q24;q32)	<5	*myc*	*IgH*
t(9;14)(p13;q32)	<5	*PAX5*	*IgH*
t(1;8)(p11~13;q32)	<5	?	*myc*
t(14;18)(q32;q21)	?	*IgH*	*bcl-2*
Deletions	**Frequency (%)**	**Involved genes**	
del(13)(q14~25)	15–50	Rb, DBM	
del(17)(p13)	30–50	*p53*	

including t(4;14)(p16.3;q32.3), t(6;14)(p25;q32), and t(14;16)(q32.3;q23).[23–26] Several of these aberrations are similar to those seen in other B-cell disorders involving a large array of exchange partners with the *IgH* locus. Therefore it remains unclear if any of these aberrations are of primary importance in myeloma.

A long latency phase prior to diagnosis may be one reason for the evolution of structural aberrations resulting in complex karyotypes. Additional secondary structural changes are observed following treatment, which tend to obscure the identification of early events.

The search for a single 'primary' cytogenetic aberration has proven unsuccessful, since the IgH locus appears to allow a promiscuous array of exchange partners with subtle differences in molecular phenotypes.

UNTREATED PATIENTS VERSUS TREATED PATIENTS

The variation in the number of abnormal karyotypes reported is at least in part due to the stage of the disease when patients are studied.

More advanced disease is associated with higher frequencies of chromosome aberrations,[8] and chromosome aberrations accumulate in treated patients.[5,10,12] Typically, previously treated and relapsing patients have a higher frequency of chromosomal abnormalities; 35–60% compared with 20–35% in newly diagnosed patients.[8, 14–18]

The most striking feature among untreated patients with abnormal karyotypes is the finding of either full or partial monosomy for chromosome 13 and/or chromosome 16.[8,14] Treated patients also show hypodiploidy and monosomy for chromosome 13 as the single most common chromosome loss. Half of the treated patients showed complete or partial monosomy for chromosome 13, including deletion of the chromosome band 13q14, known to be the locus of the retinoblastoma (*Rb*) tumor suppressor gene.

In a study of 79 previously untreated patients Seong et al[27] reported abnormal karyotypes in 46% (64% hyperdiploidy and 31% hypodiploid). Trisomies of chromosomes 9 and 15, and monosomy or deletion of chromosome 13 were the most common numerical aberrations.

CYTOGENETIC STUDIES IN MGUS

While MGUS often has a benign clinical course, some patients progress to myeloma or other lymphoproliferative disorders. Metaphase cytogenetic studies have not been reported in MGUS until recently, because the very low proliferative capacity of these cells has precluded successful karyotyping.

Calasanz et al[18] found mostly structural abnormalities in a group of 11 MGUS patients. Interestingly, all showed modal chromosome numbers near 46 with structural aberrations similar to those found in myeloma, including add(14)(q32), del(16)(q22), and del(22)(q11). The metaphase chromosome analysis, however, found none of the trisomies that have previously been reported by fluorescence in situ hybridization (FISH).[28] The discrepancy between the high level of aneuploidy found by FISH and the near-normal modal number found in association with the structural aberrations by these two different methods of analysis may be partially explained by different proliferative activity of cytogenetically heterogeneous subpopulations. A growing number of studies suggest that standard cytogenetics underestimates numerical abnormalities revealed by FISH techniques.[29]

EVOLUTION OF CHROMOSOME ABERRATIONS IN MYELOMA: CHROMOSOME INSTABILITY

The evolution of chromosome aberrations and related genomic instability in myeloma is most clearly evidenced by chromosome 1q aberrations. B-cell hematologic malignancies with aggressive disease can show decondensation of 1qh pericentromeric regions, resulting in unstable 'jumping translocations' of chromosome 1 (Figure 5.3).[30]

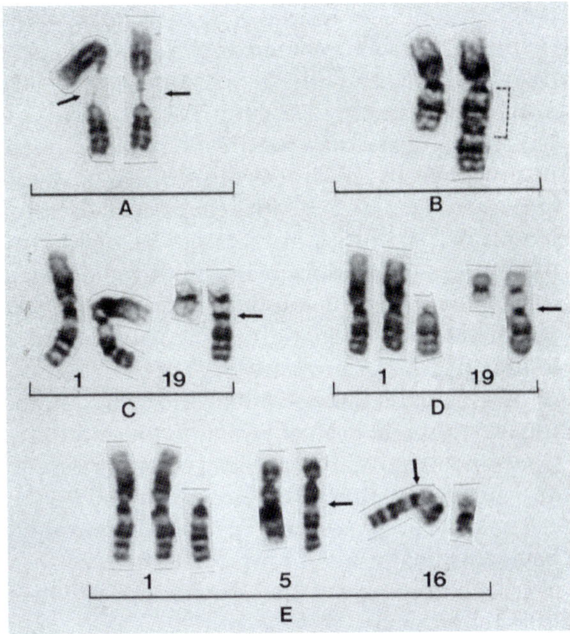

Figure 5.3 Partial G-banded karyotypes of chromosomes 1 from five different cells from five different patients showing the various types of chromosome 1 instability seen in aggressive plasma cell disorders. These cells illustrate the typical pattern of progression of 1q aberrations in myeloma. (A) Chromosomes 1 showing pericentromeric decondensation of both homologues. (B) Chromosomes 1 showing a duplication of the entire long arm [brackets]. (C) Whole-arm translocation of 1q to 19q (arrow). This cell is thus trisomic for 1q. (D) This cell shows two normal 1s, a free 1q, and a 1q whole-arm translocation to 19p (arrow, the 19s are inverted). (E) This partial karyotype shows a total of five copies of 1q, including two normal 1s, a free 1q, and whole-arm 1q translocations to 5q15 and to 16pter (arrows). This cell thus illustrates the 'jumping 1q' translocation to multiple chromosomes.

Chromosome 1 aberrations are common in most hematologic malignancies, and constitute the most common structural aberration in myeloma. The primary numerical chromosome aberrations seen in myeloma karyotypes apparently evolve over an extended period of time as a subclinical phenomenon. In later stages of progression, cytogenetic evolution takes place, resulting in secondary chromosomal aberrations commonly involving chromosome 1. Structural aberrations of chromosome 1 have been reported in about 40% of patients with myeloma showing abnormal karyotypes,[4] and a relationship between aberrations in the short arm of chromosome 1 and N-*ras* mutations has been suggested.[31] Interstitial deletions occur in the short arm of chromosome 1; however, it is the long arm of chromosome 1 that not only is involved in structural rearrangements but also is trisomic in many patients. Trisomy for the long arm of chromosome 1 is common in many types of cancer[32–33] and has been reported previously in myeloma by several groups,[5,8,17] who found between 30% and 50% of their patients trisomic for all or part of 1q. Two types of apparently interrelated aberrations of chromosome 1q occur during karyotype evolution in myeloma. The more common aberration is the duplication of region 1q21~31.[5] In many patients, duplication of this region is the only aberration of 1q noted; however, in a subset of patients, these duplications become unstable and lead to more complex aberrations involving the movement 1q.

The decondensation of the centromeric heterochromatin of 1q associated with these aberrations suggests that hypomethylation of this region may play a role in the somatic pairing, fragility and formation of the aberrations involving the long arm of chromosome 1 (Figure 5.3A).[30] These events are apparently the cytogenetic precursors to the subsequent 'jumping translocations'. The striking similarity between chromosome 1q aberrations in myeloma patients and those with high-grade lymphomas suggests the possibility of a common mechanism in a number of malignancies. The correlation of trisomy for 1q with the progression of malignancy has been correlated with the metastatic potential in colon and renal cell carcinomas, including the involvement of the *SKI* oncogene located at 1q21.[34–35]

Several different recurring translocations of the whole arm of 1q are found in myeloma.[15,17,30,38] The two most common ones are der(15)t(1;15)(q10;p10) and der(16)t(1;16)(q10;p10). der(15)t(1;15) is a rare but nonrandom change also associated with myelodysplastic syndrome and myeloproliferative disorders. This aberration has been reported as the sole aberration in most patients.[36–37] The der(16)t(1;16) has been reported in myeloma[17,38] and a wide variety of other malignancies, including breast cancer, Ewing's sarcoma, and Wilms' tumor. This aberration has also been reported as the sole aberration in some cases, but as a secondary aberration in most patients.[39–43] It may be that the probability of recombination of these centromeric repeats is favored by the sequence homology shared in the regions corresponding to the t(1;16) exchange points. The derivative der(5)t(1;5)(q10;q15) has been found in conjunction with other 1q aberrations, and thus may constitute a further sign of the progressive chromosome instability in the evolution of the myeloma karyotype.[30] Since this unbalanced translocation results in the loss of most of 5q, it may represent a new variant type of myelodysplasia-associated translocation.

An additional recurring translocation involving chromosome 1 breakpoints at 1q21 has also been identified in myeloma by routine banding.[30] The recent cloning of a novel gene (*bcl-9*) involving t(1;14)(q21;q32) indicates this may be an important breakpoint in some B-cell neoplasia.[44] The function of the *bcl-9* gene is not yet known, but some translocations of 1q21 result in overexpression of *bcl-9*. Several patients have been identified with 1q21 breakpoints, including the variant translocations t(1;14)(q21;q32), t(1;22)(q21;q11), and t(1;16)(q21;q11,22); suggesting that these recurring breakpoints may also play a role in the progression of myeloma. Shortened telomeres have been implicated in the jumping translocations involving the 1q21 breakpoint.[45]

A hypothetical model of the clonal evolution of tumor cell populations suggests that during the cytogenetic progression of cancer, acquired genetic lability permits the stepwise selection of variant subclones.[46] During this evolution tumor cell populations emerge that may or may not be viable. Nearly all variants are apparently eliminated, but occasionally one has a selective advantage and becomes the predominant subpopulation. It is likely that the complex karyotypes found in myeloma are induced by a variety of mechanisms. Hypomethylation appears to be one possible mechanism associated with chromosome instability in myeloma. It could be that hypomethylation may also have an as yet unknown effect on other centromeric regions. It is possible that global hypomethylation may affect the segregation of other chromosomes in a more subtle fashion than dramatic decondensation of chromosome 1, and thus play a role in aneuploidy involving other chromosomes.

MOLECULAR CYTOGENETICS OF PLASMA CELL DISORDERS

FISH is a powerful adjunct to traditional G-banding because it allows the identification of abnormal clones in interphase nuclei and cryptic translocations in metaphase cells. FISH allows detection of chromosome aberrations in specimens with no mitotic index.

The use of chromosome-specific centromeric probes identifies numerical aberrations in interphase cells (Figure 5.4A–C). FISH procedures are now in routine use, and allow the identification of multiple trisomies in a single interphase nucleus (Figure 5.4B). Locus-specific probes are available that can identify cryptic translocations or deletions in interphase or metaphase cells (Figure 5.4D).

Methods for chromosome painting such as Multicolor FISH (M-FISH) and multicolor spectral karyotyping (SKY), have greatly enhanced the ability to resolve the complex translocations so commonly associated with plasma cell dyscrasias. SKY provides the power to simultaneously analyze multiple genetic rearrangements with a combination of up to 24 different chromosome painting probes in a single hybridization procedure (Figure 5.5).

Interphase FISH for chromosome aneuploidy in MGUS

The advantage of FISH analysis is the ability to assess chromosomal abnormalities independent of proliferative capacity of the tumor cells. This is especially important in myeloma, where a number of patients have few or no analyzable metaphase spreads. With this approach, a number of important findings have resulted.

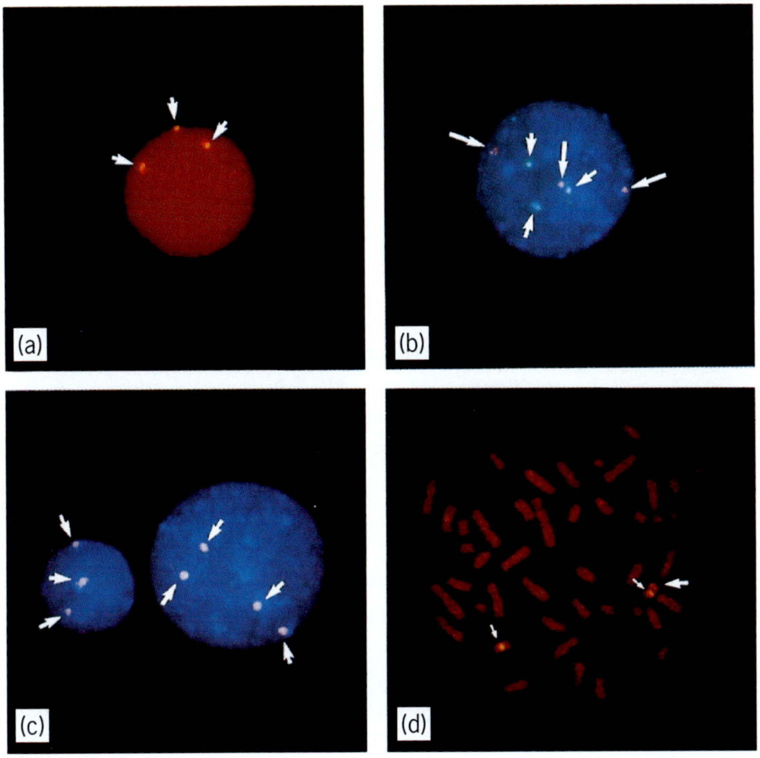

Figure 5.4 Fluorescence in situ hybridization (FISH) to interphase and metaphase cells. (a) Interphase FISH of a centromeric probe of chromosome 11, showing detection of trisomy 11 (arrows) in interphase. (b) Two-color FISH showing detection of two trisomies simultaneously in an interphase cell. Green signals indicate trisomy of chromosome 11 (small arrows), while red signals indicate trisomy for chromosome 15 (large arrows). (c) FISH detection of extra copies of chromosome 1q in interphase cells. (d) Metaphase FISH showing cryptic translocation of an *IgH* probe at 14q32 (large arrow) to chromosome 16 (chromosome 16 centromeres are indicated by small arrows).

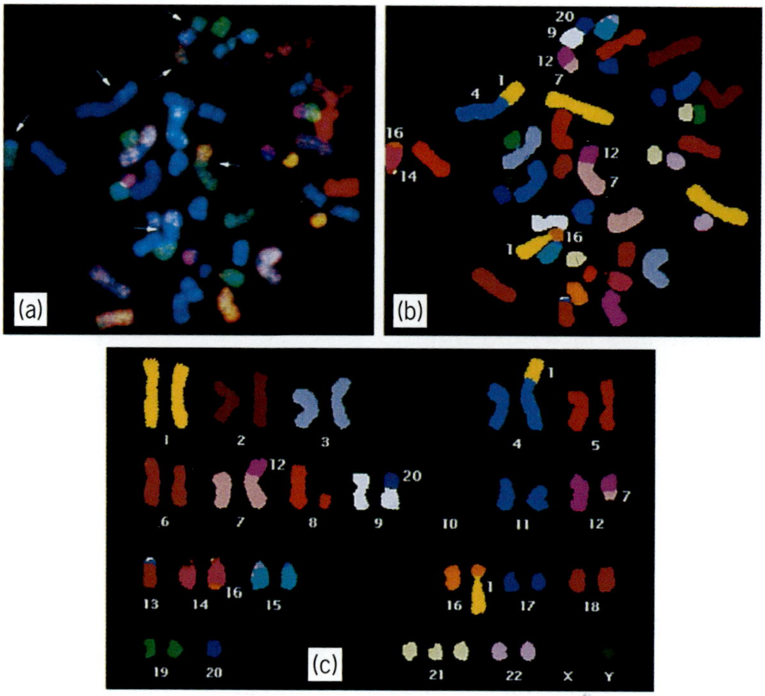

Figure 5.5 Spectral karyotype of myeloma bone marrow chromosomes. (a) Demonstration of simultaneous hybridization of 24 combinatorially labeled chromosome painting probes shown in display colors. Aberrant chromosomes are indicated by arrows. (b) Spectra-based classification of the display colors shown of the same metaphase chromosomes. Numbers beside chromosomes denote origin of translocated material. (c) Karyotype of classification-colored chromosomes. From: Sawyer JR, Lukacs JL, Mumski N et al. Identification of new nonrandom translocations in multiple myeloma with multicolor spectral karyotyping. *Blood* 1998; **92**: 4269–78. Copyright Americal Society of Hermatology, used by permission.

Aneuploidy in MGUS and myeloma has for many years been detected by abnormal DNA content on flow cytometry.[28,47–48] It is not surprising that, as in myeloma, chromosome aneuploidy is found by FISH in MGUS. Drach et al[28] have reported aneuploidy in over 50% of the patients with MGUS studied with centromeric probes. Gains of chromosome 3 (39%), 11 (25%) and 7 (17%) were the commonest abnormalities; similar to myeloma. They found that the chromosomal abnormalities were confined to a subpopulation of bone marrow plasma cells in patients with MGUS, suggesting that these aberrations may be secondary changes occurring as a consequence of some other primary transforming event. Zandecki et al[49] have also identified cytogenetic subclones in patients with MGUS by interphase FISH. They also suggest the chromosome changes in the various clones are acquired slowly and distributed within several related subclones.

Interphase FISH for chromosome aneuploidy in myeloma

FISH analysis has greatly increased the level of chromosomal aneuploidy detected in myeloma. Using 10 alpha-satellite DNA probes, Drach et al[50] were able to demonstrate the presence of cytogenetic abnormalities in approximately 80–90% of patients, regardless of disease status. This is significantly more frequent than the level of aneuploidy reported by conventional banding techniques. Tabernero et al,[51] using FISH with 15 different probes on a series of 52 patients, found trisomy in 84% and monosomy in 16% of the cases. Chromosomes 9 and 15 were most frequently hyperdiploid, while hypodiploidy for chromosome 13 was identified in 26% of patients. More recently, Perez-Simon et al[52] analyzed 63 patients with a combination of 15 different probes, and found numerical chromosome aberrations in 81% of patients when seven or more chromosome probes were used for the analysis.

One limitation of interphase FISH with alpha-satellite probes, pointed out by Drach et al,[50] is that rearrangements occurring in the pericentromeric regions of chromosomes can give rise to extra hybridization signals because the alpha-satellite probes could be split in cases where a whole-arm translocation has taken place. Therefore a gain in copy numbers observed by FISH may not necessarily be associated with numerical aberrations in all cases.

Locus-specific FISH analysis

In addition to the ability to identify numerical chromosome aberrations, both interphase and metaphase FISH can identify structural aberrations such as translocations and deletions. M-FISH can be used as a tool to analyze chromosome translocations in interphase and metaphase cells by labeling specific gene loci or chromosome breakpoints with different colors. Yeast artificial chromosome (YAC) clones are excellent FISH probes, because they provide superior hybridization and signals after Alu-polymerase chain reaction (PCR) amplification of human specific sequences.[53]

Nahishida et al[54] identified translocations of 14q32 with dual-color FISH in 34 (74%) of 46 patients with myeloma and other plasma cell disorders (including 3 with MGUS): t(11;14) was the commonest, followed by t(8;14) and t(14;18). More recently, Avet-Loiseau et al[55] found illegitimate *IgH* recombination in 57% of 141 patients examined by FISH. The most common translocation was t(11;14), occurring in 16%, followed by t(4;14) occurring in 12%. These results reinforce previous findings of the frequency of the t(11;14) translocation in plasma cell malignancies. However, since these chromosomal changes are not found in most patients and the number of translocation partners is large, these *IgH* translocations probably cannot be regarded as the primary event in the genetic evolution of plasma cell malignancies.

Rb deletions by FISH

The *Rb* gene maps to 13q14 and is the prototype for the tumor suppressor gene model. Monosomy for chromosome 13 or deletions of *Rb* (or genes in close proximity) may be very frequent in myeloma, and may be associated with poor prognosis.[56] The *Rb* gene product (Rb) has been shown to suppress tumorigenesis in neoplastic cell lines, inhibit apoptosis, and facilitate differentiation. In myeloma, Rb is believed to downregulate IL-6 gene expression, an important growth factor in myeloma. The absence of Rb may induce an autocrine IL-6 expression in myeloma cells and contribute to autonomous growth in myeloma.[57] Although monoallelic deletions are very common, biallelic deletions of *Rb* are infrequent. Monoallelic deletions of *Rb* apparently do not modulate Rb expression. Therefore, complex interactions of Rb with other growth factors and transcription factors such as E2F are not fully understood.

The biological significance of −13/13q− aberrations is also not understood. Although *Rb* is deleted in at least 50% of patients by interphase FISH analysis,[58] there is apparently no correlation between *Rb* gene deletion and Rb protein levels. Although 30% of patients with B-cell chronic lymphocytic leukemias (B-CLL) have hemizygous deletions of *Rb*, most of them have a functional *Rb* allele.

The D13S25 locus located just telomeric to the *Rb* gene is more frequently deleted than *Rb*, and often the deletions are homozygous.[59] *BRCA2* may also be a candidate gene whose somatic inactivation could play a role in initiation and progression of B-CLL as well as myeloma. The association of monosomy or deletions of chromosome 13 and poor prognosis has also recently been reported by Dallinger et al,[60] who found loss of *Rb* by FISH in 49% of patients. Shaughnessy et al,[61] using a panel of 11 probes spaced along the long arm of chromosome 13, have found deletions of chromosome 13 by interphase FISH in most patients with myeloma, suggesting a putative tumor suppressor gene on this chromosome.

p53 deletions by FISH

The *p53* tumor suppressor gene maps to 17p13, and is believed to be involved in the control of normal cellular proliferation, differentiation, and apoptosis.[62] In addition, *p53* apparently functions in DNA replication and repair mechanisms, and therefore has been called the 'guardian of the genome'.[63] *p53* is the most commonly mutated gene in human malignancies. In response to DNA damage, *p53* induces growth arrest at the G_1 phase of the cell cycle. In case of sublethal damage, *p53*-induced G_1 arrest enables the cell to undergo DNA repair. However, if the damage is extensive, the cell undergoes apoptosis.

p53 mutations have been thought to be rare at the time of diagnosis in myeloma, and are considered a late event in the progression.[64–69] However, Drach et al[70] have reported the presence of monoallelic chromosomal deletions of *p53* in one-third of newly diagnosed myeloma patients. These findings indicate that deletions of 17p involving the *p53* gene locus are much more common than previously found by routine metaphase cytogenetics. Most of the chromosomal deletions of *p53* are apparently submicroscopic interstitial deletions and are only detectable by FISH. *p53* deletions were associated with shorter survival after conventional chemotherapy.[70]

SPECTRAL KARYOTYPING

Newer molecular cytogenetic techniques such as M-FISH and multicolor SKY (Figure 5.5) make the analysis of complex chromosomal rearrangements possible.[71–73] These techniques, in conjunction with FISH probes for single genes, hold the promise of helping bridge the gap between traditional banding techniques and molecular genetic analysis.

SKY is a chromosome painting technique that allows the simultaneous display of each chromosome in a different colour. This technique makes possible the identification of chromosomal bands of unknown origin, including translocations, insertions, complex rearrangements, and small marker chromosomes. The SKY technique holds great promise, but is limited, in some respects, by the inability to detect chromosomal inversions, very small deletions, insertions, or translocations.

SKY enables the identification of hidden chromosome abnormalities in hematologic malignancies.[73] Several new recurring translocations have been found in myeloma with SKY, and several translocations that had previously been incorrectly identified have been refined. Rao et al.[74] were the first to report SKY in myeloma; detecting two cases with a novel t(14;20) and three regions involving recurring translocations, including 3q27~29,17q24~25, and 20q11.2~12.

The t(14;16)(q32.3;q22~23) translocation recently identified as a recurring aberration in myeloma cell lines by molecular techniques has now also been found by SKY in bone marrow samples.[75] This translocation has been shown to be associated with c-*maf* overexpression.[26] The 16q23 breakpoints in these cell lines appear to be dispersed over approximately 100 kb and appear to be separated from c-*maf* by less than 500 kb. The dispersion of breakpoints and distance from the oncogene appear to be compatible with dysregulation of c-*maf* by the strong 3′ *IgH* enhancer.[26] At the chromosome banding level, variants of this translocation appear to involve a range of breakpoints on chromosome 16 from q22~q23. In some patients, the breakpoint appears at 16q22, which makes the add(14)(q32) appear larger; in other patients, the breakpoint appears more distal at q23, so that the add(14)(q32) segment looks smaller. SKY probe cocktails can identify the add(14)(q32) material as chromosome 16 in all cases, suggesting a reciprocal translocation, but are unable to identify any exchange of chromosome 14 material to the chromosome 16. In these cases, a FISH probe for the IgH locus (14q32.3) can be used in conjunction with an alpha-satellite probe to chromosome 16 or other chromosome 16 markers to determine if 14q32 has translocated to 16. Indeed, the 14q32 probe signals can be shown to be translocated to chromosome 16 by FISH, thus confirming the reciprocal translocation in all patients (Figure 5.4D). The reports of add(14)(q32) chromosomes in the same G-band karyotypes with deletions of 16q22~24, indicates that the t(14;16)(q32.3;q22~23) translocation is below the resolution of conventional techniques in most cases.[15,18] It is conceivable that analysis of more cases with add(14)(q32) and/or del(16)(q22) may reveal hitherto unrecognized recurring translocations.

An additional reciprocal translocation to emerge from SKY analysis of the add(14)(q32) chromosomes is the t(9;14)(p13;q32) translocation.[75] The SKY technique can identify the add(14)(q32) as a t(9;14)(p13;q32). However, the 14q32 segment that is translocated to 9p13 is too small to be resolved by SKY. Again in this case, the 14q32 translocations can be identified at 9p13 by FISH probes for the 14q32.3 locus. The t(9;14)(p13;q32) translocation has been associated with lymphoplasmacytoid lymphoma and Waldenström's macroglobulinemia.[76] The translocation in this case juxtaposes the *PAX-5* gene at 9p13 with the *Ig* regulatory elements at 14q32, apparently deregulating *PAX-5* and causing overexpression of *PAX-5* mRNA.[77]

One of the great advantages of the SKY technique in bone marrow chromosome analysis is the ability to overcome the poor chromosome morphology associated with short and poorly banded chromosomes found in some studies. In this regard, the identification of new 8q24 translocations and redesignation of different 8q24 translocations by SKY suggests that this technique may be able to refine the number and types of translocations found at this breakpoint. Some of the t(8;14)(q24;q32) translocations reported in myeloma studies have in fact been incorrectly identified, while other 8q24 translocations may have been missed.[75]

The increased c-Myc protein levels found in most myeloma patients have to date not been supported by a high number of c-*myc* translocations.[78] c-Myc is a transcription factor associated with cell cycle progression, and in interaction with Rb and other factors regulates transformation, proliferation, and apoptosis.[79] At the molecular level, c-Myc is involved in the transcriptional activation of cell cycle progression by involvement with genes such as those encoding for cyclin D1 and ornithine deoxycarboxylase. In the classic paradigm, one c-*myc* allele is dysregulated by translocation to an *Ig* locus. The translocated allele is expressed at a high level, whereas the expression of the non-translocated allele is not detected. It has been hypothesized that c-*myc* is *cis*-dysregulated by a structural chromosome aberration of the c-*myc* locus at 8q24 in myeloma.[80] Therefore, the finding of new recurring 8q24 translocations or redesignations of hitherto cryptic translocations may eventually alter this seeming paradox of high c-Myc expression and the apparent rare occurrence of c-*myc* translocations. A new recurring translocation t(1;8)(p11~13;q24) has been identified by G-banding and SKY,[75] which suggests an alternative translocation for the dysregulation of c-*myc* in myeloma, as does the possibility that the complex evolution of the t(8;22)(q24;q11) translocation may also be detected more frequently by the SKY technique.[81]

Although spectral karyotyping identifies additional rearrangements in most cases, the technique does have limitations. The main drawback appears to be the limits of resolution of the painting probe cocktails, which are reported to be between 500 and 1500 kb.[72] Therefore, the technique is unable to completely resolve the very subtle translocations of less than 500 kb. It appears clear that multiple techniques in addition to G-banding, including both FISH and SKY, are necessary to resolve the complex karyotypes seen in myeloma.

COMPARATIVE GENOMIC HYBRIDIZATION

Comparative genomic hybridization (CGH) is a technique used to analyze chromosome copy-number changes. CGH uses small amounts of tumor DNA hybridized to normal chromosome preparations, rather than relying on metaphase tumor cells as in traditional studies. CGH appears to be more sensitive in detecting chromosome copy-number changes than conventional G-banding.

Using CGH, Avet-Loiseau et al[82] found that the loss of 13q and 14q and gain of 1q and chromosome 7 occurred in 50–60% of primary tumors and cell lines. In order of prevalence, they found that increases in 1q12qter and loss of 13q were the most common. In a group of 30 patients with MGUS, myeloma, or Waldenström's macroglobulinemia, Cigudosa et al[83] found 70% of patients to show clonal changes. The most common recurrent changes they reported were gain of chromosome 19 or 19p, and monosomy or deletion of chromosome 13.

PROGNOSTIC ROLE OF CYTOGENETICS IN MYELOMA

The standard prognostic indicators amongst myeloma patients receiving conventional chemotherapy include β_2-microglobulin, C-reactive protein, and plasma cell labeling index.[84–87]

The use of cytogenetic studies of myeloma in identifying patients who have a poor prognosis has been established since the early chromosome banding studies,[5,8,12,13] and suggests that patients with abnormal karyotypes have a poorer prognosis than those with normal karyotypes.[27] However, not until recently has poor prognosis been attributed to specific chromosome aberrations. A number of studies have now shown a correlation between monosomy or deletion of chromosome 13 and poor prognosis in myeloma.[27,56,88,89] This manifests as poorer response rates, and lower event-free and overall survival. See Chapter 19 for a discussion of the adverse impact of chromosome 13 abnormalities in patients undergoing high-dose chemotherapy.

The detection by FISH of *p53* deletions in myeloma patients has also been shown to be a predictor of short survival after conventional chemotherapy due to poor response to chemotherapy.[64] The presence of so many complex translocations in myeloma is an expression of profound genomic instability, and may be related to alterations in p53 function. Cells with defective p53 function are more prone to additional mutations – leading to further tumor progression. Mouse embryonic fibroblasts that lack p53 protein show multiple copies of centrosomes, resulting in unequal segregation of chromosomes[19] and the amplification of 20q DNA, which has been found in a number of malignancies.[21] The generation of multiple centrosomes by loss of *p53* or amplifications of 20q may be a source of the genomic instability commonly associated with myeloma.

PRACTICAL APPLICATION OF CYTOGENETIC STUDIES IN PLASMA CELL DYSCRASIAS

Frequency of testing

Because of the difficulty in detecting chromosomal abnormalities in myeloma, G-banding may have to be performed repeatedly after the initial diagnostic study to obtain analyzable metaphases. This is not necessary in patients in whom an abnormal karyotype has already been identified, and will be less important when interphase FISH is more widely available.

Diagnosis

Karyotyping rarely helps with diagnosis in plasma cell disorders. We have seen exceptional patients with high-grade disease who had very atypical cell morphology and high lactate dehydrogenase (LDH) levels in whom the distinction between lymphoma and myeloma was based upon the detection of complex, multiple cytogenetic abnormalities, including chromosome 13 abnormalities.

Fine-needle aspirate studies

In patients whose marrow cytogenetic studies are uninformative, computed tomography-guided fine-needle aspiration of material from bony lesions identified on magnetic resonance imaging (see Chapter 17) may yield abnormal karyotypes. This may allow the biologic nature of the disease (more or less aggressive) to be identified better.

Prognosis

As mentioned earlier, the presence of any or certain (−13 or 13q−) cytogenetic abnormalities has been associated with poorer prognosis. The prognostic value of cytogenetic abnormalities has been derived from cohorts of relatively uniformly treated patients. An important corollary of determining prognosis is to select more appropriate (individualized) therapy for patients with more aggressive disease.

Selection of therapy

Patients with high-risk disease, identified on the basis of −13/13q−, have poorer overall and event-free survival. It is possible that these patients may benefit from further intensification of therapy, such as early use of allogeneic hematopoietic stem cell transplantation or post-autograft periodic consolidation chemotherapy.

Monitoring for myelodysplasia

The development of myelodysplastic syndrome (MDS) or secondary acute myeloid leukemia is an important potential complication of the therapy of myeloma. The incidence of morphologically detectable MDS ranges from 2–5%. However, the true incidence could be considerably higher – of the order of 10–15% – as has been detected in patients who have undergone cytogenetic studies regularly and frequently.[90] This was in a population of patients who had undergone tandem autotransplantation in Arkansas. The exceedingly high rate of myelodysplasia may be the consequence of two transplants. We advocate regular monitoring for MDS in myeloma patients who have undergone tandem autotransplantation.

REFERENCES

1. Klein B, Xue-Guang Z, Lu ZL, Bataille R. Interleukin-6 in human multiple myeloma. *Blood* 1995; **85**: 863–72.
2. Barlogie B, Epstein J, Selvanayagam P, Alexanian R. Plasma cell myeloma – new biological insights and advances in therapy. *Blood* 1989; **73**: 865–79.
3. Hallek M, Bergsagel PL, Anderson KC. Multiple myeloma: increasing evidence for a multistep transformation process. *Blood* 1998; **91**: 3–21.
4. Heim S, Mitelman F. Chronic lymphoproliferative disorders. In: *Cancer Cytogenetics*, 2nd edn. New York: Wiley-Liss, 1995; 237–65.
5. Philip P, Drivsholm A, Hansen NE et al. Chromosomes and survival in multiple myeloma: a banding study of 25 cases. *Cancer Genet Cytogenet* 1980; **2**: 243–57.
6. Van den Berghe H, Vermaelen K, Louwagie A et al. High incidence of chromosome abnormalities in IgG3 myeloma. *Cancer Genet Cytogenet* 1984; **11**: 381–7.
7. Ferti A, Panani A, Arapakis G, Raptis S. Cytogenetic studies in multiple myeloma. *Cancer Genet Cytogenet* 1984; **12**: 247–53.
8. DeWald GW, Kyle RA, Hicks GA, Greipp PR. The clinical significance of cytogenetic studies in 100 patients with multiple myeloma, plasma cell leukemia or amyloidosis. *Blood* 1985; **66**: 380–90.
9. Chen KC, Bevan PC, Mathews JG. Analysis of G banded karyotypes in myeloma cells. *J Clin Pathol* 1986; **39**: 260–6.
10. Gould J, Alexanian R, Goodacre A et al. Plasma cell karyotype in multiple myeloma. *Blood* 1988; **71**: 453–6.
11. Lisse MI, Drivsholm A, Christoffersen P. Occurrence and type of chromosomal abnormalities in consecutive malignant monoclonal gammopathies: correlation with survival. *Cancer Genet Cytogenet* 1988; **35**: 27–36.
12. Clark RE, Geddes AD, Whittaker JA, Jacobs A. Differences in bone marrow cytogenetic characteristics between treated and untreated myeloma. *Eur J Cancer Clin Oncol* 1989; **25**: 1789–93.

13. Jonveauz P, Berger R. Chromosome studies in plasma cell leukemia and multiple myeloma in transformation. *Genes Chromosomes Cancer* 1992; **4**: 321–5.
14. Weh HJ, Gutensohn K, Selbacj J et al. Karyotype in multiple myeloma and plasma cell leukemia. *Eur J Cancer* 1993; **29A**: 1269–73.
15. Sawyer JR, Waldron JA, Jagannath S, Barlogie B. Cytogenetic findings in 200 patients with multiple myeloma. *Cancer Genet Cytogenet* 1995; **82**: 41–9.
16. Lai JL, Zandecki M, Mary JY et al. Improved cytogenetics in multiple myeloma: a study of 151 patients including 117 patients at diagnosis. *Blood* 1995; **85**: 2490–7.
17. Smadja NV, Louvet C, Isnard F et al. Cytogenetic study in multiple myeloma at diagnosis: comparison of two techniques. *Br J Haematol* 1995; **90**: 619–24.
18. Calasanz MJ, Cigudosa JC, Odero MD et al. Cytogenetic analysis of 280 patients with multiple myeloma and related disorders: primary breakpoints and clinical correlations. *Genes Chromosomes Cancer* 1997; **18**: 84–93.
19. Fukasawa K, Choi T, Kuriyama R et al. Abnormal centrosome amplification in the absence of p53. *Science* 1996; **271**: 1744–7.
20. Pihan GA, Purohit A, Wallace J et al. Centrosome defects and genetic instability in malignant tumors. *Cancer Res* 1998; **58**: 3974–85.
21. Zhou H, kuang J, Zhong L et al. Tumor amplified kinase STK15/BTAK induces centrosome amplification, aneuploidy and transformation. *Nature Genet* 1998; **20**: 189–93.
22. Chesi M, Bergsagel P, Brents L et al. Dysregulation of cyclin D1 by translocation into an IgH gamma switch region in two multiple myeloma cell lines. *Blood* 1996; **88**: 674–81.
23. Bergsagel PL, Chesi M, Nardini E et al. Promiscuous translocations into immunoglobulin heavy chain switch regions in multiple myeloma. *Proc Natl Acad Sci USA* 1996; **93**: 13931–6.
24. Chesi M, Nardini E, Breants LA et al. Frequent translocation of t(4;14)(p16.3;q32) in multiple myeloma is associated with increased expression and activating mutations of fibroblast growth factor receptor 3. *Nature Genet* 1997; **16**: 260–4.
25. Iida S, Rao PH, Butler M et al. Deregulation of MUM1/IRF4 by chromosomal translocation in multiple myeloma. *Nature Genet* 1997; **17**: 226–30.
26. Chesi M, Bergsagel PL, Shonukan OO et al. Frequent dysregulation of the c-maf protooncogene at 16q23 by translocation to an Ig locus in multiple myeloma. *Blood* 1998; **91**: 4457–63.
27. Seong C, Delasallie K, Hayes K et al. Prognostic value of cytogenetics in multiple myeloma. *Br J Haematol* 1998; **101**: 189–95.
28. Drach J, Angerler J, Schuster J et al. Interphase fluorescence in situ hybridization identifies chromosomal abnormalities in plasma cells from patients with monoclonal gammopathy of undetermined signficance. *Blood* 1995; **86**: 3915–21.
29. Dohner H, Stilgenbauer S, James M et al. 11q deletions identify a new subset of B-cell chronic lymphocytic leukemia characterized by extensive nodal involvement and inferior prognosis. *Blood* 1997; **89**: 2516–22.
30. Sawyer JR, Tricot G, Mattox S et al. Jumping translocations of chromosome 1q in multiple myeloma: evidence for a mechanism involving decondensation of heterochromatin. *Blood* 1998; **91**: 1732–41.
31. Neri A, Murphy JP, Cro L et al. Ras oncogene mutation in multiple myeloma. *J Exp Med* 1989; **170**: 1715–25.
32. Atkin NB. Chromosome 1 aberrations in cancer. *Cancer Genet Cytogenet* 1986; **21**: 279–85.
33. Olah E, Balogh E, Kovacs I, Kiss A. Abnormalities of chromosome 1 in relation to human malignant disease. *Cancer Genet Cytogenet* 1989; **43**: 179–94.
34. Gagos S, Hopwood VL, Iliopoulos D et al. Chromosomal markers associated with metastasis in two colon cancer cell lines established from the same patient. Anticancer Res 1995; **15**: 369–78.
35. Gronwald J, Storkel S, Holtgreve-Grez H et al. Comparison of DNA gains and losses in primary renal clear cell carcinomas and metastatic sites: importance of 1q and 3p copy number changes in metastatic events. *Cancer Res* 1997; **57**: 481–7.
36. Mitelman F, Kaneko Y, Trent J. Report of the committee on chromosome changes in neoplasia. *Cytogenet Cell Genet* 1990; **55**: 358–86.
37. Wong, KF, Hayes KJ, Glassman AB, der(1;15)(q10;q10). A nonrandom chromosomal abnormality of myloid neoplasia. *Cancer Genet Cytogenet* 1995; **83**: 144–6.
38. Mugneret F, Sidaner I, Favre B et al. Der(16)t(1;16)(q10;p10) in multiple myeloma: a new nonrandom abnormality that is frequently associated with Burkitt's type translocations. *Leukemia* 1995; **9**: 277–81.

39. Pandis N, Heim S, Bardi G et al. Whole-arm t(1;16) and i(1q) as sole anomalies identify gain of 1q as a primary chromosomal abnormality in breast cancer. *Genes Chromosomes Cancer* 1992; **5**: 235–8.
40. Pandis N, Teixeira MR, Gerdes AM et al. Chromosome abnormalities in bilateral breast carcinomas. *Cancer* 1995; **76**: 250–8.
41. Mugneret F, Lizard S, Aurias A, Turc-Carel C. Chromosomes in Ewing's sarcoma: nonrandom additional changes, trisomy 8 and der(16)t(1;16). *Cancer Genet Cytogenet* 1988; **32**: 239.
42. Kondo G,Chilcote RR, Mauer HS, Rowley JD. Chromosome abnormalities in tumor cells from patients with sporadic Wilms' tumor. *Cancer Res* 1984; **44**: 5376–81.
43. Kokalj-Vokac N, Almeida A, Gerbault-Seureau M et al. Two color FISH characterization of i(1q) and der(1;16) in human breast cancer cells. *Genes Chromosomes Cancer* 1993; **7**: 8.
44. Willis TG, Zalcberg IR, Coignet LJA et al. Molecular cloning of translocation t(1;14)(q21;q32) defines a novel gene (BCL9) at chromosome 1q21. *Blood* 1998; **91**: 1873–81.
45. Hatakeyama S, Jujita K, Mori H et al. Shortened telomeres involved in a case with a jumping translocation at 1q21. *Blood* 1998; **91**: 1514–19.
46. Nowell PC. The clonal evolution of tumor cell populations. *Science* 1976; **194**: 23–8.
47. Latreille J, Barlogie B, Gohde W et al. Cellular DNA content as a marker of human multiple myeloma. *Blood* 1980; **55**: 403–8.
48. Tsuchiya H, Epstein J, Selvanayagam P et al. Correlated flow cytometric analysis of H-rap p21 and nuclear DNA in multiple myeloma. *Blood* 1988; **72**: 796–800.
49. Zandecki M, Lai JL, Genevieve F et al. Several cytogenetic subclones may be identified within plasma cells from patients with monoclonal gammopathy of undetermined significance, both at diagnosis and during the indolent course of this condition. *Blood* 1997; **90**: 3682–90.
50. Drach J, Schuster J, Nowotny H et al. Multiple myeloma: high incidence of chromosomal aneuploidy as detected by interphase fluorescence in situ hybridization. *Cancer Res* 1995; **55**: 3854–9.
51. Tabernero D, San Miguel JF, Garcia-Sanz M et al. Incidence of chromosome numerical changes in multiple myeloma: fluorescence in situ hybridization analysis using 15 chromosome-specific probes. *Am J Pathol* 1996; **149**: 153–61.
52. Perez-Simon JA, Garcia-Sanz, Tabernero MD et al. Prognostic value of numerical chromosome aberrations in multiple myeloma : a FISH analysis of 15 different chromosomes. *Blood* 1998; **91**: 3366–71.
53. Taniwaki M, Matsuda F, Jauch A et al. Detection of 14q32 translocations in B-cell malignancies by in situ hybridization with yeast artificial chromosome clones containing the human IgH locus. *Blood* 1994; **83**: 2962–9.
54. Nishida K, Tamura A, Nakazawa N et al. The Ig heavy chain gene is frequently involved in chromosomal translocations in multiple myeloma and plasma cell leukemia as detected by in situ hybridization. *Blood* 1997; **90**: 526–34.
55. Avet-Loiseau H, Brigaudeau C, Morineau N et al. High incidence of cryptic translocations involving the Ig heavy chain gene in multiple myeloma, as shown by fluorescence in situ hybridization. *Genes Chromosomes Cancer* 1999; **24**: 9–15.
56. Tricot G, Barlogie B, Jagannath S et al. Poor prognosis in multiple myeloma is associated only with partial or complete deletions of chromosome 13 or abnormalities involving 11q and not with other karyotype abnormalities. *Blood* 1995; **86**: 4250–6.
57. Juge-Morineau N, Harousseau JL, Amiot M, Bataille R. The retinoblastoma susceptibility gene RB-1 in multiple myeloma. *Leuk Lymphoma* 1997; **24**: 229–37.
58. Dao D, Sawyer J, Epstein J et al. Deletion of retinoblastoma in multiple myeloma. *Leukemia* 1994; **8**: 1280–4.
59. Lui Y, Grander D, Soderhall S et al. Retinoblastoma gene deletions in B-cell chronic lymphocytic leukemia. *Genes Chromosomes Cancer* 1992; **4**: 250–6.
60. Dallinger S, Kaufmann H, Zojer J et al. Interphase fluorescence in situ hybridization confirms the poor prognosis of patients with multiple myeloma and deletion of 13q. *Blood* 1998; **92**: 259A.
61. Shaughnessy J Jr, Erming T, Sawyer J et al. High incidence of chromosome 13 deletion in multiple myeloma detected by multicolor FISH. *Blood* 2000; **96**: 1505–11.
62. Vogelstein B, Kinzler KW. p53 function and dysfunction. *Cell* 1992; **70**: 523–6.
63. Lane DP. p53, guardian of the genome. *Nature* 1992; **358**: 15–16.
64. Porterier M, Moles JP, Mazars GR et al. p53 and RAS gene mutations in multiple myeloma. *Oncogene* 1992; **7**: 2539.

65. Preudhomme C, Facon T, Zandecki M et al. Rare occurrence of P53 gene mutation in multiple myeloma. *Br J Hematol* 1992; **81**: 440–3.
66. Willems PMW, Kuypers A, Meijerink J et al. Sporadic mutation of p53 gene in multiple myeloma and no evidence for germline mutations in three myeloma pedigrees. *Leukemia* 1993; **7**: 986.
67. Neri A, Baldini L, Trecca D et al. p53 gene mutations in multiple myeloma are associated with advanced forms of malignancy. *Blood* 1993; **81**: 128–35.
68. Corradini P, Inghirami G, Astolfi M et al. Inactivation of tumor suppressor genes, p53, and Rb1, in plasma cell dyscrasias. *Leukemia* 1994; **8**: 758.
69. Owen RG, Davis SAA, Randerson J et al. p53 gene mutations in multiple myeloma. *J Clin Pathol: Mol Pathol* 1997; **50**: 18.
70. Drach J, Ackermann J, Fritz E et al. Presence of p53 gene deletion in patients with multiple myeloma predicts for short survival after conventional-dose chemotherapy. *Blood* 1998; **92**: 802–9.
71. Speicher MR, Ballard SG, Ward DC. Karyotyping human chromosomes by combinatorial multifluor FISH. *Nature Genet* 1996; **14**: 368–75.
72. Schrock E, duManoir S, Veldman T et al. Multicolor spectral karyotyping of human chromosomes. *Science* 1996; **273**: 494–7.
73. Veldman T, Vignon C, Schrock E et al. Hidden chromosome abnormalities in hematological malignancies detected by multicolour spectral karyotyping. *Nature Genet* 1997; **15**: 406–10.
74. Rao PH, Cigudosa JC, Ning Y et al. Multicolor spectral karyotyping identifies new recurring breakpoints and translocations in multiple myeloma. *Blood* 1998; **92**: 1743–8.
75. Sawyer JR, Lukacs JL, Munshi N et al. Identification of new nonrandom translocations in multiple myeloma with multicolor spectral karyoytping. *Blood* 1998; **92**: 4269–78.
76. Offit K, Parsa NZ, Filippa D et al. t(9;14)(p13;q32) denotes a subset of low-grade non-Hodgkin's lymphoma with plasmacytoid differentiation. *Blood* 1992; **80**: 2594–9.
77. Iida S, Rao PH, Nallasivam P et al. The t(9;14)(p13;q32) chromosomal translocation associated with lymphoplasmacytoid lymphoma involves the PAX-5 gene. *Blood* 1996; **88**: 4110–17.
78. Bergsagel PL, Nardini E, Breants L et al. IgH translocations in multiple myeloma: a nearly universal event that rarely involves c-myc. *Curr Top Microbiol Immunol* 1997; **224**: 283–7.
79. Ryan KM, Birnie GD. Myc oncogenes: the enigmatic family. *Biochem J* 1996; **314**: 713–21.
80. Shou Y, Gabrea A, Martelli ML et al. Dysregulation on one C-myc allele in multiple myeloma. *Blood* 1998; **92**: 259A.
81. Sawyer JR, Lukacs JL, Thomas EL et al. Multicolour spectral karyotyping identifies new translocations and a recurring pathway for chromosome loss in multiple myeloma. *Br J Haematol* 2001; **112**: 167–74.
82. Avet-Loiseau H, Andree-Ashley LE, Moore D et al. Molecular cytogenetic abnormalities in multiple myeloma and plasma cell leukemia measured using comparative genomic hybridization. *Genes Chromosomes Cancer* 1997; **19**: 124–33.
83. Cigudosa JC, Rao PH, Calasanz MJ et al. Characterization of nonrandom chromosomal gains and losses in multiple myeloma by comparative genomic hybridization. *Blood* 1998; **91**: 3007–10.
84. Bataille R, Boccadoro M, Klein B et al. C-reactive protein and β2 microglobulin produce a simple and powerful myeloma staging system. *Blood* 1992; **80**: 733–7.
85. Greipp PR, Lust JA, O'Fallon WM et al. Plasma cell labeling index and β_2–microglobulin predict survival independent of thymidine kinase and C-reactive protein in multiple myeloma. *Blood* 1993; **81**: 3382–7.
86. San Miguel JF, Garcia-Sanz R, Gonzalez M et al. A new staging system for multiple myeloma based on the number of S-phase plasma cells. *Blood* 1995; **85**: 448–55.
87. Ffrench M, Ffrench P, Remy F et al. Plasma cell proliferation in monoclonal gammopathy: relations with other biologic variables – diagnostic and prognostic significance. *Am J Med* 1995; **98**: 61–6.
88. Tricot G, Sawyer JR, Jagannath S et al. Unique role of cytogenetics in the prognosis of patients with myeloma receiving high-dose therapy and autotransplants. *J Clin Oncol* 1997; **15**: 2659–66.
89. Barlogie B, Sawyer J, Ayers D et al. Chromosome 13 myeloma is a distinct entity with poor prognosis despite tandem autotransplants. *Blood* 1998; **92**: 259A.
90. Drach J, Ayers D, Govindarajan R et al. MDS-associated cytogenetic abnormalities (CGA) in both hematopoietic and neoplastic cells after autotransplants (AT) in 868 patients with multiple myeloma (MM). *Blood* 1998; **92**(Suppl 1): 97a.

6

Immunoregulatory mechanisms and immunotherapy

Qing Yi

CONTENTS • **Immunoregulatory mechanisms in myeloma** • **Immunotherapy in B-cell malignancies**

IMMUNOREGULATORY MECHANISMS IN MYELOMA

Clonogenic B cells and idiotype

Plasma cell disorders are characterized by a proliferation of clonal B lymphocytes at various stages of maturation and by plasma cell infiltration of the bone marrow. The monoclonal immunoglobulin (Ig) (the 'M component') produced by the clonal B cells has unique variable regions in the heavy and light chains. B cells belonging to the tumor clone can be identified by their cell surface expression of the monoclonal Ig that carries the same idiotype as the M component.[1] Such monoclonal B cells are present in the bone marrow as well as in peripheral blood. The presence of circulating monoclonal B cells in the peripheral blood in myeloma and monoclonal gammopathy of undetermined significance (MGUS) has been confirmed by cytogenetic analysis.[2] Clonal rearrangement of Ig heavy- and light-chain genes has been demonstrated in blood lymphocytes and bone marrow plasma cells by Southern blot analysis.[3] Using highly sensitive polymerase chain reaction (PCR) techniques, circulating clonal B lymphocytes have been detected in almost all patients with myeloma, although the reported frequencies differ significantly.[4–6]

Idiotype structures present on the secreted M component and on the surface Ig of clonal B cells are tumor-specific antigens; as such, they are potential targets for specific anti-idiotype immunity.[7] Myeloma B lymphocytes are mature B cells. They may express, on the cell surface, idiotypic Ig as well as major histocompatibility complex (MHC) class I and II molecules, and are sensitive to regulatory signals provided by cellular and humoral components of the idiotype-specific immune network (Figure 6.1). The majority of the tumor cells in myeloma, however, are the bone marrow plasma cells, which may not express surface Ig. Myeloma plasma cells secrete the M component and express cytoplasmic Ig (cIg). It has been shown that cIg in mouse B-cell lymphoma and plasmacytoma cells is processed intracellularly, and that degraded idiotypic peptides are presented on the cell surface in the context of MHC molecules.[8] Moreover, myeloma plasma cells may express MHC class I antigens,[9,10] adhesion molecules (e.g. CD44, CD56, CD54 and VLA-4),[11,12] and the signaling or co-stimulatory molecules CD40 and

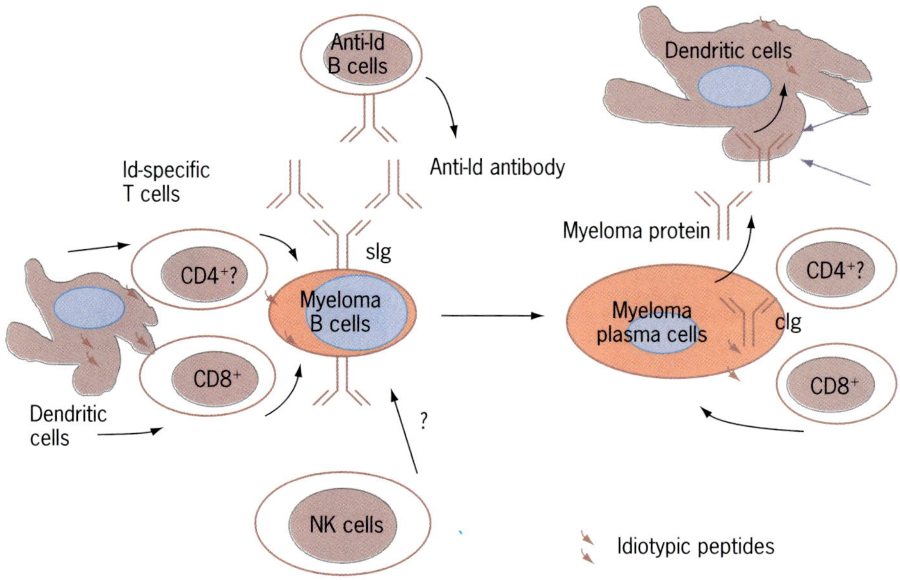

Figure 6.1 Schematic model of an immune network in myeloma, showing idiotype (Id) as myeloma-specific tumor antigen and idiotype-specific cellular and humoral immune responses. The immune responses may be initiated by professional antigen-presenting dendritic cells and, once primed, are able to regulate the growth and differentiation of myeloma cells. sIg, surface Ig; cIg, cytoplasmic Ig; NK, natural killer.

CD28,[10,13,14] as well as the Fas antigen (CD95).[15] Some of the plasma cells also express HLA-DR, CD80, and CD86.[10] A recent study has shown that myeloma plasma cells were able to activate alloreactive T cells and present the recalled antigens, purified protein derivative (PPD) and tetanus toxoid (TT), to autologous T cells.[10] Therefore, it is conceivable that myeloma plasma cells are also be subject to immune regulation, at least by the cellular components of the immune network (Figure 6.2).

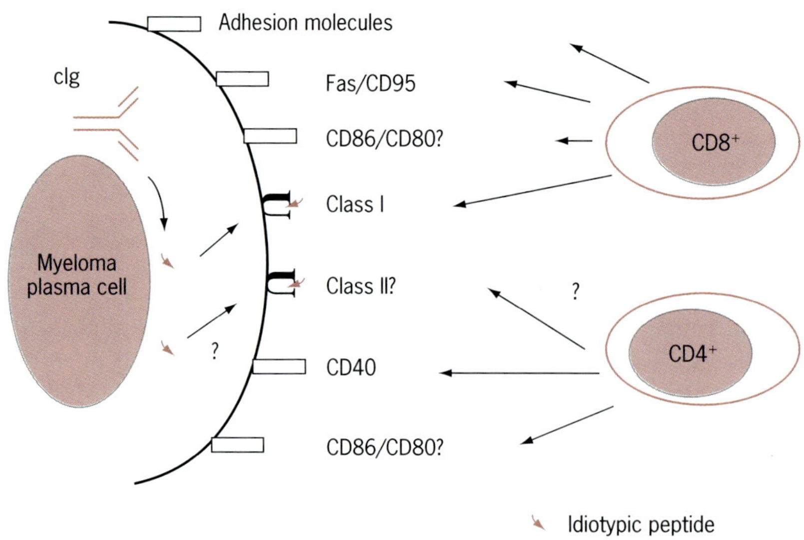

Figure 6.2 Possible interactions between myeloma plasma cells and idiotype-specific CD4+ and CD8+ T cells. Myeloma plasma cells express HLA-ABC, adhesion molecules, CD40, and Fas antigens.[9–14] Some of the cells may also express HLA-DR and B7 (CD80 and CD86) molecules.[10] Although it has been shown in mouse B-cell lymphoma and plasmacytoma that endogenously produced idiotypic peptides can be presented on MHC class II molecules,[8] it is not known whether this is the case for of human myeloma cells.

Immune regulation in murine myeloma

Early evidence of immune regulation on idiotype-expressing malignant B cells came from animal studies. Both antibodies (humoral response) and T cells (cellular response) regulating the growth of the myeloma clone by specific recognition of the idiotype antigen were described.[7,16–18] Immunization of mice with soluble idiotype protein coupled to an adjuvant led to production of antibodies specific for idiotype protein and protected the animals against a subsequent challenge with idiotype-positive but not idiotype-negative, tumor cells.[7,16] Anti-idiotypic antibodies inhibited plasmacytoma cell growth as well as the production of the idiotype-positive Ig.[18] However, as the excess of circulating M component may function as an immunological barrier by blocking anti-idiotypic antibodies, the anti-idiotypic antibodies are less likely to be efficient effectors in vivo. In fact, Daley and co-workers[19] demonstrated in mice that specific myeloma transplantation resistance was eliminated by post-immunization thymectomy, providing convincing evidence that T cells mediated the resistance. Similarly, idiotype-specific T cells were found to inhibit myeloma cell growth in vitro,[20] as well as differentiation and Ig secretion of myeloma B cells.[21]

Immune regulation in human myeloma

T-cell abnormalities or changes have been demonstrated in patients with myeloma (Table 6.1). A consistent finding was a low CD4/CD8 ratio, which was most pronounced in patients with advanced disease.[22,23] An increase in the $CD4^+CD45^+$ subset (previously defined as suppressor/inducer T cells) in MGUS[24] and a low number of these cells in myeloma[25] have also been described. More recently, investigators have demonstrated decreased $CD4^+$ cells (both native and memory $CD4^+$ cells) in myeloma[26,27] and an increase in or shift to $CD8^+CD57^+$ T cells, which may have immunosuppressive effects.[28–30] In addition, a lower expression of T-cell receptor/CD3-associated signaling molecules, such as PKC-α, has been described in myeloma T cells.[31] Thus, T-cell abnormalities in myeloma involve changes in the number and activation status of T-cell subsets as well as in their functions in terms of signal transduction. These abnormalities may be among the mechanisms contributing to tumor escape.

Some early studies described myeloma-reactive T cells in patients. Paglieroni and MacKenzie[32] demonstrated blood cells cytotoxic for autologous plasma cells in a chromium-release assay. Hoover and co-workers[33] reported an increased number of $CD8^+$ T cells with Fc receptors for the myeloma Ig isotype. The presence of activated (HLA-DR^+) T cells in myeloma patients was also reported.[34,35] These T cells produced large amounts of interleukin (IL)-2 and interferon-γ (IFN-γ) and generated anti-plasma-cell activity in vitro after CD3 stimulation. More recently, this same group of investigators examined the susceptibility of T cells to apoptosis in myeloma patients by determining the surface

Table 6.1 T-cell abnormalities or changes in myeloma

- Elevated $CD8^+$ cells, reduced $CD4^+/CD8^+$ ratio[22]
- Elevated $CD8^+CD57^+$ and HLA-DR^+ cells and enhanced susceptibility to apoptosis[28,30]
- Elevated $CD8^+CD11b^+$ Leu-8^- (memory) T cells[29]
- Reduced $CD4^+$ cells and correlation with relapse[115,116]
- Reduced $CD4^+CD45RA^+$ and $CD45RO^+$ cells[25,27]
- Reduced $CD4^+$ cells (both percentage and absolute number) and correlation with advanced disease and shorter survival[23,26]
- Hyperreactive T cells and dysregulated Fas and Bcl-2 expression[34,36]
- Reduced T-cell signaling molecule PKC-α[31]
- T-cell expansion in both $CD4^+$ and $CD8^+$ subsets, oligoclonality of expanded T cells[37–39]

expression of Fas and Bcl-2 antigens.[36] They found that Fas^+ cells were significantly higher, whereas Bcl-2^+ cells were significantly lower, in myeloma patients compared with disease-free controls. The percentage of cells undergoing spontaneous or triggered apoptosis was higher in myeloma patients, and was mainly restricted to the HLA-DR^+ T cells. These findings suggest that T cells may have a dysregulated expression of Fas and Bcl-2 molecules that is associated with an enhanced susceptibility to apoptosis in myeloma.

There is indirect evidence of T-cell regulation of human myeloma from studies examining T-cell receptor (TCR) usage of peripheral blood T cells in myeloma patients. Using a panel of eight monoclonal antibodies covering about 25% of the TCR repertoire, Janson and co-workers[37] found a predominant usage of V_α and V_β gene segment products within the $CD4^+$ and $CD8^+$ T cells in 40% of patients. In some patients, up to 50% of all $CD8^+$ or $CD4^+$ T cells were stained with one antibody. Similar results were reported in two other studies.[38,39] By TCR CDR3 length analysis, determination of J_β gene usage, and nucleotide sequencing, the clonality of expansion was determined, and oligoclonal expansions within $CD4^+$ or $CD8^+$ subsets were noted.[38,39] In one study,[39] reactivity to the autologous idiotype antigen of expanded T cells was examined. Two expansions within the $CD8^+$ population ($V_{\beta 3}$ and $V_{\beta 5.2}$) displayed no reactivity against the antigen. Instead, idiotype recognition was confined to a $CD8^+$ non-expanded $V^+_{\beta 22}$ T-cell population with a highly restricted TCR usage. Based on these results, it is believed that the T-cell expansions may be induced and maintained by chronic conventional antigenic stimulation since a superantigen-driven T-cell expansion should be polyclonal and confined to both $CD4^+$ and $CD8^+$ subsets.[40] Thus, a possible role for common, but not yet identified, tumor antigens in the generation of the expansions is suggested. In chronic lymphocytic leukemia and solid tumors, expanded T cells with specific antitumor activity have been reported.[41,42] Further work to identify the relevance of such T cells to the B-cell malignancy is warranted.

As depicted in Figure 6.1, idiotype proteins are myeloma-specific antigens and should evoke an immune response.[43] However, this response may be weak and has obviously failed to control the growth of tumor cells in patients. To prove this point, various approaches have been used. By isolating T cells that bind to idiotype protein, Dianzani and co-workers[44] were able to detect idiotype-reactive T cells with an activated phenotype ($CD8^+$HLA-DR^+) in the peripheral blood of myeloma patients. Using the same approach, another group reported the generation of idiotype-reactive T-cell clones.[45] However, it is not clear whether the cells were truly idiotype-specific or bound to the constant regions of the Ig molecule. Studies in both murine plasmacytoma[46] and human myeloma[47] have clearly shown that idiotype-induced T-cell stimulation requires the presence of antigen-presenting cells, such as monocytes or B cells, and is MHC-restricted. Idiotype-specific T cells recognize only processed idiotypic peptides in the context of MHC molecules.

The presence of idiotype-specific T cells in the peripheral blood of patients with myeloma or MGUS has been studied by detecting idiotype-induced T-cell proliferation and cytokine secretion. The number of cells secreting certain cytokines, such as IFN-γ or IL-2, after antigen stimulation can be enumerated in an enzyme-linked immunospot (ELISPOT) assay.[48,49] By using the ELISPOT assay, we were able to detect idiotype-specific T cells in 90% of patients with myeloma or MGUS.[49] We confirmed these results using two independent in vitro assays, a proliferation assay and an ELISPOT assay for IFN-γ and IL-2, as well as an in vivo test (delayed-type hypersensitivity, DTH).[50] Based on the number of idiotype-induced IFN-γ- or IL-2-secreting cells, the median number of idiotype-specific T cells in the patients was calculated to be about 20 per 10^5 peripheral blood mononuclear cells (PBMC), corresponding to 1 per 5000 PBMC.[49] Consistent with these results, we and others have shown that T cells in myeloma patients responded to peptides corresponding to CDRI-III of heavy and light chains of the autologous M component.[51,52]

These findings provide evidence to support the notion that an idiotype-specific T-cell response can be detected in most patients and emphasize the importance of using different readout assays to detect such low-frequency idiotype-specific T cells in the peripheral blood.

Attempts have also been made to detect the humoral response against idiotype protein. The search for anti-idiotypic antibodies in the serum of patients has been unsuccessful, presumably due to the blocking effect of clonal Ig. However, by using Epstein–Barr virus transformation of peripheral blood lymphocytes from patients, B-cell lines were obtained that produced IgM anti-idiotypic antibodies directly against the autologous, but not allogeneic or polyclonal, Ig molecules.[53] It was found, in a subsequent study, that the prevalence of such B cells was higher in MGUS and in early (stage I) myeloma than in advanced (stage III) myeloma.[54] The presence of anti-idiotypic B cells in myeloma and MGUS was confirmed by using the ELISPOT assay to detect the number of B cells secreting anti-idiotypic IgM antibodies.[55] As expected, the frequency of such B cells in peripheral blood was low (1 per 6×10^4 PBMC).

Human $CD4^+$ T helper (Th) cells may be subdivided into subsets based on their cytokine-secretion profile and function.[56–58] Th1 cells secrete IFN-ψ and IL-2, but not IL-4, whereas Th2 cells secrete IL-4 and IL-10.[56] Most Th1 cells, but only a minority of Th2 cells, exhibit cytolytic activity against autologous antigen-presenting B cells. Th2 cells are more efficient in providing help to B cells to differentiate and produce antibodies.[57,58] A similar subdivision of $CD8^+$ cytotoxic T (Tc) cells, based on their cytokine secretion profile and function, has been described.[59,60] Cells with cytotoxic activity are mainly of the Th1 and Tc1 subsets, while cells that provide help to B cells may be Th2 and Tc2.

The presence of idiotype-specific T-cell subsets in patients with stage I myeloma has been studied.[61] We found that idiotype-induced T-cell stimulation was mainly confined to the $CD4^+$ subsets in most of the patients examined and was MHC class II-restricted (Figure 6.3a, b). Idiotype-specific $CD8^+$ T cells were also demonstrated at a lower frequency. One patient showed a strong and dominating activation of $CD8^+$ T cells, which was MHC class I-restricted (see Figure 6.4a, b). Idiotype-specific $CD4^+$ and

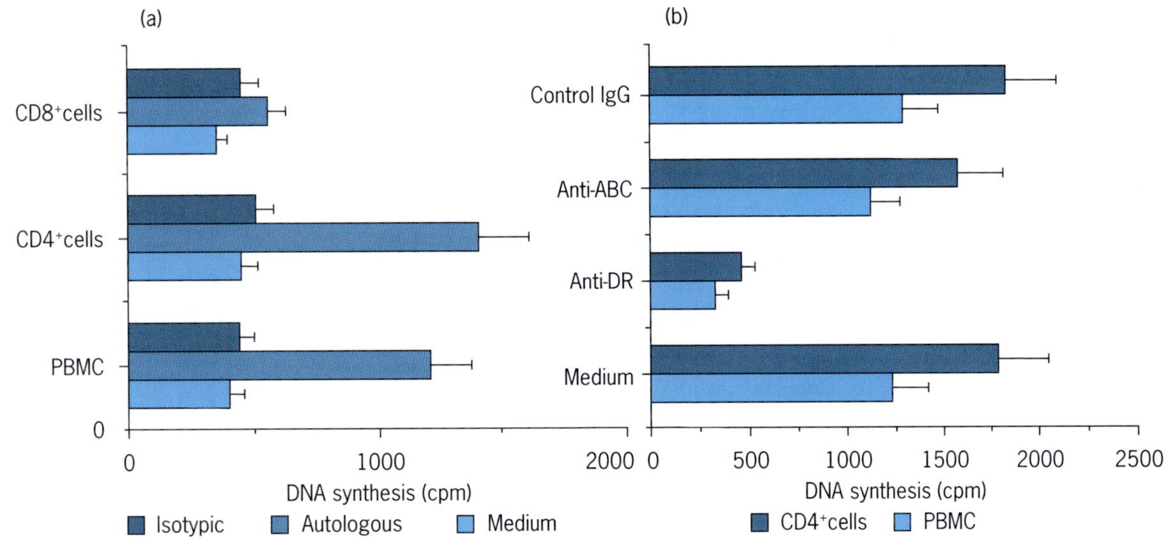

Figure 6.3 (a) Cell proliferation (DNA synthesis) in PBMC and enriched $CD4^+$ and $CD8^+$ T cells in medium or induced by idiotypic or isotypic proteins. (b) Inhibition of cell proliferation in PBMC and enriched $CD4^+$ T cells, with or without the addition of a control IgG, anti-HLA-DR, or anti-HLA-ABC antibodies.

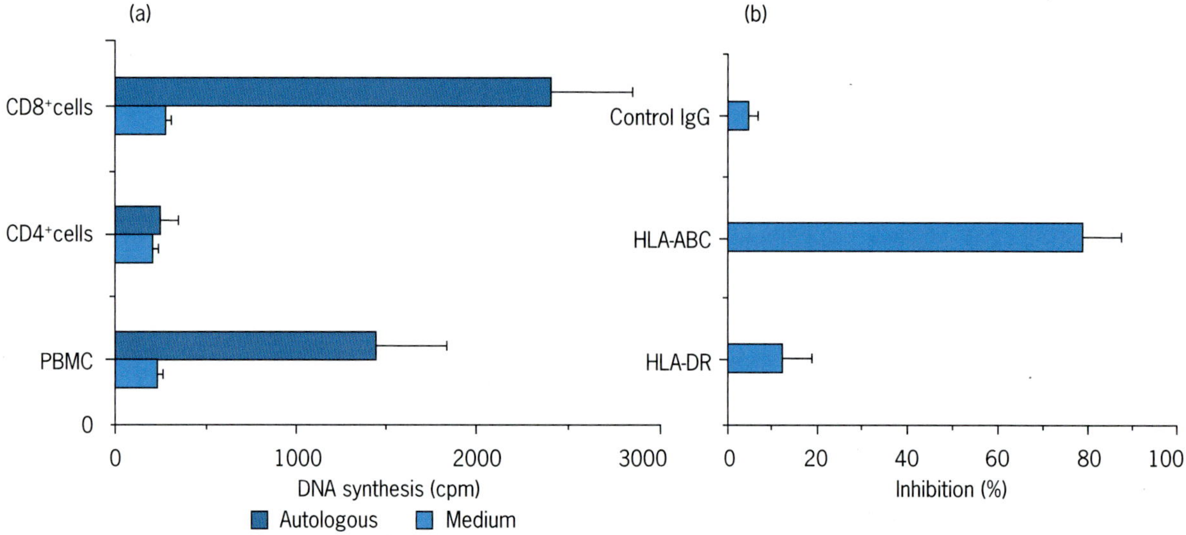

Figure 6.4 (a) Cell proliferation (DNA synthesis) in PBMC and enriched $CD4^+$ and $CD8^+$ T cells in medium or induced by idiotypic protein in one patient. (b) Inhibition of cell proliferation in PBMC with the addition of a control IgG, anti-HLA-DR or anti HLA-ABC antibodies.

$CD8^+$ T cells were mainly of the type 1 subsets, as judged by their secretion of IFN-γ and IL-2. In another study, we examined Th subsets and their relation to tumor load in patients with MGUS and myeloma.[62] As shown in Figure 6.5, the proportion of individuals who had an idiotype-specific response of the Th1 type (IFN-γ- and/or IL-2-secreting cells) was significantly higher in patients with indolent disease (MGUS and myeloma stage I) compared with those with advanced myeloma (stage II/III). In contrast, cells secreting the Th2-subtype cytokine profile (IL-4 only) were seen more frequently in patients with advanced myeloma (stage II/III). A similar pattern of cytokine secretion was also reported by others.[63] Collectively, these findings indicate that a shift may occur from an idiotype-specific type 1 response (Th1 and Tc1) in early myeloma to a type 2 response, (Th2 and probably Tc2) in advanced disease. These studies provide indirect evidence that idiotype-specific T cells may have a regulatory impact on human tumor B cells.

Experiments in murine plasmacytoma revealed that idiotype-specific $CD4^+$ T-cell clones were of both the Th1 and Th2 subtypes.[64] In vivo and in vitro experiments showed that although both the Th1 and Th2 clones had suppressive effects, only the Th1 clones were cytotoxic to the tumor cells.[65] It is also conceivable that the type 2 T cells may promote the growth of tumor B cells and support their differentiation into plasma cells.[66,67] The fact that the type 2 T-cell-derived cytokines, such as IL-6 and IL-10, are growth factors for myeloma cells, whereas the type 1 T-cell-derived cytokines, such as IFN-γ and tumour necrosis factor α (TNF-α) inhibit the growth of myeloma cells,[68] supports this notion. It may be speculated that T-cell perturbations in myeloma might precede the development of the expanding B-cell clone.[69] Therefore, it is important to examine in detail the roles of idiotype-specific T subsets on tumor B cells.

For the generation of an immune response in vitro and in vivo, professional antigen-presenting cells are required. Dendritic cells (DC) are the most potent antigen-presenting cells, and have attracted the attention of investigators for their initiation and expansion of antitumor responses. DC express high densities of MHC, adhesion, and co-stimulatory molecules on the surface.[70] By secreting IL-12, they may be able to

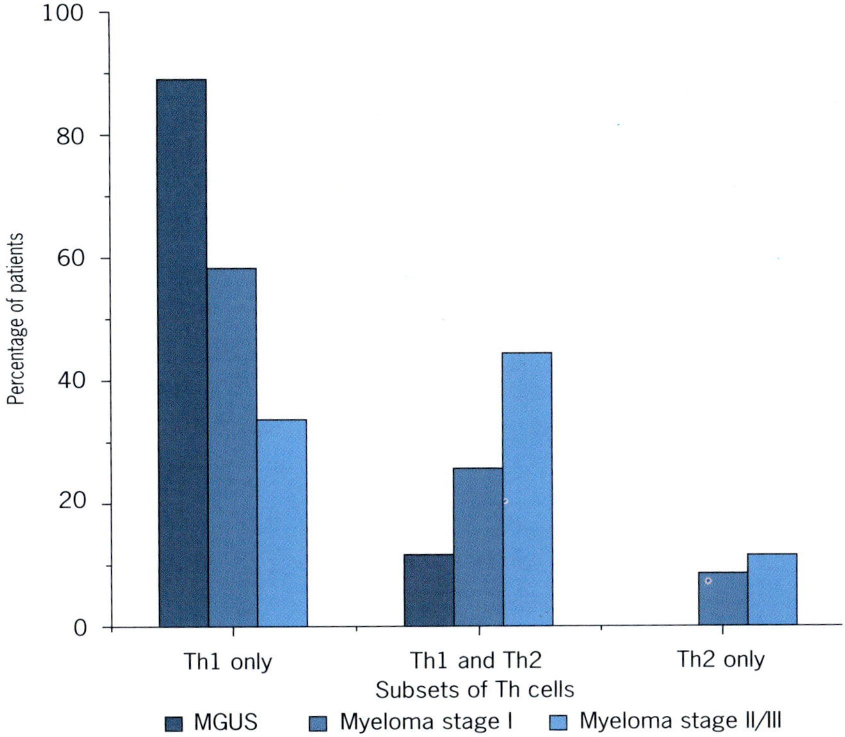

Figure 6.5 Percentage of patients with MGUS, myeloma stage I, or myeloma stage II/III who had cells secreting cytokines corresponding to different Th subsets.

direct the immune response to a Th1-type cell.[71] In addition, DC may directly stimulate the CD8$^+$ CTL.[72] The efficiencies of DC and monocytes in presenting idiotypic antigens to T cells and inducing T-cell activation have been evaluated.[73] DC were generated from blood adherent cells (monocytes) in a 7–day culture with granulocyte–macrophage colony-stimulating factor (GM-CSF) and IL-4. The results showed that DC induced a significantly stronger idiotype-specific immune response than monocytes (Figure 6.6). Moreover, with DC as antigen-presenting cells, a predominant IFN-γ (type 1 T-cell) response was seen in all patients tested. Both IFN-γ and IL-4 (type 1 and type 2 T-cell) responses were noted when monocytes were used (Figure 6.7). These results indicate that DC pulsed with idiotypic protein can be used for the induction of type 1 anti-idiotypic response in patients with myeloma.

Conclusions

Based on the studies described above, it can be concluded that an idiotype-specific immune response involving both humoral and cellular components exists in human myeloma, and idiotype-specific type 1 T cells may have a regulatory effect on tumor B cells. Nevertheless, it is also obvious that the immune response evoked is too weak to control the growth of tumor cells. This may be due to several factors. First, idiotypes are weak auto-antigens, and the high amount of circulating M component may induce T-cell tolerance or depletion.[74] These mechanisms may have contributed to the low numbers of idiotype-specific T and B cells detected in patients. Second, myeloma plasma cells have low, if any, expression of MHC class II and co-stimulatory molecules,[10,75] which renders the cells unable to prime native T cells and resistant

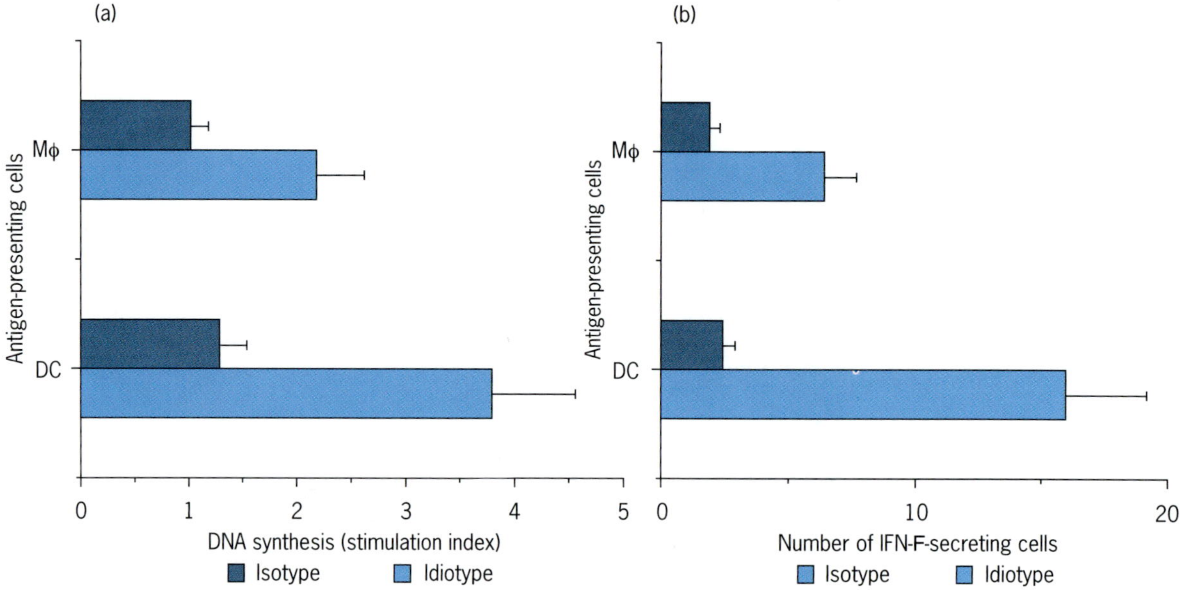

Figure 6.6 Proliferation (DNA synthesis) (a) and number of IFN-γ-secreting T cells (b) (mean ± SEM of five patients) induced by idiotypic or isotypic proteins presented by dendritic cells (DC) or monocytes (Mϕ).

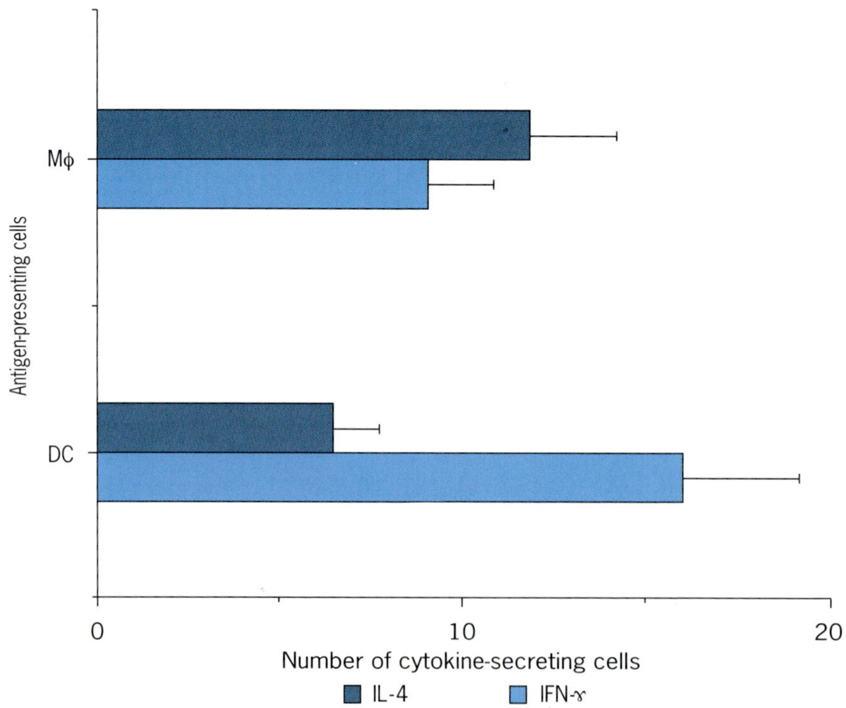

Figure 6.7 Numbers of IFN-γ- and IL-4-secreting T cells (mean ± SEM of five patients) induced by idiotypic proteins presented by dendritic cells (DC) or monocytes (Mϕ).

to the attack mediated by $CD4^+$ T cells. Third, the expression of Fas ligand (FasL)[76] and some immunosuppressive cytokines, such as IL-10 and transforming growth factor β (TGF-β),[77,78] by myeloma cells could induce apoptosis and/or downregulate the function of the specific T cells. The mutations in the Fas antigen in myeloma[79] may be another way of protecting the tumor cells from FasL-induced apoptosis.

IMMUNOTHERAPY IN B-CELL MALIGNANCIES

Idiotype-based immunotherapies

Since idiotypes may serve as tumor-specific antigens, an intervention aimed at expanding idiotype-specific T cells with cytotoxic or suppressive effects on the tumor B-cell clone may be a feasible immunotherapeutic approach. Active immunization against idiotypic determinants on malignant B cells has produced resistance to tumor growth in transplantable murine B-cell lymphoma and myeloma.[16,79–82] A study of active immunization of B-cell lymphoma patients with autologous idiotype proteins conjugated to a carrier protein, keyhole-limpet hemocyanin (KLH), was reported in 1992.[83] Seven of nine immunized patients developed idiotype-specific humoral and/or cellular responses. Tumor regression was observed in two patients who had measurable disease. It was shown in subsequent studies that cell-mediated cytolytic immune responses may be an important determinant of vaccine efficacy[84] and that the ability to evoke such a specific immune response is correlated with a more favorable clinical outcome.[85] These studies clearly demonstrate that idiotype protein can be formulated and used as a tumor-specific immunogen in humans with B-cell malignancies.

In myeloma, pilot studies of active immunization of patients with idiotype proteins have been reported. In one study, we repeatedly immunized five patients with stage I–III disease, who were previously untreated, with the autologous M component precipitated in aluminum phosphate suspension.[86] In three patients, an anti-idiotypic T-cell response was amplified 1.9- to 5-fold during the immunization. The number of B cells secreting anti-idiotypic antibodies also increased in these three patients, and two of the three patients had a gradual decrease of blood $CD19^+$ B cells (Table 6.2). However, the induced T-cell response was transient, and it was eliminated during repeated immunization. In another of our studies, immunization was performed by injection of the M component combined with GM-CSF.[87] Five patients with IgG myeloma were treated, and all the patients developed an idiotype-specific type 1 T-cell response. The response involved both $CD8^+$ and $CD4^+$ subsets and was mainly MHC class I-restricted. There was a transient rise in B cells producing IgM anti-idiotypic antibodies in all patients (Table 6.3). One of the patients had a clinical response, defined by a significant

Table 6.2 Enhancement of anti-idiotype T- and B-cell responses and decrease in the number of $CD19^+$ B cells in five myeloma patients during immunization

	Patient				
Responses	**1**	**2**	**3**	**4**	**5**
Anti-Id T cells	+	+	–	–	+
Anti-Id B cells	+	+	–	–	+
Decrease of $CD19^+$ B cells	+	+	–	–	–

Table 6.3 Summary of immunological responses in five myeloma patients immunized with the autologous idiotype protein combined with GM-CSF

	Patient				
Responses	**1**	**2**	**3**	**4**	**5**
T-cell type 1 response[a]	+	+	+	+	+
T-cell type 2 response[a]	±	−	−	±	±
MHC restriction[b]	I/II	I	I	I	I
DTH[c] reaction	−	−	−	−	−
B-cell response	+	+	+	+	+

[a] Type 1 or 2 T-cell responses were defined by pattern of cytokine secretion (type 1: IFN-γ and/or IL-2; type-2: IL-4)
[b] MHC restriction was examined by anti-MHC (HLA-DR for class II; HLA–ABC for class I) antibody-induced inhibition on T-cell response and based on >60% inhibition induced by corresponding blocking antibodies. I represents class I–restricted and II class–II restricted.
[c] Delayed-type hypersensitivity.

decrease in serum M component (from 20 g/l to 7 g/l) and normalization of serum Ig levels, which lasted for more than a year after commencement of immunization. Also, a study from Massaia and co-workers[88] has shown that immunization of myeloma patients with idiotype-KLH conjugate in combination with GM-CSF induces a strong idiotype-specific cellular immunity in most patients. Collectively, these results indicate that immunization of myeloma patients using the autologous M component together with GM-CSF might be a promising immunotherapy.

Idiotype immunization may also be used in allogeneic bone marrow transplantation. Kwak and co-workers[89] immunized an HLA-identical sibling marrow donor with the patient's (i.e. the recipient's) M component, and showed that idiotype-specific T-cell immunity was successfully transferred to the recipient. The transferred anti-idiotype T-cell immunity was transient (<60 days), indicating that booster immunization of the recipient may be required to maintain the antitumor immunity.

DC are the most potent antigen-presenting cells, and are ideally suited to serve as natural adjuvants for purposes of vaccination and immunotherapy.[90,91] Methods have been developed to obtain substantial numbers of DC from proliferating $CD34^+$ progenitors in bone marrow and in peripheral blood, as well as from non-proliferating precursor cells, such as monocytes, in human blood.[92–94] Animal studies have demonstrated that DC pulsed with tumor antigens can be used to induce protective immunity against tumor challenge.[95–97] Antigen-pulsed DC have been used to vaccinate patients with B-cell malignancies. Hsu and co-workers[98] reported a pilot study in which four patients with B-cell lymphoma were immunized with idiotype-pulsed DC isolated from peripheral blood. All patients developed measurable antitumor cellular immune responses, and clinical responses were observed in three of the four patients.

Wen and co-workers[99] reported vaccinating a myeloma patient with autologous idiotype protein-pulsed DC generated from blood adherent cells. Enhanced idiotype-specific cellular and humoral responses were observed in the patient. The immune responses were associated with a transient minor fall in the serum idiotype protein level. In their subsequent study,[100] six additional patients were treated using the same protocol. An immune response against idiotype was demonstrated in most of the patients. A minor clinical response (25% reduction in the M component) was observed in one patient and stable disease in the remaining patients. More recently, Reichardt and co-workers[101] reported their experience of using idiotype-pulsed DC in 12 myeloma patients after autologous peripheral blood stem cell transplantation. Their study showed that myeloma patients could make strong anti-KLH responses despite recent high-dose therapy and that DC-based idiotype vaccination was feasible after transplantation and could induce idiotype-specific T-cell responses in certain patients. It is expected that additional studies will examine the efficacy of idiotype-pulsed DC as vaccines in B-cell malignancies.

In addition to active immunization with purified idiotype proteins or idiotype-pulsed DC, DNA vaccines containing genes encoding idiotypic epitopes and carrier protein may be a convenient alternative vaccine delivery system. A study by King and co-workers[102] has described the use of DNA vaccines with single-chain Fv fused to fragment C of TT in murine lymphoma and myeloma. The vaccines promoted an anti-idiotypic response and induced strong protection against B-cell lymphoma, which was likely antibody-mediated. The same fusion design also induced protective immunity against a surface Ig-negative myeloma. This strategy may have implications for immunotherapy in human diseases.

Other immunotherapies

Other methods of immunotherapy for B-cell malignancies involve the use of monoclonal antibodies as adoptive immunization. Levy and co-workers[103,104] used anti-idiotypic antibody to treat patients with B-cell lymphoma and demonstrated that the majority of the patients responded (18% complete response rate and 66% complete and partial response rate). About 13% of these patients experienced prolonged complete remission up to 10 years. In the patients with complete remission, the malignant tumor cells were detectable, suggesting that the treatment may induce tumor dormancy rather than tumor eradication.

Anti-idiotypic antibodies can be genetically modified to contain the IL-2 domain, which may augment the therapeutic effect of such antibodies. These fusion proteins have been made and tested in a B-cell lymphoma mouse model.[105] The results showed that an anti-idiotype–IL-2 fusion protein retained the biological activities IL-2, induced tumor cell lysis in vitro, and inhibited tumor growth in vivo. However, such antibodies are unlikely to work in myeloma, since as myeloma plasma cells do not express surface Ig and the existence of high amounts of M component in serum may have a blocking effect on anti-idiotypic antibodies.

IL-6 is an important growth factor for myeloma cells.[68] Thus, monoclonal antibodies against IL-6 may have a myeloma-suppressive effect. Bataille and co-workers[106] have treated 10 patients with advanced myeloma with a murine anti-IL-6 antibody. Although an inhibition of myeloma cell proliferation was observed in vivo, none of the patients had improved outcome or achieved remission.

For the purpose of enhancing the activity of T cells, natural killer (NK) cells, and lymphokine-activated killer (LAK) cells, Peest and co-workers[107] administered low-dose recombinant IL-2 subcutaneously to treat advanced myeloma. Of 18 patients, 6 experienced tumor response, defined as objective tumor mass reduction or long-lasting stable disease following tumor progress before initiation of treatment. During therapy, activated $CD4^+$ T cells, expanded NK cells, and enhanced NK- and LAK-cell activities were observed. The severe side-effects associated with IL-2 given intravenously were not noted in this study.

Allogeneic bone marrow transplantation is associated with a graft-versus-leukemia effect because of the antileukemia action of donor lymphocytes.[108] A graft-versus-myeloma effect, which can be evoked using donor leukocytes with or without cytokines, has been observed.[109–113] The published data, especially that from the Dutch group,[113] indicate a close correlation between the development of graft-versus-host disease and graft-versus-myeloma effect, as well as a high treatment-related toxicity. These observations strongly support the existence of a graft-versus-myeloma effect in the post-allograft relapse setting, and demonstrate the powerful antitumor effect mounted by a relatively low number of donor cells.

Conclusions

Various immunotherapy treatment strategies have been tested in B-cell malignancies, including myeloma. Most of these have focused on targeting idiotype-specific immunity.

When idiotype-based vaccines are used, induction or enhancement of idiotype-specific immunity has been observed, indicating that the vaccines are able to elicit a specific immune response. However, clinical response is still a rare event, occurring in a minority of treated patients, suggesting that the elicited or enhanced immunity is still too weak to cause significant tumor destruction. Alternatively, a non-beneficial immune response (such as the type 2 T-cell response)[114] may also be generated by immunization, which may enhance tumor B-cell growth and facilitate differentiation into plasma cell tumors.[66,67]

Ideally, a tumor-specific immunotherapy should induce or expand only the beneficial immune responses mediated by CTL (Th1 and Tc1 subsets) that have sufficient cytotoxic effects toward tumor cells. Further studies are warranted so that we can better understand the immune regulation mechanism in B-cell malignancies.

REFERENCES

1. Mellstedt H, Holm G, Björkholm M. Multiple myeloma, Waldenström's macroglobulinemia, and benign monoclonal gammopathy: characteristics of the B cell clone, immunoregulatory cell populations and clinical implications. *Adv Cancer Res* 1984; **41**: 257–89.
2. MacKenzie MR, Lewis JP. Cytogenetic evidence that the malignant event in multiple myeloma occurs in a precursor lymphocyte. *Cancer Genet Cytogenet* 1985; **17**: 13–20.
3. Berenson J, Wong R, Kim K et al., Evidence of peripheral blood B lymphocyte but not T lymphocyte involvement in multiple myeloma. *Blood* 1987; **70**: 1550–3.
4. Billadeau D, Quam L, Thomas W et al. Detection and quantitation of malignant cells in the peripheral blood of multiple myeloma patients. *Blood* 1992; **80**: 1818–24.
5. Chen BJ, Epstein J. Circulating clonal lymphocytes in myeloma constitute a minor subpopulation of B cells. *Blood* 1996; **87**: 1972–6.
6. Szczepek AJ, Seeberger K, Wizniak J et al. A high frequency of circulating B cells share clonotypic Ig heavy-chain VDJ rearrangements with autologous bone marrow plasma cells in multiple myeloma, as measured by single-cell and in situ reverse transcriptase-polymerase reaction. *Blood* 1998; **92**: 2844–55.
7. Lynch RG, Graff RJ, Sirisinha S et al. Myeloma proteins as tumor-specific transplantation antigens. *Proc Natl Acad Sci USA* 1972; **69**: 1540–4.
8. Bogen B, Weiss S. Processing and presentation of idiotypes to MHC-restricted T cells. *Int Rev Immunol* 1993; **10**: 337–55.
9. Duperray C, Klein B, Durie BGM et al. Phenotypic analysis of human myeloma cell lines. *Blood* 1989; **73**: 566–72.
10. Yi Q, Dabadghao S, Österborg A et al. Myeloma bone marrow plasma cells: evidence for their capacity as antigen-presenting cells. *Blood* 1997; **90**: 1960–7.
11. Leo R, Boeker M, Peest D et al. Multiparameter analyses of normal and malignant human plasma cells: $CD38^{++}$, $CD56^{+}$, $CD54^{+}$, cIg^{+} is the common phenotype of myeloma cells. *Ann Hematol* 1992; **64**: 132–9.
12. Barker HF, Hamilton MS, Ball J et al. Expression of adhesion molecules IFA-3 and N-CAM on normal and malignant human plasma cells. *Br J Haematol* 1992; **81**: 331–5.
13. Westendorf JJ, Ahmann GJ, Armitage RJ et al. CD40 expression in malignant plasma cells. Role in stimulation of autocrine IL-6 secretion by a human myeloma cell line. *J Immunol* 1994; **152**: 117–28.
14. Pellat-Deceunynck C, Bataille R, Robillard N et al. Expression of CD28 and CD40 in human myeloma cells: a comparative study with normal plasma cells. *Blood* 1994; **84**: 2597–603.
15. Hata H, Matsuzaki H, Takeya M et al. Expression of Fas/Apo-1 (CD95) and apoptosis in tumor

cells from patients with plasma cell disorders. *Blood* 1995; **86**: 1939–45.
16. Sirisinha S, Eisen HN. Autoimmune-like antibodies to the ligand-binding sites of myeloma proteins. *Proc Natl Acad Sci USA* 1971; **68**: 3130–5.
17. Stevenson FK, George AJT, Glennie MJ. Anti-idiotypic therapy of leukemias and lymphomas. *Chem Immunol* 1990; **48**: 126–66.
18. Mahony J, Bose A, Cowdrey D et al. A monoclonal antiidiotypic antibody to MOPC 315 IgA inhibits the growth of MOPC 315 myeloma cells in vitro. *J Immunol* 1981; **126**: 113–17.
19. Daley MJ, Gebel HM, Lynch RG. Idiotype-specific transplantation resistance to MOPC-315: abrogation by post-immunization thymectomy. *J Immunol* 1978; **120**: 1620–4.
20. Flood PM, Philipps C, Taupier MA et al. Regulation of myeloma growth in vitro by idiotype-specific T lymphocytes. *J Immunol* 1980; **124**: 424–30.
21. Lynch RG, Immunoglobulin-specific suppressor T cells. *Adv Immunol* 1987; **40**: 135–51.
22. Mellstedt H, Holm G, Pettersson D et al. T cells in monoclonal gammopathies. *Scand J Immunol* 1982; **29**: 57–64.
23. San Miguel JF, Caballero MD, Gonzalez M. T-cell subpopulations in patients with monoclonal gammopathies: essential monoclonal gammopathy, multiple myeloma, and Waldenström's macroglobulinemia. *Am J Hematol* 1985; **20**: 267–73.
24. Shapira R, Froom P, Kinarty A et al. Increase in the suppressor-inducer T cell subset in multiple myeloma and monoclonal gammopathy of undetermined significance. *Br J Haematol* 1989; **71**: 223–5.
25. Serra HM, Mant MJ, Ruether BA et al. Selective loss of $CD4^+CD45^+$ T cells in peripheral blood of multiple myeloma patients. *J Clin Immunol* 1988; **8**: 259–65.
26. San Miguel JF, Gonzalez M, Gascon A et al. Lymphoid subsets and prognostic factors in multiple myeloma. *Br J Haematol* 1992; 80: 305–9.
27. Kay NE, Leong T, Bone N et al. T-helper phenotypes in the blood of myeloma patients on ECOG phase III trials E9486/E3A93. *Br J Haematol* 1998; **100**: 469–77.
28. Gonzalez M, San Miguel JF, Gascon A et al. Increased expression of natural-killer-associated and activation antigens in multiple myeloma. *Am J Hematol* 1992; **39**: 84–9.
29. Frassanito MA, Silvestris F, Cafforio P et al. $CD8^+/CD57^+$ cells and apoptosis suppress T-cell functions in multiple myeloma. *Br J Haematol* 1998; **100**: 469–77.
30. Van den Hove LE, Meeus P, Derom A et al. Lymphocyte profiles in multiple myeloma and monoclonal gammopathy of undetermined significance: flow-cytometric characterization and analysis in a two-dimensional correlation biplot. *Ann Hematol* 1998; **76**: 249–56.
31. Bianchi A, Mariani S, Beggiato E et al. Distribution of T-cell signaling molecules in human myeloma. *Br J Haematol* 1997; **97**: 815–20.
32. Paglieroni T, MacKenzie MR. In vitro cytotoxic response to human myeloma plasma cells by peripheral blood leukocytes from patients with multiple myeloma and benign monoclonal gammopathy. *Blood* 1979; **54**: 226–37.
33. Hoover RG, Hickman S, Gebel HM et al. Expansion of Fc receptor-bearing T lymphocytes in patients with immunoglobulin G and immunoglobulin A myeloma. *J Clin Invest* 1981; **67**: 308–11.
34. Massaia M, Bianchi A, Attisano C et al. Detection of hyperreactive T cells in multiple myeloma by multivalent cross-linking of the CD3/TCR complex. *Blood* 1991; **78**: 1770–80.
35. Massaia M, Attisano C, Peola S et al. Rapid generation of antiplasma cell activity in the bone marrow of myeloma patients by CD3-activated T cells. *Blood* 1993; **82**: 1787–97.
36. Massaia M, Borrione P, Attisano C et al. Dysregulated Fas and bcl-2 expression leading to enhanced apoptosis in T cells of multiple myeloma patients. *Blood* 1995; **85**: 3679–87.
37. Janson CH, Grunewald J, Österborg A et al. Predominant T cell receptor V gene usage in patients with abnormal clones of B cells. *Blood* 1991; **77**: 1776–80.
38. Moss P, Gillespie G, Frodsham P et al. Clonal populations of $CD4^+$ and $CD8^+$ T cells in patients with multiple myeloma and paraproteinemia. *Blood* 1996; **87**: 3297–306.
39. Halapi E, Werner Å, Wahlström J et al. T cell repertoire in patients with multiple myeloma and monoclonal gammopathy of undetermined significance: clonal $CD8^+$ T cell expansions are found preferentially in patients with a low tumor burden. *Eur J Immunol* 1997; **27**: 2245–52.
40. Shu S, Krinock RA, Matsumura T et al. Stimulation of tumor-draining lymph node cells with superantigenic staphylococcal toxins leads

to the generation of tumor-specific effector T cells. *J Immunol* 1994; **152**: 1277–88.
41. Farace F, Orlanducci F, Dietrich PY et al. T cell repertoire in patients with B chronic lymphocytic leukemia. *J Immunol* 1994; **153**: 4281–90.
42. Sensi ML, Parmiani G, Analyses of TCR usage in human tumors: a new tool for assessing tumor specific immune responses. *Immunol Today* 1995; **16**: 588–95.
43. Holm G, Bergenbrant S, Lefvert AK et al. Anti-idiotypic immunity as a potential regulator in myeloma and related diseases. *Ann NY Acad Sci* 1991; **636**: 178–83.
44. Dianzani U, Pileri A, Boccadoro M et al. Activated idiotype-reactive cells in suppressor/cytotoxic subpopulations of monoclonal gammopathies: correlation with diagnosis and disease status. *Blood* 1988; **72**: 1064–8.
45. Österborg A, Masucci M, Bergenbrant S et al. Generation of T cell clones binding $F(ab')_2$ fragments of idiotypic immunoglobulin in patients with monoclonal gammopathy. *Cancer Immunol Immunother* 1991; **34**: 157–62.
46. Bogen B, Malissen B, Haas W. Idiotype-specific T cell clones that recognize syngeneic immunoglobulin fragments in the context of class II molecules. *Eur J Immunol* 1986; **16**: 1373–8.
47. Yi Q, Holm G, Lefvert AK. Idiotype-induced T cell stimulation requires antigen presentation in association with HLA-DR molecules. *Clin Exp Immunol* 1996; **104**: 359–65.
48. Czerkinsky CC, Andersson G, Ekre HP et al. Reverse ELISPOT assay for clonal analysis of cytokine production. I. Enumeration of gamma-interferon-secreting cells. *J Immunol Meth* 1988; **110**: 29–36.
49. Yi Q, Bergenbrant S, Österborg A et al. T-cell stimulation induced by idiotypes on monoclonal immunoglobulins in patients with monoclonal gammopathies. *Scand J Immunol* 1993; **38**: 529–34.
50. Österborg A, Yi Q, Bergenbrant S et al. Idiotype-specific T cells in multiple myeloma stage I: an evaluation by four different functional tests. *Br J Haematol* 1995; **89**: 110–16.
51. Wen YJ, Ling M, Lim SH. Immunogenicity and cross-reactivity with idiotypic IgA of VH CDR3 peptide in multiple myeloma. *Br J Haematol* 1998; **100**: 464–8.
52. Fagerberg J, Yi Q, Gigliotti D et al. T cell epitope mapping of the idiotypic monoclonal IgG heavy and light chains in multiple myeloma. *Int J Cancer* 1999; **80**: 671–80.
53. Andersson M, Holm G, Lefvert AK et al. Anti-idiotypic B cell lines from a patient with monoclonal gammopathy of undetermined significance. *Scand J Immunol* 1989; **130**: 489–92.
54. Bergenbrant S, Österborg A, Holm G et al. Anti-idiotypic antibodies in patients with monoclonal gammopathies. Relation to tumor load. *Br J Haematol* 1991; **78**: 66–70.
55. Bergenbrant S, Yi Q, Ösby E et al. Anti-idiotypic B lymphocytes in patients with monoclonal gammopathies. *Scand J Immunol* 1994; **40**: 216–20.
56. Romagnani S. Human Th1 and Th2 subsets: doubt no more. *Immunol Today* 1991; **12**: 256–8.
57. Del Prete GF, De Carli M, Ricci M et al. Helper activity for immunoglobulin synthesis of T helper type 1 (Th1) and Th2 human T cell clones: the help of Th1 clones is limited by their cytolytic capacity. *J Exp Med* 1991; **174**: 809–13.
58. Mosmann TM, Sad S. The expanding universe of T-cell subsets: Th1, Th2 and more. *Immunol Today* 1996; **17**: 138–46.
59. Kemany DM, Noble A, Holmes BJ et al. Immune regulation: a new role for the $CD8^+$ T cell. *Immunol Today* 1994; **15**: 107–10.
60. Seder RA, Gros GGL. The functional role of $CD8^+$ T helper type 2 cells. *J Exp Med* 1995; **181**: 5–7.
61. Yi Q, Eriksson I, He W et al. Idiotype-specific T lymphocytes in monoclonal gammopathies. Evidence for the presence of $CD4^+$ and $CD8^+$ subsets. *Br J Haematol* 1997; **96**: 338–45.
62. Yi Q, Österborg A, Bergenbrant S et al. Idiotype-reactive T subsets and tumor load in monoclonal gammopathies. *Blood* 1995; **86**: 3043–9.
63. Walchner M, Wick M. Elevation of $CD8^+CD11b^+Leu\text{-}8^-$ T cells is associated with the humoral immunodeficiency in myeloma patients. *Clin Exp Immunol* 1997; 109: 310–16.
64. Lauritzsen GF, Bogen B. Idiotype-specific, major histocompatibility complex restricted T cells are of both Th1 and Th2 type. *Scand J Immunol* 1991; **33**: 647–56.
65. Lauritzsen GF, Weiss S, Bogen B. Anti-tumor activity of idiotype-specific, MHC-restricted TH1 and Th2 clones in vitro and in vivo. *Scand J Immunol* 1993; **37**: 77–85.
66. Clark EA, Ledbetter JA. How B and T cells talk to each other. *Nature* 1994; **367**: 425–8.
67. Hilbert DM, Shen MY, Rapp UR et al. T cells induce terminal differentiation of transformed B cells to mature plasma cell tumors. *Proc Natl Acad Sci USA* 1995; **92**: 649–53.

68. Hallek M, Bergsagel PL, Anderson KC. Multiple myeloma: increasing evidence for a multistep transformation process. *Blood* 1998; **91**: 3–21.
69. Paglieroni T, Caggiano V, MacKenzie M. Abnormalities in immune regulation precede the development of multiple myeloma. *Am J Hematol* 1992; **40**: 51–5.
70. Steinman RM. The dendritic cell system and its role in immunogenicity. *Ann Rev Immunol* 1991; **9**: 271–96.
71. Macatonia SE, Hosken NA, Litton M et al. Dendritic cells produce IL-12 and direct the development of Th1 cells from native $CD4^+$ T cells. *J Immunol* 1995; **154**: 5071–9.
72. Young J, Inaba K. Dendritic cells as adjuvants for class I major histocompatibility complex-restricted anti-tumor responses. *J Exp Med* 1996; **183**: 7–11.
73. Dabadghao S, Bergenbrant S, Anton D et al. Anti-idiotypic T-cell activation in multiple myeloma induced by M-component fragments presented by dendritic cells. *Br J Haematol* 1998; **100**: 647–54.
74. Bogen B. Peripheral T cell tolerance as a tumor escape mechanism: deletion of $CD4^+$ T cells specific for a monoclonal immunoglobulin idiotype secreted by a plasmacytoma. *Eur J Immunol* 1996; **26**: 2671–9.
75. Epstein J, Hoover R, Kornbluth J et al. Biological aspects of multiple myeloma. *Baillière's Clin Haematol* 1995; **8**: 721–34.
76. Villunger A, Egle A, Marschitz I et al. Constitutive expression of Fas (Apo-1/CD95) ligand on multiple myeloma cells: a potential mechanism of tumor-induced suppression of immune surveillance. *Blood* 1997; **90**: 12–20.
77. Portier M, Zhang XG, Ursule E et al. Cytokine gene expression in human multiple myeloma. *Br J Haematol* 1993; **85**: 514–20.
78. Gu ZJ, Costes V, Lu ZY et al. Interleukin-10 is a growth factor for human myeloma cells by induction of an oncostatin M autocrine loop. *Blood* 1996; **88**: 3972–86.
79. Landowski TH, Qu N, Buyuksal I et al. Mutations in the Fas antigen in patients with multiple myeloma. *Blood* 1997; **90**: 4266–70.
80. Stevenson FK, Gordon J. Immunization with idiotypic immunoglobulin protects against development of B lymphocytic leukemia, but emerging tumor cells can evade antibody attack by modulation. *J Immunol* 1983; **130**: 970–3.
81. Kaminski MS, Kitamura K, Maloney DG et al. Idiotype vaccination against murine B cell lymphoma: inhibition of tumor immunity by free idiotype protein. *J Immunol* 1987; **138**: 1289–96.
82. Campbell MJ, Esserman L, Byars NE et al. Idiotype vaccination against murine B cell lymphoma: humoral and cellular requirements for the full expression of antitumor immunity. *J Immunol* 1990; **145**: 1029–36.
83. Kwak L, Campbell MJ, Czerwinski DK et al. Induction of immune responses in patients with B-cell lymphoma against the surface-immunoglobulin idiotype expressed by their tumors. *N Engl J Med 1992*; **327**: 1209–15.
84. Nelson EL, Li X, Hsu FJ et al, Tumor-specific, cytotoxic T-lymphocyte response after idiotype vaccination for B-cell, non-Hodgkin's lymphoma. *Blood* 1996; **88**: 580–9.
85. Hsu FJ, Caspar CB, Czerwinski D et al, Tumor-specific idiotype vaccines in the treatment of patients with B-cell lymphoma: long-term results of a clinical trial. *Blood* 1997; **89**: 3129–35.
86. Bergenbrant S, Yi Q, Österborg A et al. Modulation of anti-idiotypic immune response by immunization with the autologous M-component protein in multiple myeloma patients. *Br J Haematol* 1996; **92**: 840–6.
87. Österborg A, Yi Q, Henriksson L et al. Idiotype immunization combined with granulocyte-macrophage colony-stimulating factor in myeloma patients induced type I, major histocompatibility complex-restricted, CD8- and CD4-specific T-cell responses. *Blood* 1998; **91**: 2459–66.
88. Massaia M, Borrione P, Battaglio S et al. Idiotype vaccination in human myeloma: generation of tumor-specific immune responses after high-dose chemotherapy. *Blood* 1999; **94**: 673–83.
89. Kwak LW, Taub DD, Duffey PL et al. Transfer of myeloma idiotype-specific immunity from an actively immunised marrow donor. *Lancet* 1995; **345**: 1016–20.
90. Grabbe S, Beissert S, Schwartz T et al. Dendritic cells as initiators of tumor immune response: a possible strategy for tumor immunotherapy? *Immunol Today* 1995; **16**: 117–21.
91. Girolomoni G, Ricciardi-Castagnoli P. Dendritic cells hold promise for immunotherapy. *Immunol Today* 1997; **118**: 102–4.
92. Reid CD, Stackpoole A, Meager A et al. Interactions of tumor necrosis factor with granulocyte-macrophage colony-stimulating factor and other cytokines in the regulation of dendritic cell

growth in vitro from early bipotent CD34+ progenitors in human bone marrow. *J Immunol* 1992; **149**: 2681–8.
93. Sallusto F, Lanzavecchia A. Efficient presentation of soluble antigen by cultured human dendritic cells is maintained by granulocyte/macrophage colony-stimulating factor plus interleukin 4 and down-regulated by tumor necrosis factor α. *J Exp Med* 1994; **179**: 1109–18.
94. Romani N, Gruner S, Brang D et al. Proliferating dendritic cell progenitors in human blood. *J Exp Med* 1994; **180**: 83–93.
95. Flamand V, Sornasse T, Thielemans K et al. Murine dendritic cells pulsed in vitro with tumor antigen induce tumor resistance in vivo. *Eur J Immunol* 1994; **24**: 605–10.
96. Mayordomo JI, Loftus DJ, Sakamoto H et al. Therapy of murine tumors with p53 wild-type and mutant sequence peptide-based vaccines. *J Exp Med* 1996; **183**: 1357–65.
97. Celluzzi CM, Mayordomo JI, Storkus WJ et al. Peptide-pulsed dendritic cells induce antigen-specific, CTL-mediated protective tumor immunity. *J Exp Med* 1996; **183**: 283–7.
98. Hsu FJ, Benike C, Fagnini F et al. Vaccination of patients with B-cell lymphoma using autologous antigen-pulsed dendritic cells. *Nature Med* 1996; **2**: 52–8.
99. Wen YJ, Ling M, Bailey-Wood R et al. Idiotypic protein-pulsed adherent peripheral blood mononuclear cell-derived dendritic cells prime immune system in multiple myeloma. *Clin Cancer Res* 1998; **4**: 957–62.
100. Lim SH, Bailey-Wood R. Idiotypic protein-pulsed dendritic cell vaccination in multiple myeloma. *Int J Cancer* 1999; **83**: 215–22.
101. Reichardt VL, Okada CY, Liso A et al. Idiotype vaccination using dendritic cells after autologous peripheral blood stem cell transplantation for multiple myeloma – a feasibility study. *Blood* 1999; **93**: 2411–19.
102. King CA, Spellerberg MB, Zhu D et al. DNA vaccines with single-chain Fv fused to fragment C of tetanus toxin induce protective immunity against lymphoma and myeloma. *Nature Med* 1998; **4**: 1281–6.
103. Maloney DG, Brown S, Czerwinski DK et al. Monoclonal anti-idiotype antibody therapy of B-cell lymphoma: the addition of a short course of chemotherapy does not interfere with the antitumor effect nor prevent the emergence of idiotype-negative variant cells. *Blood* 1992; **80**: 1502–10.
104. Davis TA, Maloney DG, Czerwinski DK et al. Anti-idiotype antibodies can induce long-term complete remissions in non-Hodgkin's lymphoma without eradicating the malignant clone. *Blood* 1998; **92**: 1184–90.
105. Liu SJ, Sher YP, Ting CC et al. Treatment of B-cell lymphoma with chimeric IgG and single-chain Fv antibody-interleukin-2 fusion proteins. *Blood* 1988; **92**: 2103–12.
106. Bataille R, Barlogie B, Lu ZY et al. Biological effects of anti-interleukin-6 murine monoclonal antibody in advanced multiple myeloma. *Blood* 1995; **86**: 685–91.
107. Peest D, Leo R, Bloche S et al. Low-dose recombinant interleukin-2 therapy in advanced multiple myeloma. *Br J Haematol* 1995; **89**: 328–37.
108. Kolb HJ, Mittermuller J, Clemm CH et al. Donor leukocyte transfusions for treatment of recurrent chronic myelogenous leukemia in marrow transplant patients. *Blood* 1990; **76**: 2462–5.
109. Or R, Mehta J, Naparstek E et al. Successful T cell-depleted allogeneic bone marrow transplantation in a child with recurrent multiple extramedullary plasmacytomas. *Bone Marrow Transplant* 1992; **10**: 381–2.
110. Collins RH Jr, Pineiro LA, Nemunaitis JJ et al. Transfusion of donor buffy coat cells in the treatment of persistent or recurrent malignancy after allogeneic bone marrow transplantation. *Transfusion* 1995; **35**: 891–8.
111. Tricot G, Vesole DH, Jagannath S et al. Graft-versus myeloma effect: proof of principal. *Blood* 1996; **87**: 1196–8.
112. Verdonck LF, Lokhorst HM, Dekker AW et al. Graft-versus-myeloma effect in two cases. *Lancet* 1996; **347**: 800–1.
113. Lokhorst HM, Schattenberg A, Cornelissen JJ et al. Donor leukocyte infusions are effective in relapsed multiple myeloma after allogeneic bone marrow transplantation. *Blood* 1997; **90**: 4206–11.
114. Hu HM, Urba WJ, Fox BA. Gene-modified tumor vaccine with therapeutic potential shifts tumor-specific T cell response from a type 2 to a type 1 cytokine profile. *J Immunol* 1998; **161**: 3033–41.
115. Bergmann L, Mitrou PS, Kelker W et al. T-cell subsets in malignant lymphomas and monoclonal gammopathies. *Scand J Haematol* 1985; **34**: 170–6.
116. Hicks MJ, Durie BGM, Slymen DJ. Low circulating T-helper cells in relapsing multiple myeloma. *J Clin Lab Anal* 1989; **3**: 202–8.

7

Bone disease in myeloma

James R Berenson

CONTENTS • **Introduction** • **Biology** • **Bone resorbing factors** • **Assessment of myeloma bone disease** • **Treatment of myeloma bone disease** • **Radiotherapy** • **Surgery** • **Drug therapy**

INTRODUCTION

Some of the major clinical manifestations of myeloma are related to osteolytic bone destruction.[1] Even patients responding to chemotherapy may have progression of skeletal disease,[2,3] and recalcification of osteolytic lesions is rare. Bone disease can lead to pathologic fractures, spinal cord compression, hypercalcemia, and pain, and is a major cause of morbidity and mortality.[4]

These complications result from asynchronous bone turnover wherein increased osteoclastic bone resorption is not accompanied by a comparable increase in bone formation. The increase in osteoclast activity in myeloma is mediated by the release of osteoclast-stimulating factors.[5,6] These factors are produced locally in the bone marrow microenvironment by cells of tumor and non-tumor origin.[6,7] The enhanced bone loss results from the interplay between the osteoclasts, tumor cells, and other, non-malignant, cells in the bone marrow microenvironment.

Bisphosphonates are specific inhibitors of osteoclastic activity and are effective in the treatment of hypercalcemia associated with malignancies.[8,9,10] These agents have been evaluated alone and as adjunctive therapy to primary anticancer treatment in patients with cancers involving the bone, including myeloma.[11–15] Oral etidronate given daily showed no clinical benefit,[3] while the use of oral clodronate daily showed variable clinical results in three randomized trials.[12,16] Oral administration of pamidronate was ineffective in reducing the skeletal complications of these patients.[17] A large randomized double-blind study was conducted in which stage III myeloma patients received either pamidronate (90 mg) or placebo as a 4-hour infusion every 4 weeks for 21 cycles in addition to antimyeloma chemotherapy.[18,19] This intravenously administered bisphosphonate significantly reduced the development of skeletal complications, and improved the survival of patients who had failed first-line chemotherapy. Ongoing studies are evaluating newer and more potent bisphosphonates such as ibandronate and zoledronic acid. A number of other types of new anti-bone-resorptive agents are also in early clinical development.

BIOLOGY

Much progress has been made over the past few years in better defining the biological basis of bone loss in myeloma patients. Using bone histomorphometry, increased bone resorption with both increased eroded surfaces and mean erosion depth has been clearly demonstrated in myeloma patients.[20,21] This excessive bone resorption has been shown to occur in the proximity of the tumor cells themselves, even in patients without obvious lytic bone disease.[22] Patients in remission and the uninvolved marrow of patients with solitary plasmacytomas do not show this excessive bone resorption.[7] This observation points to the importance of the bone marrow microenvironment in causing local destruction of bone, and suggests that this may be mediated by direct intercellular means as well as local release of bone resorbing factors. Even patients presenting with early myeloma show this phenomenon. In patients with monoclonal gammopathy of undetermined significance (MGUS), the presence of increased bone resorption is associated with a greater likelihood of developing full-blown myeloma.[23]

Although osteoclast size appears to be normal in these patients, there appears to be increased recruitment, survival and activation of these cells.[24] Obviously, enhanced osteoclastic activity would not be associated with enhanced bone loss if there were no accompanying loss in bone formation.[7,23] This uncoupling of bone process (i.e. increased bone resorption in the presence of a reduction in bone formation) is the hallmark of myeloma patients with osteolytic bone disease. Interestingly, in the one-fourth of patients who present without these lesions, this uncoupling process has not been observed.[25] These patients often have both enhanced bone resorption and bone formation. In addition, osteocalcin, a marker of bone formation activity, has been shown to be decreased in patients with lytic bone disease, whereas those patients without evidence of lytic disease had higher osteocalcin levels.[26] In support of the important relationship of bone disease to overall outcome in these patients, serum osteocalcin levels were shown to be inversely related to survival in one study.[27]

BONE RESORBING FACTORS

The landmark studies of Mundy and colleagues[28] suggested the presence of osteoclast activating factors in the supernatants derived from cultures of both human myeloma cell lines and freshly obtained myeloma bone marrow. Although early work suggested that interleukin (IL)-1β and lymphotoxin (tumor necrosis factor (TNF)-β) were these factors, more recent studies have implicated other factors, including IL-6, IL-11, transforming growth factor β (TGF-β), macrophage colony-stimulating factor (M-CSF), hepatocyte growth factor (HGF), matrix metalloproteinases (MMPs), macrophage inflammatory protein 1α (MIP-1α), and a receptor for activation of NF-κB (RANK – a new member of the TNF receptor family) and its ligand (RANKL). See Table 7.1.

IL-1β

Controversy exists as to the importance of IL-1β in myeloma bone resorption as well as that of the cells that produce this cytokine in the myeloma microenvironment. Although IL-1β is clearly increased in supernatants from unseparated fresh myeloma bone marrow samples,[29] recent attempts to determine whether the malignant cells themselves were producing this factor have produced conflicting results.[30–34] The role of IL-1β in stimulating bone resorption has been shown in some studies using bone organ cultures, and this activity has been blocked by antibodies to this cytokine.[31–33] The inhibitors of IL-1β function, the soluble IL-1 receptor and IL-1 receptor antagonist, have been shown to be able to completely inhibit the bone resorption generated by supernatants derived from unfractionated myeloma bone marrow.[35] However, other workers have not confirmed the importance of IL-1β in stimulating bone resorption in myeloma patients.[36]

TNF-α and TNF-β

Early studies suggested that TNF-β was an important factor in enhancing bone resorption in myeloma patients.[37] However, more recent studies have failed to confirm these initial

Table 7.1 Cytokines in myeloma bone disease

Protein[a]	Source	Effect on		
		Growth	Apoptosis	Bone disease
IL-1β	Stroma/ ? tumor			+++
TNF-α	Stroma	+/−	−	+
IL-6	Stroma/occasionally tumor	++	−−	+
HGF	Tumor	++		++
TGF-β	Stroma			+
M-CSF	Stroma			+
MMPs	Stroma/tumor			+
Sydecan-1	Tumor	−	+	−
MIP-1α	Stroma/tumor			+++
RANKL	Stroma/tumor	+?	+?	+++

[a] See text for explanation of abbreviations.

results, and have not even shown increased secretion of this cytokine from bone marrow cells derived from myeloma patients.[29,30] TNF-α has been shown to be an important bone-resorbing cytokine, and has been found in increased amounts in the supernatants from unfractionated myeloma bone marrow,[29,30] and other studies have also suggested its production by the malignant cells.[35]

The effects of TNF-α and several other cytokines, including IL-1, are mediated by stimulation of the proteolytic breakdown of IκB, which leads to the release of NF-κB. This enhancer translocates into the nucleus, where it induces transcription of specific genes, some of which are involved in enhancing bone resorption as well as increasing myeloma tumor burden. The importance of NF-κB in bone resorption is supported by studies showing that NF-κB-knockout mice show osteopetrotic bones.[38] A number of other proteins involved in bone resorption, including RANK (see below), also utilize the NF-κB signaling pathway. This enhancer protein represents a new therapeutic target for reducing tumor burden as well as bone loss in myeloma patients.

IL-6

IL-6 has been shown to be a critical factor in stimulating growth and preventing apoptosis of the malignant cells in myeloma[39]. Although early studies suggested that tumor cells in myeloma produced IL-6,[40] most studies have shown that IL-6 is largely produced by the bone marrow stromal cells and that this production is enhanced by adhesion of tumor cells.[41] In addition, IL-6 has been shown to play a major role in bone disease.[42] IL-6 has been shown to inhibit bone formation.[43] It stimulates the development of osteoclasts[42] but also has been shown to promote osteoblasts. Interestingly, IL-6 is produced in large quantities by both of these cell types.[42,44] The use of anti-IL-6 antibodies clinically has demonstrated the importance of this cytokine in stimulating bone loss in myeloma patients.[45] It has also been shown that both IL-1 and TNF-α stimulate IL-6,[46] and that IL-6 is capable of synergizing with IL-1 in the stimulation of osteoclasts.[47] In addition to IL-6, its soluble receptor (gp80) is also important in this process. Specifically, when gp80 that is present in large amounts in the myeloma bone marrow becomes associated with IL-6, it stimulates myeloma growth[48] as well as osteoclast formation.[49] Thus, IL-6 and gp80 together play dual roles in increasing both tumor burden and bone loss in myeloma patients.

TGF-β

TGF-β has been shown to be produced by both tumor cells and stromal cells in myeloma bone marrow.[50] It plays an important role in the pathogenesis of metastatic bone disease in breast cancer.[51] In the bone milieu, TGF-β is capable of stimulating parathyroid hormone-related peptide (PTHRP) release from breast cancer cells, which in turn stimulates bone resorption and more TGF-β release from the bone microenvironment. TGF-β greatly increases the differentiation of osteoclast precursors from monocyte precursors by RANKL and M-CSF (see below).[52] In myeloma, TGF-β has been shown to stimulate IL-6 production by tumor cells and stromal cells, which may similarly enhance bone resorption in addition to stimulating tumor growth.[50] Interestingly, another member of the TGF-β family, bone morphogenetic protein 2 (BMP-2), has been shown to be capable of both enhancing bone formation[53] and inducing apoptosis of myeloma cells.[54] However, this protein may also enhance osteoclast function.[55]

RANK and RANKL

A recently identified receptor for activation of NF-κB (RANK), which is a member of the TNF receptor family, and its ligand (RANKL) have been shown to be key players in the development of osteoclasts.[56] Unlike other soluble bone-resorbing factors, the activity of these molecules requires direct cell-to-cell contact. It has been known for some time that osteoclastogenesis requires the direct interaction of osteoblasts or stromal cells with osteoclasts. The identification of RANK expressed on the surface of osteoclasts and RANKL on osteoblasts and stromal cells explains how this interaction leads to osteoclast development. TNF-α itself is capable of stimulating osteoblasts to increase expression of RANKL, although TNF-α may stimulate osteoclast differentiation by a mechanism that is independent of the RANKL–RANK interaction.[57] Malignant plasma cells from myeloma patients have been shown to express RANKL,[58,59] so that it is possible that the tumor cells themselves may directly stimulate osteoclast development in the myeloma bone marrow environment.

Importantly, there is a soluble decoy receptor called osteoprotegerin (OPG) that binds RANKL and prevents the binding of the ligand to RANK.[56] In fact, animals lacking OPG show profound osteoporosis.[60] It is the delicate balance between soluble OPG and RANKL that determines the amount of bone loss. In two separate studies involving murine models, OPG prevented and reversed hypercalcemia of malignancy[61] and blocked cancer-induced bone destruction and bone pain without obvious toxicity.[62] Because of these promising preclinical results, OPG is now being evaluated in early clinical trials in myeloma and breast cancer patients with bone metastases. Since myeloma tumor cells express RANKL, it is possible that blockage of the RANKL–RANK interaction may not only reduce osteoclast stimulation but also have inhibitory effects on the tumor cells themselves. Indeed, two recent studies show that inhibition of the RANK–RANKL interaction by either RANK-Fc or TR-Fc (TRANCE antagonist) reduces both bone loss as well as tumor burden in SCID–hu murine models of myeloma.[63,64]

Other factors

M-CSF is present in increased amounts in the serum of myeloma patients, and correlates with tumor load.[65,66] This cytokine is capable of attracting osteoclast precursors as well as enhancing survival of osteoclasts.[67,68,69] Although M-CSF along with RANKL (see below) are all that is required for osteoclastogenesis to occur in vitro, the role of M-CSF in myeloma bone disease remains unclear.

IL-11 stimulates osteoclastogenesis and inhibits bone formation.[70] It has been shown to be produced by osteoblasts, and is present in culture supernatants of bone marrow cells from myeloma patients.[71] It stimulates RANKL expression by osteoblasts. In addition, recent studies have shown that HGF, which has been shown to be produced by malignant plasma cells,[72] may also induce IL-11 secretion by osteoblasts.[71] HGF is a potent stimulator of bone resorption.[73,74] Other cytokines, such as IL-1, are capable of potentiating the effect of HGF on IL-11 secretion. High serum levels of HGF are associated with a poor prognosis in myeloma patients.[75]

Matrix metalloproteinases (MMPs) have been shown to play an important role in stimulating bone resorption, since their inhibitors, called TIMPs (tissue inhibitors of metalloproteinases), can prevent bone resorption.[76–78] Specifically, MMP-9 has been shown to be expressed by the tumor cells in myeloma patients, whereas the bone marrow stromal cells produce MMP-1 and MMP-2.[79] In addition, co-culture of stromal cells with myeloma cells upregulates MMP-1 secretion. These specific MMPs have been shown to play a critical role in directly degrading matrix and promoting metastasis.[80] The amount of MMP-2 secretion predicted the progression of myeloma in one clinical study.[81]

Syndecan-1, a heparan sulfate proteoglycan, has been shown to be expressed on the surface of myeloma cells.[82] This molecule is actively released from the cell surface of the tumor cells, and has been demonstrated to reduce both tumor burden and bone destruction in animal and in vitro myeloma models.[83] Syndecan-1 inhibits osteoclast differentiation while stimulating osteoblast formation, and SCID mice injected with the human myeloma cell line ARH-77 transfected with this gene were less likely to develop lytic bone disease.

Recently, MIP-1α has been identified as an important factor involved in myeloma bone disease.[84] Levels of this cytokine are also elevated in the bone marrow of patients with myeloma. It is capable of inducing osteoclast formation in vitro, and antibodies to it block the induction of osteoclast formation by fresh bone marrow plasma from myeloma patients. The importance of MIP-1α in inducing myeloma bone loss has been reinforced by a recent study showing that an antisense construct to this molecule reduces bone loss in SCID mice containing a human myeloma cell line.[85] In addition, this chemokine attracts and activates monocytes, and is a potent inhibitor of early hematopoiesis.

There is evidence for an increasing role of angiogenesis in the pathogenesis of myeloma.[81,86] It is clear that vascular endothelial growth factor (VEGF) is produced by malignant plasma cells, and the receptors that bind this factor are expressed on bone marrow stromal cells.[87] In fact, recent results show that VEGF increases IL-6 production by bone marrow stromal cells from myeloma patients.[88] This may indirectly lead to increased bone loss in these patients. Until recently, it was not clear that VEGF had any direct role in bone resorption. However, it is now clear that VEGF can replace M-CSF in leading to early osteoclast development.[89]

ASSESSMENT OF MYELOMA BONE DISEASE

Plain radiographs and bone scans

Because the major clinical manifestations of myeloma are related to bone disease, the importance of assessing its status cannot be overestimated. A variety of techniques have been used to evaluate bone disease in myeloma (Table 7.2). Early detection of lesions at risk of fracture or of leading to cord compression allows prompt use of prophylactic surgery or radiotherapy. In addition, determination of changes in bone disease is an important part of assessing the patient's response to systemic treatment. The gold standard has been the use of plain radiographs of the skull, spine, pelvis, and long bones of the upper and lower extremities. One study has shown that patients with normal X-rays have the worst prognosis, whereas those with minimal lytic changes have the longest survival.[90] Patients with either osteoporosis alone or extensive lytic lesions had an intermediate prognosis.[90] Although older studies suggest that the

Table 7.2 Assessing myeloma bone disease

Plain radiographs – skeletal survey
Bone scan
Magnetic resonance imaging (MRI)
Bone densitometry
^{99m}Tc-MIBI scan (experimental)
Positron emission tomography (PET) scan
Bone resorption markers: pyridinoline, deoxypyridinoline, ICTP,[a] N-telopeptide
Bone formation markers: alkaline phosphatase, osteocalcin, PINP[b]

[a] C-terminal telopeptide of type I collagen. [b] N-terminal propeptide of type I procollagen.

lytic lesions that make up myeloma bones are not well demonstrated using bone scans,[91,92] a recent study suggests that this modality may be useful, especially in lesions in the ribs, vertebral bodies and sternum.[93] On the other hand, the skull, the extremities, and the pelvic bones were better evaluated with plain radiographs in this study. In most cases, bone scans are unnecessary as part of the routine evaluation of myeloma bone disease.

Bone histomorphometry

Although bone histomorphometry may be effective in assessing the extent of bone loss at individual sites,[8] its usefulness is limited by both the invasiveness of the procedure and the heterogeneous nature of bone involvement in these patients. The expertise of an experienced bone pathologist is required for interpretation of the results.

Bone densitometry

In order to gain a better idea of general bone status in these patients, the use of dual-energy X-ray absorptiometry (DEXA) has now been evaluated in some centers.[94,95] This technique has clearly provided important information in patients with osteoporosis with respect to risk of fractures and response to therapeutic interventions.[96] Early studies in myeloma patients have shown marked bone loss, and have suggested that changes in bone density correlate with clinical stage and risk of fractures.[94,95] Although treatment with oral glucocorticoids effectively lowers tumor burden in these patients, its use has also been shown to be associated with loss of bone mineral density.[95] DEXA has been used to assess changes in bone density in myeloma patients treated with bisphosphonates, and has shown marked increases in patients receiving intravenous pamidronate alone as their antimyeloma therapy in an ongoing phase II trial.[97] In addition, a recently completed randomized phase II clinical trial evaluating pamidronate and three dose levels of zoledronic acid for 280 patients with myeloma and breast cancer with osteolytic bone disease showed marked increases in bone mineral density among patients receiving either bisphosphonate.[98] Among patients receiving zoledronic acid, those individuals receiving the lowest dose (0.4 mg) showed the smallest increases in bone density and were more likely to develop skeletal-related bone complications. These studies have begun to suggest the usefulness of evaluating bone densitometry in patients receiving bisphosphonate treatment for myeloma bone disease. However, whether bone densitometry will be predictive of the efficacy of bisphosphonate treatment or of the risk of developing skeletal complications during the course of an individual's disease still remains to be determined.

Magnetic resonance imaging (MRI)

MRI techniques are increasingly being used in assessing myeloma patients. These procedures are much more sensitive in detecting lesions that are not identified by plain radiographs. In the small subset of patients (approximately 20%) with normal MRI scans, the clinical features suggest earlier-stage disease and the prognosis appears to be better.[99] When the MRI scan is abnormal, it generally demonstrates three patterns, including diffuse involvement without the appearance of normal marrow signal, nodular or focal areas of replacement of normal marrow, or multiple tiny areas of replacement.[100] Studies demonstrate that patients with diffuse involvement have the worst outlook, with decreased hemoglobin and increased plasma cell loads.[99] MRI may be particularly useful in determining which patients with early myeloma will develop active disease.[101] Approximately 2% of patients with plasma cell dyscrasias present with a solitary bony lesion. Although radiotherapy may effectively eliminate this tumor, most patients eventually develop myeloma.[102] It is in these patients that MRI may be especially useful in predicting outcome. The presence of other bone lesions on the MRI scan is associated with an earlier progression to myeloma than in those patients with normal MRI scans.[103] However, no studies have shown that additional interventions at the time of diagnosis in this subset of patients change the clinical outcome.

In patients with more advanced myeloma, MRI is particularly useful in the evaluation of spinal cord compression, but its use as a routine procedure in these patients has not been well established. However, the presence of more than 10 focal lesions or diffuse involvement in the spine predicted the earlier development of vertebral compression fractures in these patients.[104,105] On the other hand, another study showed a lack of correlation between MRI-identified lesions and the risk of vertebral fractures.[106]

With the increasing use of MRI in evaluating myeloma patients at diagnosis, the modality has also been used to assess response to treatment. Despite effective chemotherapy, most MRI scans remain abnormal, although there does appear to be an improvement in their appearance in responding patients.[106–108] However, until the cost of this procedure is reduced, it is unlikely to gain widespread use in the routine follow-up of myeloma patients.

Other radionuclide scans

Recently, a new radionuclide tracer has been shown to predict overall disease status in these patients. Patterns of uptake of a new radionuclide tracer, technetium-99m 2-methoxyisobutylisonitrile (^{99m}Tc-MIBI, ^{99m}Tc-sestamibi), have been shown useful in predicting the stage of disease and current clinical status of myeloma patients.[109,110] The use of position emission tomography (PET) scans to evaluate patients with myeloma bone disease is now being undertaken, but its role remains unknown.

Markers of bone resorption and bone formation

A variety of markers of bone resorption and formation have been used to assess bone disease in myeloma patients. Patients with myeloma show the expected increases in bone resorption markers such as the C-terminal telopeptide of type I collagen (ICTP), pyridinoline, and deoxypyridinoline, and decreases in bone formation markers such as osteocalcin.[26,27,111,112] In addition, a decrease in osteocalcin level or higher ICTP concentrations predict a shortened survival in myeloma. In a placebo-controlled randomized Finnish clinical trial involving oral clodronate,[113] higher baseline levels of the N-terminal propeptide of type I procollagen (PINP – a product of growing osteoblasts), ICTP, and alkaline phosphatase (AP) were associated with a worse survival. PINP and ICTP levels decreased dramatically during clodronate treatment. Similarly, treatment with oral risedronate reduced urinary pyridinoline/creatinine and deoxypyridinoline/creatinine ratios as well as the bone formation markers AP and osteocalcin plasma levels.[114] Monthly administration of intravenous pamidronate is also associated with a decrease in both bone resorption and bone formation markers.[18] In the Finnish clodronate trial, a decrease in these markers during clodronate therapy was associated with better survival. In current clinical trials evaluating newer bisphosphonates, it is being determined whether baseline values or changes in these markers predict for the development of new skeletal complications and whether these agents will be clinically effective in individual cases. In a recent study conducted in myeloma patients undergoing high-dose therapy and autologous transplantation, bone resorption markers were elevated even among patients in remission pre transplant.[115] However, bone resorption markers normalized in most patients several months following the transplant procedure.

TREATMENT OF MYELOMA BONE DISEASE

Until the early 1950s, radiotherapy and surgery were the only treatment modalities available to the myeloma patient. Although both could effectively palliate the majority of patients, these interventions had little impact on the overall course of the disease. With the development of effective chemotherapy, the role of these modalities became of secondary importance in the overall management of the myeloma patient. With the advent of hemibody irradiation, total-body irradiation, and bone-seeking radionuclides as part of high-dose therapy regimens, radiation treatment may become recognized as an important part of the systemic management of myeloma (see Chapter 21 for a detailed discussion).

RADIOTHERAPY

Early studies showed the exquisite sensitivity of myeloma cells to radiation.[116] This treatment modality may be curative in some patients with solitary plasmacytoma of bone or extramedullary sites, although the majority of these patients will eventually progress to myeloma. Most patients with myeloma will require radiotherapy at some time in the course of their disease. The most common indication for radiotherapy is a painful lesion.[117,118] The vast majority of patients achieve pain relief with local radiotherapy at a dose of approximately 3000 cGy given in 10–15 fractions.[116] Occasional patients with more extensive bone pain may benefit from more extensive hemibody irradiation.[119,120] Other indications for radiotherapy may include treatment of impending or actual pathologic fractures, spinal cord compression, tumors causing local neurologic problems, and large soft tissue plasma cell tumors.[119] Approximately 10% of patients with myeloma will develop spinal cord compression, and the immediate use of systemic glucocorticoids and radiotherapy is important to prevent the development of a permanent neurologic deficit. Radiotherapy has also been evaluated in preventing the development of new vertebral fractures in myeloma patients with neurologic complications.[121] In this small non-randomized study, there was some suggestion that fewer vertebral fractures occurred in irradiated vertebrae than in unirradiated ones as assessed by MRI. However, caution must be used in the application of radiotherapy, since this will result in permanent bone marrow damage in the treated areas. The importance of this point cannot be overemphasized in the case of a patient whose overall clinical status depends upon the ability to tolerate chemotherapeutic agents that cause loss of bone marrow function. A study has shown that irradiation of the entire shaft of the long bone is probably not necessary in most cases.[122] Even in the few cases showing recurrence outside the previously irradiated field, palliation with radiotherapy was effective.

A novel radiotherapeutic approach for myeloma patients based on the bone-seeking nature of phosphonates has been recently initiated in the context of high-dose therapy and autologous peripheral blood stem cell transplantation (PBSCT).[123] Specifically, the radionuclide holmium-166 has been attached to a tetraphosphonate and given to myeloma patients prior to high-dose melphalan with or without total-body irradiation followed by PBSCT. Preliminary results evaluating its antimyeloma effect are encouraging, with high complete remission rates, although its specific role in managing bone disease was not evaluated.

SURGERY

Surgical intervention may be required in patients with an impending or actual fracture or a destabilized spine. Several recent reports have suggested that this modality is underutilized in myeloma patients with either long bone or vertebral fractures. In some patients, the presence of disease that is not evident radiographically in areas adjacent to the surgical site may impede the success of the procedure. Most patients also require radiotherapy in conjunction with the surgical procedure. Importantly, consideration must be given to the patient's overall clinical status in decisions regarding the timing of surgery.

DRUG THERAPY

Earlier attempts to reduce the skeletal complications of myeloma involving large randomized trials with sodium fluoride either alone or in combination with calcium, and androgenic steroids proved unsuccessful.[3,124,125] In addition, gallium nitrate was evaluated in one published study that suggested both a decrease in bone pain and loss of total body calcium with this treatment, but this trial was open-label, involving only 13 patients.[126]

Bisphosphonates

Most of the recent studies have evaluated whether a variety of bisphosphonates administered either orally or intravenously have an impact on skeletal disease as well as its clinical manifestations. Bisphosphonates are specific inhibitors of osteoclastic activity, and are effective in the treatment of hypercalcemia associated with malignancies.[10,127]

Pharmacology of bisphosphonates

Pyrophosphates are compounds that contain two phosphonate groups bound to a common oxygen, and are potent inhibitors of bone resorption in vitro. However, when used in vivo, they are readily hydrolyzed and are ineffective at reducing bone resorption.[9,10] By simply replacing the oxygen with a carbon, the molecules become resistant to hydrolysis and yet remain active as inhibitors of bone resorption. With the carbon substitution, these synthetic compounds, known as bisphosphonates, contain two additional chains of variable structure (called R1 and R2) that have given rise to a large number of different drugs (Figure 7.1). Most bisphosphonates contain a hydroxyl group at R1, which allows high affinity for calcium crystals and bone mineral. Marked differences in anti-resorptive potency result from differences at the R2 site (Table 7.3). Most of the recently developed newer agents, which are more potent, contain a nitrogen-containing R2 moiety, in contrast to the earlier agents with simple halide or methyl R2 side-chains. In addition, the nitrogen-containing bisphosphonates also have different mechanisms of action than the older first-generation agents that lack a nitrogen atom in their R2 substituent (see below).

These drugs are poorly absorbed orally (usually <1%) and also poorly tolerated orally, with significant gastrointestinal toxicity (particularly esophagitis and esophageal ulcers). The bisphosphonates are almost exclusively eliminated through renal excretion, and significant nephrotoxicity can occur with these compounds. Because bisphosphonates have high affinity for

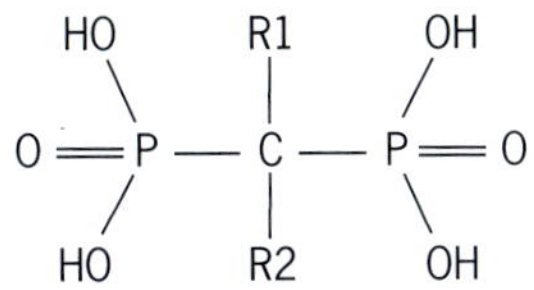

Figure 7.1 Backbone chemical structure of a bisphosphonate.

Table 7.3 Relative potency of bisphosphonates evaluated in multiple myeloma patients

Drug	N-containing	Potency
Etidronate	No	1
Clodronate	No	10
Pamidronate	Yes	100
Ibandronate	Yes	1000–10 000
Zoledronic acid	Yes	10 000–100 000

bone mineral, they are highly concentrated in bone. Once the drug becomes a part of the bone that is not remodeling, it is biologically inactive. As a result, continued administration of bisphosphonates is required to achieve the desired lasting inhibition of bone resorption.

Mechanisms of action of bisphosphonates

The inhibition of bone resorption occurs as a result of the effect of these drugs on osteoclasts both directly and indirectly. However, emerging data also suggest that these drugs may have an antimyeloma effect both directly and indirectly (Figure 7.2). Bisphosphonates were first shown to reduce development of osteoclasts from their precursors, inhibit movement of osteoclasts to the bone surface where they would normally resorb bone, and induce apoptosis of osteoclasts.[128] These drugs are also capable of inducing apoptosis of tumor cells from myeloma patients.[129] Interestingly, the induction of apoptosis in myeloma cells and osteoclasts has been shown to occur as a result of inhibition of the mevalonic acid pathway, particularly with nitrogen-containing bisphosphonates.[130,131] Interestingly, the statin drugs that lower cholesterol also block enzymes in this same pathway. Both types of drugs prevent prenylation of a number of proteins, including guanidine triphosphatases such as Ras, Rac, and Rho. Specifically, the addition of geranylgeranylated derivatives rather than farnesylated compounds is able to

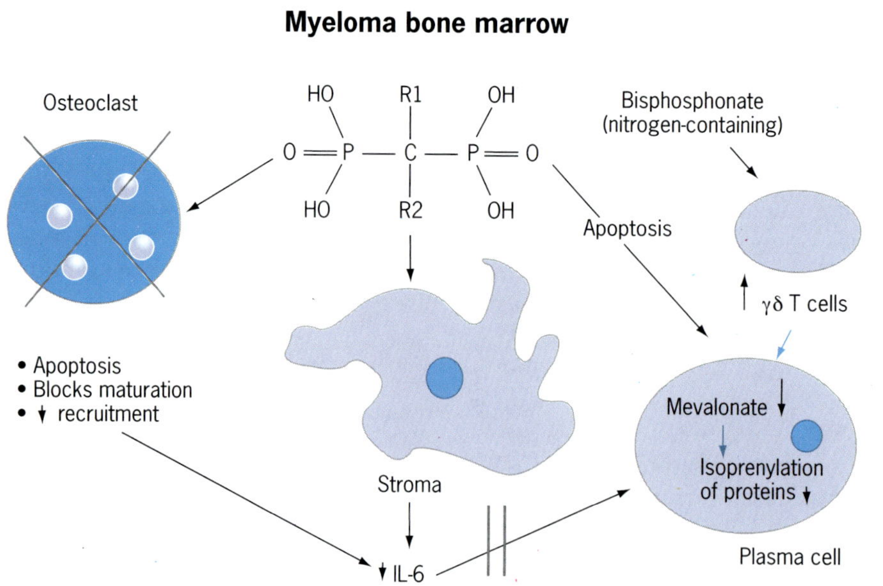

Figure 7.2 Possible mechanisms of the antitumor effect of bisphosphonates in myeloma bone marrow.

overcome the apoptosis-inducing effects of aminobisphosphonates and statin derivatives.[130] The nitrogen-containing bisphosphonates such as pamidronate have also been shown to enhance the differentiation and bone-forming activities of osteoblasts.[132] A potential indirect anti-bone-resorptive effect has recently been found for the nitrogen-containing bisphosphonates. These drugs reduce the production of the cytokine IL-6 from myeloma bone marrow stromal cells.[133,134] Studies have shown similar effects of bisphosphonates on IL-6 production by osteoblasts,[135] which are normally potent producers of IL-6. Not only is this cytokine capable of stimulating bone resorption but it is also an important growth factor and anti-apoptotic factor in myeloma.[39] Thus, reducing the availability of IL-6 in the bone microenvironment by exposure to bisphosphonates may not only reduce bone loss but also have an antimyeloma effect. Inhibition of the proteolytic activity of MMPs involved in bone destruction has been shown to occur in the presence of nitrogen-containing bisphosphonates.[134] Animal studies have shown that the nitrogen-containing bisphosphonates also have potent anti-angiogenic activity.[136] Anti-angiogenesis agents such as thalidomide have been shown to be effective antitumor agents in myeloma.[137] Thus, the anti-angiogenic effect of the bisphosphonates may contribute to the anti-bone-resorptive effect of these drugs (see above) as well as providing additional mechanisms by which they may have antimyeloma effects.

Another potential antitumor mechanism for these compounds was recently reported for pamidronate.[138] This drug was shown to induce expansion of $\gamma\delta$ T cells in myeloma patients receiving it intravenously, and to enhance the cytotoxic action of these cells against of malignant plasma cells. Thus, there is increasing in vitro evidence that bisphosphonates, especially the nitrogen-containing compounds, can have direct and indirect effects that result not only in less bone loss but also in less tumor burden in myeloma patients. In the murine 5T2 in vivo myeloma model, Radl and colleagues[139] showed that pamidronate reduced the tumor burden in the bone marrow of treated mice. Epstein and colleagues[140] have shown a reduction in both lytic bone metastases and improvement in survival in SCID mice implanted with fresh human myeloma bone marrow and fetal bone that received pamidronate. Zoledronic acid has been shown to produce similar effects in this animal model.[63] However, treatment with ibandronate in a murine model of myeloma showed only a reduction in lytic bone disease, without an impact on tumor burden.[141]

Bisphosphonates in myeloma bone disease

These agents have been evaluated alone and as adjunctive therapy to primary anticancer treatment in patients with cancers involving the bone, including myeloma.[2,12–19,142] Recent large placebo-controlled clinical trials have shown the efficacy of bisphosphonates in reducing skeletal complications in myeloma patients, and have suggested that these agents may also alter the overall course of the disease.

Although early studies involving bisphosphonates in myeloma patients suggested a reduction in bone pain and healing of lytic lesions, the trials involved relatively few patients.[13,14] Six large randomized trials of long-term bisphosphonate use have now been published, and involved the use of either the first-generation bisphosphonates etidronate or clodronate or the second-generation aminobisphosphonate pamidronate.[2,12,16–19,142]

Etidronate

In the Canadian study involving etidronate,[2] 173 newly diagnosed patients all received intermittent oral melphalan and prednisone as primary chemotherapy, and 166 were then randomized to receive either daily oral etidronate (5 mg/kg) or placebo until death or stopping the treatment due to side-effects. Although significant height loss occurred in both placebo and etidronate-treated patients, no difference was found between the two arms. Similarly, the other outcome measures (new fractures, hypercalcemic episodes, and bone pain) showed no differences between the two arms.

Clodronate

In a small study involving only 13 patients, use of daily oral clodronate was associated with a reduction in bone pain and lack of progression of bone lesions, in contrast to the clinical deterioration that occurred in the patients treated with placebo.[143] Histomorphometric analysis of bone biopsies showed decreases in osteoclast numbers with clodronate treatment, whereas patients receiving placebo showed a slight increase in these cells. Intravenously administered clodronate was evaluated in a randomized Italian study, which involved only 30 patients with active bone disease.[144] There was a reduction in new lytic lesions and pathologic fractures with the bisphosphonate therapy.

Three large randomized trials have been published using oral clodronate in myeloma patients. In the Finnish trial,[12] 350 previously untreated patients were entered, and 336 were randomized to receive either clodronate (2.4 g) or placebo daily for two years. All patients were also treated with intermittent oral melphalan and prednisolone. Only a little more than half of patients had radiographs completed at both study entry and two years. Given this limitation, the proportion of patients with progression of lytic lesions was less in the clodronate-treated group (12%) than in the placebo group (24%). However, the progression of overall pathologic fractures, as well as both vertebral and non-vertebral fractures, was not different between the arms. In addition, the number of patients developing hypercalcemia was similar in the two arms. Changes in pain index and use of analgesics were similar in both arms.

Clodronate has also been evaluated in an open-label randomized German trial involving 170 previously untreated patients.[142] In addition to intermittent intravenous melphalan and oral prednisone, these patients were randomized to receive either no bisphosphonate or oral clodronate (1.6 g) daily for a year. Unfortunately, premature termination occurred in more than half of the patients despite the short length of the study. The results showed no difference in progression of bone disease as assessed by plain radiographs in the two arms. However, there was a trend toward a reduction in the number of new progressive sites in the clodronate-treated group after 6 and 12 months, although this did not reach statistical significance. Although the proportion of patients without pain or analgesic requirement was higher in the clodronate group, the open-label design of this trial made it difficult to interpret these findings.

The UK Medical Research Council (MRC) has published the results of a large trial involving 536 recently diagnosed myeloma patients randomized to receive oral clodronate 1.6 g daily or placebo in addition to alkylating-agent-based chemotherapy.[16] The primary endpoints of the trial were unclear. However, after combining the proportion of patients developing either non-vertebral fractures or severe hypercalcemia, including those leaving the trial due to severe hypercalcemia, there were fewer clodronate-treated patients experiencing these combined events than placebo patients. However, the numbers of patients developing hypercalcemia were similar in the two arms. The number of patients experiencing non-vertebral fractures was lower in the clodronate group. Although vertebral fractures reportedly occurred in significantly fewer clodronate-treated patients than placebo patients, only half of the patients obtained at least one post-baseline radiograph. Back pain and poor performance status were not significantly different between the two groups, except at one time point (24 months). The proportions of patients requiring radiotherapy were similar in the two arms. There was no difference in time to first skeletal event or overall survival.

Pamidronate

In a randomized, double-blinded trial, a Danish–Swedish cooperative group evaluated daily oral pamidronate (300 mg/day) compared with placebo in 300 newly diagnosed myeloma patients also receiving intermittent melphalan and prednisone.[17] After a median duration of 18 months, there were no significant differences in the primary endpoint, defined as skeletal-related morbidity (bone fracture, surgery for impending fracture, vertebral collapse, or increase in number and/or size of lytic lesions), hypercalcemic episodes, or survival between the arms. Fewer episodes of severe pain and less height loss were observed in the oral pamidronate-treated patients, however.

Results of small open-label trials lasting up to 24 months suggested that infusional pamidronate disodium might be effective in reducing skeletal complications of myeloma.[13,14] Therefore, a large randomized, double-blinded study was conducted to determine whether monthly 90 mg infusions of pamidronate compared with placebo for 21 months reduced skeletal events in patients with myeloma who were receiving chemotherapy.[18,19] This study included patients with Durie–Salmon stage III myeloma and at least one osteolytic lesion. Unlike the etidronate and clodronate trials, which involved untreated patients, patients were required to receive an unchanged chemotherapy regimen for at least two months before enrolment. Patients were stratified according to their antimyeloma therapy at trial entry: stratum 1, first-line chemotherapy; stratum 2, second-line or greater chemotherapy. The primary endpoint, skeletal events (pathologic fractures, spinal cord compression associated with vertebral compression fracture, surgery to treat or prevent pathologic fracture or spinal cord compression associated with vertebral compression fracture, or radiation to bone) and secondary endpoints (hypercalcemia, bone pain, analgesic drug use, performance status, and quality of life) were assessed monthly. Importantly, although the chemotherapeutic regimen was not uniform at study entry, the types and numbers of chemotherapeutic regimens in the two groups were similar at study entry and during the trial.

At the preplanned primary endpoint after nine cycles of therapy,[18] the proportion of patients having any skeletal event was 41% in the placebo group but only 24% in the pamidronate group (Figure 7.3). In addition, the number of skeletal events per year in the patients treated with pamidronate was half of that in those receiving placebo. The proportion of pamidronate-treated patients with skeletal events was lower in both stratum 1 (first-line therapy) and stratum 2 ($\geqslant$ second-line therapy). The patients who received pamidronate also had significant decreases in bone pain and no increase in analgesic usage, and showed no deterioration in performance status and quality of life at the end of nine months. Similar to the results after nine cycles of therapy, the proportions of patients developing any skeletal event and the skeletal morbidity rate continued to remain significantly lower in the pamidronate group than the placebo group during the additional 12 cycles of treatment.[19] However, there were no differences between the treatment groups in the percentage of patients with healing or progression of osteolytic lesions.

Although overall survival in all patients was not significantly different between the two treatment groups, in patients who failed first-line chemotherapy (stratum 2) the median survival time was 21 months for pamidronate patients compared with 14 months for placebo patients (Figure 7.4).

These results show that the adjunctive use of bisphosphonates in addition to chemotherapy is superior to chemotherapy alone for myeloma patients with respect to bone complications. Bisphosphonate treatment should now be considered for all patients with myeloma and at least one osteolytic lesion.

The three large randomized studies with clodronate show inconsistent results with oral administration of this first-generation bisphosphonate.[12,16,142] Curiously, the Finnish trial using a larger daily dose[12] shows less effect than the MRC trial using a smaller amount of clodronate.[16] In addition, in the latter trial, although the drug had some effect in reducing fractures and severe hypercalcemia in these patients, it did not affect the time to first skeletal event or use of radiotherapy. Similarly, oral pamidronate has also not been effective in reducing the skeletal complications of myeloma.[17] Given the clinical results and the poor tolerability of oral agents, this route of administration for bisphosphonates is unlikely to be of much benefit in these patients. Clearly, intravenous pamidronate reduces skeletal complications as well as improving the quality of life of these patients.[18,19] Although 90 mg monthly is efficacious, the

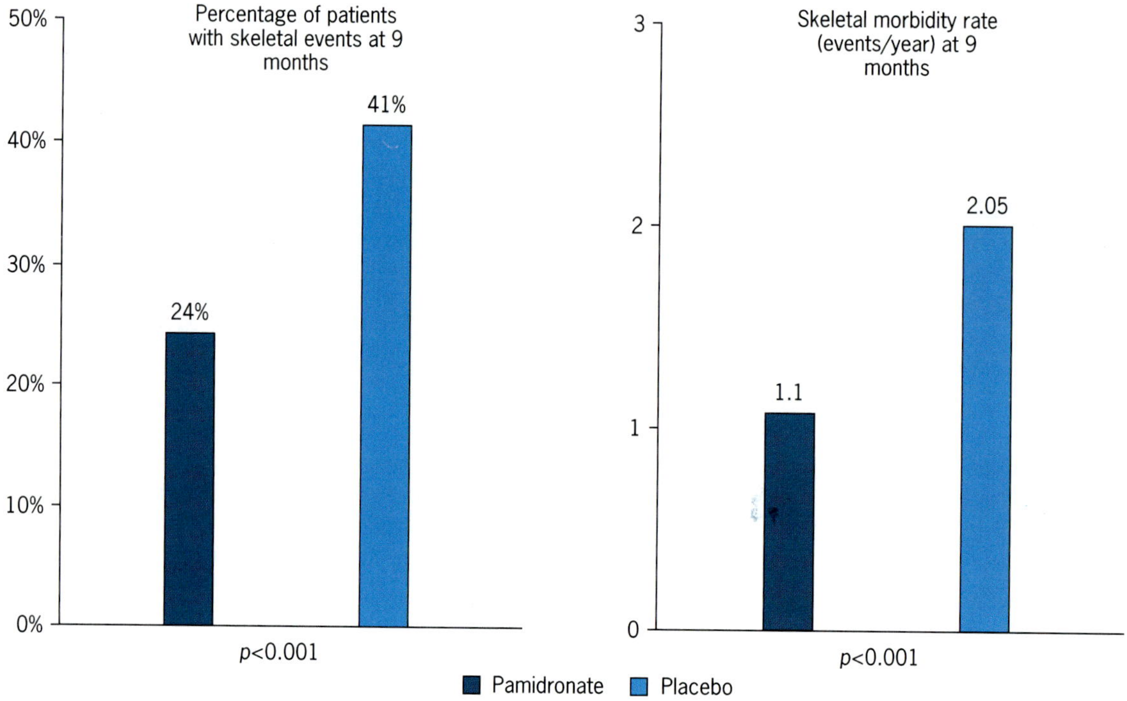

Figure 7.3 Time to first skeletal-related event (SRE) and mean number of SREs per year in myeloma patients treated with intravenous pamidronate or placebo (intent-to-treat patients).

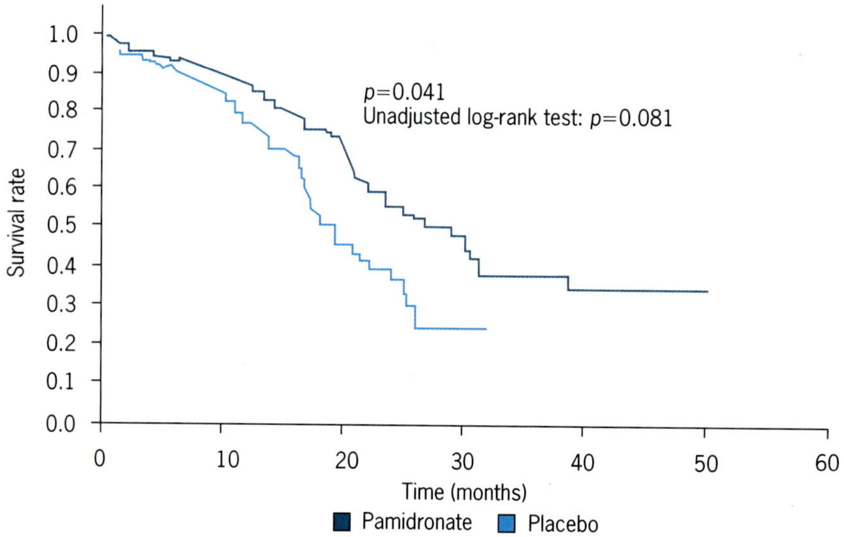

Figure 7.4 Kaplan–Meier estimates of survival in stratum 2 patients with myeloma treated with intravenous pamidronate or placebo. Survival was measured from randomization date to 1 February 1995. The median survival was 21 and 14 months in pamidronate ($n = 66$) and placebo ($n = 65$) patients, respectively. The log-rank test was adjusted for ECOG performance status and β_2-microglobulin level, which were the only prognostic variables significantly influencing survival.

optimal duration and dose of pamidronate are unknown, but patients should receive at least 21 months of treatment, based on the results of the published trial. Whether this drug is effective in earlier-stage disease or in patients without bone disease is unknown. The role of pamidronate in myeloma may go beyond simply inhibiting bone resorption and the resulting skeletal complications. Some preclinical studies suggest that it may have an antimyeloma effect either directly or indirectly (Figure 7.2), and the results of the large randomized clinical trial evaluating intravenous monthly pamidronate have shown that administration of this drug improves survival among patients who have failed first-line chemotherapy.

Newer bisphosphonates

The third-generation bisphosphonates zoledronic acid and ibandronate are more than 100 times as potent as second-generation aminobisphosphonates according to in vitro and animal in vivo studies.[145,146] They have recently entered clinical trials. Very small doses of these agents effectively restore normocalcemia in patients with tumor-induced hypercalcemia.[147,148] Recent results of a randomized study show the superiority of zoledronic acid (at either 4 or 8 mg) compared with pamidronate (90 mg) in reversing tumor-induced hypercalcemia in 287 patients.[127] Clinical evaluation of zoledronic acid and ibandronate in the treatment of bone metastases is in progress. Zoledronic acid can be given safely monthly over several minutes and produce similar antiresorptive effects at doses of 1.5 mg or more (as assessed by bone resorption marker) as 90 mg of monthly pamidronate.[149,150] The results from a randomized phase II study comparing monthly infusions of zoledronic acid (0.4, 2, or 4 mg as a five-minute infusion) compared with pamidronate (90 mg as a two-hour infusion) in 280 patients with lytic bone metastases (109 with myeloma) have been reported.[98] The proportion of patients with any skeletal-related event (SRE) was lower in the 2 mg and 4 mg zoledronic acid groups and the pamidronate group (30–35%) compared with the 0.4 mg zoledronic acid group (46%). These results are consistent with the two phase I trials suggesting that doses of less than 1.5 mg do not effectively suppress bone resorption markers. This phase II trial was not 'powered' to show superiority of zoledronic acid compared with pamidronate. It should be noted that the current recommended infusion time for zoledronate is 15 minutes.

An ongoing, larger phase III randomized trial is comparing higher doses of monthly infusional zoledronic acid with 90 mg pamidronate in patients with myeloma or breast cancer with osteolytic bone disease.

Ibandronate is another newer potent bisphosphonate. A phase III placebo-controlled trial of 214 stage II–III myeloma patients has been completed.[151] Patients received either monthly bolus injections of 2 mg of ibandronate or placebo injections in addition to their antineoplastic therapy. Ninety-nine patients in each group were evaluable for efficacy. The mean number of events per patient-year on treatment was similar in both groups (ibandronate 2.13 versus placebo 2.05). However, in the subgroup of ibandronate-treated patients showing a sustained reduction in bone resorption markers, there were fewer SREs per year. There was no difference in overall survival. Thus, this dose of ibandronate is inadequate to show significant effects in preventing skeletal complications in myeloma. As studies of both zoledronic acid and ibandronate are performed at higher doses of these newer agents, it is possible that these drugs not only may be more effective in palliating the devastating effects of bone disease in these patients but also may hold the promise of being able to improve overall survival while also improving quality of life.

REFERENCES

1. Mundy GR, Bertoline DR. Bone destruction and hypercalcemia in plasma cell myeloma. *Semin Oncol* 1986: **13**: 291–9.
2. Belch AR, Bergsagel DE, Wilson K et al. Effect of daily etidronate on the osteolysis of multiple myeloma. *J Clin Oncol* 1991; **9**: 1397–402.

3. Kyle RA, Jowsey J, Kelly PJ et al. Multiple myeloma bone disease. The comparative effect of sodium fluoride and calcium carbonate or placebo. *N Engl J Med* 1975; **293**: 1334–8.
4. Kyle RA. Multiple myeloma, review of 869 cases. *Mayo Clin Proc* 1975; **50**: 29–40.
5. Stashenko P, Dewhirst FE, Peros WJ et al. Synergistic interactions between interleukin 1, tumor necrosis factor, and lymphotoxin in bone resorption. *J Immunol* 1987; **138**: 1464–8.
6. Mundy GR, Mechanisms of osteolytic bone destruction. Bone 1991; **12**(Suppl 1): S1–6.
7. Bataille R, Chappard D, Basle M. Excessive bone resorption in human plasmacytomas: direct induction by tumor cells in vivo. *Br J Haematol* 1995; **90:** 721–4.
8. Berenson JR, Lipton A. Bisphosphonates in the treatment of malignant bone disease. *Annu Rev Med* 1999; **50**: 237–48.
9. Kanis JA, McCloskey EV, Taube T, et al: Rationale for the use of bisphosphonates in bone metastases. *Bone* 1991; **12**(Suppl 1): S13–18.
10. Fleisch H. Bisphosphonates: a new class of drugs in diseases of bone and calcium metabolism. In: *Recent Results in Cancer Research*, Vol 116: *Bisphosphonates and Tumor Osteolysis* (Brunner KW, Fleisch H, Senn H-J, eds). Berlin: Springer-Verlag, 1989: 1–28.
11. Lahtinen R, Laakso M, Palva I et al. Randomized, placebo-controlled multicentre trial of clodronate in multiple myeloma. *Lancet* 1992; **340**: 1049–52.
12. Man Z, Otero AB, Rendo P et al. Use of pamidronate for multiple myeloma osteolytic lesions. *Lancet* 1990; **335**: 663.
13. Thiebaud D, Leyuraz S, Von Fliedner V et al. Treatment of bone metastases from breast cancer and myeloma with pamidronate. *Eur J Cancer* 1991; **27**: 37–41.
14. Purohit OP, Anthony C, Radstone CR et al. High-dose intravenous pamidronate for metastatic bone pain. *Br J Cancer* 1994; **70**: 554–8
15. van Holten-Verzantvoort AATM, Kroon HM, Bijvoet OLM et al. Palliative treatment in patients with bone metastases from breast cancer. *J Clin Oncol* 1993; **11**: 491–8.
16. McCloskey, EV, MacLennan, CM, Drayson, MT et al. A randomized trial of the effect of clodronate on skeletal morbidity in multiple myeloma. *Br J Haematol* 1998; **101**: 317–25.
17. Brincker H, Westin J, Abildgaard N et al. Failure of oral pamidronate to reduce skeletal morbidity in multiple myeloma: a double-blind placebo-controlled trial. *Br J Haematol* 1998; **101**: 280–6.
18. Berenson JR, Lichtenstein A, Porter L et al. Efficacy of pamidronate in reducing the skeletal events in patients with advanced multilpe myeloma. *N Engl J Med* 1996; **334**: 488–93.
19. Berenson J, Lichtenstein A, Porter L et al. Long-term pamidronate treatment of advanced multiple myeloma patients reduces skeletal events. *J Clin Oncol* 1998; **16**: 593–602.
20. Bataille R, Chappard D, Alexandre C et al. Importance of quantitative histology of bone changes in monoclonal gammopathy. *Br J Cancer* 1986; **53**: 805–10.
21. Valentin-Opran A, Charhon SA , Meunier PJ et al. Quantitative histology of myeloma-induced bone changes, *Br J Haematol* 1982; **52**: 601–10.
22. Taube T, Beneton MNC, McCloskey EV et al. Abnormal bone remodelling in patients with myelomatosis and normal biochemical indices of bone resorption. *Eur J Haematol* 1992; **49**: 192–8.
23. Bataille R, Chappard D, Basle M. Quantifiable excess of bone resorption in monoclonal gammopathy is an early symptom of malignancy: a prospective study of 87 biopsies. *Blood* 1996; **87**: 4762–9.
24. Chappard D, Rossi JF, Bataille R et al. Cytomorphometry of osteoclasts demonstrates an abnormal population in B-cell malignancies but not in multiple myeloma. *Calcif Tissue Int* 1991; **48**: 13–17.
25. Bataille R, Chappard D, Marcelli C et al. Mechanism of bone destruction in multiple myeloma. The importance of an unbalanced process in determining the severity of myeloma. *J Clin Oncol* 1989; **7**: 1909–14.
26. Bataille R, Delmas PD, Chappard D, Sany J. Abnormal serum bone Gla protein levels in multiple myeloma. *Cancer* 1990; **66**: 167–72.
27. Carlson K, Ljunghall S, Simonsson B et al. Serum osteocalcin concentrations in patients with multiple myeloma – correlation with disease stage and survival. *J Intern Med* 1992; **231**: 133–7.
28. Mundy GR, Raisz LG, Cooper RA et al. Evidence for the secretion of an osteoclast stimulating factor in myeloma. *N Engl J Med* 1974; **291**: 1041–6.
29. Lichtenstein A, Berenson J, Norman D et al. Production of cytokines by bone marrow cells obtained from patients with multiple myeloma. *Blood* 1989; **74**: 1266–73.

30. Cozzolino F, Torcia M, Aldinucci D et al. Production of interleukin-1 by bone marrow myeloma cells. *Blood* 1989; **74**: 380–7.
31. Kawano M, Yamamoto I, Iwato K et al. Interleukin-1 beta rather than lymphotoxin as the major bone resorbing activity in human multiple myeloma. *Blood* 1989; **73**: 1646–9.
32. Yamamoto I, Kawano M, Sone T et al. Production of interleukin-1β, a potent bone resorbing cytokine, by cultured human myeloma cells. *Br J Haematol* 1989; **49**: 4242–6.
33. Bakkus MHC, Bakel-Van Peer KMJ, Adriaansen HJ et al. Detection of interleukin-1β and interleukin-6 in human multiple myeloma by fluorescent in situ hybridisation. *Leuk Lymphoma* 1991; **4**: 389–95.
34. Sati HIA, Greaves M, Apperley JF et al. Expression of Il-1β and TNFα mRNA by neoplastic plasma cells, detected by dual colour fluorescence in situ hybridisation. *Bone* 1997; **20**(Suppl): 63S.
35. Torcia M, Lucibello M, Vannier E et al. Modulation of osteoclast-activating factor activity of multiple myeloma bone marrow cells by different interleukin-1 inhibitors. *Exp Hematol* 1996; **24**: 868–74.
36. Alsina M, Boyce B, Devlin RD et al. Development of an in vivo model of human multiple myeloma bone disease. *Blood* 1996; **87**: 1495–501.
37. Garrett IR, Durie BGM, Nedwin GE et al. Production of lymphotoxin, a bone-resorbing cytokine, by cultured human myeloma cells. *N Engl J Med* 1987; **317**: 526–32.
38. Iotsova V, Caamano J, Loy J et al. Ostepetrosis in mice lacking NF-κ B1 and NF-κ B2. *Nature Med* 1997; **3**: 1285–9.
39. Klein B, Zhang XG, Lu Z-Y, Bataille R. Interleukin-6 in multiple myeloma. *Blood* 1995; **85**: 863–72.
40. Kawano M, Hirano T, Matsuda T et al. Autocrine generation and requirement of BSF-2/IL-6 for human multiple myelomas. *Nature* 1988; **332**: 83–5.
41. Uchiyama H, Barut BA, Mohrbacher A et al. Adhesion of human myeloma-derived cell lines to bone marrow stroma stimulates IL-6 secretion. *Blood* 1993; **82**: 3712–20.
42. Ishimi Y, Mijaura C, Jin CH et al. IL-6 is produced by osteoblasts and induces bone resorption. *J Immunol* 1990; **145**: 3297–303.
43. Hughes FJ, Howells GL, Interleukin-6 inhibits bone formation in vitro. *Bone Miner* 1993; **21**: 21–8.
44. Linkhart TA, Linkhart SG, McCharles DC et al. Interleukin-6 messager RNA expression and interleukin-6 protein secretion in cells isolated from normal human bone: regulation by interleukin-1. *J Bone Miner Res* 1991; **6**: 1285–94.
45. Bataille R, Barlogie B, Lu ZY et al. Biologic effects of anti-interleukin-6 murine monoclonal antibody in advanced multiple myeloma. *Blood* 1995; **86**: 685–91.
46. Dinarello CA. The biology of interleukin-1 and comparison to tumor necrosis factor. *Immunol Lett* 1987; **16**: 227–32.
47. Lacey DL, Grosso LE, Moser SA et al. IL-1-induced murine osteoblast IL-6 production is mediated by the type 1 IL-1 receptor and is increased by 1,25 dihydroxyvitamin D_3. *J Clin Invest* 1993; **91**: 1731–42
48. Gaillard JP, Bataille R, Brailly H et al. Increased and stable levels of functional soluble interleukin-6 receptor in sera of patients with monoclonal gammopathy, *Eur J Immunol* 1993; **23**: 820.
49. Tamura T, Udagawa N, Takahashi N et al. Soluble interleukin-6 receptor triggers osteoclast formation by interleukin-6. *Proc Natl Acad Sci USA* 1993; **90**: 11924–8.
50. Urashima M, Ogata A, Chauhan D et al. Transforming growth factor-β1: differential effects on multiple myeloma versus normal B cells. *Blood* 1996; **87**: 1928–38
51. Yoneda T. Cellular and molecular mechanisms of breast and prostate cancer metastasis to bone. *Eur J Cancer* 1998; **34**: 240–5.
52. Kaneda T, Nojima T, Nakagawa M et al. Endogenous production of TGF-β is essential for osteoclastogensis induced by a combination of receptor activator of NF-κB ligand and macrophage-colony stimulating factor. *J Immunol* 2000; **165**: 4254–63.
53. Rosen V, Thies RS. The BMP proteins in bone formation and repair. *Trends Genet* 1992; **8**: 97–102.
54. Kawamura C, Kizaki M, Yamato K et al. Bone morphogenetic protein-2 induces apoptosis in human myeloma cells with modulation of STAT3. *Blood* 2000; **96**: 2005–11.
55. Kaneko H, Arakawa T, Mano H et al. Direct stimulation of osteoclastic bone resorption by bone morphogenetic protein (BMP)-2 and expression of BMP receptors in mature osteoclasts. *Bone* 2000; **27**: 479–86.

56. Hofbauer LC. Osteoprotegerin ligand and osteoprotegerin: novel implications for osteoclast biology and bone metabolism. *Eur J Endocrinol* 1999; **141**: 195–210.
57. Kobayashi K, Takahashi N, Jimi E et al. Tumor necrosis factor α stimulates osteoclast differentiation by a mechanism independent of the ODF/RANKL–RANK interaction. *J Exp Med* 2000; **191**: 275–85.
58. Altamirano CV, Ma HJ, Parker KM et al. RANKL is expressed in malignant multiple myeloma (MM) cell lines. *Blood* 2000; **96**: 365a.
59. Shipman CM, Holen I, Lippitt JM et al. Tumor cells isolated from patients wiuth multiple myeloma express the critical osteoclastogenic factor, RANKL. *Blood* 2000; **96**: 360a.
60. Bucay N, Saroosi I, Dunstan CR et al. Osteoprotegerin-deficient mice develop early onset osteoporosis and arterial calcification. *Genes Dev* 1998; **12**: 1260–8.
61. Capparelli C, Kostenuik PJ, Morony S et al. Osteoprotegerin prevents and reverses hypercalcemia in a murine model of humoral hypercacemia of malignancy. *Cancer Res* 2000; **60**: 783–7.
62. Honore P, Luger NM, Sabino MAC et al. Osteoprotegerin blocks bone cancer-induced skeletal destruction, skeletal pain and pain-related neurochemical reorganization of the spinal cord. *Nature Med* 2000; **6**: 521–8.
63. Yaccoby S, Pearse R, Epstein J et al. Reciprocal relationship between myeloma-induced changes in the bone marrow microenvironment and myeloma cell growth. *Blood* 2000; **96**: 549a.
64. Pearse RN, Sordillo EM, Yaccoby S et al. Administration of the TRANCE-antagonist TR-Fc limits myeloma-induced bone destruction. *Blood* 2000; **96**: 549a.
65. Nakamura M, Merchav S, Carter A et al. Expression of a novel 3–5-kb macrophage colony-stimulating factor transcript in human myeloma cells. *J Immunol* 1989; **143**: 3543–7.
66. Janowska-Wieczorek A, Belch AR, Jacobs A et al. Increased circulating colony-stimulating factor-1 in patients with preleukemia, leukemia, and lymphoid malignancies. *Blood* 1991; **77**: 1796–803.
67. MacDonald BR, Mundy GR, Clark S et al. Effects of human recombinant CSF-GM and highly purified CSF-1 on the formation of multinucleated cells with osteoclast characteristics in long-term marrow cultures. *J Bone Miner Res* 1986; **1**: 227–33.
68. Sarma U, Flanagan AM, Macrophage colony-stimulating factor induces substantial osteoclast generation and bone resorption in human bone marrow cultures. *Blood* 1996; **88**: 2531–2540.
69. Fuller K, Owens JM, Jagger CJ et al. Macrophage colony-stimulating factor stimulates survival and chemotactic behaviour in isolated osteoclasts. *J Exp Med* 1993; **189**: 1733–44.
70. Girasole G, Passeri G, Jilka RL et al. Interleukin-11: a new cytokine critical for osteoclast development. *J Clin Invest* 1994; **93**: 1516.
71. Hjertner O, Torgersen ML, Seidel C et al. Hepatocyte growth factor (HGF) induces interleukin-11 secretion from osteoblasts: a possible role for HGF in myeloma-associated osteolytic bone disease. *Blood* 1999; **94**: 3883–8.
72. Borset M, Hjorth-Hansen H, Seidel C et al. Hepatocyte growth factor and its receptor c-Met in multiple myeloma. *Blood* 1996; **88**: 3998–4004.
73. Fuller K, Owens J, Chambers TJ. The effect of hepatocyte growth factor on the behaviour of osteoclasts. *Biochem Biophys Res Commun* 1995; **212**: 334–40.
74. Grano M, Galimi F, Zambonin G et al. Hepatocyte growth factor is a coupling factor for osteoclasts and osteoblasts in vitro. *Proc Natl Acad Sci USA* 1996; **93**: 7644–8.
75. Seidel C, Borset M, Turesson I et al. Elevated serum concentrations of hepatocyte growth factor in patients with multiple myeloma. *Blood* 1998; **91**: 806–12.
76. Conway JG, Wakefield JA, Brown RH et al. Inhibition of cartilage and bone destruction in adjuvant arthritis in the rat by a matrix metalloproteinase inhibitor. *J Exp Med* 1995; **182**: 449.
77. Hill PA, Docherty AJP, Bottomley KMK et al. Inhibition of bone resorption in vitro by selective inhibitors of gelatinase and collagenase. *Biochem J* 1995; **308**: 167.
78. Yoneda T, Sasaki A, Dunstan C et al. Inhibition of osteolytic bone metastasis of breast cancer by combined treatment with the bisphosphonate ibandronate and tissue inhibitor of the matrix metalloproteinase-2. *J Clin Invest* 1997; **99**: 2509–17.
79. Barille S, Akhoundi C, Collette M et al. Metalloproteinases in multiple myeloma: Production of matrix metalloproteinase-9 (MMP-9), activation of proMMP-2, and induction of MMP-1 by myeloma cells. *Blood* 1997; **90**: 1649–55.
80. Ray J, Stetler-Stevenson W. Gelatinase A activity directly modulates melanoma cell adhesion and spreading. *EMBO J* 1995; **14**: 908.
81. Vacca A, Ribatti D, Preta M et al. Bone marrow neovascularization, plasma cell angiogenic

potential, and matrix metalloproteinase-2 secretion parallel progression of human multiple myeloma. *Blood* 1999; **93**: 3064–73.

82. Ridley RC, Xiao H, Hata H et al. Expression of syndecan regulates human myeloma plasma cell adhesion to type I collagen. *Blood* 1993; **81**: 767–74
83. Dhodapkar MV, Abe E, Theus A et al. Syndecan-1 is a multifunctional regulator of myeloma pathobiology: control of tumor cell survival, growth, and bone cell differentiation. *Blood* 1998; **91**: 2679–88.
84. Choi SJ, Cruz JC, Craig F et al. Macrophage inflammatory protein 1-alpha is a potential osteoclast stimulatory factor in multiple myeloma. *Blood* 2000; **96**: 671–5.
85. Choi SJ, Alsina M, Oba Y et al. Antisense construct to MIP-1-alpha blocks bone destruction in an in vivo model of myeloma. *Blood* 2000; **96**: 549a.
86. Vacca A, Ribatti D, Roncalli L et al. Bone marrow angiogenesis and progression in multiple myeloma. *Br J Haematol* 1994; **87**: 505–8.
87. Bellamy WT, Richer L, Frutiger Y et al. Expression of vascular endothelial growth factor and its receptors in hematopoietic malignancies. *Cancer Res* 1999; **59**: 728–33.
88. Dankbar B, Padro T, Leo R et al. Vascular endothelial growth factor and interleukin-6 in paracrine tumor–stromal cell interactions in multiple myeloma. *Blood* 2000; **95**: 2630–6.
89. Niida S, Kaku M, Amano H et al. Vascular endothelial growth factor can substitute for macrophage colony-stimulating factor in the support of osteoclastic bone resorption. *J Exp Med* 1999; **190**: 293–8.
90. Smith DB, Scarffe JH, Eddleston B. The prognostic significance of X-ray changes at presentation and reassessment in patients with multiple myeloma. *Hematol Oncol* 1988; **6**: 1–6.
91. Bataille R, Chevalier J, Rossi M et al. Bone scintigraphy in plasma-cell myeloma. *Radiology* 1982; **145**: 801–4.
92. Woolfenden JM, Pitt MJ, Durie BGM et al. Comparison of bone scintigraphy and radiography in multiple myeloma. *Radiology* 1980; **134**: 723–8.
93. Agren B, Lonnqvist B, Bjorkstrand B et al. Radiography and bone scintigraphy in bone marrow transplant multiple myeloma patients. *Acta Radiol* 1997; **38**: 144–50.
94. Abildgaard N, Brixen K, Kristensen JE et al. Assessment of bone involvement in patients with multiple myeloma using bone densitometry. *Eur J Haematol* 1996; **57**: 370–6.
95. Diamond T, Levy S, Day P et al. Biochemical, histomorphometric and densitometric changes in patients with multiple myeloma: effects of glucocorticoid therapy and disease activity. *Br J Haematol* 1997; **97**: 641–8.
96. Cummings SR, Black DM, Thompson DE et al. Effect of alendronate on risk of fracture in women with low bone density but without vertebral fractures. *JAMA* 1998; **280**: 2077–82.
97. Berenson J, Webb I, Hennick K et al. A phase II dose-ranging trial of single-agent pamidronate for relapsed/refractory multiple myeloma. *Blood* 1998; **92**(Suppl 1): 107a.
98. Berenson J, Rosen LS, Howell A et al. Zoledronic acid reduces skeletal related events in patients with osteolytic metastases: a double-blind, randomized dose–response study. *Cancer* 2001; **91:** 1191–200.
99. Kusumoto S, Jinnai I, Itoh K. Magnetic resonance imaging patterns in patients with multiple myeloma. *Br J Haematol* 1997; **99**: 649–55.
100. Moulopoulos LA, Dimopoulos MA. Magnetic resonance imaging of the bone marrow in hematologic malignancies. *Blood* 1997; **90**: 2127–47.
101. Moulopoulos LA, Dimopoulos MA, Smith TL et al. Prognostic significance of magnetic resonance imaging in patients with asymptomatic multiple myeloma. *J Clin Oncol* 1995; **13**: 251–6.
102. Frassica DA, Frassica FJ, Schray MF et al. Solitary plasmacytoma of bone: Mayo Clinic experience. *Int J Radiat Oncol Biol Phys* 1989; **16**: 43–8.
103. Moulopoulos LA, Dimopoulos MA, Weber D et al. Magnetic resonance imaging in the staging of solitary plasmacytoma of bone. *J Clin Oncol* 1993; **11**: 1311–15.
104. Rahmouni A, Divine M, Mathieu D et al. MR appearance of multiple myeloma of the spine before and after treatment. *AJR* 1993; **160**: 1053–7.
105. Agren B, Rudberg U, Isberg B et al. MR imaging of multiple myeloma patients with bone-marrow transplants. *Acta Radiol* 1998; **39**: 36–42.
106. Lecouvet FE, Vande Berg BC, Michaux Ł. Development of vertebral fractures in patients with multiple myeloma: Does MRI enable recognition of vertebrae that will collapse? *J Comput Assist Tomogr* 1998; **22**: 430–6.
107. Moulopoulos LA, Dimopoulos MA, Alexanian R et al. Multiple myeloma: MR patterns of response to treatment. *Radiology* 1994; **193**: 441–6.

108. Rahmouni A, Divine M, Mathieu D et al. Appearance of multiple myeloma of the spine before and after treatment. *AJR* 1993; **160**: 1053–7.
109. Tirovola EB, Biassoni L, Britton KE et al. The use of ^{99m}Tc-MIBI scanning in multiple myeloma. *Br J Cancer* 1996; **74**: 1815–20.
110. Pace L, Catalano L, Pinto A et al. Different patterns of technetium-99m sestamibi uptake in multiple myeloma. *Eur J Nucl Med* 1998; **25**: 714–20.
111. Nawawi H, Samson D, Apperley J et al. Biochemical bone markers in patients with multiple myeloma. *Clin Chim Acta* 1996; **253**: 61–77.
112. Abildgaard N, Bentzen SM, Nielsen JL et al. Serum markers of bone metabolism in multiple myeloma: prognostic significance of the carboxy-terminal telopeptide of type 1 collagen (ICTP). *Br J Haematol* 1997; **96**: 103–10.
113. Elomaa I, Risteli L, Laakso M et al. Monitoring the action of clodronate with type I collagen metabolites in mutliple myeloma. *Eur J Cancer* 1996; **32A**: 1166–70.
114. Roux C, Ravaud P, Cohen-Solal M et al. Biologic, histologic and densitometric effects of oral risedronate on bone in patients with multiple myeloma. *Bone* 1994; **15**: 41–9.
115. Clark RE, Flory AAJ, Ion EM et al. Biochemical markers of bone turnover following high-dose chemotherapy and autografting in multiple myeloma. *Blood* 2000; **96**: 2697–702.
116. Rowell NP, Tobias JS. The role of radiotherapy in the management of multiple myeloma. *Blood Rev* 1991; **5**: 84–9.
117. Bosch A, Frias Z. Radiotherapy in the treatment of multiple myeloma. *Int J Radiat Oncol Biol Phys* 1988; **15**: 1363–9.
118. Adamietz IA, Schober C, Schulte RWM et al. Palliative radiotherapy in plasma cell myeloma. *Radiother Oncol* 1991; **20**: 111–16.
119. Rostom AY. A review of the place of radiotherapy in myeloma with emphasis on whole body irradiation. *Hematol Oncol* 1988; **6**: 193–8.
120. Giles FJ, McSweeney EN, Richards JDM et al. Prospective randomized study of double hemibody irradiation with and without subsequent maintenance recombinant alpha 2b interferon on survival in patients with relapsed multiple myeloma. *Eur J Cancer* 1992; **28A**: 1392–5.
121. Lecouvet F, Richard F, Vande Berg B et al. Long-term effects of localized spinal radiation therapy on vertebral fractures and focal lesions appearance in patients with multiple myeloma. *Br J Haematol* 1997; **96**: 743–5.
122. Catell D, Kogen Z, Donahue B et al. Multiple myeloma of an extremity: Must the entire bone be treated? *Int J Radiat Oncol Biol Phys* 1998; **40**: 117–19.
123. Giralt S, Champlin R, Goodman M et al. Preliminary results of a phase I/II study of multiple myeloma (MM) patients treated with ^{166}holmium-DOTMP in combination with high dose melphalan +/− total body irradiation (TBI) with autologous stem cell transplant (ASCT). *Blood* 2000; **96**: 558a.
124. Cohen HJ, Silberman HR, Tornyos K et al. Comparison of two long-term chemotherapy regimens, with or without agents to modify skeletal repair, in multiple myeloma. *Blood* 1984; **63**: 639–48.
125. Acute Leukemia Group B, Eastern Cooperative Oncology Group B. Ineffectiveness of fluoride therapy in multiple myeloma. *N Engl J Med* 1972; **286**: 1283–8.
126. Warrell RP, Lovett D, Dilmanian A et al. Low-dose gallium nitrate for prevention of osteolysis in myeloma: results of a pilot randomized study. *J Clin Oncol* 1993; **11**: 2443–50.
127. Major P, Lortholary A, Hon J et al. Zoledronic acid is superior to pamidronate in the treatment of hypercalcemia of malignancy: a pooled analysis of two randomized controlled clinical trials. *J Clin Oncol* 2001; **19:** 558–67.
128. Fleisch H. Bisphosphonates: mechanisms of action. *Endocrinol Rev* 1998; **19**: 80–100.
129. Aparicio A, Gardner A, Tu Y et al. In vitro cytoreductive effects on multiple myeloma cells induced by bisphosphonates. *Leukemia* 1998; **12**: 220–9.
130. Shipman CM, Croucher PI, Russell GG et al. The bisphosphonate incadronate (YM175) causes apoptosis of human myeloma cells in vitro by inhibiting the mevalonate pathway. *Cancer Res* 1998; **58**: 5294–7.
131. Luckman SP, Hughes DE, Coxon FP et al. Nitrogen-containing bisphosphonates inhibit the mevalonic pathway and prevent post-translational prenylation of GTP-binding proteins, including ras. *J Bone Miner Res* 1998; **13**: 581–9.
132. Reinholz GG, Getz B, Pederson L et al. Bisphosphonates directly regulate cell proliferation, differentiation, and gene expression in human osteoblasts. *Cancer Res* 2000; **60**: 6001–7.
133. Savage AD, Belson DJ, Vescio RA et al. Pamidronate reduces IL-6 production by bone marrow stroma from myeloma patients. *Blood* 1996; **88**: 105a.

134. Derenne S, Amiot M, Barille S et al. Zoledronate is a potent inhibitor of myeloma cell growth and secretion of IL-6 and MMp-1 by the tumoral environment. *J Bone Miner Res* 1999; **14**: 2048–56.
135. Giuliani N, Pedrazzoni M, Passeri G et al. Bisphosphonates inhibit IL-6 production by human osteoblast-like cells. *Scand J Rheumatol* 1998; **27**: 38.
136. Wood J, Schnell C, Greeen J. Zoledronic acid (Zometa), a potent inhibitor of bone resorption, inhibits proliferation and induces apoptosis in human endothelial cells in vitro and is anti-angiogenic in a murine growth factor implant model. *Proc Am Soc Clin Oncol* 2000; **19**: 664a.
137. Singhal S, Mehta J, Desikan R et al. Antitumor activity of thalidomide in refractory multiple myeloma. *N Engl J Med* 1999; **341**: 1565–1.
138. Kunzmann V, Bauer E, Feurle J et al. Stimulation of γδT cells by aminobisphosphonates and induction of antiplasma cell activity in multiple myeloma. *Blood* 2000; **96**: 384–92.
139. Radl J, Croese JW, Zurcher C et al. Influence of treatment with APD-bisphosphonate on the bone lesions in the mouse 5T2 multiple myeloma. *Cancer* 1985; **55**: 1030–40.
140. Yaccoby S, Barlogie B, Epstein J. Pamidronate inhibits growth of myeloma in vivo in the SCID–hu system. *Blood* 1998; **92**: 106a.
141. Dallas SL, Garrett IR, Oyajobi BO et al. Ibandronate reduces osteolytic lesions but not tumor burden in a murine model of myeloma bone disease. *Blood* 1999; **93**: 1697–706.
142. Heim ME, Clemens MR, Queisser W et al. Prospective randomized trial of dichloromethylene bisphosphonate (clodronate) in patients with multiple myeloma requiring treatment. A multicenter study. *Onkologie* 1995; **18**: 439–48.
143. Delmas PD, Charhon S, Chapuy MC et al. Long-term effects of dichloromethylene diphosphonate (C12MDP) on skeletal lesions in multiple myeloma. *Metabol Bone Dis Rel Res* 1982; **4**: 163–8.
144. Merlini G, Parrinello GA, Piccinini L et al. Long-term effects of parenteral dichloromethylene bisphosphonate (C12MDP) on bone disease of myeloma patients treated with chemotherapy. *Hematol Oncol* 1990; **90**: 2127–47.
145. Muhlbacher RC, Bauss F, Schenk R et al. BM.21.0955, a potent new bisphosphonate to inhibit bone resorption. *J Bone Miner Res* 1991; **6**: 1003
146. Green JR, Muller K, Jaeggi KA. Preclinical pharmacology of CGP 42′446, a new, potent heterocyclic bisphosphonate compound. *J Bone Miner Res* 1994; **9**: 745–50.
147. Percherstorfer M, Hermann Z, Body et al. Randomized phase II trial comparing different doses of the bisphosphonate idbandronate in the treatment of hypercalcemia of malignancy. *J Clin Oncol* 1996; **14**: 268–76.
148. Body JJ, Lortholary A, Romieu G et al. A dose-finding study of zoledronate in hypercalcemic cancer patients. *J Bone Miner Res* 1999; **14**: 1557–61.
149. Berenson J, Vescio R, Henick K et al. A phase I, open label, dose ranging trial of intravenous bolus zoledronic acid, a novel bisphosphonate, in cancer patients with metastatic bone disease. *Cancer* 2001; **91**: 144–54.
150. Berenson JR, Vescio RA, Rosen LS et al. A phase I dose-ranging trial of monthly infusions of zoledronic acid for the treatment of osteolytic bone metastases. *Clin Cancer Res* 2001; **7**: 478–85.
151. Fontana A, Hermann Z, Menssen HD et al. Effects of intravenous ibandronate therapy on skeletal related events (SRE) and survival inpatients with advanced multiple myeloma. *Blood* 1998; **92**: 106a.

8

Angiogenesis and thalidomide in plasma cell disorders

Angelo Vacca, Seema Singhal, Domenico Ribatti, Franco Dammacco

INTRODUCTION

Angiogenesis, the formation of new blood vessels, is seen physiologically in utero during fetal growth, during wound healing, and cyclically in the menstruating endometrium.[1] Normally, the microvasculature remains in a quiescent state, with very low proliferation and turnover of the endothelial cells.[2] Endothelial cells rest on a specialized extracellular matrix (ECM) – the basement membrane – the main constituents of which are laminin and type IV collagen.[3]

Angiogenesis develops through five steps:[4]

1. Basement membrane degradation through the action of proteolytic enzymes such as matrix metalloproteinases and plasminogen activators secreted by endothelial cells, resulting in the formation of tiny sprouts, which penetrate into the perivascular stroma.
2. Migration of the endothelial cells at the sprout tip towards the angiogenic stimulus.
3. Proliferation of the endothelial cells below the sprout.
4. Canalization, branching and formation of vascular loops, leading to the development of a functioning circulatory network.
5. Perivascular apposition of pericytes, and synthesis of basement membrane constituents by endothelial cells and pericytes.

Tumour angiogenesis goes through the same steps, but is uncontrolled and not limited in time. It is characterized by a 30- to 40-fold increase in the proliferative activity of endothelial cells.[5] It is essential for tumour progression in the form of growth, invasion, and metastasis, because these develop through the transition from the avascular to the vascular phase.[6]

The avascular phase has been studied using tumour spheroids in agar[7] and tumour implants into the anterior chamber of the rabbit eye.[8] In the spheroid, the increase in cell mass is proportional to the cube of its radius, whereas the surface area increases in proportion to the square of the radius. The tumour growth reaches a steady state when the area becomes too small to allow nutritional material to be supplied to the deep regions of the tumour and to permit the removal of catabolites. The spheroid is nourished solely by diffusible substances in the culture medium, and thus reaches a steady state when its volume is very small (of order (1 mm^3) with (0.2–1) × 10^6 cells. Cells that proliferate and enter the system at the surface overlap those lost in depth by apoptosis and necrosis.[9] The tumour has no metastatic potential, and may remain in this 'dormant' phase indefinitely.[10] In situ carcinoma and melanoma are clinical examples of tumours in an avascular phase.[6]

Conversely, if the tumour is implanted onto a site with angiogenic potential, such as the rabbit iris, it is soon permeated by new vessels and its proliferative activity increases exponentially. Proliferating (S-phase) cells replace those lost from the system, resulting in a rapid growth in the mass. The steady state is reached at high volumes (4000–16 000 times the original volume). Clinically, fast-growing, locally invasive, and metastatic tumours are examples of tumours in the vascular phase.[8] The tumour proliferative activity is enhanced because the neovaculature conveys oxygen and nutrients and removes catabolites, while endothelial cells secrete paracrine growth factors for tumour cells, such as insulin-like growth factor 1 (IGF-1) and basic fibroblast growth factor (FGF-2).[11] New vessels facilitate invasion because endothelial cells at their sprout tips secrete proteolytic enzymes that allow tumour cells to spread into and through the stroma.[12] Neovaculature permits metastasis, because the expanding endothelial surface offers tumour cells more opportunities to enter the circulation.[13]

The vascular phase also parallels tumour progression in terms of neoplastic changeover.[14] In all these systems, the neoplastic or preneoplastic cell capable of inducing angiogenesis is ultimately responsible for the transition from the avascular to the vascular phase.[15]

CELL KINETICS IN MYELOMA: THE GOMPERTZIAN GROWTH

In myeloma, the neoplastic cell population consists of three clonally related compartments:[16] a small stem cell compartment containing totipotent malignant cells, an expansion compartment or 'growth fraction' (GF) whose proliferative activity expands the small population of totipotent cells entering the GF, and a differentiation compartment, the largest of the three, where proliferation stops and differentiation into mature plasma cells takes place. Cell loss by apoptosis and necrosis occurs in the differentiation compartment.

The kinetics of the stem cell compartment are unknown. The GF contains cells in the G_1, S, G_2, and M phases, as well as resting G_0 cells, which are not in the proliferative cycle but are capable of rejoining it following appropriate stimuli. The balance between GF cell production and cell loss from the differentiation compartment determines growth, steady state, or reduction of the myeloma cell mass.

GF proliferative activity is measured by the plasma cell labelling index (LI), which identifies the S-phase cell fraction.[17] LI at diagnosis is usually low (median 1%, range 0–5%) when expressed as a fraction of the entire tumour burden. When expressed as a proportion of the GF, which is generally small (mean <1%), LI is much higher (median 30%, range 15–100%), implying very active proliferation. The tumour doubling time in myeloma is relatively short (5–15 months), despite a huge cell loss (>90%, given the large size of the differentiation compartment), indicating that cell production by the GF is very high.

Myeloma is clinically diagnosed when the tumour mass is greater than 10^{12} cells – a stage reached following Gompertzian growth.[17] The initial exponential growth progressively reduces (decline in LI and GF) until the steady state is reached about 5–25 months after neoplastic changeover. This duration differs between patients, and determines the steady-state tumour burden. At diagnosis, the plasma cell proliferative activity is variable, depending on the steady-state level.[16] If the steady state has been reached, further growth is moderate (low LI and GF, which are balanced by the apoptosis) and the disease is not aggressive ('non-active'). If the steady state is still a long way ahead, even though the cell mass is large enough (>10^{12}) to elicit clinical symptoms, growth is exponential (high LI and GF, low apoptosis and cell loss), the tumour mass expands rapidly, and the disease is aggressive ('active'). In relapse, which is usually diagnosed when the cell mass is less than 10^{12} cells, growth is exponential because the steady state is distant and the disease is active.[16] In the plateau phase, the cell mass has been reduced to a level beyond which no further cytoreduction occurs, most cells are in G_0 and growth is limited (LI $< 1\%$, GF $\leq 0.5\%$), resulting in quiescent, non-active disease.[16] While on therapy, responsive patients display growth conditions close to the plateau phase.[17] The neoplastic population in monoclonal gammopathy of undetermined significance (MGUS) reaches the steady state at very low cell mass levels (10^{10}–10^{11} cells) and growth is very slow (LI $< 1\%$).[17]

Growth characteristics of active myeloma are similar to those of tumours in the vascular phase, and those of non-active myeloma and MGUS to those of tumours in the avascular phase.

BONE MARROW ANGIOGENESIS IN MYELOMA

We have investigated bone marrow microvessel density in patients with active myeloma, non-active myeloma, and MGUS.[18] Deparaffinized 6 μm sections were sequentially incubated with a murine monoclonal antibody to the endothelial cell marker factor VIII, a biotin-labelled horse anti-mouse IgG, and avidin–peroxidase conjugate, followed by red staining with a 3-amino-9-ethylcarbazole solution and counterstaining with haematoxylin. Among all the stained vessels, microvessels (capillaries and small venules) were identified on 250× fields within a superimposed 484-point square mesh 0.125 mm^2 in size. The area they occupied ('microvessel area') was calculated by using the planimetric method of 'point counting', according to which the area equals the sum of points that hit microvessels. The microvessel area was normalized to the cellular area (mesh area minus dense connective tissue, bone lamellae, fat, necrosis, and haemorrhagic area) by using a computerized image analysis system. The few megakaryocytes stained with the factor VIII were easily distinguishable from microvessels by their morphology and size.

Figure 8.1 shows that the microvessel area of patients with active myeloma was five- to sixfold higher than that of patients with non-active myeloma or MGUS. Rapidly progressive disease was associated with the highest microvessel area. The area of patients with non-active myeloma differed only marginally from that of patients with MGUS. The area correlated tightly with the proliferative activity as evaluated by plasma cell LI.[19]

The differences in microvessel area between patients with active myeloma and other patient groups are shown in Figure 8.2, from which it can be seen that microvessels in patients with active myeloma are thin, winding, often without visible lumina, and characterized by single or clustered endothelial cells and small endothelial 'sprouts' without lumina. In contrast, vessels are straight without sprouts in patients with non-active myeloma and MGUS. As progression from in situ to invasive and metastatic solid tumours is accompanied and enhanced by the switch from the prevascular to the vascular phase, these findings suggest that active myeloma may represent the 'vascular phase' of plasma cell tumours, and non-active myeloma and MGUS their 'prevascular phase'. Bone marrow angiogenesis may therefore favour progression from MGUS or non-active myeloma to active myeloma.

THE VASCULAR PHASE OF OTHER LYMPHOPROLIFERATIVE DISEASES

Excessive angiogenesis is seen in the lymph nodes of patients with hyperplastic and dysplastic disorders of B cells, such as Castleman's disease,[20] and in the marrows of patients with acute lymphoblastic leukaemia.[21] Lymph node angiogenesis correlates with disease progression in B-cell non-Hodgkin's lymphomas.[22–24] In patients with mycosis fungoides, the microvessel area increases with disease progression from the eczematous stage to the plaque and nodule stages.[25] As in active myeloma, neovascularization in these

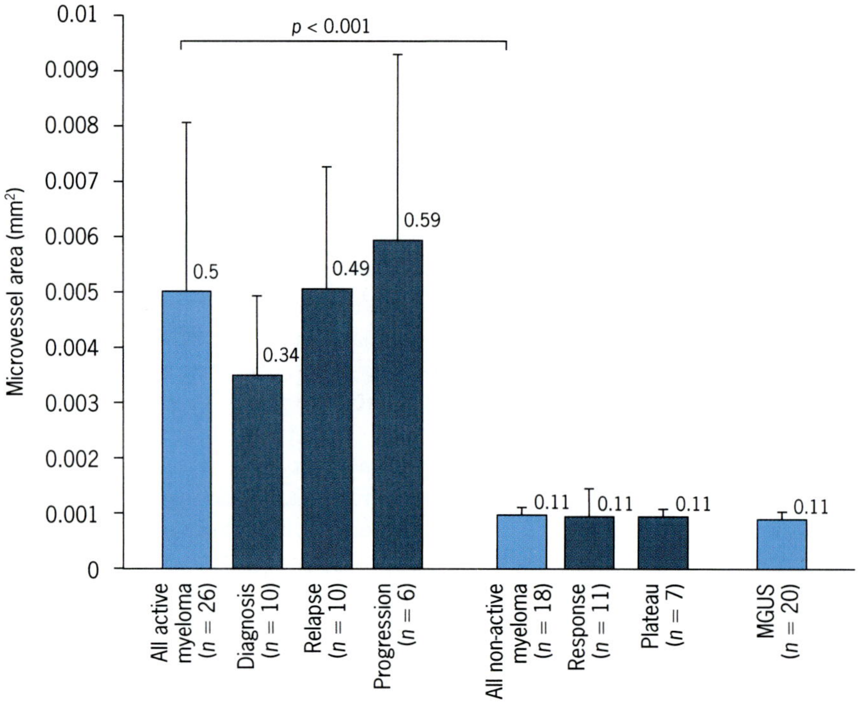

Figure 8.1 Significantly higher bone marrow microvessel area in patients with active myeloma compared with non-active myeloma and MGUS.

diseases consists of thin, winding, branching, mutually anastomosed microvessels and endothelial cell clusters.[26]

MECHANISMS CONTROLLING THE SWITCH TO THE VASCULAR PHASE

Various regulatory elements control the switch to the vascular phase:

1. *Genetic factors*. In transgenic mice containing an oncogene in the beta cells of the pancreatic islets, angiogenic activity was observed in a subset of hyperplastic islet cells before the onset of tumour formation.[14] In a tumour model of transgenic mice containing the genome of the bovine papilloma virus type 1, the switch to the angiogenic phenotype was associated with the ability to export the angiogenic cytokine FGF-2 from the cell.[27] Angiogenesis in human fibroblasts is controlled by the suppressor gene *p53*, which regulates the synthesis of thrombospondin-1. Thrombospondin-1 is a potent inhibitor of angiogenesis, and is downregulated during tumorigenesis.[28]
2. *Secretion by tumour cells of various growth factors*. These include cytokines that stimulate proliferation, chemotaxis, and chemoinvasion of endothelial cells, such as FGF-2, [29] vascular endothelial growth factor (VEGF),[30] hepatocyte growth factor/scatter factor (HGF/SF),[31] nitric oxide,[32] angiogenin,[33] platelet-derived growth factor (PDGF),[34] and placenta growth factor.[35] These also include cytokines that induce vessel differentiation such as transforming growth factors α and β (TGF-α and TGF-β).[36]
3. *Recruitment of inflammatory cells by chemotactic factors*[37] *released by tumour cells and release of angiogenic factors by them*. Activated macrophages release tumour necrosis factor α (TNF-α) and interleukin (IL)-8,[38] mast cells release heparin, histamine, tryptase, FGF-2,

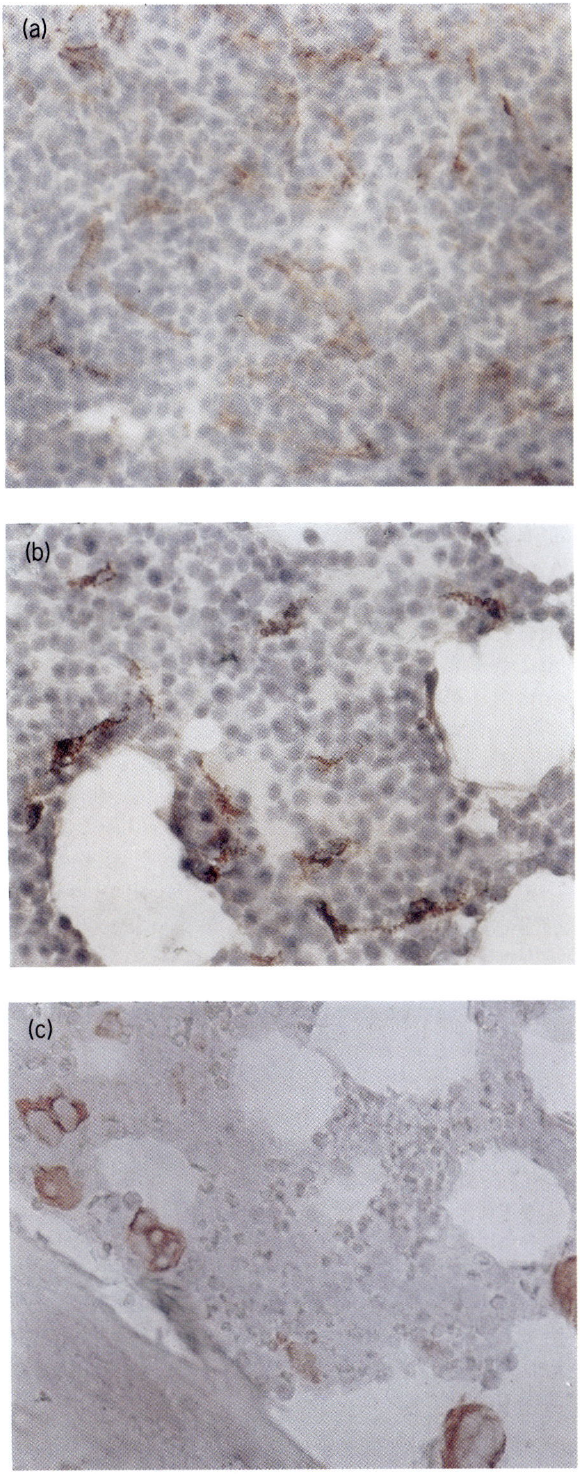

Figure 8.2 Demonstration of bone marrow microvasculature by staining with factor VIII in patients with (a) active myeloma (relapse), (b) non-active myeloma (response), and (c) MGUS. 250× fields of mm^2 (the bar represents 10 μm). The cellular areas were 0.12 mm^2 in (a), 0.097 mm^2 in (b), and 0.084 mm^2 in (c) and the microvessel areas were 0.082 mm^2 in (a) and 0.002 mm^2 in (b). Note in (c) the lack of vessels and the presence of strongly stained megakaryocytes.

and VEGF,[39] and other cells release IL-1, IL-6, IL-15, granulocyte colony-stimulating factor (G-CSF), and granulocyte–macrophage colony-stimulating factor (GM-CSF).[40]

4. *Mobilization of angiogenic cytokines such as FGF-2, VEGF, and TGF-β*, which are stored in the heparin-like glycosaminoglycans of ECM following its degradation by proteinases secreted by tumour cells and inflammatory cells.[12] Tumour and inflammatory cells also secrete proteinase inhibitors. Thus, the degree of ECM degradation and angiogenesis stimulation by the released cytokines depends on the level of proteinase/inhibitor equilibrium,[41] and the serum levels of matrix metalloproteinase-2 (MMP-2)/tissue inhibitor of MMP-2 (TIMP-2) complexes or of free MMP-9 are markers of angiogenesis and invasive capability.[42,43]
5. *Interaction of adhesion receptor $\alpha_v\beta_3$ with a specific integrin of the ECM*. The receptor is selectively expressed on growing blood vessels, but not on quiescent vessels.[44] The integrin binds activated MMP-2 to the surface of endothelial cells, facilitating ECM degradation.[45] Thus, the receptor and its integrin act cooperatively with MMP-2 to promote endothelial cell functions necessary for angiogenesis (cell adhesion and migration), as well as ECM degradation, which results in tumour cell invasion.
6. *Upregulation of angiopoietin-2*. This occurs in endothelial cells at the sprout tips in response to the production of FGF-2, VEGF, and angiopoietin-1 by tumour cells.[46] Angiopoietin-2 disrupts interactions between endothelial cells, pericytes, and smooth muscle cells, making endothelial cells susceptible to mitogenic and chemotactic signals from FGF-2, VEGF, and angiopoietin-1.[47]

ANGIOGENIC ABILITY OF PLASMA CELLS

We have shown that plasma cells from patients with myeloma are capable of inducing an angiogenic phenotype in cultured human endothelial cells, and also stimulate angiogenesis in vivo.[48] Figure 8.3(a) shows that 14 out of 26 (53%) active myeloma patients stimulated human umbilical vein endothelial cell (HUVEC) proliferation as against only 2 out of 18 (11%) non-active myeloma patients and 3 out of 20 (15%) MGUS patients. Figure 8.3(b) shows that there was more proliferation with exposure to active myeloma. Similarly, Figure 8.3(c–f) show that a greater proportion of patients with active myeloma stimulated HUVEC and monocyte chemotaxis and to a greater extent. Plasma cells from 20 of 26 patients (77%) with active myeloma could induce angiogenesis in a chick embryo chorioallantoic membrane (CAM) sponge system (Figure 8.3g) compared with 33% and 22% of non-active myeloma and MGUS patients,[49] and the extent of the microvessel area was larger with active myeloma (Figure 8.3h). The bone marrow microvessel area and CAM microvessel area correlated significantly ($r = 0.81$; $p < 0.001$).

We have shown[48] that levels of FGF-2 are significantly higher in the plasma cell lysates of patients with active myeloma compared with non-active myeloma and MGUS patients (Figure 8.4). Inhibition of FGF-2 by means of a polyclonal anti-FGF-2 antibody suppressed the angiogenic potential of plasma cells from patients with active myeloma, as reflected by inhibition of HUVEC proliferation and chemotaxis, monocyte chemotaxis and CAM angiogenesis (Figure 8.5). Partial rather than complete inhibition (Figure 8.5) with anti-FGF-2 antibody, as well as the lack of correlation between plasma cell FGF-2 levels and the extent of angiogenesis in the bone marrow (unpublished data), suggest that FGF-2 is not the only factor capable of inducing bone marrow angiogenesis in myeloma. VEGF is perhaps not involved directly, since its levels in plasma cell lysates of patients with active myeloma, non-active myeloma, and MGUS are low and comparable (Figure 8.4). Nevertheless, VEGF may act synergistically with FGF-2.[50]

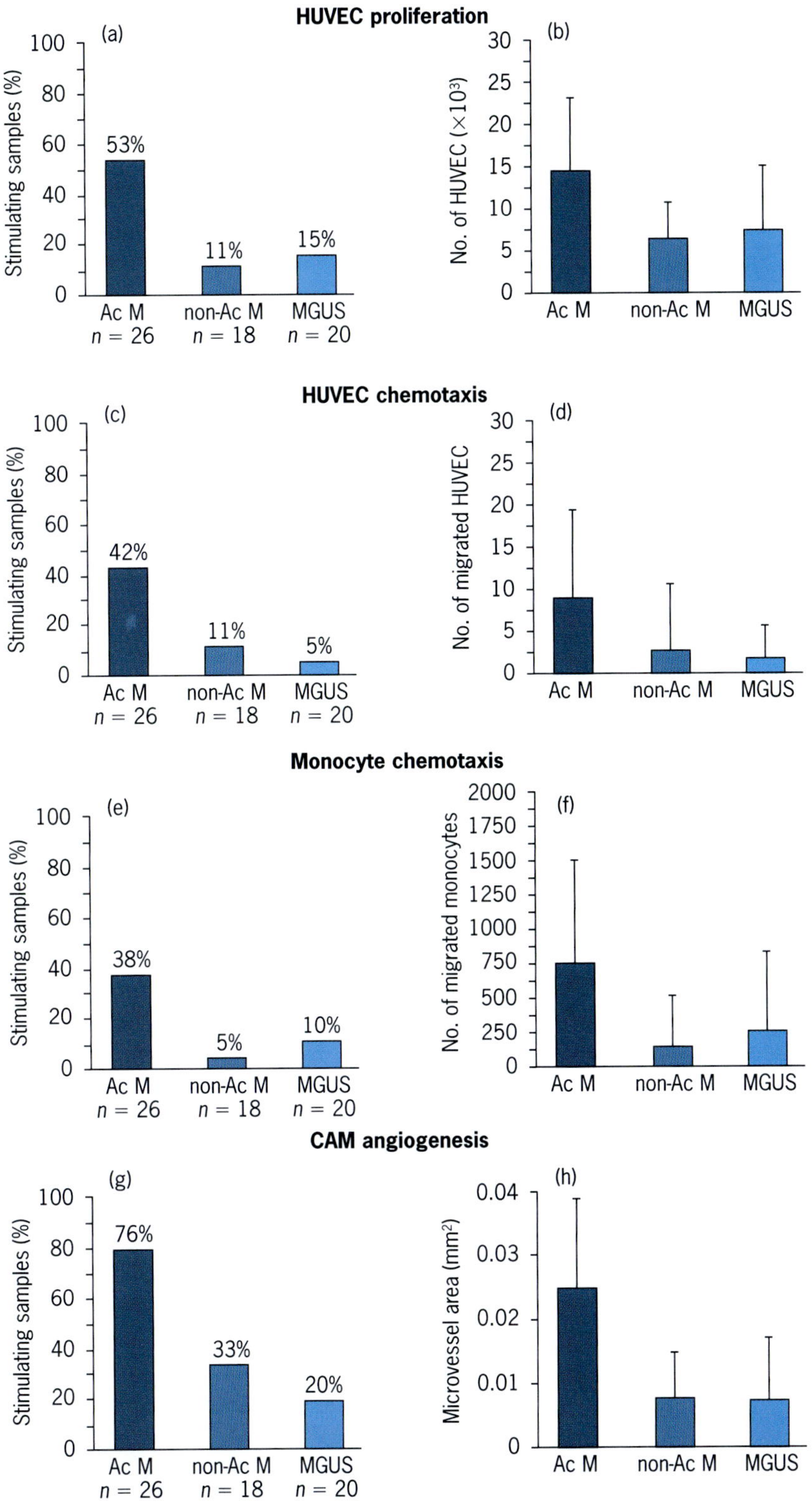

Figure 8.3 The effect of bone marrow plasma cells from patients with active myeloma (Ac M), non-active myeloma (non-Ac M), and MGUS on human umbilical vein endothelial cell (HUVEC) proliferation, HUVEC chemotaxis, human monocyte chemotaxis, and chick embryo chorioallantoic membrane (CAM) angiogenesis.

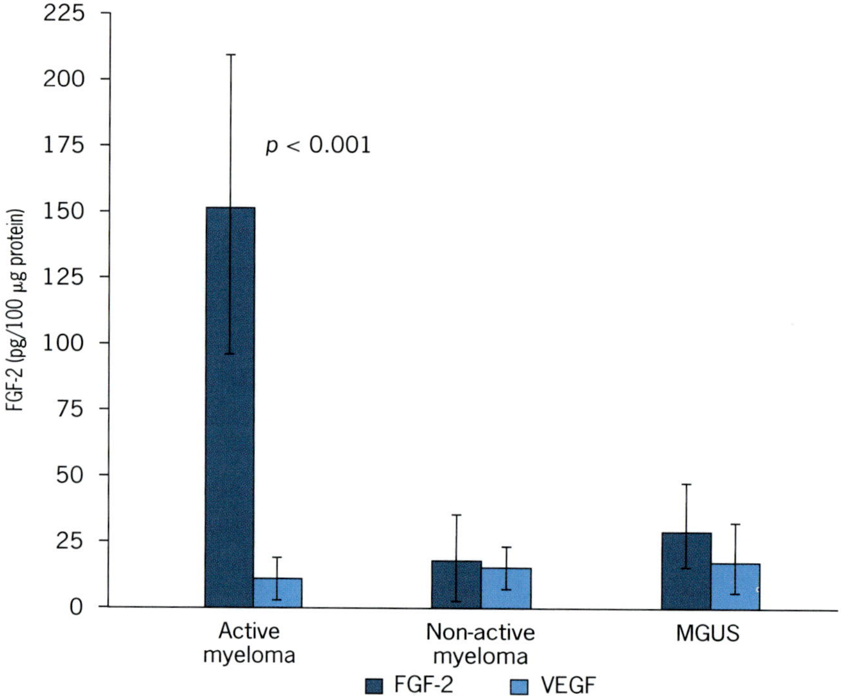

Figure 8.4 Quantification of FGF-2 and VEGF in bone marrow plasma cell lysates by enzyme-linked immunosorbent assay (ELISA). FGF-2 levels in patients with active myeloma are significantly higher.

OTHER ANGIOGENIC CYTOKINES IN MYELOMA

Hepatocyte growth factor/scatter factor (HGF/SF) is an angiogenic cytokine that has been identified in human myeloma cell lines [51] and in freshly isolated myeloma cells.[52] Serum levels of this factor are high in approximately 40% of patients at diagnosis and decline to normal levels as there is response to induction therapy. There is no decline if the therapy is ineffective, and the levels become high again upon relapse.[53] Based on these observations and on the fact that the levels fluctuate concordantly with the serum/urine M-component levels, HGF/SF is probably secreted by plasma cells. A number of other factors may be responsible for bone marrow angiogenesis in myeloma. Plasma cells secrete TGF-β and IL-1β;[54] the latter stimulates the marrow microenvironment to secrete IL-6 and the platelets to secrete PDGF.[55] IL-6, IL-8, G-CSF, GM-CSF, and TNF-α are secreted by the marrow microenvironment.[56] IL-6, IL-8, GM-CSF, and IL-1β are secreted mostly in the active phase of myeloma.[57] Our hypothesis on the induction of bone marrow angiogenesis in myeloma is illustrated in Figure 8.6.

Bone marrow plasma cells of patients with myeloma and MGUS express mRNA for MMP-2 and MMP-9. Usually, MMP-2 expression is stronger. Both MMPs are expressed more intensely in patients with active myeloma than in patients with non-active myeloma and MGUS, who show a much lower expression (Figure 8.7). A number of myeloma cell lines and freshly isolated bone marrow plasma cells of myeloma patients produce MMP-9, although correlation with disease activity has not been assessed.[58] It has been shown that bone marrow stromal cells (e.g. fibroblasts and osteoblasts) of myeloma patients constitutively produce MMP-1 and the MMP-2 proenzyme, which is converted into active MMP-2 in co-cultures with plasma cells.[58] Given the ability of MMP-1 to degrade

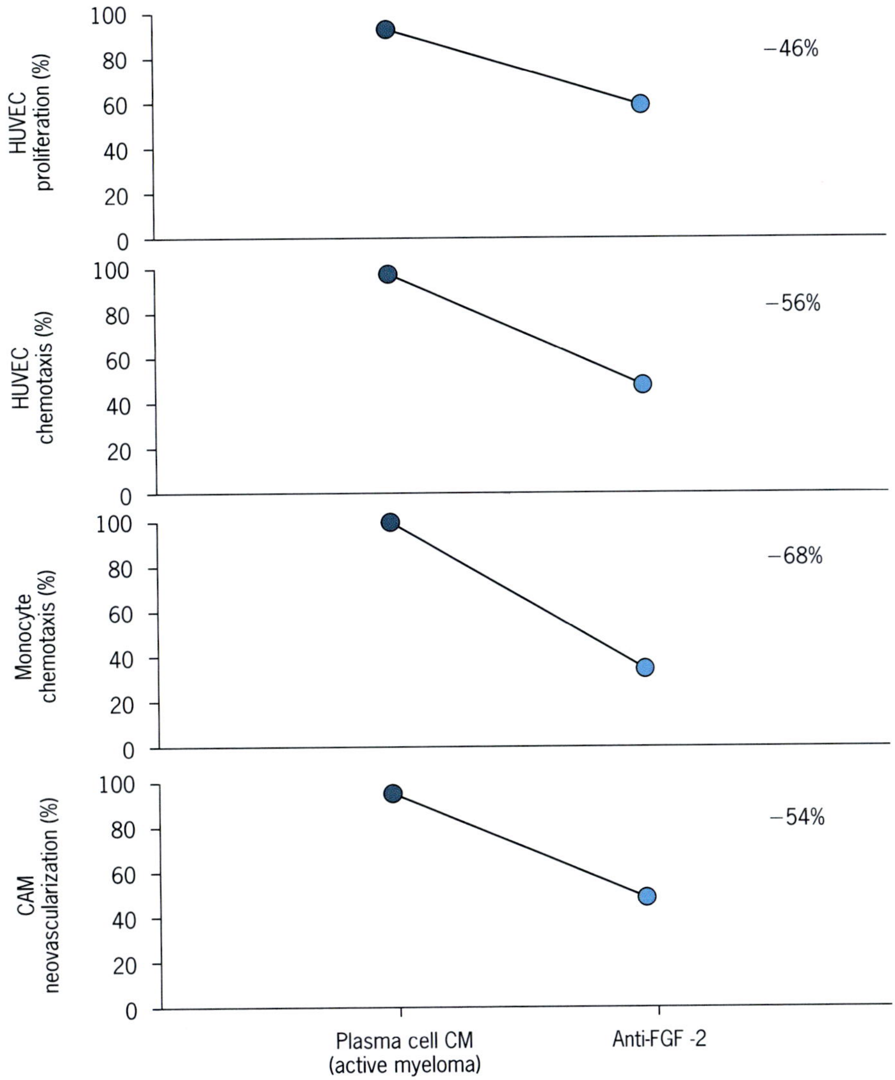

Figure 8.5 Decline in angiogenic processes (Figure 8.3) as a result of the antagonism of FGF-2 by the addition of a polyclonal anti-FGF-2 antibody (400 μg/ml) to plasma cells from patients with active myeloma (CM, conditioned medium).

type I collagen, and of MMP-2 and MMP-9 to degrade type IV, V, VII, and X collagens as well as fibronectin,[12] plasma cells of active myeloma patients are capable of invading both the stroma and the basement membrane. In addition, as already mentioned, the degradation of the ECM brings about the release of angiogenic factors that are stored inside it (Figure 8.6). Thus, the data suggest that proteolytic activity and angiogenesis occur together in close vicinity of plasma cells, and this establishes suitable conditions for intra- and extramedullary dissemination of plasma cells.

INVOLVEMENT OF HOST INFLAMMATORY CELLS

In parallel with increased angiogenesis, mast cell density increases in the bone marrow of

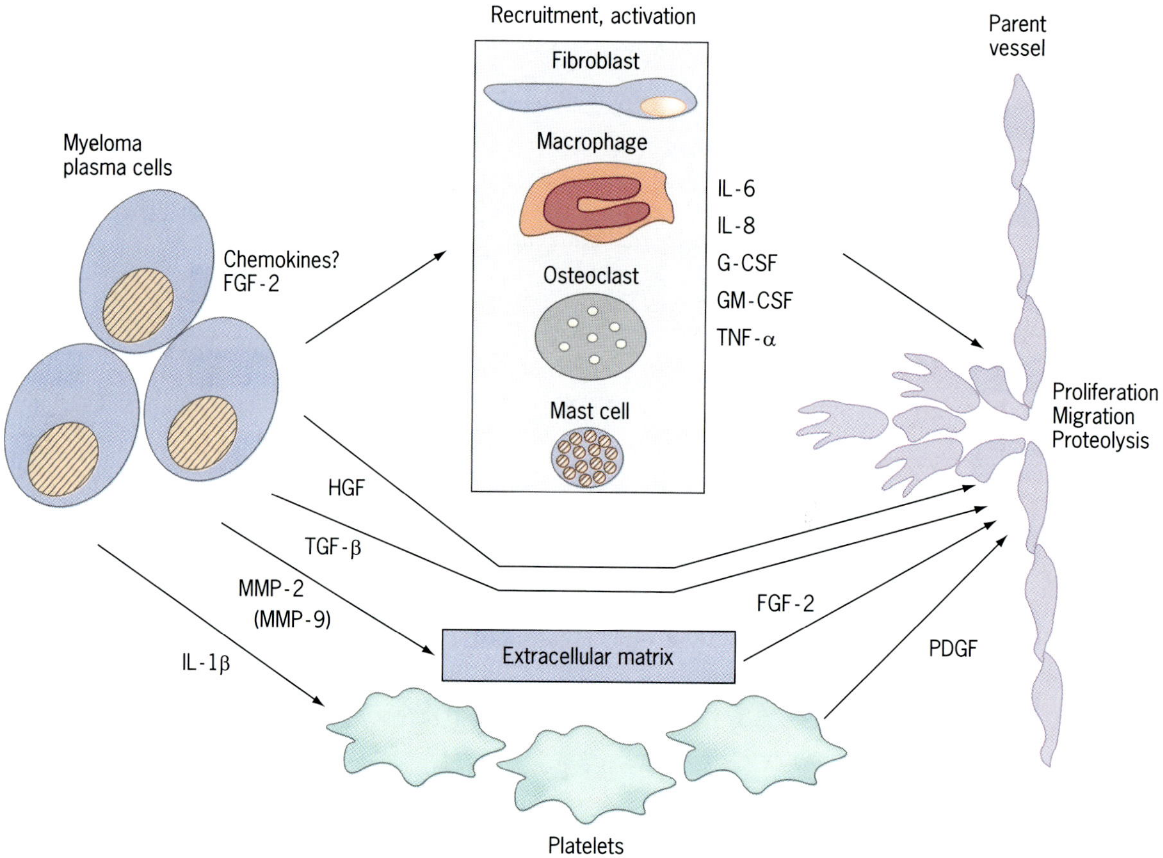

Figure 8.6 Hypothetical mechanism of angiogenesis induction in myeloma. Plasma cells could recruit and activate cells of the bone marrow microenvironment (fibroblasts, macrophages, osteoclasts, and mast cells) to release angiogenic cytokines, secrete angiogenic cytokines themselves, and degrade the extracellular matrix with the release of angiogenic cytokines.

patients with active myeloma.[59] At the ultrastructural level, the majority of cells display semilunar aspects of cytoplasmic granules, suggesting a chronic and slow release of mediators in response to a degranulatory stimulus. We hypothesize that mast cells are recruited and activated in the bone marrow by malignant plasma cells, and that angiogenesis is mediated, at least partly, by the angiogenic factors contained in their secretory granules. These results are similar to those demonstrating bone marrow angiogenesis in the SCID–hu myeloma model in close association with a dense stromal cell infiltrate.[60]

PROGNOSTIC VALUE OF BONE MARROW ANGIOGENESIS IN MYELOMA

In breast, lung, colon, head and neck, and prostate carcinoma, increased microvessel density is associated with poorer prognosis.[61] Bone marrow angiogenesis in patients with myeloma and MGUS correlates with the proliferative capacity of plasma cells measured by their LI. LI is an important prognostic factor, with shorter mean survival in patients with LI $\geq$ 1% (15 months) than in those with LI $<$ 1% (40 months) irrespective of the cell mass.[16] In the Gompertzian pattern of growth, myeloma patients with a high LI are

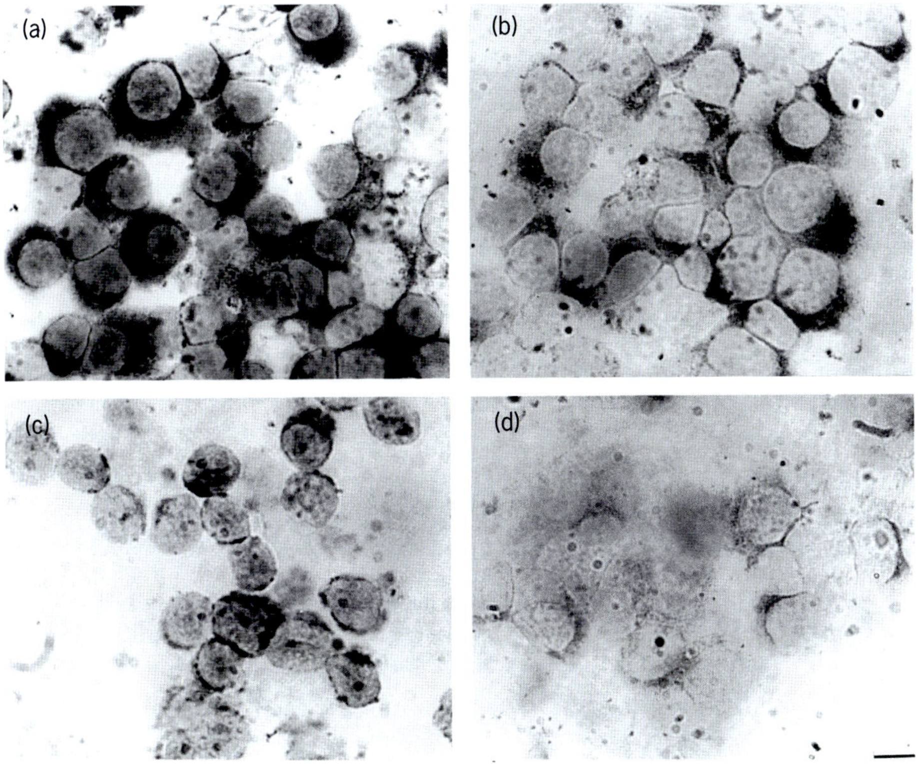

Figure 8.7 In situ hybridization for MMP-2 and MMP-9 mRNA in bone marrow plasma cells. There is strong MMP-2 (a) and MMP-9 (b) mRNA expression in plasma cells isolated from a patient with active myeloma, weak MMP-2 expression in a patient with MGUS (c), and negative control for MMP-2 mRNA in active myeloma (d). The bar represents 16 μm.

still far from steady state, since their tumour is in the exponential portion of the growth curve. They respond rapidly to induction chemotherapy (the so-called 'early responders'), but the response is short-lived and is followed by a rapid relapse due to a massive recruitment of G_0 plasma cells into the cell cycle. Since we have shown that bone marrow angiogenesis and LI are correlated closely with the various phases of the disease, it may well be that risk of progression in myeloma may be predicted on the basis of bone marrow angiogenesis.

Increased bone marrow microvascularity at the time of presentation is predictive of shorter overall and event-free survival as well as shorter remission duration in myeloma patients, despite high-dose chemotherapy.[62] The observation that some patients with myeloma who are in remission after high-dose chemotherapy still show persistent marrow angiogenesis[63] may allow identification of patients at early risk of relapse.

THERAPEUTIC ANGIOGENESIS INHIBITION IN MYELOMA

Dexamethasone is one of the most active agents in the treatment of myeloma (see Chapter 18). While it has several mechanisms of action in myeloma,[64] it is possible that inhibition of angiogenesis could be one of them.[65] Interferon is also active in myeloma to a limited extent (see Chapter 22) and is an inhibitor of angiogenesis.[66] However, the first drug to be used in myeloma primarily for its angiogenesis-inhibiting activity was thalidomide.[67]

While a number of agents with potential for angiogenesis inhibition (etanercept, infliximab, pirfenidone, PS-341, neovastat, CC 5013) are being evaluated by us at the Myeloma Program of the Northwestern University Medical School (NUMS), Chicago, the mainstay of non-conventional therapy is thalidomide.

THALIDOMIDE IN MYELOMA

The use of thalidomide in patients with end-stage, refractory myeloma by Singhal et al[67] was based on the work of Vacca et al[18,19] showing increased marrow microvascularity in myeloma and on the observation that thalidomide could induce apoptosis of neovasculature and inhibit angiogenesis in animal models.[68,69].

Eighty-four patients with refractory myeloma, most having relapsed after at least one preceding cycle of high-dose chemotherapy and transplantation, were treated with thalidomide.[67] The starting dose was 200 mg daily, and this was increased by 200 mg every two weeks to a maximum of 800 mg per day. The serum or urine levels of paraprotein decreased by 90% or more in eight patients (two achieving complete remission), by 75% or more in six patients, by 50% or more in seven patients, and by 25% or more in six patients; the total response rate being 32%. The median time to response was one month, and 80% of the responses were apparent within two months. Responses were associated with decreased marrow plasmacytosis. The median response duration was six months.

These encouraging results have now been confirmed by a number of other groups.[70–76] Currently available data suggest that between 30% and 60% of patients with previously treated myeloma, including those who have relapsed after a preceding transplant, respond to thalidomide. Responses are characterized by decreases in paraprotein, marrow plasmacytosis, β2-microglobulin, creatinine, and C-reactive protein, and increases in haemoglobin, albumin, and uninvolved immunoglobulins (unpublished observations).

Mechanism of action

While angiogenesis inhibition[68,69] remains an attractive potential mechanism of action, thalidomide has a number of other properties that could explain its activity in myeloma. These include alteration of adhesion molecule expression,[77] modulation of TNF-α production,[78] increasing the in vivo production of IL-10,[79] and enhancement of cell-mediated immunity by direct co-stimulation of T cells.[80] No consistent relationship was found between microvessel density and response in the original study,[67] but limited data from other groups suggest a relationship between bone marrow microvasculature and response to thalidomide.[81,82].

Dose

Thalidomide was started at the dose of 200 mg daily at bedtime and increased in 200 mg steps every two weeks to a maximum of 800 mg daily in the original study.[67] Others have started the drug at doses as low as 50 mg daily[71] and have escalated the dose much more slowly in 50–100 mg steps. The optimum dose is still undefined. Until formal dose-escalation studies have been performed, the approach we have adopted at the NUMS is to start the drug at the dose of 100 mg daily and escalate this by 50 mg every week to the maximum tolerated dose. There appears to be a dose–response relationship – at least in individual instances: responding patients whose disease recurred after the dose was lowered have often achieved response again when the higher dose was re-instituted (unpublished observations).

Duration of therapy

Paraprotein decline on thalidomide therapy is gradual. The median time to response is approximately one month, and some patients take several months to show response. However, most patients respond within four months. One month therefore is a minimum reasonable trial of therapy and four months is adequate. Patients who have not responded within four months should receive alternative treatments (including thalidomide-containing combinations; see below). Thalidomide should be continued indefinitely in responding patients in the absence of intolerable side-effects.

Adverse effects

Adverse effects, while common (75% of the patients at 200 mg), are usually WHO grade 1–2. The commonest toxicities are somnolence, constipation, weakness, and fatigue. Bone marrow suppression is uncommon. Symptoms of peripheral neuropathy are seen in a third of the patients, but less than half of those tested show evidence of neuropathy on electrophysiologic studies. Pyridoxine 100 mg daily given concomitantly may help prevent development of neuropathic symptoms, and help those with symptoms at the dose of 200 mg daily. One-quarter of patients develop a skin rash. This is usually an itchy, maculopapular rash which subsides when the drug is stopped or the dose decreased. A Stevens– Johnson syndrome-like picture can be seen rarely, and is a contraindication to restarting the drug. Bradycardia, possibly as a result of autonomic neuropathy, is seen in a minority of patients. Thrombotic phenomena have been of concern, especially when the thalidomide is used in conjunction with other agents.

Relapse

Like all therapeutic interventions in myeloma, thalidomide is probably not curative. With a median follow-up of a year,[67] 40% of the responding patients have relapsed at a median of six months. One of the two patients who started thalidomide in December 1997 for terminal disease and went into near-complete remission eventually relapsed in September 1999. Despite having disease that had never responded to dexamethasone in the past, he responded promptly to the combination of dexamethasone and thalidomide. He eventually relapsed and died almost 2½ years after thalidomide was initially started. The likelihood is that all responding patients will eventually relapse, but a number will respond to thalidomide-containing salvage combinations.

Approach to non-responders or relapse

There may be synergy between thalidomide and chemotherapy, because patients who have not responded to either individually do respond to the combination. The combinations that have been utilized include thalidomide–dexamethasone[76] as well as thalidomide with other forms of standard chemotherapy.[83,84]

Thalidomide in newly diagnosed myeloma

Formal comparative studies are required to evaluate thalidomide in previously untreated patients. Limited, anecdotal experience suggests excellent response rates to thalidomide as a single agent, with 50% decline in paraprotein in two-thirds of patients (unpublished data). Thalidomide in combination with standard chemotherapy in newly diagnosed patients may impair peripheral blood stem cell mobilization and collection somewhat.[85]

Thalidomide as maintenance therapy after autografting

Our usual approach to maintenance therapy after autotransplantation is interferon, dexamethasone, or a combination of the two. However, there are circumstances under which we have started using thalidomide. These include intolerance of interferon and/or dexamethasone, disease known to be unresposive to dexamethasone, diabetes, and myelosuppression. We also employ a six- to eight-week therapeutic trial of thalidomide before the transplant. Responders receive thalidomide post transplant as maintenance, and non-responders receive dexamethasone and/or interferon.

The place of thalidomide in the treatment of myeloma

Much work needs to be done to determine the exact place of thalidomide in myeloma. It is

Table 8.1 Use of thalidomide in myeloma patients at the Myeloma Program of the Northwestern University Medical School, Chicago

Treatment approach	Stage of the disease	Activity
Thalidomide alone	Relapsed	+++
	Primary refractory	+++
	Post-autograft maintenance	???
	Newly diagnosed	+++
Thalidomide and dexamethasone	Relapsed	+++
	Primary refractory	+++
	Responding (pre-autograft therapeutic trial)	+++
	Post-autograft maintenance	???
	Newly diagnosed	+++
	No response to thalidomide alone	++
	Relapse on thalidomide alone	++
Thalidomide with combination chemotherapy	No response to thalidomide alone	++
	Relapse on thalidomide alone	++
	No response to thalidomide and dexamethasone	+
	Relapse on thalidomide and dexamethasone	+

useful at all stages of the disease, and is active by itself and in combination with other agents. Table 8.1 shows the way in which thalidomide is currently employed at NUMS, either as routine practice or as part of ongoing clinical trials. Our approach to the use of thalidomide or thalidomide-containing combination therapy, as well as the manangement of side-effects, has been outlined in depth elswhere recently.[86,87]

REFERENCES

1. Folkman J. Angiogenesis in cancer, vascular, rheumatoid and other disease. *Nature Med* 1995; **1**: 27–31.
2. Pepper MS. Positive and negative regulation of angiogenesis: from cell biology to the clinic. *Vasc Med* 1996; **1**: 259–66.
3. Grant DS, Kibbey MC, Kinsella JL et al. The role of basement membrane in angiogenesis and tumor growth. *Pathol Res Pract* 1994; **190**: 854–63.
4. Risau W. Mechanism of angiogenesis. *Nature* 1997; **386**: 671–4.
5. Ausprunk DH, Folkman J. Migration and proliferation of endothelial cells in preformed and newly formed blood vessel during tumor angiogenesis. *Microvasc Res* 1977; **14**: 53–65.
6. Folkman J. What is the evidence that tumors are angiogenesis-dependent? *J Natl Cancer Inst* 1990; **82**: 4–6.
7. Sutherland RM, McCredie JA, Inch WR. Growth of multicell spheroids in tissue culture as a model of nodular carcinomas. *J Natl Cancer Inst* 1971; **46**: 113–17.
8. Gimbrone MA Jr, Leapman S, Cotran RS, Folkman J. Tumor dormancy in vivo by prevention of neovascularization. *J Exp Med* 1972; **136**: 261–7.
9. Folkman J, Greenspan HP. Influence of geometry on control of cell growth. *Biochim Biophys Acta* 1975; **417**: 211–36.
10. Uhr JW, Scheuermann RH, Street NE, Vitetta ES. Cancer dormancy: opportunities for new therapeutic approaches *Nature Med* 1997; **3**: 505–9.
11. Hamada J, Cavanaugh PG, Lotan O. Separable growth and migration factors for large-cell lymphoma cells secreted by microvascular endothelial cells derived from target organs for metastasis. *Br J Cancer* 1992; **66**: 349–54.
12. Mignatti P, Rifkin DB. Biology and biochemistry of proteinases in tumor invasion. *Physiol Rev* 1993; **73**: 161–95.

13. Zetter BR. Angiogenesis and tumor metastasis. *Annu Rev Med* 1998; **49**: 407–24.
14. Folkman J, Watson K, Ingber D, Hanahan D. Induction of angiogenesis during the transition from hyperplasia to neoplasia. *Nature* 1989; **339**: 58–61.
15. Hanahan D, Folkman J. Patterns and emerging mechanisms of the angiogenic switch during tumorigenesis, *Cell* 1996; **86**: 353–64.
16. Hallek M, Bergsagel PL, Anderson KC. Multiple myeloma: increasing evidence for a multistep transformation process. *Blood* 1998; **91**: 3–21.
17. Durie BGM. Staging and kinetics of multiple myeloma. In: *Neoplastic Diseases of the Blood*, Vol I, 2nd edn (Wiernik PH, Canellos GP, Kyle RA, Schiffer CA, eds). New York: Churchill Livingstone, 1991: 439–51.
18. Vacca A, Di Loreto M, Ribatti D et al. Bone marrow of patients with active multiple myeloma: angiogenesis and plasma cell adhesion molecules LFA-1, VLA-4, LAM-1 and CD44. *Am J Hematol* 1995; **50**: 9–14.
19. Vacca A, Ribatti D, Roncali L et al. Bone marrow angiogenesis and progression in multiple myeloma. *Br J Haematol* 1994; **87**: 503–8.
20. Frizzera G. Castleman's disease and related disorders. *Semin Diagn Pathol* 1988; **5**: 346–64.
21. Perez-Atayde AR, Sallan SE, Tedrow U et al. Spectrum of tumor angiogenesis in the bone marrow of children with acute lymphoblastic leukemia *Am J Pathol* 1997; **150**: 815–21.
22. Ribatti D, Vacca A, Nico B et al. Angiogenesis spectrum in the stroma of B-cell non-Hodgkin's lymphomas. An immunohistochemical and ultrastructural study. *Eur J Haematol* 1996; **56**: 45–53.
23. Vacca A, Ribatti D, Fanelli M et al. Expression of tenascin is related to histologic malignancy and angiogenesis in B-cell non-Hodgkin's lymphomas. *Leuk Lymphoma* 1996; **22**: 473–81.
24. Vacca A, Ribatti D, Fanelli M et al. Lymph node angiogenesis in lymphoproliferative disorders: type II mixed cryoglobulinemia as a model. *Clin Exp Rheumatol* 1995; **13**(Suppl 13): 115–18.
25. Vacca A, Moretti S, Ribatti D et al. Progression of mycosis fungoides is associated with changes in angiogenesis and expression of the matrix metalloproteinase-2 and -9. *Eur J Cancer* 1997; **33**: 1685–92.
26. Vacca A, Ribatti D, Roncali L, Dammacco F. Angiogenesis in B-cell lymphoproliferative diseases. Biological and clinical studies. *Leuk Lymphoma* 1995; **20**: 27–38.
27. Kandel J, Bossy-Wetzel E, Raduvanyi F et al. Neovascularization is associated with a switch to export of FGF-2 in the multistep development of fibrosarcoma. *Cell* 1991; **66**: 1095–104.
28. Dameron KM, Volpert OV, Tainsky MA, Bouck N. Control of angiogenesis in fibroblasts by p53 regulation of thrombospondin-1, *Science* 1994; **265**: 1582–4.
29. Schultz HS, Haghaye GHS. Beta fibroblast growth factor expression in human and murine squamous cell carcinomas and its relationship to regional endothelial proliferation. *Cancer Res* 1993; **53**: 1444–9.
30. Fontanini G, Vignati S, Boldrini L et al. Vascular endothelial growth factor is associated with neovascularization and influences progression of non-small cell lung carcinoma. *Clin Cancer Res* 1997; **3**: 861–5.
31. To CT, Tsao MS., The roles of hepatocyte growth factor/scatter factor and met receptor in human cancers. *Oncol Rep* 1998; **5**: 1013–24.
32. Gallo O, Masini E, Morbidelli L et al. Role of nitric oxide in angiogenesis and tumor progression in head and neck cancer. *J Natl Cancer Inst* 1998; **90**: 587–96.
33. Shimoyama S, Gansauge F, Gansauge S et al. Increased angiogenin expression in pancreatic cancer is related to cancer aggressiveness. *Cancer Res* 1996; **56**: 2703–6.
34. Barnhill RL, Xiao M, Graves D, Antoniades HN. Expression of platelet-derived growth factor (PDGF)-A, PDGF-B and the PDGF-alpha receptor, but not the PDGF-beta receptor, in human malignant melanoma in vivo. *Br J Dermatol* 1996; **135**: 898–904.
35. Viglietto G, Romano A, Maglione D et al. Neovascularization in human germ cell tumors correlates with a marked increase in the expression of the vascular endothelial growth factor but not the placenta-derived growth factor. *Oncogene* 1996; **13**: 577–87.
36. Ray Chaudhury A, D'Amore PA., Endothelial cell regulation by transforming growth factor-beta. *J Cell Biochem* 1991; **47**: 224–9.
37. Rollins BJ, Chemokines. *Blood* 1997; **90**: 909–28.
38. Leek RD, Lewis CE, Harris AL. The role of macrophages in tumour angiogenesis. In: *Tumour Angiogenesis* (Bicknell R, Lewis CE, Ferrara N, eds). Oxford: Oxford University Press, 1997: 81–9.
39. Norrby K, Whooley D. Role of mast cells in mitogenesis and angiogenesis in normal tissues and tumour tissues. *Adv Biosci* 1993; **89**: 71–136.

40. Polverini PF. How the extracellular matrix and macrophages contribute to angiogenesis-dependent diseases. *Eur J Cancer* 1996; **32A**: 2430–7.
41. Pepper MS, Vassalli JD, Wilks JW et al. Modulation of bovine microvascular endothelial cell proteolytic properties by inhibitors of angiogenesis. *J Cell Biochem* 1994; **55**: 419–34.
42. Zucher S, Lysik RM, Zarrabi MH, Moll U. *M(rr)* 92000 type IV collagenase is increased in plasma of patients with colon cancer and breast cancer. *Cancer Res* 1993; **53**: 140–6.
43. Liabakk NB, Talbot I, Smith RA et al. Matrix metalloprotease 2 (MMP-2) and matrix metalloprotease-9 (MMP-9) type IV collagenases in colorectal cancer. *Cancer Res* 1996; **56**: 190–6.
44. Brooks PC, Clark RAF, Cheresh DA. Requirement of vascular integrin avb3 for angiogenesis. *Science* 1994; **264**: 569–71.
45. Brooks PC, Stromblad S, Sanders LC et al. Localization of matrix metalloproteinase MMP-2 to the surface of invasive cells by interaction with integrin $\alpha_v\beta_3$, *Cell* 1996; **85**: 683–93.
46. Lauren J, Gunji Y, Alitalo K. Is angiopoietin-2 necessary for the initiation of tumor angiogenesis? *Am J Pathol* 1998; **153**: 1333–9.
47. Stratmann A, Risau W, Plate KH. All type-specific expression of angiopoietin-1 and angiopoietin-2 suggest a role in glioblastoma angiogenesis. *Am J Pathol* 1998; **153**: 1459–66.
48. Vacca A, Ribatti D, Presta M et al. Bone marrow neovascularization, plasma cell angiogenic potential and matrix metalloproteinase-2 secretion parallel progression of human multiple myeloma. *Blood* 1999; **93**: 3064–73.
49. Ribatti D, Gualandris A, Bastaki M et al. New model for the study of angiogenesis and antiangiogenesis in the chick embryo chorioallantoic membrane: the gelatin sponge/chorioallantoic membrane assay. *J Vascular Res* 1997; **34**: 455–63.
50. Goto F, Goto K, Weindel K, Folkman J. Synergistic effects of vascular endothelial growth factor and basic fibroblast growth factor on the proliferation and cord formation of bovine capillary endothelial cells within collagen gels. *Lab Invest* 1993; **69**: 508–17.
51. Børset M, Lien E, Espevik T et al. Concomitant expression of hepatocyte growth factor/scatter factor and the receptor c-MET in human myeloma cell lines. *J Biol Chem* 1996; **271**: 24655–61.
52. Børset M, Hjorth-Hansen H, Seidel C et al. Hepatocyte growth factor and its receptor c-met in multiple myeloma. *Blood* 1996; **88**: 3998–4004.
53. Seidel C, Børset M, Turesson I et al. Elevated serum concentrations of hepatocyte growth factor in patients with multiple myeloma. *Blood* 1998; **91**: 806–12.
54. Portier M, Zhang XG, Ursule E et al. Cytokine gene expression in human multiple myeloma. *Br J Haematol* 1993; **85**: 514–20.
55. Mantovani A, Bussolino F, Dejana E. Cytokine regulation of endothelial cell function. *FASEB J* 1992; **6**: 2591–9.
56. Klein B, Cytokines, cytokine receptors, transduction signals and oncogenes in multiple myeloma. *Semin Hematol* 1995; **32**: 4–19.
57. Merico F, Bergui L, Gregoretti MG et al. Cytokines involved in the progression of multiple myeloma. *Clin Exp Immunol* 1993; **92**: 27–31.
58. Barillé S, Akhoundi C, Collette M et al. Metalloproteinases in multiple myeloma: production of matrix metalloproteinase-9 (MMP-9), activation of proMMP-2, and induction of MMP-1 by myeloma cells. *Blood* 1997; **90**: 1649–55.
59. Ribatti D, Vacca A, Nico B et al. Bone marrow angiogenesis and mast cell density increase simultaneously with progression of human multiple myeloma. *Br J Cancer* 1999; **79**: 451–5.
60. Yaccoby S, Barlogie B, Epstein J. Primary myeloma cells growing in SCID–hu mice: a model for studying the biology and treatment of myeloma and its manifestations. *Blood* 1998; **92**: 2908–13.
61. Weidner N. Tumoural vascularity as a prognostic factor in cancer patients: the evidence continues to grow. *J Pathol* 1998; **184**: 119–22.
62. Munshi N, Wilson C, Penn J et al. Angiogenesis in newly diagnosed multiple myeloma (MM): poor prognosis with increased microvessel density (MVD) in bone marrow biopsies (BMBX). *Blood* 1998; **92**(Suppl 1): 98a.
63. Rajkumar SV, Fonseca R, Witzig TE et al. Bone marrow angiogenesis in patients achieving complete response after stem cell transplantation for multiple myeloma. *Leukemia* 1999; **13**: 469–72.
64. Hardin J, MacLeod S, Grigorieva I et al. Interleukin-6 prevents dexamethasone-induced myeloma cell death. *Blood* 1994; **84**: 3063–70.
65. Brown RA, Rees JA, McFarland CD et al. Microvascular invasion of rabbit growth plate cartilage and the influence of dexamethasone. *Bone Miner* 1990; **9**: 35–47.
66. Maheshwari RK, Srikantan V, Bhartiya D et al. Differential effects of interferon gamma and

alpha on in vitro model of angiogenesis. *J Cell Physiol* 1991; **146**: 164–9.
67. Singhal S, Mehta J, Desikan R et al. Antitumor activity of thalidomide in refractory multiple myeloma. *N Engl J Med* 1999; **341**: 1565–71.
68. D'Amato RJ, Loughnan MS, Flynn E, Folkman J. Thalidomide is an inhibitor of angiogenesis. *Proc Natl Acad Sci USA* 1994; **91**: 4082–5.
69. Kenyon BM, Browne F, D'Amato RJ. Effects of thalidomide and related metabolites in a mouse corneal model of neovascularization. *Exp Eye Res* 1997; **64**: 971–8.
70. Desikan R, Munshi N, Zeldis J et al. Activity of thalidomide (thal) in multiple myeloma (MM) confirmed in 180 patients with advanced disease. *Blood* 1999; **94**(Suppl 1): Abst 2685.
71. Durie BGM, Stepan DE. Efficacy of low dose thalidomide (T) in multiple myeloma. *Blood* 1999; **94**(Suppl 1): Abst 1413.
72. Juliusson G, Celsing F, Turesson I et al. Thalidomide frequently induces good partial remission and best response ever in patients with advanced myeloma and prior high dose melphalan and autotransplant. *Blood* 1999; **94**(Suppl 1): Abst 546.
73. Rajkumar SV, Fonseca R, Dispenzieri A et al, Thalidomide in the treatment of relapsed and refractory myeloma. *Blood* 1999; **94**(Suppl 1): Abst 1414.
74. Sabir T, Raza S, Anderson L, Jagannath S. Thalidomide is effective in the treatment of recurrent, refractory multiple myeloma (MM). *Blood* 1999; **94**(Suppl 1): Abst 548.
75. Schiller G, Vescio R, Berenson J. Thalidomide for the treatment of multiple myeloma relapsing after autologous peripheral blood progenitor cell transplant. *Blood* 1999; **94**(Suppl 1): Abst 1417.
76. Weber DM, Gavino M, Delasalle K et al. Thalidomide alone or with dexamethasone for multiple myeloma. *Blood* 1999; **94**(Suppl 1): Abst 2686.
77. Geitz H, Handt S, Zwingenberger K. Thalidomide selectively modulates the density of cell surface molecules involved in the adhesion cascade. *Immunopharmacology* 1996; **31**: 213–21.
78. Sampaio EP, Sarno EN, Galilly R et al. Thalidomide selectively inhibits tumor necrosis factor alpha production by stimulated human monocytes. *J Exp Med* 1991; **173**: 699–703.
79. Haslett PA, Corral LG, Albert M, Kaplan G. Thalidomide costimulates primary human T lymphocytes, preferentially inducing proliferation, cytokine production, and cytotoxic responses in the CD81 subset. *J Exp Med* 1998; **187:** 1885–92.
80. McHugh SM, Rifkin IR, Deighton J et al. The immunosuppressive drug thalidomide induces T helper cell type 2 (Th2) and concomitantly inhibits Th1 cytokine production in mitogen- and antigen-stimulated human peripheral blood mononuclear cell cultures. *Clin Exp Immunol* 1995; **99**: 160–7.
81. Cheng D, Kini AR, Rodriguez J et al. Microvascular density and cytotoxic T cell activation correlate with response to thalidomide therapy in myeloma patients. *Blood* 1999; **94** (Suppl 1): Abst 1408.
82. Neben K, Hawighorst H, Moehler TM. Clinical response to thalidomide monotherapy correlates with improvement in dynamic magnetic resonance (d-MRI) angiogenesis parameters. *Blood* 1999; **94**(Suppl 1): Abst 545.
83. Moehler TM, Neben K, Egerer G et al. Thalidomide plus CED-chemotherapy in patients with poor prognosis multiple myeloma. *Blood* 1999; **94**(Suppl 1): Abst 547.
84. Munshi N, Desikan R, Zangari M et al. Chemoangiotherapy with DT-PACE for previously treated multiple myeloma (MM). *Blood* 1999; **94**(Suppl 1): Abst 540.
85. Munshi N, Desikan R, Anaissie E et al. Peripheral blood stem cell collection (PBSC) after CAD 1 G-CSF as part of Total Therapy II in newly diagnosed multiple myeloma (MM): influence of thalidomide (thal) administration. *Blood* 1999; **94**(Suppl 1): Abst 2577.
86. Singhal S, Mehta J. Thalidomide in cancer: potential uses and limitations. *BioDrugs* 2001; **15:** 163–72.
87. Singhal S, Mehta J. Thalidomide in cancer. *Biomed Pharmacother* 2001; in press.

Part 2

Clinical Aspects

9

Epidemiology of plasma cell disorders

Douglas E Joshua, John Gibson

INTRODUCTION

Although an uncommon diagnosis in the general population, myeloma accounts for 10–15% of all haematological malignancies. It is the best recognized of the monoclonal gammopathies, and the frequent presence of a preneoplastic clonal proliferation, monoclonal gammopathy of undetermined significance (MGUS), before overt malignant transformation, has created a unique opportunity for large-scale population studies, which have provided insight into both the etiology and epidemiology of myeloma. The hallmark of the disease is the presence of a serum or urine paraprotein, the detection and monitoring of which has contributed much to our understanding of the disease and its clinical features and progression. However, the increasing diagnostic sensitivity of detection of paraproteins, from protein electropheresis to immunoelectropheresis to immunofixation, have created some difficulties in the interpretation of epidemiological studies, particularly when one compares studies performed at different time points.

WHAT IS THE CAUSE OF MYELOMA?

This question is currently unanswerable. It was anticipated that epidemiological research would shed some light on the etiology of the disease. Despite extensive studies over almost five decades, however, there are still many unresolved issues and controversies. Epidemiological associations such as exposure to ionizing radiation and benzene, previously thought to be significant, are now questionable, whilst the list of other possible associations remains largely unexplained. Epidemiological studies, quoted below, provide limited information regarding occupational exposure and are frequently only of small size. Case–control studies are also often restricted, since there are only a few subjects who contract the disease in the occupations and industries of interest and usually only an abbreviated toxic exposure history has been obtained. A number of occupations have previously been related to disease occurrence, and these, together with a variety of environmental factors such as radiation exposure, will be discussed in more detail below. However, none of these associations has so far fulfilled the criteria of strength of association, consistency of association, specificity of association, and close temporal relationship (i.e. exposure–risk relationship) that would be required for definitive proof. It would be fair to say that in the vast majority of patients, no obvious explanation for the occurrence of the disease is available. Thus myeloma must still be regarded as being of unknown etiology.

NATURE OF THE DISEASE AND THE RELATIONSHIP WITH MGUS

Attempts to unravel both the epidemiology and etiology of myeloma, and for that matter other haematological malignancies, are also confounded by the fact that these diseases are clearly not the result of one single event but represent the cumulative result of a number of genetic and environmental events. That one single oncogenic event does not lead to neoplastic transformation was recognized in the early 1990s.[1] In vitro experiments clearly demonstrated that combinations of several oncogenes or 'cooperation' between oncogenes and tumour viruses were required for expression of the malignant phenotype. Thus, in myeloma for example, a number of events, which could presumably include some of the currently identified potential risk factors, would clearly be required for ultimate phenotypic expression of the disease.

The best recognized and most common risk factor for the development of myeloma is the presence of a monoclonal gammopathy of undetermined significance (MGUS). Patients with MGUS develop myeloma at an incidence of roughly 1.5% per year.[2,3] A number of studies have characterized the prevalence of MGUS, and have shown an age-related increase in the prevalence of monoclonal gammopathies reaching up to 5% in persons over the age of 80 years.[4,5] Men are 1.5–2 times more likely to have the condition than women. It must be stressed that earlier studies, which did not use immunofixation techniques, only detected monoclonal gammopathies of fairly large size (usually >15 g/l). The outlook for patients with small paraproteins detected by more sensitive immunofixation techniques is not well documented. It seems likely that the overall incidence of these smaller paraproteins may be higher and their outlook may be better than for patients with paraproteins of more than 15 g/l detected by earlier methods.[6]

The etiology of monoclonal gammopathies remains unknown. Their relationship to chronic disease and infection has had only limited study. There is some evidence of monoclonal protein production being stimulated by infection with cytomegalovirus and *Leishmania*, but not Epstein–Barr virus. The relationship of these findings to the development of myeloma is unclear.[7]

DESCRIPTIVE EPIDEMIOLOGY

Incidence data have been collected by a number of large studies in the USA and Europe. Data from the US Surveillance Epidemiology and End Results Programme (SEER) demonstrates that the incidence increases rapidly with age, with higher rates in males than females.[8] Incidence and mortality rates are consistently higher in the African-American population than in Caucasians, whilst its incidence is relatively low amongst Asian populations. In Caucasians, the incidence is approximately 5 per 100 000 in males and 3 per 100 000 in females rising to 10 per 100 000 and 7 per 100 000 respectively in African-Americans. The incidence in the Oriental population is approximately 2 per 100 000. Geographical data show similar rates of incidence around the world, although this is confounded by varying sensitivities and accuracies of diagnosis. The high incidence in African-American compared with Caucasian, and males compared with females, in the USA has been a consistent finding over the last decade, whilst similar results have also been reported in Brazil[9] and the Caribbean.[10] The incidence in New South Wales, Australia in 1995 was 5.8 per 100 000 in males and 3.7 per 100 000 in females, giving a lifetime risk of developing myeloma of 1 in 201 for males and 1 in 351 for females.[11]

A predominant feature of myeloma is the increasing incidence with age. From the SEER data, the disease is rare prior to the age of 30 years, but thereafter age-specific incidences rise almost exponentially.[8] Comparisons of cancer registries elsewhere show a similar effect, but any such comparisons should be made with caution. Inaccuracies of diagnosis, pathological versus clinical diagnosis, and the availability of appropriate investigations and medical care may limit the usefulness of certain comparisons. This is especially so in the elderly, where death may be due to disease complications (i.e. infection or renal failure) without the underlying disease being recognized.

The age-specific incidence in New South Wales in 1995 is illustrated in Table 9.1. Myeloma represents approximately 1% of all cancers.[11]

Myeloma in the younger age group is infrequent. In a series of 4081 patients from the Mayo Clinic, with a median age of 63 years, 12% were younger than 50 years and only 2% younger than 40 years.[12] Estimates of disease frequency in those less than 30 years old have ranged from 0.18% (US National Cancer Institute, NCI)[13] to 0.3% (Mayo Clinic).[14] Many of the clinical and laboratory features of the younger age group are similar to those of the total population, although some apparent differences have been highlighted. For instance, there appears to be a higher incidence of extramedullary involvement: 20% and 40% in those less than 40 and 30 years old, respectively. In addition, a doubling of the proportion of light-chain and IgD disease is also reported, occurring in 33% and 4% of those less than 40 years old, compared with frequencies of 15% and 2% in the total population. In general, younger myeloma patients are believed to respond to therapy at a rate similar to the whole population. An exception may be the unusual combination of multiple skeletal lesions, extraosseus spread, few bone marrow plasma cells and a small paraprotein that has been likened to multiple solitary plasmacytomata. This has been reported to be apparently more common in younger patients, who appear to have a relatively prolonged survival. A bias in reporting both younger and atypical cases cannot, however, be excluded.[12]

There is considerable uncertainty as to whether temporal changes in the incidence of myeloma have occurred. In areas where high levels of diagnostic accuracy are available, it does not seem that there has been a dramatic rise in the overall incidence of myeloma over time, other than what might be expected from improved diagnostic sophistication. Three major studies in Olmstead County, Minnesota.[15] Malmö, Sweden[16] and Switzerland,[17] together with other studies in the USA, do not suggest a change in the incidence of myeloma over the last two to three decades. In Olmstead County, the annual age-standardized incidence of myeloma has remained steady for over four decades. In Malmö, although the incidence rate in males increased between 1950 and 1980, there was no increase in the rate of females. In Switzerland, no changes have been noted in the last decade. Finally, the incidence of myeloma in four geographic areas in the USA rose by only a small amount between 1970 and 1990.[18]

In contrast, other studies have suggested an increasing incidence of myeloma, at least over some time periods. For instance, in Denmark, the reported annual incidence increased in males from 1.3 per 100 000 to 3.3 per 100 000 between 1943 and 1962 . No subsequent increase

Table 9.1 Age–specific incidence rates per 100 000 population by sex New South Wales, 1995

Age (years):	<35	35–9	40–5	45–9	56–4	55–9	60–4	65–9	70–4	75–9	80–4	85+
Males	0	0.4	2.7	3.7	5.9	10.7	21.0	29.6	26.0	44.6	39.0	52.5
Females	0	0	0.4	2.4	3.7	7.3	14.3	13.4	15.5	35.6	30.9	25.5

was, however, observed in the following two decades.[19] It has been suggested (and in fact appears highly likely) that the reported rate increase relates to improved laboratory diagnosis, since many of the reported increases have occurred in the elderly, in whom a diagnosis might have previously less commonly been sought. Apart from age and race, no other demographic factors have been shown to have a consistent relationship with myeloma. In particular, socio-economic status does not appear to be a significant factor. Any increased incidence reported in the higher socio-economic group relate to better access to sensitive diagnostic methods.

CHRONIC ANTIGENIC STIMULATION AND AUTOIMMUNE DISORDERS

Does chronic immunostimulation in situations such as autoimmune disorders predispose to myeloma?

Antigen exposure appears to be crucial to the development of this disease. For instance germ-free BALB/c mice do not develop plasmacytomas following injection of mineral oil. It could be postulated that chronic immunostimulation with overproduction of interleukin-6 (IL-6) may be responsible for polyclonal B-cell and plasma cell expansion, or perhaps even selection of a 'premalignant' clone.[20] In the murine plasmacytoma model, pristane-induced polyclonal granulomas are a prerequisite for the development of plasmacytomas. The reports from some laboratories of the HHV-8/KSHV γ-herpesvirus in association with myeloma and the possibility that a viral IL-6 may play a role has added further weight to this question.[21] A variety of states in which chronic antigen stimulation is thought to occur have been studied to examine this hypothesis. These include exposure to silicone gel in mice, asthma, allergy treatments, chronic and acute infections, and immunization protocols.[22–25] Both population-based case–control and tumour-registry-based case–control studies have been employed. One difficulty with these analyses is that no specific techniques were used to measure a dose relationship between incidence and the extent or duration of the putative chronic antigenic stimulation.

Given the available data, however, there seems to be little evidence that chronic immune stimulation is likely to significantly increase the risk of myeloma. One exception may be rheumatoid arthritis, in which there does seem to be an increased frequency of myeloma. A consistent relationship between rheumatoid arthritis and myeloma was documented both in a Finnish Study and in the Mayo Clinic cohort, as well as in a number of other studies.[26–27] As a possible explanation for this observation, it has been suggested that the idiotypes of paraproteins associated with myeloma have a high incidence of antibodies to autoimmune antigens.[28]

LIFESTYLE FACTORS

A variety of lifestyle factors have been evaluated as possible risk factors for myeloma. Cigarette smoking and alcohol consumption in particular have been studied extensively without any evidence of increased risk.[29–33] Cigarette smoking has historically often been used as a surrogate marker for benzene exposure, which is further discussed below.

Does benzene exposure cause myeloma?

Benzene exposure has been linked to the etiology of a number of haematological malignancies, including myeloma. With respect to myeloma, the majority of studies and authorities have until recently appeared to support this association.[34–36] For instance a review by Goldstein[34] concluded that 'it is more likely than not that benzene exposure is an etiological factor in multiple myeloma'.

More recently, however, this association has been questioned, with futher analyses casting doubt on the association of benzene exposure with myeloma. A cohort mortality study was conducted by epidemiologists from the US

National Institute for Occupation Safety and Health, among workers exposed to benzene during the manufacture of pliofilm. An initial report[36] had suggested a fourfold increase in myeloma amongst workers exposed to benzene from 1950 to 1981. No pattern of risk with cumulative levels of benzene exposure was, however, apparent. When subsequently updated in 1994,[37] no additional deaths from myeloma were found, and it was then concluded that the risk of developing myeloma after benzene exposure was no longer statistically significant. In the final update of this cohort, published in 1995,[38] the lack of relationship to myeloma was confirmed, although a definite relationship was shown between cumulative exposure of benzene and the development of acute myeloid leukaemia (AML). This lack of an association between exposure to benzene and myeloma has also been supported by other large-scale studies. For instance, a large-cohort study of petroleum and transport workers exposed to petrol containing 2–5% benzene detected no relationship between benzene exposure and the development of myeloma.[39]

In an analysis of published case–control literature by Bezabeh et al,[40] evidence for the relationship of benzene exposure to myeloma was critically reviewed. This study reviewed 13 case–control population or hospital-based myeloma studies, and employed odds-ratio or risk-ratio analysis for occupational exposure. Neither exposure to benzene nor exposure to benzene surrogates were documented as having a relationship to myeloma. Similarly, an analysis of employment-based exposure history failed to reveal a definite association. In the absence of analysis of specific benzene exposure, analysis of surrogates of benzene exposure were also reviewed. Odds ratio for exposure to petroleum products, with one exception, were not significantly increased. This exception was exposure to petroleum combustion products. Combustion products consist of a wide range of carcinogenic and non-carcinogenic constituents, and no particular constituent was positively distinguished. Furthermore, the absence of relationship to cigarette smoking, which is often considered a surrogate for benzene exposure, and the positive relationship to AML were confirmed, further reinforcing that benzene exposure is unlikely to be a significant causal agent for myeloma.

Thus the literature on benzene is contradictory, and does not fulfil the criteria of consistency, dose relationship, and specificity that would be required to conclude that benzene is a definite cause of myeloma.

IONIZING RADIATION: OCCUPATIONAL, ATMOSPHERIC, AND CLINICAL

Like exposure to benzene, radiation exposure is a well-recognized leukaemogen. However, also like the benzene association, the relationship of radiation exposure to myeloma remains highly controversial. Two early studies reporting the risk of myeloma in Japanese survivors of atomic bombs supported a statistically significant relationship between the incidence of myeloma at radiation dose estimates of more than 1 Gy. Relative risk ratios were given as 3.29, with 90% confidence interval (CI) 1.67–6.13.[41,42] A follow-up study by Preston et al[43] ascertained 59 persons whose first cancer diagnosis was myeloma and whose dose estimates were less than 4 Gy. The relative risk observed by Preston et al was, however, now only 1.25, which was not considered to be significant. The difference between the earlier data sets and the latest data has been evaluated in an attempt to determine why different conclusions were obtained. It may be related to a more complete follow-up, more stringent diagnostic criteria, and exclusion of myeloma cases defined as second primaries. The frequency of monoclonal gammopathy does not appear to be increased in survivors of the atom bombs, and nor is the relative risk of an M protein significantly increased with increasing radiation dose.[44]

Other studies have shown an increased risk of myeloma in workers at nuclear processing plants,[45] and an excess of myeloma deaths among American radiologists was also reported three decades ago.[46] In contrast, a survey of Chinese diagnostic X-ray workers showed no increased incidence of myeloma over a 30-year period,[47] whilst other studies evaluating employment at nuclear facilities have shown a lower rate of myeloma than that observed in the general population.[48]

Arguing against a significant relationship between radiation and myeloma are studies demonstrating no evidence of an increased risk of myeloma in relation to residential proximity to nuclear facilities,[49–50] and although an increase in myeloma incidence has been observed amongst British military personnel who participated in atmospheric nuclear tests, no increase was seen amongst New Zealand military participants in the same tests.[51,52] Similarly, it does not appear that diagnostic or therapeutic X-ray use or exposure is related to the incidence of myeloma, although again there is some disagreement in the literature. For instance, follow-up studies of patients with ankylosing spondylitis, who received a single course of X-ray treatment, and of patients treated for cervical cancer, revealed no significant elevated risk of myeloma.[53–54]

Exposure to ionizing radiation therefore cannot be confirmed as a definitive cause of myeloma. The many inconsistencies in the literature are in clear contrast to the relationship of AML to radiation exposure, which is clear and definitive.

HUMAN IMMUNODEFICIENCY VIRUS AND MYELOMA

The report of the novel human herpesvirus-8 (HHV-8; also known as Kaposi sarcoma herpesvirus, KSHV) in the dendritic cells of patients with myeloma has raised considerable interest in the possibility that myeloma may be an HIV-associated disease.[21] Plasma cell dyscrasias have been reported in patients with HIV infection.[55–58] In one series, a serum M protein was seen in 11 out of 341 asymptomatic HIV-positive patients. In 7 of these patients, the protein disappeared after a median follow-up time of 50 months, and the presence of the M protein did not appear to influence outcome.[59] In one HIV-positive patient, the IgGκ M protein recognized the HIV p24 Gag antigen, suggesting that an antigen-driven response to the viral infection played a role in the pathogenesis of myeloma in this patient.[60]

In a study of AIDS-associated malignant disorders, the risk of myeloma in patients with AIDS compared with the normal population was 4.5-fold, compared with 113-fold for non-Hodgkin's lymphoma.[61] It is possible that myeloma in the setting of HIV will have unusual features, with a higher frequency of extramedullary involvement, whilst the differentiation of anaplastic myeloma from immunoblastic lymphoma or body cavity lymphoma may add to the confusion.

OCCUPATIONAL EXPOSURES

Do various occupations put individuals at risk for the development of myeloma?

As with the benzene and radiation issues, the answer to this question is also quite uncertain. As mentioned previously, the rarity of myeloma gives cohort studies limited weight owing to the small number of individuals employed in any single occupation, and given the few cases of myeloma identified (sometimes only two or three), absolute risk ratios are unlikely to be significant. Analysis by industry type may provide some specific clues, but the information is not usually specific enough to identify a definite relationship between individual products and myeloma. Another confounding observation is that in cases in which positive exposure to chemicals has apparently been identified (particularly those agents known to be hazardous), patients recall these exposures better than control patients.

Two of the best case–control studies are those reported by Heineman et al[62] and Pottern et al,[63] which were based on work histories obtained in large population-based case–control studies from Denmark. One of these large studies evaluated occupational exposures in over 1000 Danish males diagnosed with myeloma from 1970 to 1984 and in over 4000 age- and gender-matched controls alive at the time of case diagnosis.[62] Informational histories were obtained from the supplementary pension fund that recorded employment of all adult Danish males. A similar study was performed for myeloma in females, using the Danish Cancer Registry datalink system.[63]

In males, myeloma risks were found to be significantly elevated in road and railroad workers, metal workers, and workers in transportation and community industries. After adjusting for multiple exposures and disregarding exposures within 10 years of diagnosis, exposure to vinyl chloride was associated with the highest risk. Exposure to agriculture (see below) was not confirmed as a risk.

For females, an increased risk of myeloma was found in those patients not in the pension fund who had an occupation title coded as 'Mrs Homemaker'. No other significant risks were found. The strongest, but not statistically significant, association was with employment in the agriculture industry.

These data serve to reinforce the difficulty of making conclusions regarding occupational exposures and myeloma. The majority of general occupational exposures do not fulfil the criteria of consistency and dose response such that we can confirm that they are definitively related to myeloma. Specific occupational industries are discussed below.

Agricultural exposure

The risk of the occurrence of myeloma in agricultural workers has frequently been reported to be increased, albeit often only to a very limited extent.[64,65] Agriculture-related exposures include those to fuels and pesticides.[66] Individual studies on the incidence of pesticide exposure have been conducted. In the dioxin industrial accident in Italy, the risk of myeloma in the subsequent 10 years was elevated in both men (relative risk 3.2; 95% CI 0.8–13.3) and in women (relative risk 5.2; 95% CI 1.2–22.6).[67] However, other studies including those by Le Vecchia et al[68] and Pearce et al[64] have not confirmed a relationship between a history of exposure to pesticides and myeloma. Thus, while there appears to be some suggestion that those involved in agricultural occupations may well have an increased risk of myeloma, the specific agents responsible for this remain unknown.

Metalworkers

Statistical links have been made between employment in metal industries and myeloma.[69–71] Significantly elevated risks have been observed amongst smelter and nickel workers in some, but not all, studies. Of note, the large Danish studies did not find this risk to be significant.[62,63]

Rubber and plastics

The rubber and plastics industries have been another area in which it has been suggested that industrial exposure may lead to an increased risk of myeloma. Female, but not male, workers from a cohort of rubber workers in the USA were observed to have an increased incidence of myeloma. This risk was, however, not seen in the male members, thus casting doubt upon the significances of the association.[72,73] It is important to note that in the large studies by Heineman, Pottern et al,[62,63] no association between a history of work in the rubber or plastic manufacturing industries and myeloma was observed. Thus one can only conclude that, given the current evidence, such an association is also unlikely to be very significant.

Petroleum refining

Workers in the petroleum industry are exposed to a variety of known carcinogens, including polycyclic aromatic hydrocarbons. The vast majority of studies, including three out of four case–control studies, indicate that petroleum workers do not have an increased risk of death from myeloma.[25,65,74] A large Australian Institute of Petroleum health surveillance programme did not find a significant increase in myeloma in its subjects, although it did document an overall increase in the lympho-haematopoietic cancers in petroleum workers, particularly leukaemias and, within the leukaemias, particularly myeloid leukaemias.[75]

Wood, leather, and textile industries

As with many of the industries cited above, studies of workers in these industries are inconsistent, although the majority of studies suggest little or no altered risk.[25,62,63,68,76]

Beauty industry

An increase risk of myeloma has been associated with the use of hair dyes in some, but not all, studies. Some studies, for example the American Cancer Society cohort, show no relationship between the duration of the use of permanent hair dyes for less than 20 years and deaths from myeloma.[77] In the Nurses Health Study, there was an inverse association between ever having used a permanent hair dye and the subsequent incidence of myeloma.[78] However, other studies have reported an increased risk of myeloma according to the personal use of hair dyes in both women and men.[79,80] The relationship therefore remains uncertain. The exact substances that might be responsible are also uncertain.

Asbestos: mining and industrial-use exposure, and industries involved in mining

Asbestos is a recognized carcinogen. A number of epidemiological studies have examined the relationship between the history of asbestos exposure and myeloma, and vary in their results. Most case–control studies have found no association,[29,62,81] although one positive study has been reported.[82]

Painters

Painters and workers in the paint industry are exposed to a variety of toxins, including aromatic hydrocarbons. A relationship between the history of exposure to paints and solvents and myeloma has been reported by some.[83,84] There is also some evidence of a dose response, with duration of employment of over 10 years and high exposures apparently being associated with a higher risk.[84] Significantly, however, the large Danish studies did not confirm such a relationship.[62,63]

FAMILIAL MYELOMA

In a population-based case–control study from Sweden, the occurrence of myeloma in relatives was investigated. Data from 239 cases with myeloma and 220 controls were analysed, and an increased risk was found in first-degree relatives, in whom the relative risk was 5.64 (95% CI 1.16–27.51). An increased risk was also seen if close relatives had experienced a brain tumour (relative risk 6.61; 95% CI 1.41–30.67).[85] There have been over 50 reported incidents of myeloma occurring in more than one family member, and in four of these reports more than three siblings have been affected.[86] The isotype has varied in different family members, and no clear genomic mutation has been identified.[87] M-protein idiotypes were also different, and in a familial case of two sisters with plasma cell dyscrasia, anti-idiotypic antibodies against one patient's λ light-chain showed no cross reactivity with her sister's λ light-chain.[88]

Thus an increased incidence of myeloma in certain families does appear to be a real finding even though the risk is relatively small. Some family members have inherited identical HLA haplotypes, suggesting that the tendency may be HLA-linked. In a large population study of 46 African-American males and 85 Caucasian males with myeloma, increased gene frequencies for Bw65, Cw2, and DRw14 were identified in the former population and A3 and CRw2 in the latter, suggesting that

Cw2 or closely related loci confer susceptibility to myeloma.[89]

Another possibility is that the increased incidence in certain families and the occurrence of myeloma in spouses (unpublished observations) may reflect a similar environmental factor. Differentiation between environmental and hereditary causes is, at this stage, not possible.

CONCLUSIONS

Although the descriptive epidemiology of myeloma is currently well documented, causation and etiology remain enigmatic. The high risk of developing myeloma in those patients who have MGUS may provide us with an understanding of the transformation from a benign to a malignant proliferation, but it still does not elucidate the etiology of the initial autonomous clone.

A number of case–control and cohort studies have suggested occupation and workplace exposures, but these have not been consistent. In general, risk ratios are relatively low and confidence intervals are large.

Given the current evidence, it seems likely that some forms of occupational exposure in the agricultural workforce may increase the risk of developing myeloma. This may be related to exposure to pesticides, but the exact agents responsible are unclear. Whilst benzene exposure and radiation exposure have traditionally been thought as being etiologically significant in the causation of myeloma, recent data have cast considerable doubt on such associations, and these agents can no longer be definitively associated with this disease.

REFERENCES

1. Cooper GM. *Oncogenes*, 2nd edn. Boston: Jones & Bartlett, 1995.
2. Kyle RA. 'Benign' monoclonal gammopathy – after 20 to 35 years of follow-up. *Mayo Clin Proc* 1993; **68**: 26–36.
3. Blade J, Lopez-Guilllermo A, Rozman C et al. Malignant transformation and life expectancy in monoclonal gammopathy of undertermined significance. *Br J Haematol* 1992; **81**: 91–4.
4. Kyle RA, Finkelstein S, Elseback LR et al. Incidence of monoclonal proteins in a Minnesota community with a cluster of multiple myeloma. *Blood* 1972; **40**: 719–24.
5. Saleun JP, Vicariot M, Deroff P et al. Monoclonal gammopathies in the adult population of Finistere, France. *J Clin Pathol* 1982; **35**: 63–8.
6. Axelsson U, Bachmann R, Hallen J. Frequency of pathological proteins (M-components) in 6995 sera from an adult population. *Acta Med Scand* 1966; **179**: 235–47.
7. Haas H, Anders S, Bornkamm GW et al. Do infections induce monoclonal immunoglobulin components? *Clin Exp Immunol* 1990; **81**: 435–40.
8. Miller BA, Ries LAG, Hankey BF et al. *SEER Cancer Statistics Review 1973–1990.* NIH Publication 93–2789. Bethseda, MD: National Cancer Institute, 1993.
9. Bouchardy C, Mirra AP, Khlat M et al. Ethnicity and cancer risk in Sao Paulo, Brazil. *Cancer Epidemiol Biomark Prev* 1991; **1**: 21–7.
10. Grulich A, Swerdlow AJ, Head J et al. Cancer mortality in African and Caribbean migrants to England and Wales. *Br J Cancer* 1992; **66**: 905–11.
11. Coates M, Armstrong B. *Cancer in New South Wales – Incidence and Mortality*. Sydney: NSW Cancer Council, 1998.
12. Blade J, Kyle RA. Multiple myeloma in young patients: clinical presentation and treatment approach. *Leuk Lymphoma* 1998; **30**: 493–501.
13. Young JL, Percy CL, Asire AJ. *Surveillance, Epidemiology, and End-Results. National Cancer Institute Monograph 57.* Bethesda, MD: US Department of Health and Human Services, 1981.
14. Blade J, Kyle RA, Greipp PR. Multiple myeloma in patients younger than 30 years. Report of 10 cases and review of the literature. *Arch Intern Med* 1996; **156**: 1463–8.
15. Kyle RA, Beard CM, O'Fallon M et al. Incidence of monoclonal proteins in a Minnesota community with a cluster of multiple myeloma. *Blood* 1972; **40**: 719–24.
16. Turesson I, Zettervall O, Cuzick J et al. Comparison of trends in the incidence of multiple myeloma in Malmo, Sweden, and other countries 1950–1979. *N Engl J Med* 1984; **310**: 421–4.
17. Levi F, La Vecchia C. Trends in multiple myeloma. *Int J Cancer* 1990; **46**: 755–6.
18. Devesa SS, Silverman DT, Young JL et al. Cancer incidence and mortality trends among Whites in

the United States 1947–84. *J Natl Cancer Inst* 1987; **79**: 701–70.
19. Hansen NE, Karle H, Olsen JH. Trends in the incidence of multiple myeloma in Denmark 1943–1982: a study of 5500 patients. *Eur J Haematol* 1989; **41**: 72–6.
20. Riedel DA, Pottern LM. The epidemiology of multiple myeloma. *Hematol Oncol Clin North Am* 1992; **6**: 225–47.
21. Rettig MB, Ma HJ, Vescio RA et al. Kaposi's sarcoma-associated herpesvirus infection of bone marrow dendritic cells from multiple myeloma patients. *Science* 1997; **276**: 1851–4.
22. Gallagher RP, Spinelli JJ, Elwood JM et al. Allergies and agricultural exposure and risk factors for multiple myeloma. *Br J Cancer* 1983; **48**: 853–7.
23. Lewis DR, Pottern LM, Brown LM et al. Multiple myeloma among blacks and whites in the United States: the role of chronic antigenic stimulation. *Cancer Causes Control* 1995; **5**: 529–39.
24. Linet MMS, Harlow SD, McLaughlin JK. A case–control study of multiple myeloma in whites: chronic antigenic stimulation, occupation, and drug use. *Cancer Res* 1987; **47**: 2978–81.
25. Cuzick J, De Stavola B. Multiple myeloma – a case–control study. *Br J Cancer* 1988; **57**: 516–20.
26. Katusic S, Beard CM, Kurland LT et al. Occurrence of malignant neoplasms in the Rochester, Minnesota, rheumatoid arthritis cohort. *Am J Med* 1985; **78**: 50–5.
27. Isomaki HA, Hakulinen T, Joutsenlaht U. Excess risk of lymphomas, leukemia and myeloma in patients with rheumatoid arthritis. *J Chron Dis* 1978; **31**: 6916.
28. Hardiman KL, Horn S, Manoharan A et al. Rheumatic autoantibodies in the sera of patients with paraproteins. *Clin Exp Rheumatol* 1994; **12**: 363–8.
29. Boffetta P, Stellman SD, Garfinkel L. A case–control study of multiple myeloma nested in the American Cancer Society prospective study. *Int J Cancer* 1989; **43**: 554–9.
30. Brown LM, Everett GD, Gibson R et al. Smoking and risk of non-Hodgkin's lymphoma and multiple myeloma. *Cancer Causes Control* 1992; **3**: 49–55.
31. Brownson RC. Cigarette smoking and risk of myeloma. *J Natl Cancer Inst* 1991; **83**: 1036–7.
32. Friedman GD. Cigarette smoking, leukaemia and multiple myeloma. *Ann Epidemiol* 1993; **3**: 425–8.
33. Brown LM, Gibson R, Burmeister LF et al. Alcohol consumption and risk of leukemia, non-Hodgkin's lymphoma and multiple myeloma. *Leuk Res* 1992; **16**: 979–84.
34. Goldstein BD. Is exposure to benzene a cause of human multiple myeloma? *Ann NY Acad Sci* 1990; **609**: 225–30.
35. Aksov M, Erdem S, Dincol G et al. Clinical observations showing the role of some factors in the etiology of multiple myeloma. A study in 7 patients. *Acta Haematol* 1984; **71**: 116–20.
36. Rinsky RA, Smith AB, Hornung R et al. Benzene and leukemia. An epidemiologic risk assessment. *N Engl J Med* 1987; **316**: 1044–50.
37. Paxton MB, Chinchilli VM, Brett SM et al. Leukemia risk associated with benzene exposure in the pliofilm cohort: I. Mortality update and exposure distribution. *Risk Anal* 1994; **14**: 147–54.
38. Wong O. Risk of acute myeloid leukaemia and multiple myeloma in workers exposured to benzene. *Occup Environ Med* 1995; **52**: 380–4.
39. Yin SN, Hayes RB, Linet MS et al. Cohort study of cancer among workers exposed to benzene in China: I. General methods and resources. *Am J Ind Med* 1994; **26**: 383–400.
40. Bezabeh S, Engel A, Morris CB et al. Does benzene cause multiple myeloma? An analysis of the published case–control literature. *Environ Health Perspect* 1996; **104** (Suppl 6): 1393–8.
41. Shimizu Y, Kato H, Schull W. Studies of the mortality of A-bomb survivors. 9. Mortality, 1950–1985: Part 2. Cancer mortality based on the recently revised doses (DS86). *Radiat Res* 1990; **121**: 120–41.
42. Ichimaru M, Ishimaru T, Mikami M et al. Multiple myeloma among atomic bomb survivors in Hiroshima and Nagasaki 1950–76: relationship to radiation dose absorbed by marrow. *J Natl Cancer Inst* 1982; **69**: 323–8.
43. Preston DL, Kusumi S, Tomonaga M et al. Cancer incidence in atomic bomb survivors. Part III: Leukemia, lymphoma and multiple myeloma, 1950–87. *Radiat Res* 1994; **137**: S68–97.
44. Neriishi K, Yoshimoto Y, Carter RL et al. Monoclonal gammopathy in atomic bomb survivors. *Radiat Res* 1993; **133**: 351–9.
45. Gilbert ES, Fry SA, Wiggs LD et al. Analyses of combined mortality data on workers at the Hanford site, Oak Ridge National Laboratory, and Rocky Flats Nuclear Weapons Plant. *Radiat Res* 1989; **120**: 19–35.
46. Lewis EB. Leukemia, multiple myeloma, and aplastic anemia in American radiologists. *Science* 1963; **142**: 1492–4.

47. Wang JX, Boice JD, Li BX et al. Cancer among medical diagnostic x-ray workers in China. *J Natl Cancer Inst* 1988; **80**: 344–50.
48. Kendall GM, Muirhead CR, MacGibbon BH et al. Mortality and occupational exposure to radiation: first analysis of National Registry for Radiation Workers. *BMJ* 1992; **304**: 220–5.
49. Cook-Mozaffari PJ, Darby SC, Doll R et al. Geographical variation of mortality from leukemia and other cancers in England and Wales in relation to proximity to nuclear installations 1969–78. *Br J Cancer* 1989; **59**: 476–85.
50. Dousset M. Cancer mortality around La Hague nuclear facilities. *Health Physician* 1989; **56**: 875–84.
51. Darby SC, Kendall GM, Fell TP et al. A summary of mortality and incidence of cancer in men from the United Kingdom who participated in the United Kingdom's atmospheric nuclear weapon tests and experimental programmes. *BMJ Clinical Research Ed* 1988; **296**: 332–8.
52. Pearce N, Prior I, Methven D et al. Follow up of New Zealand participants in British atmospheric nuclear weapons tests in the Pacific. *BMJ* 1990; **300**: 1161–6.
53. Darby SC, Doll R, Gill SK et al. Long term mortality after a single treatment course with X-rays in patients treated for ankylosing spondylitis. *Br J Cancer* 1987; **55**: 179–90.
54. Boice JD Jr, Day NE, Andersen A et al. Second cancers following radiation treatment for cervical cancer. An international collaboration among cancer registries. *J Natl Cancer Inst* 1985; **74**: 955–75.
55. Karnad AB, Martin AW, Koh HK et al. Nonsecretory multiple myeloma in a 26-year-old man with acquired immunodeficiency syndrome, presenting with multiple extramedullary plasmacytomas and osteolytic bone disease. *Am J Hematol* 1989; **32**: 305–10.
56. Voelkerding KV, Sandhaus LM, Kim HC et al. Plasma cell malignancy in the acquired immune deficiency syndrome: association with Epstein–Barr virus. *Am J Clin Pathol* 1989; **92**: 222–8.
57. Gold JE, Schwam L, Castella A et al. Malignant plasma cell tumors in human immunodeficiency virus-infected patients. *Cancer* 1990; **66**: 363–8.
58. Kumar S, Kumar D, Schnadig VJ et al. Plasma cell myeloma in patients who are HIV-positive. *Am J Clin Pathol* 1994; **102**: 633–9.
59. Lefrere JJ, Debbia M, Lambin P. Prospective follow-up of monoclonal gammopathies in HIV-infected individuals. *Br J Haematol* 1993; **84**: 151–5.
60. Konrad RJ, Kricka LJ, Goodman DB et al. Myeloma-associated paraprotein directed against the HIV-1 p24 antigen in an HIV-1 seropositive patient. *N Engl J Med* 1993; **328**: 1817–19.
61. Goedert JJ, Cote TR, Virgo P et al. Spectrum of AIDS-associated malignant disorders. *Lancet* 1998; **351**: 1833–9.
62. Heineman EF, Olsen JH, Pottern LM et al. Occupational risk factors for multiple myeloma among Danish men. *Cancer Causes Control* 1992; **3**: 555–68.
63. Pottern LM, Heineman EF, Olsen JH et al. Multiple myeloma among Danish women: employment history and workplace exposures. *Cancer Causes Control* 1992; **3**: 427–32.
64. Pearce NE, Smith AH, Howard JK et al. Case–control study of multiple myeloma and farming. *Br J Cancer* 1986; **54**: 493–500.
65. Eriksson M, Karlsson M. Occupational and other environmental factors and multiple myeloma: a population based case-control study. *Br J Ind Med* 1992; **49**: 95–103.
66. Alavanja MCR, Blair A, Merkle S et al. Mortality among agricultural extension agents. *Am J Ind Med* 1988; **14**: 167–76.
67. Bertazzi PA, Pesatori AC, Consonni D et al. Cancer incidence in a population accidentally exposed to 2,3,7,8-tetrachlorodibenzo-*para*-dioxin. *Epidemiology* 1993; **4**: 398–406.
68. La Vecchia C, Negri E, D'Avanzo B et al. Occupation and lymphoid neoplasms. *Br J Cancer* 1989; **60**: 385–8.
69. Morris PD, Koepsell TD, Daling JR et al. Toxic substance exposure and multiple myeloma: a case–control study. *J Natl Cancer Inst* 1986; **76**: 987–94.
70. Egedahl RD, Coppock E, Homik R. Mortality experience at a hydrometallurgical nickel refinery in Fort Saskatchewan, Alberta between 1954 and 1984. *J Soc Occup Med* 1991; **41**: 29–33.
71. Gallagher RP, Threlfall WJ. Cancer mortality in metal workers. *Can Med Assoc J* 1983; **129**: 1191–4.
72. Andjelkovich D, Taulbee J, Symons M. Mortality experience of a cohort of rubber workers, 1964–73. *J Occup Med* 1978; **20**: 409–13.
73. Andjelkovich D, Taulbee J, Blum S. Mortality of female workers in a rubber manufacturing plant. *J Occup Med* 1978; **20**: 409–13.
74. Demers PA, Vaughan TL, Koepsell TD et al. A case–control study of multiple myeloma and occupation. *Am J Ind Med* 1992; **23**: 629–39.
75. *Health Watch: the Australian Institute of Petroleum Health Surveillance Program Nine Report.*

Melbourne: Department of Public Health and Community Medicine, 1993.

76. Nandakumar A, Armstrong BK, DeKlerk NH. Multiple myeloma in Western Australia: a case–control study in relation to occupation, father's occupation, socio-economic status and country of birth. *Int J Cancer* 1986; **37**: 223–6.
77. Thun MJ, Altekruse SF, Namboodiri MM et al. Hair dye use and risk of fatal cancers in US women. *J Natl Cancer Inst* 1994; **86**: 210–5.
78. Grodstein F, Hennekens CH, Colditz GA et al. A prospective study of permanent hair dye use and hematopoietic cancer. *J Natl Cancer Inst* 1994; **86**: 1466–70.
79. Zahm SH, Weisenburger DD, Babbitt PA et al. Use of hair coloring products and the risk of lymphoma, multiple myeloma and chronic lymphocytic leukaemia. *Am J Public Health* 1992; **82**: 990–7.
80. Herrinton LJ, Weiss NS, Koepsell TD et al. Exposure to hair-coloring products in relation to risk of multiple myeloma. *Am J Public Health* 1994; **84**: 1142–4.
81. Schwartz DA, Vaughan TL, Heyer NJ et al. B cell neoplasms and occupational asbestos exposure. *Am J Ind Med* 1988; **14**: 661–71.
82. Raffn E, Lynge E, Juel K et al. Incidence of cancer and mortality among employees in the asbestos cement industry in Denmark. *Br J Ind Med* 1989; **46**: 90–6.
83. Lundberg I. Mortality and cancer incidence among Swedish paint industry workers with long term exposure to organic solvents. *Scand J Work Environ Health* 1986; **12**: 108–13.
84. Bethwaite PB, Pearce N, Fraser J. Cancer risks in painters: study based on the New Zealand Cancer Registry. *Br J Ind Med* 1990; **47**: 742–6.
85. Eriksson M, Hallberg B. Familial occurrence of hematologic malignancies and other disease in multiple myeloma: a case–control study. *Cancer Causes Control* 1992; **3**: 63–7.
86. Roddie PH, Dang R, Parker AC. Multiple myeloma in three siblings. *Clin Lab Haematol* 1998; **20**: 191–3.
87. Willems PM, Kuypers AW, Meijerink JP et al. Sporadic mutations of the p53 gene in multiple myeloma and no evidence for germline mutations in three familial myeloma pedigrees. *Leukaemia* 1993; **7**: 986–91.
88. Loth TS, Perrotta AL, Lima J et al. Genetic aspects of familial multiple myeloma. *Mil Med* 1991; **156**: 430–3.
89. Pottern LM, Gart JJ, Nam JM et al. HLA and multiple myeloma among black and white men: evidence of a genetic association. *Cancer Epidemiol Biomark Prev* 1992; **1**: 177–82.

10

Clinical features and diagnostic criteria

Henk Lokhorst

CONTENTS • **Introduction** • **Epidemiology** • **Diagnosis and staging** • **Diagnostic criteria** • **Presenting symptoms in myeloma**

INTRODUCTION

Myeloma, the most common malignancy of plasma cells, accounts for about 1% of all malignant diseases and 10% of haematological malignancies.[1] It is the result of a clonal proliferation of plasma cells, which produce a homogeneous immunoglobulin fraction detectable in the serum and/or urine. Bone destruction due to the production of osteoclastic factors by the malignant plasma cells is the most characteristic feature of the disease, and bone pain is the predominant presenting symptom. The incidence of bone problems has decreased over the last 30 years.[2] This is probably due to more intensive healthcare management and a greater awareness of the disease, with a considerable proportion of patients now being diagnosed during routine investigations. Other presenting symptoms include anaemia, uraemia, recurrent infections, and, less commonly, hypercalcaemia, hyperviscosity, polyneuropathy, spinal cord compression, and amyloidosis.

EPIDEMIOLOGY

The incidence of multiple myeloma increases with age, and it is typically found in middle-aged and elderly patients (Figure 10.1). The annual incidence is around 4 per 100 000, and is slightly higher in men then in women (Table 10.1 and Figure 10.1). The incidence among Blacks is twice that among Whites.[2,3] Long-term records in the Netherlands indicate that the incidence of myeloma is not increasing with time.[4] The disease is rarely found in patients under 40 years of age. The proportion of myeloma patients younger than 40 and 30 years out of 3278 patients seen at the Mayo Clinic was 2.2% and 0.3% respectively.[5] Although some reports suggested a more aggressive course in younger patients, this was not confirmed by Blade et al,[5] who found that symptoms and prognostic factors in 72 patients diagnosed with myeloma under the age of 40 years were no different from those seen in older patients.

DIAGNOSIS AND STAGING

When the diagnosis of myeloma is suspected, accurate diagnostic and staging procedures should be performed (Figure 10.2); see Chapter 15. These include qualitative and quantitative measurement of serum/and urine M protein, and routine laboratory investigations such as peripheral blood picture, renal function, serum calcium, and lactate dehydrogenase (LDH).

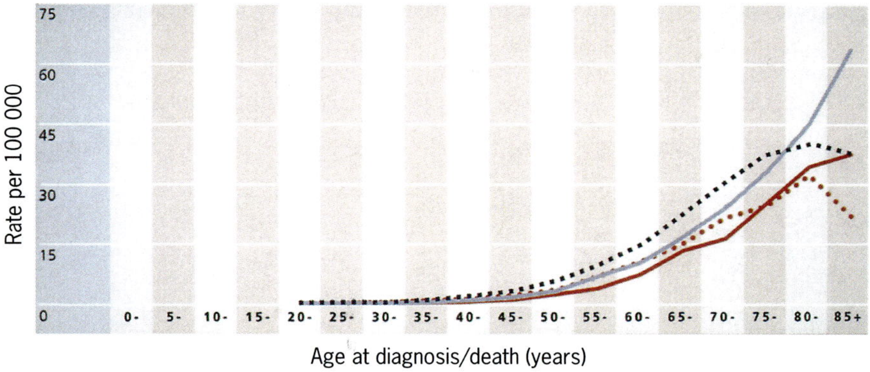

Figure 10.1 Age-specific incidence of and mortality from multiple myeloma, 1989–95. Dots represent incidence, lines mortality, blue males, and red females.

Table 10.1 Incidence and gender/age distribution of multiple myeloma in the Netherlands (Source: Netherlands Cancer registry)

Year	Incidence				Mortality			
	Males		Females		Males		Females	
	No.	ESR[a]	No.	ESR	No.	ESR	No.	ESR
1989	345	5.2	298	3.2	293	4.4	319	3.2
1990	345	5.1	342	3.7	288	4.4	323	3.2
1991	371	5.4	331	3.5	268	3.9	301	2.9
1992	381	5.4	348	3.6	303	4.4	304	2.9
1993	384	5.4	361	3.8	316	4.6	286	2.8
1994	367	5.1	352	3.5	299	4.3	318	2.9
1995	360	4.9	360	3.6	295	4.1	313	3.0

[a] ESR, European standardized rate per 100 000 persons.

Gender			Age category (years)					
	Total		0 – 49[b]		50–69		701	
	No.	%	No.	%	No.	%	No.	%
Males	2553	100	221	9	1140	45	1192	47
Females	2392	100	135	6	843	35	1414	59

[b] Age of youngest patient 22 years.

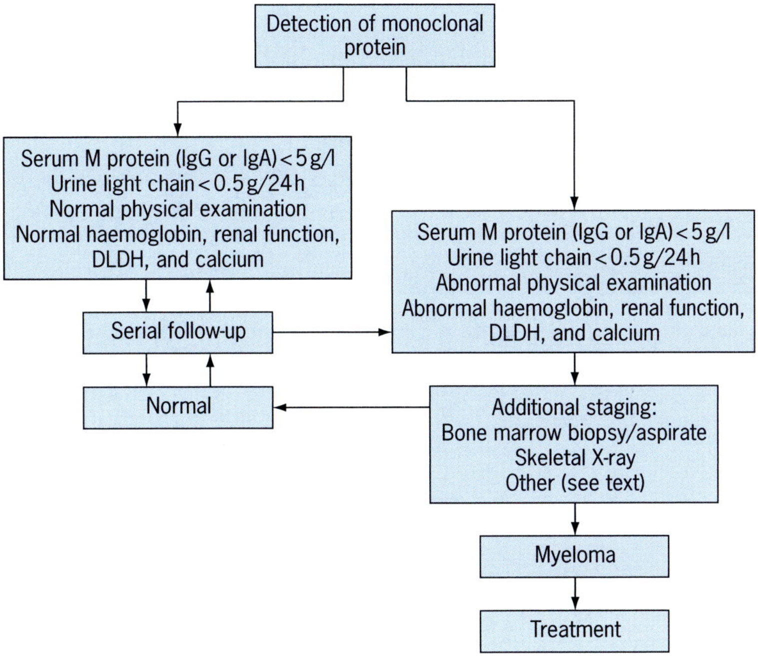

Figure 10.2 Diagnosis and staying procedures.

If the serum M-protein concentration is less than 5 g/l (IgA or IgG), the urine M-protein concentration is less than 0.5 g/l, and no abnormalities are found in the history, examination, and laboratory investigations, then no additional tests are indicated apart from regular follow-up of the M-protein concentration (guidelines from the Consensus Committee on Paraproteinaemia of the Dutch Ministry of Health, 1999). In the case of IgM paraproteinaemia, a survey for non-Hodgkin's lymphoma may be indicated.

Otherwise, additional staging procedures are performed, including bone marrow examination (see Chapter 16), radiographic studies (see Chapter 17), and determination of prognostic factors such as the plasma cell labelling index (PCLI), serum β_2-microglobulin, serum albumin, C-reactive protein (CRP), and cytogenetics (see Chapter 5). Additional tests may include magnetic resonance imaging (MRI) of the bone marrow, and a survey for amyloidosis.

Underestimation of bone marrow plasma cell infiltration may occur when only aspirates are evaluated. We compared plasma cell infiltration in biopsies and aspirates, and found that in 48% of patients, the infiltration in the aspirate was lower than in the biopsy.[6] In only two patients (4%) was a higher plasma cell infiltration found in the aspirate; 20% of patients had less than 20% plasma cells in the aspirate and more than 50% in the biopsy (Figure 10.3). Underestimation of plasma cell load in the aspirate especially seems to occur in patients with a focal growth pattern of myeloma or when significant marrow fibrosis is present.

DIAGNOSTIC CRITERIA

Several diagnostic systems are used to diagnose and classify patients with plasma cell dyscrasias. In a recent comparison of the practical usefulness of the Durie–Salmon,[7] Kyle–Greipp,[8] and British Columbia Cancer Agency (BCCA)[9] systems, few differences were found, although the BCCA criteria were thought to be the easiest to use.[10]

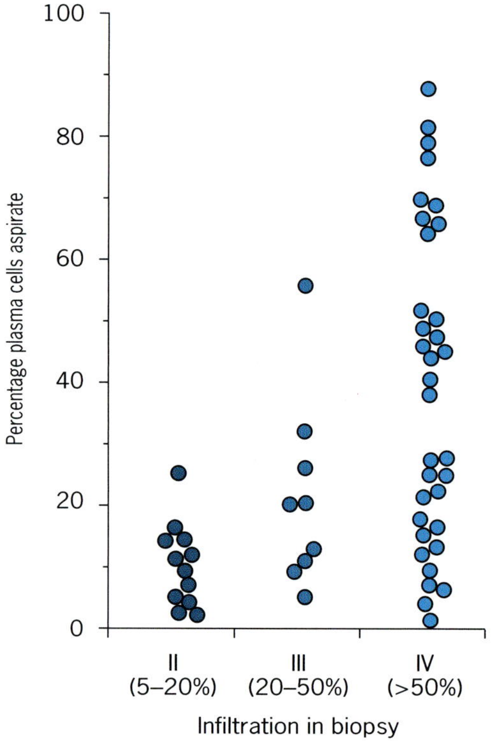

Figure 10.3 Comparison of (simultaneously obtained) plasma cell percentages in bone marrow biopsies and bone marrow aspirates.

The diagnostic criteria can be used to distinguish the following entities: myeloma, indolent myeloma (IMM), smouldering myeloma, monoclonal gammopathy of undetermined significance (MGUS), and solitary plasmacytoma.

Myeloma

In most patients presenting with symptomatic disease, the classic triad of myeloma comprising multiple lytic bone lesions, a high serum M component, and extensive (>30%) bone marrow plasmacytosis is present. Myeloma, however, may be difficult to diagnose and to distinguish from MGUS and smouldering myeloma. In 10% of cases, only light chains are produced, and in rare cases, neither a serum nor urine paraprotein is present (non-secretory myeloma).

In the Durie–Salmon system, diagnostic criteria are divided into 'major' and 'minor'. In most cases, one major criterion together with one minor criterion is sufficient to diagnose myeloma (Table 10.2). In the Kyle–Greipp classification (Table 10.3), because the presence of a paraprotein is mandatory, the diagnosis of non-secretory myeloma is not possible. The list of criteria in the easy-to-handle BCCA system is short. The whole range of possibilities is covered, and all criteria are equally important (Table 10.4). In a study including 157 patients extracted from a population-based registry of 847 patients with paraproteinaemia, differences between the systems were small, despite the fact that the diagnosis was identical according to all three systems in only 64% of the patients.[10]

In patients who satisfy the diagnostic criteria for myeloma, the Durie–Salmon criteria are commonly applied to determine the stage of disease based on the presence or absence of bone lesions, anaemia, hypercalcaemia, and paraprotein levels (Table 10.5).[7] Patients with stage I

Table 10.2 Diagnostic criteria according to Durie and Salmon

Myeloma

Major criteria
(1) Plasmacytoma on tissue biopsy
(2) Bone marrow plasmacytosis with > 30% plasma cells
(3) Monoclonal globulin spike on serum electrophoresis: IgG > 35 g/l, IgA > 20 g/l, light-chain excretion on urine electrophoresis ⩾ 1 g/24 h in the absence of amyloidosis

Minor criteria
(a) Bone marrow plasmacytosis with 10–30% plasma cells
(b) Monoclonal globulin spike present, but lower levels than defined above
(c) Lytic bone lesions
(d) Normal IgM > 500 mg/l, IgA > 1 g/l, or IgG > 6 g/l

The diagnosis of myeloma requires a minimum of one major and one minor criterion (although (1) + (a) is not sufficient) or three minor criteria that must include (a) + (b).

Indolent myeloma

Criteria as for myeloma with the following limitations:
(a) Absent or only limited bone lesions (⩽ 3 lytic lesions), no compression fractures
(b) Stable paraprotein levels IgG < 70 g/l, IgA < 50 g/l
(c) No symptoms or associated disease features: Karnofsky performance status > 70%, haemoglobin > 100 g/l, normal serum calcium normal, serum creatinine < 3 mg/dL, no infections
(d) Plasma cell labelling index ⩽ 0.5%

Table 10.3 Diagnostic criteria according to Kyle and Greipp

Myeloma

(1) Paraprotein present in serum or urine
(2) ⩾ 10% bone marrow plasma cells, or aggregates on biopsy
(3) One or more ancillary findings; must not be attributable to another cause:
    (a) anaemia
    (b) lytic bone lesions, or osteoporosis and ⩾ 30% plasma cells in bone marrow
    (c) bone marrow plasma cell labelling index > 1%
    (d) renal insufficiency (adult-acquired Fanconi syndrome or light-chain deposition disease not sufficient)
    (e) hypercalcaemia

Smouldering myeloma

(1) Serum paraprotein (usually > 30 g/l) and ⩾ 10% bone marrow plasma cells or aggregates on biopsy
(2) No anaemia, renal failure or hypercalcemia attributable to myeloma
(3) Bone lesions absent on radiographic bone survey
(4) Bone marrow plasma cell labelling index < 1%

Table 10.4 Diagnostic criteria for myeloma according to the British Columbia Cancer Agency (BCCA)

At least one of the following:
(1) Presence of a paraprotein in serum or urine
(2) Lytic bone lesion(s)
(3) Bone marrow plasma cell infiltrate in excess of 10% of the cells present

Table 10.5 The Durie and Salmon staging system for myeloma (applicable once the diagnosis of myeloma has been established based upon diagnostic criteria)

Stage I (low tumour burden)	
All of the following criteria must be satisfied:	
Haemoglobin > 10 g/dl	
Serum calcium < 12 mg/dl	
X-ray: no bone destruction (scale 0), or solitary plasmacytoma	
Low paraprotein production:	serum IgG < 5 g/dL
	serum IgA < 3 g/dL
	urine light chain < 4 g/24 h
Stage II (intermediate tumour burden)	
Laboratory and radiologic parameters intermediate between stages I and III	
Stage III (high tumour burden)	
At least one of the following criteria must be satisfied:	
Haemoglobin < 8.5 g/dl	
Serum calcium > 12 mg/dl	
X-ray: advanced lytic bone lesions (scale 3)	
Low paraprotein production:	serum IgG > 7 g/dl
	serum IgA > 5 g/dl
	urine light chain > 12 g/24 h
(A) Serum creatinine < 2 mg/dl	
(B) Serum creatinine ⩾ 2 mg/dl	

disease who have no clinical symptoms are usually not treated. These patients need careful monitoring, and treatment is started in the case of disease progression. Immediate therapy is usually indicated for patients in stages II and III.

Monoclonal gammopathy of undetermined significance

MGUS indicates the presence of M protein in serum and or/urine without evidence of a malignancy such as myeloma, related syndromes such as AL amyloidosis, or non-Hodgkin lymphomas. In patients with MGUS, the M protein is usually less than 30 g/l, bone marrow infiltration is less than 10%, and lytic bone lesions, bone pain, anaemia, hypercalcaemia and renal insufficiency are absent (Table 10.6); see Chapter 24.

An important criterion is the absence of proliferative plasma cells. This can be measured by staining with bromodeoxyuridine, which identifies actively synthesizing DNA (S-phase cells),[11] or with the monoclonal antibody Ki-67, which reacts with a nuclear antigen that is present only in proliferating cells.[12] An increased plasma cell growth fraction is present in less than 5% of patients with MGUS, while the majority of myeloma patients have an increased growth fraction at presentation. There are no other laboratory indicators as helpful in the differential diagnosis of MGUS and myeloma.[13] Serum neural cell adhesion molecule (NCAM) may help to separate myeloma from paraproteinaemias due to other causes.[14]

Smouldering myeloma

Absence of plasma cell proliferation is also an important characteristic of smouldering myeloma. These patients satisfy the criteria for myeloma, but do not have any symptoms and the disease runs an indolent course. Kyle and Greipp[15] were the first to describe patients who satisfied the criteria for smouldering myeloma (Table 10.3). These patients may remain stable for many years without requiring specific treatment. They should be followed carefully to ensure that therapy is started as soon as symptomatic disease develops.

Indolent myeloma

Indolent myeloma shares many of the features of smouldering myeloma such as the absence of symptoms, a low proliferative index of the plasma cells, and an indolent course (Table 10.2). However, a few lytic bone lesions and mild anaemia may be present. When these patients are carefully staged and monitored, the start of chemotherapy may be postponed until it is necessary.

We have followed several patients satisfying the criteria for indolent myeloma for many years without administering chemotherapy. A most impressive follow-up was seen in a patient who was diagnosed with stage II disease in 1985 on the basis of bone marrow plasma cell infiltration of 30–40% (plasma cell labelling index < 0.5%), a serum IgA κ paraprotein of 40 g/l, and mild anaemia. He had no skeletal lesions except for slight osteoporosis. After almost 15 years' follow-up in 2000, the patient presented with signs of radicular pain due to extradural spread of a myeloma mass.

It is obvious that indolent myeloma is a difficult condition with a variable clinical course, and careful monitoring of patients is necessary. As bone destruction has already occurred in some of these patients, supportive therapy with bisphosphonates may be indicated.

Table 10.6 Monoclonal gammopathy of undetermined significance (MGUS)

(1) Paraprotein levels: IgG ≤ 35 g/l, IgA ≤ 20 g/l, Bence Jones protein ≤ 1 g/24 h
(2) Bone marrow plasma cells < 10%
(3) No bone lesions
(4) No symptoms
(5) No anaemia, renal failure or hypercalcaemia
(6) Plasma cell labelling index < 0.5%

Solitary plasmacytoma of the bone

Solitary plasmacytoma of the bone (SPB) comprises between 3% and 5% of plasma cell malignancies. The usual clinical presentation is pain localized at the site of the skeletal involvement and/or neurologic dysfunction due to spinal cord or nerve root compression. In the majority of cases, the lesions occur in the vertebral column.[16–20] The thoracic vertebrae are most frequently involved. Most patients with SPB eventually develop myeloma.[16–18] In 72% of 57 patients with SPB treated with radiotherapy at the MD Anderson Cancer Center, Houston, serum and/or urine M protein was found.[18] After radiotherapy, 51% of patients developed myeloma at a median of 20 months. The likelihood of developing myeloma was directly related to the persistence of the M protein after radiotherapy.

Solitary extramedullary plasmacytoma

More than 90% of extramedullary plasmacytomas (EMP) develop in the head and neck area; usually in the nasal fossa and the paranasal sinuses. Other reported sites include the parotid gland, nasopharynx, larynx, orbit, skin, lungs, lymph nodes, spleen, and gastrointestinal tract. [21–23] Symptoms are related to local anatomical disturbances. In contrast to SPB, dissemination of EMP is rare, and response to local radiotherapy good.

Plasma cell leukaemia

Plasma cell leukaemia (PCL) is defined as an absolute plasma cell count of more than $20 \times 10^9/l$, with plasma cells also comprising more than 20% of the total leukocyte count.[24,25] Primary PCL is initial presentation with a PCL-type picture, and secondary PCL is the development of PCL in patients with known myeloma. PCL is characterized by frequent extramedullary involvement (including meningeal infiltration), a high tumour load, and a high incidence of adverse prognostic factors. A large series of 26 primary (de novo) PCL patients described by Garcia-Sanz et al[26] was characterized by a remarkably high incidence of monosomy 13. Owing to the clinical and biological aspects of the disease, it is not surprising that the overall survival of patients with PCL is considerably poorer than that of myeloma patients (8 months versus 36 months).[26,27]

PRESENTING SYMPTOMS IN MYELOMA

Clinical suspicion of myeloma based on symptomatology may be difficult owing to the great variation in presenting symptoms as well as the non-specific nature of some of the symptoms. In the elderly, symptoms such as fatigue, back pain, and height loss are quite common without any underlying plasma cell dyscrasia.

Ong et al[28] found that in 47 out of 127 (37%) patients with myeloma, myeloma was not included in the initial differential diagnosis ('delayed diagnosis') although in the group with delayed diagnosis, 51% of patients had stage III disease (Table 10.7). Table 10.7 shows the variety of symptoms that patients present with, and the non-specific nature of most of these.

Apart from the lack of specificity of the presenting symptoms, lack of symptoms may be an important reason for delayed diagnosis. About 10% of patients are completely asymptomatic and are diagnosed during routine investigations. Riccardi et al[2] compared the presentation features of three series of patients diagnosed over the periods 1960–71, 1972–86, and 1987–90, and concluded that myeloma is diagnosed earlier now than in the past. In the most recently diagnosed patients, the number of symptomatic patients decreased from 90% to 86% to 66%.[2] A greater awareness of the disease and more intensive healthcare management may be responsible for this changing clinical presentation of myeloma.

Table 10.7 Presenting symptoms and signs in myeloma[28]

	Delayed diagnosis (n = 47)	Diagnosed immediately (n = 80)	Total (n = 127)
Bone pain/fractures	11 (23%)	59 (74%)	70 (53%)
Malaise	9 (19%)	37 (46%)	46 (36%)
Infection/fever	4 (9%)	8 (10%)	12 (9%)
Anaemia	12 (26%)	47 (59%)	59 (46%)
Hypercalcaemia	1 (2%)	18 (23%)	19 (15%)
Hyperviscosity/bleeding	1 (2%)	7 (9%)	8 (6%)
Elevated erythrocyte sedimentation rate	11 (23%)	16 (20%)	27 (21%)
Other symptoms	20 (43%)	14 (18%)	34 (27%)
Cardiac/respiratory	7	0	7 (5%)
Gastrointestinal.	7	2	9 (7%)
Renal	0	7	7 (5%)
Neurologic	2	1	3 (2%)
Musculoskeletal	1	0	1 (1%)
miscellaneous	4	4	4 (3%)

Bone pain

Bone pain is the most frequently reported presenting symptom, affecting 50–90% of patients.[28–30] The pain is usually localized in the back and the ribs, and is precipitated by standing and movement. Persistent pain may indicate pathologic fractures, or compression of the spinal cord and nerve roots by local tumour growth. The pain is caused by proliferation of the myeloma tumour cells which produce osteoclast-activating factors induced by interleukin (IL)-1β, tumour necrosis factor (TNF)-β and IL-6.[31–35] This results in excessive osteoclast activity and increased bone resorption, leading to diffuse bone loss, lytic lesions, and fractures (Figure 10.4). Lahtinen et al[35] showed that over 50% of patients present with vertebral fractures and up to 30% with non-vertebral fractures. Kanis and McClosky[36] found that 60% of patients had diffuse bone loss, and in 5% this was present in the absence of lytic lesions. The extent of bone destruction is closely associated with tumour infiltration, and correlates with tumour load.

Riccardi et al[2] reported a decrease in the frequency of pain as a presenting feature. The frequency and extent of bone lesions, however, had not changed during the period considered. As already mentioned, this may be due to a greater awareness of the disease and earlier diagnosis.

Plain radiography remains the most widely used method to assess skeletal involvement at diagnosis and for staging.[37] Bone scintigraphy is less sensitive in the identification of lytic lesions, especially in the skull and in the thoraco-lumbar spine.[38,39] Dual-energy X-ray absorptiometry (DEXA), which can measure bone mass, is more sensitive than conventional radiography, and may be of value in monitoring bone status during treatment.[40,41] MRI is expensive and requires skilled personnel, and may be useful for the identification of lesions in patients with normal bone X-rays and to define the need for local/and or systemic treatment to prevent pathologic fractures and cord compression.[42–44]

Infections

Infections are a major cause of morbidity and mortality in patients with myeloma, both at

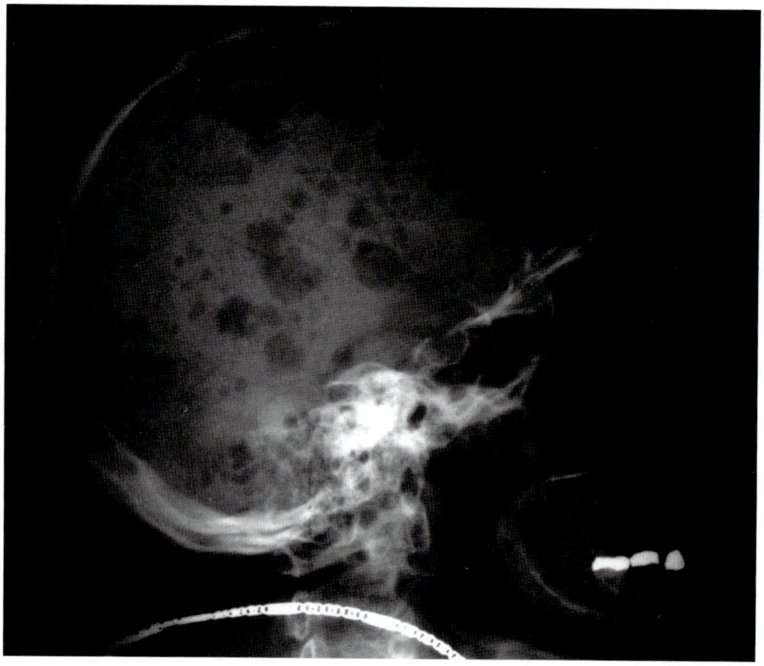

Figure 10.4 Typical punched-out lesions in the skull of a patient with myeloma.

presentation and during follow-up (see Chapter 14). Fever caused by viral and bacterial infections is the presenting symptom in about 10% of patients.[2,28–30]

Up to 25% of patients may die from infections during the first six months after diagnosis, and 70% of patients ultimately die from infection.[45–47] The incidence of infections in myeloma patients is 15 times higher than in normal individuals.

An important predisposing factor, especially for infections with encapsulated organisms such as *Streptococcus pneumoniae* and *Haemophilus influenzae*, is acquired humoral immunodeficiency.[48,49] This is present in almost all patients at presentation, and is seen to a variable extent during treatment. Deficiency in the synthesis of polyclonal immunoglobulin is restored in patients achieving good response (usually complete remission) after intensive treatment.[50]

At presentation, *S. pneumoniae* and *H. influenzae* are the most frequently isolated bacteria, and the respiratory and urinary tracts are the common sites of infection.[51–54] Later on during the course of the disease, other infections with Gram-negative organisms and with staphylococcus species become more common. This is related to the stage of disease, treatment modalities such as high-dose therapy and transplantation, which leads as in periods of neutropenia and hospitalization, the use of central venous catheters, and the use of of high-dose corticosteroids.[55–57]

Clinically obvious fungal infections are rare in myeloma patients receiving conventional chemotherapy, although their incidence is probably underestimated.[46] These patients normally have no periods of prolonged neutropenia. Fungal infections are more common in patients undergoing intensive treatment as well as in those receiving high-dose steroids.

Impairment of T-cell function is not uncommon in myeloma, although it is clinically not as important as the B-cell deficiency. Intensive corticosteroid therapy suppresses T-cell function markedly. Cutaneous herpes zoster is seen frequently in myeloma patients,[58] and there are incidental reports of *Pneumocystis carinii* infections.[59]

B symptoms

B symptoms such as fever, night sweat and unexplained weight loss are rare in myeloma patients. Only a few case reports describe patients who present with fever not associated with infection.[60,61] Kyle[29] estimated that in 'uncomplicated' myeloma, only 1% of patients have B symptoms. Patients with PCL, anaplastic/undifferentiated disease, and lymphoma-like disease with high LDH are more likely to have B symptoms.

Fatigue and wasting

Unlike the classical systemic B symptoms such as fever and night sweat, which are uncommon in myeloma, fatigue and wasting are important symptoms present in 40–50% of patients at diagnosis.[2,8,16] These symptoms are strongly correlated with the presence and severity of anaemia. Hypercalcaemia, hyperviscosity, polyneuropathy, myopathy, and renal insufficiency may also contribute to a feeling of generalized malaise.

About two-thirds of patients have anaemia at presentation.[8,61] The anaemia is usually associated with depressed erythropoietin levels. These levels are low because of a an inadequate erythropoietin response to anaemia. Impaired availability of storage iron and overproduction of cytokines such as IL-1 and TNF-α that can inhibit erythropoiesis[62–64] contribute to anaemia. Determining the level of endogenous erythropoietin may help to select patients who may benefit from treatment with recombinant erythropoietin.[65] Coombs-positive haemolytic anaemia is occasionally seen.[66,67]

Neurologic symptoms

A variety of neurologic abnormalities may be presenting symptoms in myeloma. The most well known and dramatic is the sudden onset of paraplegia due to spinal cord compression. Other neurologic complications include cauda equina syndrome, radicular pain, peripheral neuropathy, and cranial nerve palsies usually due to local encroachment by tumour cells near the exit foraminae of the skull floor. Leptomeningeal myelomatous involvement and intracerebral plasmacytomas are rarely diagnosed.[68–70]

In most studies, the reported incidence of presentation with neurologic symptoms is low (<5%).[2,16,28] Careful examination at presentation, however, may reveal a much higher incidence. Spiess et al[71] reported that signs of spinal cord compression on examination were found in 12% of newly diagnosed myeloma patients. Spinal cord and cauda equina compression, caused by collapsed vertebrae, direct extrusion of bone fragments in the spinal canal, or extradural spread of the tumour, develops in at least 20% of patients during the course of the disease. A careful neurologic history and examination is obligatory at presentation and during follow-up so that early signs of cord compression are recognized and are adequately treated.

Peripheral neuropathy associated with plasma cell dyscrasia is a well-known entity (see Chapter 12).[72–76] Most neuropathies are associated with MGUS and IgM paraproteinaemia. About 50% of patients with IgM-associated polyneuropathy have a distinctive clinical syndrome that is associated with antibodies against myelin-associated glycoprotein (MAG).[72]

Peripheral neuropathy in patients with overt myeloma is rare (<5%).[76] The neuropathy is usual axonal, mixed sensorimotor, and symptoms are usually symmetrical, distal, and progressive. The exact mechanism of axonal damage is not known. Removing the paraprotein by plasma exchange has no consistent effect on the neuropathy.[76] Differential diagnostic considerations of polyneuropathy in myeloma include amyloidosis, cryoglobulinaemia, vasculitis, direct tumorous infiltration of peripheral nerves, and the POEMS syndrome (polyneuropathy, organomegaly, endocrinopathy, M protein, skin changes).[77,78] Neuropathic symptoms developing during therapy may result from drugs such as vincristine, cisplatin, and thalidomide.

Ocular abnormalities

The dysproteinaemias can affect all ocular tissues. Most frequently, the retina is involved as part of the hyperviscosity syndrome with haemorrhages, and vascular dilatation, tortuosity and formation of microaneurysms[79,80] (Figure 10.5). Papilloedema may be due to direct infiltration of the optic nerve or may arise from elevated intracranial pressure from an extension of plasma cell proliferation in the skull. Rarely, paraprotein may be deposited in the cornea. Localized plasmacytomas may produce compression and mass effect resulting in pain, proptosis, diplopia, and visual disturbances.[81]

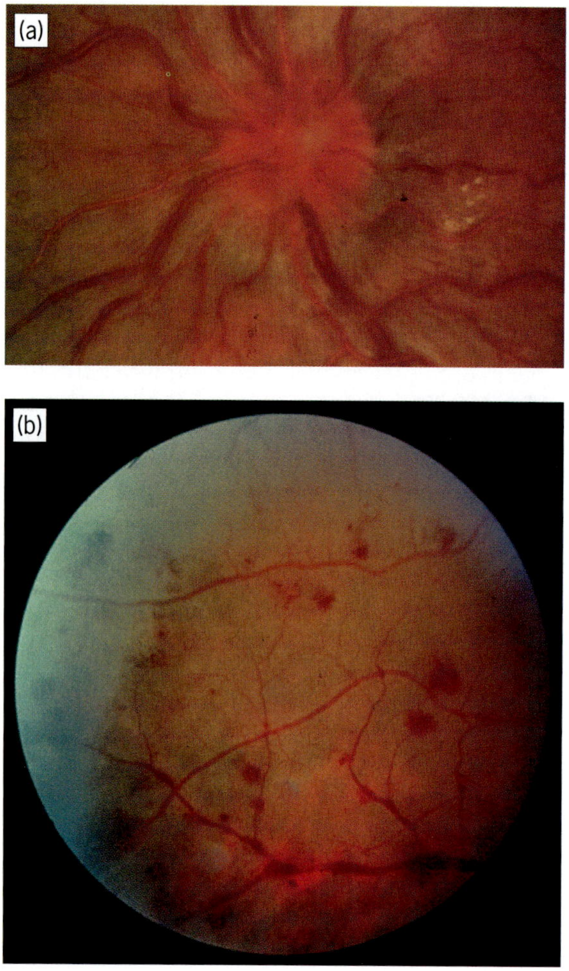

Figure 10.5 Hyperviscosity syndrome in myeloma. (a) Optic nerve head oedema with engorgement and increased tortuosity of retinal veins. (b) Multiple superficial retinal haemorrhages and sausage-like dilatation of retinal veins.

Renal involvement

Typical symptoms due to renal failure, such as polydipsia, polyuria and oedema, are relatively rare and are present in 5–10% of patients at diagnosis.[2,16,28] As the majority of patients with renal insufficiency have advanced disease symptoms, these are usually symptoms related to myeloma itself. Renal disease is common in myeloma, and its reported incidence at presentation is 20–60%[82–84] (see Chapter 13).

In a cohort of 998 patients who entered trials of the UK Medical Research Council between 1982 and 1991, 43% had abnormal renal function, defined as a serum creatinine of more than 130 μmol/l measured 48 hours after rehydration.[30] Hypercalcaemia, dehydration, and infection are the most important precipitating factors, and are found in 50–95% of myeloma patients with acute renal failure.

The use of non-steroidal anti-inflammatory drugs (NSAIDs), usually for bone pain, has been reported to be a frequent cause of acute renal insufficiency.[83] In the older literature, the use of radiographic contrast media was still a major risk factor. Contrast media are probably only a minor risk when patients are hydrated adequately.

After rehydration, treatment of hypercalcaemia, and chemotherapy, renal function becomes normal in more than 50% of patients.[85] Patients with renal failure usually have more advanced disease. Their prognosis, however, may not differ from that of other patients with comparable tumour load. Recovery of renal function is an important factor associated with survival.[85,86]

Most renal disease is found in patients who produce excess light chains; and consists of cast nephropathy, renal tubular dysfunction (acquired Fanconi syndrome), amyloidosis, and light-chain deposition disease.[87]

In myeloma cast nephropathy, the most frequent cause of renal failure in myeloma, the filtration of toxic light chains leads to both tubular dysfunction and intratubular cast formation and obstruction.[88] Clinical symptoms accompanying cast nephropathy are nonspecific, and are usually related to the myeloma itself. In the majority of patients, monoclonal light chains and relatively small amounts of albumin are found in the urine. Albuminuria of more than 1 g/day is usually associated with amyloidosis or immunoglobulin-deposition disease.

In myeloma-associated Fanconi syndrome, the toxic effect of the filtered light chains is limited to tubular dysfunction.[89] It is characterized by renal glycosuria, amino aciduria, hypophosphataemia, chronic acidosis, hypouricaemia, and hypokalaemia. It is usually accompanied by osteomalacia with pseudofractures.

In AL amyloidosis and light-chain deposition disease (heavy-chain disease is very rare), light-chain fragments are deposited in the kidney and other organs.[90,91] In amyloidosis the fragments precipitate to form the characteristic Congo-red positive, β-pleated fibrils. In light-chain deposition disease, no fibrils are formed and the deposits are Congo-red negative. Proteinuria and nephrotic syndrome are the most important presenting symptoms, rather than renal insufficiency. However, in some cases, renal function declines rapidly. Liver and cardiac involvement are the most common other manifestations of immunoglobulin-deposition disease.[92]

Cutaneous manifestations

Purpura is the most frequent skin manifestation of plasma cell disorders, and is related to thrombocytopenia, amyloidosis, cryoglobulinaemia, and hyperviscosity syndrome.[93] Apart from local plasmacytomas, rarer cutaneous manifestations are scleromyxoedema, scleroderma, cutis laxa acquisata, and necrobiotic xanthogranuloma[94–97] (Figure 10.6).

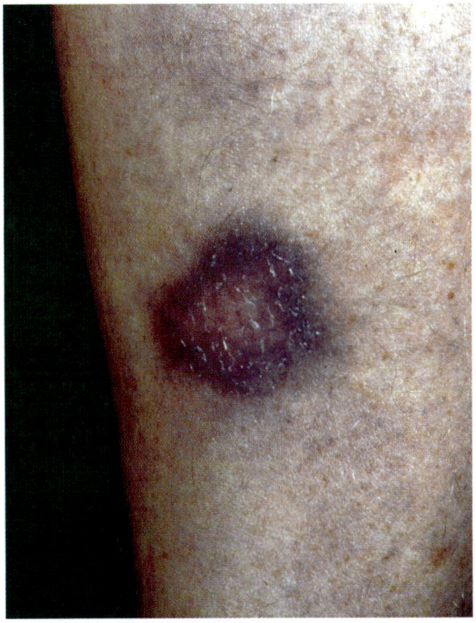

Figure 10.6 Necrobiotic xanthogranuloma in the right upper leg of a patient with myeloma.

Metabolic disturbances

Hypercalcaemia

Between 20% and 30% of patients have hypercalcaemia at presentation.[2,16,28] As many patients have a low serum albumin, the number of patients presenting with biochemical hypercalcaemia may be even higher. Typical symptoms of hypercalcaemia are polydipsia, nausea, constipation, irritability, confusion and (pre)coma. A high proportion of patients with hypercalcaemia, however, may be totally asymptomatic. Usually, the really symptomatic patient is dehydrated and has a severely impaired renal function. The mechanism of disturbed calcium metabolism and its treatment are discussed extensively in Chapter 23.

Hyperuricaemia

Hyperuricaemia is frequently found in patients with myeloma, and is related to a combination of factors, including high tumour cell turnover, tumour cell kill, and impairment of renal function. Symptomatic hyperuricaemia (gout) is rare, but prophylaxis is indicated, since a raised serum uric acid may contribute to renal impairment.

Hyperamylasaemia

All eight patients described with plasma cell dyscrasia and hyperamylasaemia were Japanese and showed the salivary amylase type.[98] Extramedullary tumour formation at diagnosis or during the course of the disease was present in all patients.

Hyperammonaemia

A few patients with central nervous system symptoms such as somnolence and precoma due to hyperammonaemia have been described. The malignant plasma cells produced the ammonia.[99,100]

Hyperviscosity syndrome

The reported incidence of hyperviscosity at the time of presentation is variable: Ong et al[28] found that 6% of patients presented with signs of hyperviscosity and bleeding, whereas symptomatic hyperviscosity was present in only 2 of 341 patients described by Riccardi et al.[2] The most common sign of hyperviscosity is a haemorrhagic diathesis resulting in gingival and mucosal bleeding, ecchymosis, and epistaxis.[78] Ophthalmic disturbances are also common, and comprise visual disturbances, diplopia, and retinal vascular abnormalities (Figure 10.5). Neurologic signs include headache, dizziness, vertigo, drowsiness, coma, and seizures. Other symptoms may include malaise, and renal and cardiac insufficiency.

IgD myeloma

This rare form of myeloma (incidence 1–2%) has some extraordinary clinical features.[28] Blade et al[101] retrospectively analysed the characteristics of 53 patients with IgD myeloma seen between 1965 and 1993 at the Mayo Clinic. Renal insufficiency (33%), hypercalcaemia (22%), extramedullary plasmacytomas (19%), and associated amyloidosis (19%) were more frequently seen than in other types of myeloma. IgD myeloma usually presents with a small or no barely detectable paraprotein, and the quantity of light chains excreted is often much more than the quantity of intact IgD. Although response to chemotherapy is similar to that reached in other patients, the overall survival may be significantly shorter.

IgE and IgM myeloma

The prevalence of IgE and IgM myeloma is very low, and is estimated at 0.01% of all myeloma cases.[102] IgE may have an especially poor prognosis, since 3 out of 11 patients described by Endo et al[102] developed plasma cell leukaemia. No specific characteristics, including adverse prognosis, were noted by de Gramont et al[103] in a review of 52 cases of IgM myeloma.

REFERENCES

1. Blattner WA. Epidemiology of multiple myeloma and related plasma cell disorders. In: *Progress in Myeloma* (Potter E, ed). Amsterdam: Elsevier/North-Holland, 1980:1–67.
2. Riccardi A, Gobbi PG, Ucci G et al. Changing clinical presentation of multiple myeloma. *Eur J Cancer* 1991; **27**: 1401–5.
3. Jacobsen RJ, Schulman G. Plasma cell myeloma and Waldenström's macroglobulinaemia in Black and White South Africans. In: *Progress in Myeloma.* (Potter E, ed). Amsterdam: Elsevier/North-Holland, 1980: 81–91.
4. Ong F, Hermans J, Noordijk EM et al. A population-based registry on paraproteinaemia in The Netherlands. *Br J Haematol* 1997; **99:** 914–20.
5. Blade J, Kyle RA, Greipp PR. Presenting features and prognosis in 72 patients with multiple myeloma who were younger than 40 years. *Br J Haematol* 1996; **93**: 345–51.
6. Terpstra WE, Lokhorst HM, Blomjous F et al. Comparison of plasma cell infiltration in bone marrow biopsies and aspirates in patients with multiple myeloma. *Br J Haematol* 1992; **82**: 46–9.
7. Durie BGM, Salmon SE. A clinical staging system for multiple myeloma. Correlation of measured myeloma cell mass with presenting clinical features, response to treatment, and survival. *Cancer* 1975; **36**: 842–54.

8. Kyle RA, Greipp RP. Plasma cell dyscrasias: current status. *Crit Rev Oncol Haematol* 1988; **8**: 93–152.
9. Lymphoma Tumour Group. Plasma cell disorders. In: *Cancer Treatment Policies*. Vancouver: British Columbia Cancer Agency, 1992: 4–6.
10. Ong F, Hermans J, Noordijk EM et al. Is the Durie and Salmon diagnostic classification system for plasma cell dyscrasias still the best choice? Application of three classification systems on a large population-based registry on paraproteinaemia and multiple myeloma. *Ann Hematol* 1995; **70:** 19–24.
11. Greipp PR, Kyle RA. Clinical, morphological and cell kinetic differences among multiple myeloma, monoclonal gammopathy of undetermined significance, and smoldering myeloma. *Blood* 1982; **62**: 161–71.
12. Lokhorst HM, Boom SE, Terpstra W et al. Determination of the growth fraction in monoclonal gammopathy with the monoclonal antibody Ki-67. *Br J Haematol* 1988; **69**: 477–81.
13. Kyle RA, Lust JA. Monoclonal gammopathies of undetermined significance. In: *Neoplastic Diseases of the Blood* (Wiernik PH, Canellos GP, Kyle RA, Schiffer CA, eds). New York: Churchill Livingstone, 1991: 571–94.
14. Ong F, Kaiser U, Seelen PJ et al. Serum Ncam differentiates multiple myeloma from paraproteinaemias due to other causes. *Blood* 1996; **87:** 712–16.
15. Kyle RA, Greipp PR. Smoldering multiple myeloma. *N Engl J Med* 1980; **302**: 1347–9.
16. Bataille R, Sarny J. Solitary myeloma: clinical and prognostic features of a review of 114 cases. *Cancer* 1981; **48**: 845–51.
17. Woodruff RK, Malpas JS, White FE. Solitary plasmacytoma. II. Solitary plasmacytoma of bone. *Cancer* 1979; **43**: 2344–7.
18. Dimopoulos MA, Goldstein J, Fuller L et al. Curability of solitary bone plasmacytoma, *J Clin Oncol* 1992; **10**: 587–90.
19. Holland J, Trenkner DA, Wasserman TH et al. Plasmacytoma: treatment results and conversion to myeloma, *Cancer* 1992; **69**:1513–17.
20. Vigliotti AP. The role of radiation therapy in the treatment of solitary plasmacytomas. *Radiother Oncol* 1990; **17**: 293–303.
21. Miller FR, Lavertu P, Wanamaker JR et al. Plasmacytomas of the head and neck, *Otolaryngol Head Neck Surg* 1998; **119**: 614–18.
22. Nofsinger YC, Mirza N, Rowan PT et al. Head and neck manifestations of plasma cells neoplasms. *Laryngoscope* 1997; **107**: 741–6.
23. Knowling MA, Harwood AR, Bergsagel DE. Comparison of extramedullary plasmacytomas with solitary and multiple plasma cell tumours of bone. *J Clin Oncol* 1983; **1**: 255–62.
24. Bennett JM, Catowsky D, Daniel MT et al. Proposals for the classification of chronic (mature) B and T lymphoid leukemias. *J Clin Pathol* 1989; **42**: 567.
25. Kyle RA, Maldonado JE, Bayrd DE. Plasma cell leukemia. Report on 17 cases. *Arch Intern Med* 1974; **133**: 813.
26. Garcia-Sanz R, Orfao A, Gonzalez M et al. Primary plasma cell leukemia: clinical, immunophenotypic, DNA ploidy, and cytogenetic characteristics. *Blood* 1999; **93**: 1032–7.
27. Dimoupoulos MA, Palumbo A, Delasalle KB et al. Primary plasma cell leukaemia. *Br J Haematol* 1994; **88**: 754.
28. Ong F, Hermans J, Noordijk EM et al. Presenting signs and symptoms in multiple myeloma: high percentages stage III in patients without apparent myeloma-associated symptoms. *Ann Hematol* 1995; **70:** 149–52.
29. Kyle RA. Multiple myeloma – review of 869 cases. *Mayo Clin Proc* 1975; **50**: 29–40.
30. MacLennan ICM, Drayson M, Dunn J. Multiple myeloma, *BMJ* 1994; **308**: 1033–6.
31. Cozzolino E, Torcia M, Aldinucci D et al. Production of interleukin-1 by bone marrow myeloma cells. *Blood* 1989; **74**: 380–7.
32. Tamura T, Udagawa N, Takahashi N et al. Soluble interleukin-6 receptor triggers osteoclast formation by interleukin-6. *Proc Natl Acad Sci USA* 1993; **90**: 11924–8.
33. Lokhorst HM, Oers R, Bloem AC. Primary tumour cells of myeloma patients induce interleukin-6 secretion in long-term bone marrow cultures. *Blood* 1994; **84**: 2269–77.
34. Bataille R, Chappard D, Basle M. Excessive bone resorption in human plasmacytomas: direct induction by tumour cells themselves. *Br J Haematol* 1995; **90**: 721–4.
35. Lahtinen R, Laakso M, Palva I. Randomised, placebo-controlled multicentre trial of clodronate in multiple myeloma. *Lancet* 1992; **340**: 1049–52.
36. Kanis JA, McCloskey EV. Disorders of calcium metabolism and their management. In: *Myeloma: Biology and Management* (Malpas JS, Bergsagel DE, Kyle RA, eds). New York: Oxford University Press, 1995: 375.
37. Croucher PI, Apperley JF. Bone disease in multiple myeloma. *Br J Haematol* 1998; **103**: 902–10.

38. Bataille R, Chevalier J, Rossi M, Sany J. Bone scintigraphy in plasma-cell myeloma, *Radiology* 1982, **145**: 801–4.
39. Woolfenden JM, Pitt MJ, Durie BGM et al. Comparison of bone marrow scintigraphy in multiple myeloma. *Radiology* 1980; **134**: 723–8.
40. Mariette X, Bergot C, Ravaud P et al. Evolution of bone densitometry in patients with myeloma treated with conventional or intensive therapy. *Cancer* 1995; **76**: 1559–63.
41. Abildgaard N, Brixen K, Kristensen JE et al. Assessment of bone involvement in patients with multiple myeloma using bone densitometry. *Eur J Haematol* 1996; **57**: 370–6.
42. Moulopoulos LA, Varma DGK, Dimopoulos MA et al. Multiple myeloma: spinal MR imaging in patients with untreated newly diagnosed disease. *Radiology* 1992; **185**: 833–7.
43. Moulopoulos LA, Dimopoulos MA, Smith TL et al. Prognostic significance of magnetic resonance imaging in patients with asymptomatic multiple myeloma. *J Clin Oncol* 1995; **13**: 251–6.
44. Terpstra WE, Lokhorst HM, Blomjous F et al. Comparison of plasma cell infiltration in bone marrow biopsies and aspirates in patients with multiple myeloma. *Br J Haematol* 1992; **82**: 46–9.
45. Oken M. Myeloma, *Med Clin North Am* 1984; **63**: 757–87.
46. Salonen J, Nikoskelainen J. Lethal infections in patients with haematological malignancies. *Eur J Haematol* 1993; **51**: 102–8.
47. Snowdon L, Gibson J, Joshua DE. Frequency of infection in plateau-phase multiple myeloma. *Lancet* 1994; **344**: 262.
48. Kyrtsonis MC, Mouzaki A, Maniatis A. Mechanisms of polyclonal hypogammaglobulinaemia in multiple myeloma. *Med Oncol* 1999; **16:** 73–7.
49. Chapel HM, Lee M, Hargreaves R et al. Randomised trial of intravenous immunoglobulin as prophylaxis against infection in plateau-phase multiple myeloma. The UK group for immunoglobulin replacement therapy in multiple myeloma. *Lancet* 1994; **343**:1059–63.
50. Selby PJ, McElwain TY, Nandi AD et al. Multiple myeloma treated with high dose intravenous melphalan. *Br J Haematol* 1987; **66**: 55–62.
51. Rodriguez-Creixems M, Munoz P, Miranda E et al. Recurrent pneumococcal bacteremia: a warning of immunodeficiency. *Arch Intern Med* 1996; **156**: 1429–34.
52. Twomey J. Infections complicating myeloma and chronic lymphocytic leukemia, *Arch Intern Med* 1973; **132**: 562–5.
53. Goranov S. Clinical problems of infectious complications in patients with myeloma, *Folica Medica* 1994; **36**: 41–6.
54. Hargreaves R, Lea J, Griffiths H et al. Immunological factors and risk of infection in plateau phase myeloma. *J Clin Pathol* 1995; **48**: 260–6.
55. Kolbe K, Domkin D, Derigs HG et al. Infectious complications during neutropenia subsequent to peripheral blood stem cell transplantation. *Bone Marrow Transplant* 1997; **19**: 143–7.
56. Lokhorst HM. Induction therapy with VAD and IDM. *Bone Marrow Transplant* 1999; **23**: 317–23.
57. McElwain TJ, Powles RL. High-dose intravenous melphalan for plasma cell leukemia and myeloma. *Lancet* 1983; **ii**: 822–4.
58. Kost R, Straus S. Postherpetic neuralgia – pathogenesis, treatment and prevention. *N Engl J Med* 1996; **335**: 32–40.
59. McKenzie R, Luther D, Goldsmith J. *Pneumocystis carinii* pneumonia complicating myeloma. *Chest* 1991; **99**: 656–9.
60. Pitz CC, Lokhorst HM, Hoekstra JB. Fever as presenting symptom of multiple myeloma. *Neth J Med* 1998; **53**: 256–9.
61. MRC Working Party on Leukemia in Adults. Prognostic features in the Third MRC Myelomatosis Trial. *Br J Cancer* 1980; **42**: 813–66.
62. Beguin Y. Erythropoiesis and erythropoietin in multiple myeloma. *Leukemia and Lymphoma* 1995; **18**: 413–21.
63. Osterborg A, Boogaerts MA, Cimino R et al. Recombinant human erythropoietin in transfusion-dependent anaemic patients with multiple myeloma and non-Hodgkin's lymphoma—a randomized multicenter study. The European Study Group of erythropoietin (epoetin beta) treatment in multiple myeloma and non-Hodgkin's lymphoma. *Blood* 1996; **87**: 2675–82.
64. Shibata K, Shimamoto Y, Nakazato S et al. Refractory anaemia with ringed sideroblasts concurrent with multiple myeloma – a brief review of the recent literature. *Haematologia* 1997; **28**: 199–205.
65. Musto P. The role of recombinant erythropoietin for the treatment of anaemia in multiple myeloma. *Leuk Lymphoma* 1998; **29**: 283–91.
66. Morado M, Canales MA, Aguado MJ et al. Association of multiple myeloma and autoimmune hemolytic anaemia. *Sangre* 1998; **43**: 467–8.

67. Vaiopoulos G, Kyriakou D, Papadaki H et al. Multiple myeloma associated with autoimmune hemolytic anaemia. *Haematologica* 1994; **79**: 262–4.
68. Leifer D, Grabowski T, Simonian N et al. Leptomeningeal myelomatosis presenting with mental status changes and other neurologic findings. *Cancer* 1992; **70**: 1899–904.
69. Olda K, Egawa H, Okuhara T et al. Meningeal involvement in Bence Jones multiple myeloma. *Cancer* 1991; **67**: 1900–2.
70. Wisniewski T, Sisti M, Inhirami G et al. Intracerebral solitary plasmacytoma. *Neurosurgery* 1990; **27:** 826–9.
71. Spiess JL, Adelstein DJ, Hines JD. Multiple myeloma presenting with spinal cord compression. *Oncology* 1988; **45**: 88–92.
72. Ropper AH, Gorson KC. Neuropathies associated with paraproteinemia. *N Engl J Med* 1998; **338**: 1601–7.
73. Notermans NC, Wokke JHJ, Lokhorst HM et al. Polyneuropathy associated with monoclonal gammopathy of undetermined significance: a prospective study of the prognostic value of clinical and laboratory abnormalities. *Brain* 1994; **117:** 1385–93.
74. Suarez GA, Kelly JJ Jr. Polyneuropathy associated with monoclonal gammopathy of undetermined significance: further evidence that IgM-MGUS neuropathies are different than IgG-MGUS. *Neurology* 1993; **43**: 1304–8.
75. Gorson KC, Allam G, Ropper AH. Chronic inflammatory demyelinating polyneuropathy: clinical features and response to treatment in 67 consecutive patients with and without a monoclonal gammopath. *Neurology* 1997; **48**: 321–8.
76. Kelly JJ Jr, Kyle RA, Miles JM et al. The spectrum of peripheral neuropathy in myeloma, *Neurology* 1981; **31**: 24–31.
77. Falk RH, Comenzo RL, Skinner M. The systemic amyloidoses. *N Engl J Med* 1997; **337**: 898–909.
78. Miralles GD, O'Fallon JR, Talley NJ. Plasma-cell dyscrasia with polyneuropathy: the spectrum of POEMS syndrome. *N Engl J Med* 1992; **327**: 1919–23.
79. Patterson WP, Caldwell CN, Doll DC. Hyperviscosity syndromes and coagulopathies. *Semin Oncol* 1990; **17**: 210–16.
80. Dobberstein H, Solbach U, Weinberger A et al. Correlation between retinal microcirculation and blood viscosity in patients with hyperviscosity syndrome. *Clin Hemorheol Microcirc* 1999; **20:** 31–5.
81. Rodman HI, Fort RL. Orbital involvement in multiple myeloma. *Arch Ophthalmol* 1972; **87**: 30–5.
82. Sanders PW, Herrera GA, Kirk KA et al. Spectrum of glomercular and tubulointerstitial renal lesions associated with monotypical immunoglobulin light chain deposition. *Lab Invest* 1991, **64**: 527.
83. Sanders PW. Pathogenesis and treatment of myeloma kidney. *J Lab Clin Med* 1994; **124**: 484.
84. Winearls CG. Acute myeloma kidney. *Kidney Int* 1995; **48**: 1347.
85. Alexanian R, Barlogie B, Dixon D. Renal failure in multiple myeloma – pathogenesis and prognostic implications. *Arch Intern Med* 1990; **150**: 1693–5.
86. Blade J, Fernandez-Llama P, Bosch F et al. Renal failure in multiple myeloma: presenting features and predictors of outcome in 94 patients from a single institution. *Arch Intern Med* 1998; **158**:1889–93.
87. Ronco PM, Auconturier P, Mougout B. Kidney involvement in plasma cell dyscrasia. In: *Oxford Textbook of Clinical Nephrology* (Davidson AM, Cameron JS, Grunfeld JP, Kerr DN, Ritz E, Winearls CG, eds). Oxford: Oxford University Press, 1988: 811–35.
88. Solomon A, Weiss DT, Kattine AA. Nephrotoxic potential of Bence Jones proteins. *N Engl J Med* 1991; **324**: 1845–51.
89. Maldonado JE, Velosa JA, Kyle RA et al. Fanconi syndrome in adults. A manifestation of a latent form of myeloma. *Am J Med* 1975; **58**: 354.
90. Buxbaum JN, Chuba JV, Hellmann GC et al. Monoclonal immunoglobulin deposition disease: light chain and light and heavy chain deposition diseases and their relation to light chain amyloidosis. Clinical features, immunopathology, and molecular analysis. *Ann Intern Med* 1990; **112**: 455.
91. Preud'homme JL, Aucouturier P, Striker L et al. Monoclonal immunoglobulin deposition disease. Relationship with structural abnormalities of immunoglobulin chains. *Kidney Int* 1994; **46**: 965–72.
92. Heilman RL, Velosa JA, Holley KE et al. Long-term follow-up and response to chemotherapy in patients with light-chain deposition disease. *Am J Kidney Dis* 1992; **20**: 34–41.
93. Piette WW., Myeloma, paraproteinaemias, and the skin. *Med Clin North Am* 1986; **70**: 155–76.
94. Dinneen AW, Dicken CH. Scleromyxedema. *J Am Acad Dermatol* 1995; **33**: 37–43.
95. Doyle JA, Connolly SM, Hoagland HC. Haematologic disease in scleroderma syndromes. *Acta Derm Venereol* 1985; **65**: 521–5.

96. Mehregan DA, Winkel RK. Necrobiotic xanthogranuloma. *Arch Dermatol* 1992; **128**: 94–100.
97. McCarty MJ, Davidson JM, Cardone JS, Anderson LL. Cutis laxa acquisita associated with multiple myeloma: a case report and review of the literature. *Cutis* 1996; **57**: 267–70.
98. Hirota K, Waga K, Nagshima S et al. Amylase-producing plasma cell dyscrasia. Genomic analysis in a case of intramuscular tumour formation and a review of the literature. *Rinsho Ketsueki* 1993; **34**: 177–82.
99. Matsuzaki H, Uchiba M, Yoshimura K et al. Hyperammonemia in multiple myeloma. *Acta Haematol* 1990; **84**: 130–4.
100. Martinelli G, Peccatori F, Ullrich B et al. Clinical manifestation of severe hyperammonaemia in patients with multiple myeloma. *Ann Oncol* 1997; **8**: 811.
101. Blade J, Lust JA, Kyle RA. Immunoglobulin D multiple myeloma: presenting features, response to therapy, and survival in a series of 53 cases. *J Clin Oncol* 1994; **12**: 2398–404.
102. Endo T, Okumura H, Kikuchi K et al. Immunoglobulin E (IgE) multiple myeloma. *Am J Med* 1981; **70**: 1127–32.
103. de Gramont A, Grasbois B, Michaux JL et al. IgM myeloma – six cases and a review of the literature. *Rev Med Interne* 1990; **11**: 13–18.

11

Prognostic factors in myeloma

Jean-Luc Harousseau, Philippe Moreau

CONTENTS • **Introduction** • **Conventional chemotherapy** • **Autologous stem cell transplantation** • **Allogeneic bone marrow transplantation** • **Conclusions**

INTRODUCTION

The survival of patients with myeloma ranges from under a year to over 10 years. This heterogeneity relates to specific characteristics both of the tumour itself and of the host. The identification of factors influencing prognosis is of major importance in order to predict outcome, to guide the choice of therapy, and to enrol homogeneous series of patients in clinical trials.

Until now, prognostic factors have been mostly evaluated in symptomatic patients treated with conventional chemotherapy. Over the last 15 years or so, high-dose therapy with autologous or allogeneic stem cell transplantation has been widely used in younger patients. The role of prognostic factors therefore needs to be reassessed in the context of high-dose therapy.

CONVENTIONAL CHEMOTHERAPY

For the last three decades, a number of clinical and biological prognostic factors have been derived from the analysis of clinical trials. They can be classified into three major subgroups: host factors, features that reflect the tumour burden, and characteristics related to intrinsic malignancy of the plasma cell and to cytokine activity.

Host factors

More than 30 years ago, Carbone et al[1] were the first to report that survival in myeloma was longer when patients had a good performance status. Younger age at presentation is also associated with a longer survival. Bladé et al[2] retrospectively studied a series of 72 patients younger than 40 years treated at the Mayo Clinic, and found that the median survival was 54 months. This survival was longer than that observed in the results of five series that included more than 2400 patients of all ages with survival ranging from 28 to 43 months. There was no explanation for this more favourable outcome in younger patients.

Another factor influencing disease progression is the immune status of the host. Immunologic changes have been described in B cells, T cells, T-suppressor/T-helper ratio, natural killer (NK) cells and soluble CD16 in patients with myeloma as compared with patients with monoclonal gammopathy of unknown significance (MGUS) or normal persons. Some authors have suggested that immunologic responses could play a role in controlling proliferation of the malignant clone and that an overt or more aggressive disease appears when the immune system is overwhelmed or fails.[3] A CD4$^+$ T-cell level less than 0.7×10^9/l has been found to be associated with a high tumour burden and a shorter duration of survival.[4] Nevertheless, few clinical trials have validated the impact of immunologic changes upon response and survival.

Tumour burden

The best way to evaluate tumour burden at diagnosis remains the clinical staging system developed at the Arizona Cancer Center by Durie and Salmon.[5] According to a combination of five factors (calcium level, haemoglobin level, concentration of monoclonal protein in the serum, proteinuria, and bone lesions), myeloma is divided into three tumour burden groups that correlate with survival: stage I (low), stage II (intermediate) and stage III (high) (see Chapter 10). In their original study of 71 cases, the median survival was over 60 months in stage I, 50 months in stage II, and 26 months in stage III.[5] Renal function independently impinging on survival was included in the staging system, with normal renal function (serum creatinine < 2 or blood urea nitrogen < 30) as substage A, and higher values as substage B. A number of other cooperative groups have now validated the Durie–Salmon myeloma staging system to evaluate survival by stage in the context of conventional chemotherapy (reviewed in reference 6, and see Table 11.1).

β_2-microglobulin (β_2M), the light chain of the class I histocompatibility antigens, is synthesized by all nucleated cells and is excreted in the urine. Renal function impairment leads to an elevation in the serum level of β_2M. Serum β_2M levels correlate with disease bulk in myeloma.[2–9] As the β_2M level in the serum depends on both myeloma cells and renal function, measurement of β_2M may be considered as an alternative to clinical staging to predict survival.[10,11] In 147 patients treated with conventional chemotherapy, 88 had β_2M values of less than 6 mg/l and 59 had values of 6 mg/l or greater. The survival rate of patients with low β_2M was 53%, at 5 years compared with 18% at 5 years in the group of patients with high β_2M ($p < 0.001$).[10]

Table 11.1 Median survival in relation to Durie–Salmon stage at diagnosis[a]

		Median survival (months)				
Series[6]	No. of cases	Stage I	Stage II	Stage III	A	B
Durie and Salmon	71	>60	50	26		
Alexanian et al	343	39	27	17		
Woodruff et al	237	64	32	6	21	2
Merlini et al	123	76	41	12		
Belpomme et al	118	>60	28	7	>60	12
Gobbi et al	91	>79	51	33		
Santoro et al	81	48	41	23	35	7
Bergsagel et al	364	46	32	23	32	11
Bladé et al	180	28	26	14		
Bataille et al	147	>80	55	23		

[a]Modified from reference 6.

An elevated serum lactate dehydrogenase (LDH) level is also a predictor of poor prognosis. In a series of 391 patients, 11% had an elevated LDH level. This was associated with extra-osseous disease, high tumour mass, and poor response to chemotherapy, and the resulting median survival was 9 months.[12]

The prognostic value of the percentage of bone marrow plasma cells (< or >50%) was analysed more than 10 years ago.[13] However, the prognostic significance of circulating plasma cells has only recently been more accurately evaluated. Their identification is possible by the expression of CD38 and syndecan-1[14] or CD38 and CD45.[15] In a large series of 254 newly diagnosed myeloma patients, Witzig et al[15] have shown that 80% of patients had blood monoclonal plasma cells (BPC) at diagnosis. Patients with 4% BPC or more (57% of patients) had a median survival of 2.4 years, versus 4.4 years for those with less than 4% PBC ($p < 0.001$), after conventional-dose chemotherapy. In a multivariate analysis, the percentage of BPC was an independent factor for survival in addition to disease stage, age, marrow plasma cell labelling index (PCLI), blood labelling index, and albumin.

Characteristics related to intrinsic malignancy of the plasma cell and to cytokine activity

Plasma cell characteristics

The morphologic characteristics of the myeloma cell have been studied for features affecting survival. In 1948, Bayrd[16] reported that none of the ten patients with myeloma who had poorly differentiated plasma cells survived a year, whereas four of seven patients with well-differentiated plasma cells were alive 2–6 years after diagnosis. Tumour cell grading (well-differentiated versus poorly differentiated plasma cells) was also an important prognostic factor among 320 patients treated with conventional-dose chemotherapy in the German Myeloma Treatment Group trial MMO1.[17]

More recently, the plasmablastic morphology of tumour cells has been identified as an independent prognostic factor in patients treated with conventional-dose chemotherapy. In the Eastern Cooperative Oncology Group (ECOG) E9486 trial comparing three chemotherapy regimens: VBMCP, VBMCP plus added cyclophosphamide, and VBMCP plus interferon-α, plasmablastic morphology at diagnosis (8.2% of 453 bone marrow aspirates reviewed among a total of 627 patients registered and eligible) was associated with a significantly lower response rate as compared with non-plasmablastic myeloma (47% versus 66.5%; $p = 0.015$) and a significantly shorter overall survival (median 1.9 years versus 3.7 years; $p < 0.0001$).[18]

Another marker of cell proliferation is the PCLI. In a series of 107 patients with newly diagnosed myeloma at the Mayo Clinic treated with conventional chemotherapy (oral melphalan and prednisone in 82% of cases), Greipp et al[19] have found that only two factors, PCLI and β_2M had independent prognostic significance. Low-risk patients (with low β_2M and low PCLI) had a median survival of 71 months, intermediate-risk patients (with only one high variable) had a median survival of 40 months, and high-risk patients (with both variables high) had a median survival of only 16 months. This indicates that a high tumour burden is associated with reduced survival; however, even a low tumour burden can rapidly reach a life-threatening level if the proliferation rate is high. As mentioned above, marrow PCLI was found to be an independent factor for survival in another large trial by Witzig et al[15] and the combination of the percentage of BPC and the bone marrow labelling index has separated the patients into low-, intermediate-, and high-risk groups, with median survivals of 52, 35, and 26 months, respectively ($p < 0.001$).

PCLI has generally been obtained after incubation of cells in the presence of tritiated thymidine or bromodeoxyurudine.[15,19] These techniques are relatively complex, time-consuming, and restricted to research laboratories. In addition, in most myeloma patients, PCLI is quite low and only 10% of cases display a PCLI above the cut-off value of 2%,[19] so that only a minority of cases are identified as high-risk. In one study, the proliferative activity of myeloma cells has been evaluated differently. San Miguel et al[20] have analysed the cell cycle distribution of bone marrow cells in 120 untreated myeloma patients using a DNA/CD38 double-straining flow cytometry technique in which plasma cells are discriminated from residual bone marrow cells based on their CD38 expression. Patients were treated with conventional chemotherapy; either melphalan and prednisone (43%) or alternating cycles of VCMP/VBAP (57%). They found that half of the patients had a low proliferative activity (S-phase plasma cells $< 3\%$). In a multivariate analysis of prognostic factors, they showed that the number of S-phase plasma cells was the best single parameter for predicting survival. This parameter, together with β_2M serum levels ($<$ or > 6 mg/l), performance status (ECOG $<$ or > 3), and age ($<$ or > 69 years) enabled them to define a simplified classification of patients into three risk groups: low (median survival > 80 months), intermediate (median survival 36 months) and high risk (median survival 9 months).

Cytogenetic studies are difficult in myeloma because of the low proliferation rate of plasma cells. In a series of 151 patients with myeloma, including 117 evaluated at diagnosis (69 of 117 were treated with conventional chemotherapy), Laï et al[21] have found that 51% of the patients had cytogenetic abnormalities (47% at diagnosis). Abnormal cytogenetics and modal chromosome number under 46 were associated with a shorter survival (survival rate 70% at 30 months in patients with normal karyotype, compared with 30% at 30 months when karyotype was abnormal; $p < 0.02$). More recently, the Spanish group has evaluated the prognostic value of numerical chromosome aberrations by fluorescence in situ hybridization (FISH) analysis of 15 different chromosomes in a group of 63 myeloma patients treated with conventional chemotherapy.[22] First, FISH studies have shown an incidence of aneuploidy of 60–90%, which is higher than that obtained by conventional cytogenetics (20–50%). Secondly, in a multivariate analysis of prognostic factors, including β_2M and C-reactive protein (CRP), they have found that monosomy of chromosome 13 occurring in 33% of cases was associated with a shorter overall survival (median 14 months versus 60 months; $p = 0.03$). Thirdly, the cytogenetic analysis also allowed them to define a favourable prognostic factor: trisomy of chromosome 6 observed in 27% of cases was associated with a prolonged survival (70 months versus 33; $p = 0.05$). The impact of cytogenetic abnormalities has to be analysed with the potential chromosomal sites at which genes have been found, such as the *Rb* tumour suppressor gene located on chromosome 13. The impact of chromosomal abnormalities is dealt with in depth in Chapter 5.

A number of small studies have looked at the prognostic significance of molecular abnormalities.[23] Although *p53* tumour suppressor gene mutations are rare events at the time of diagnosis (2–4%),[24] an analysis has shown that deletions of the *p53* gene may occur in up to 33% of patients with relapsed myeloma.[25] In a stepwise multivariate regression analysis performed on 59 patients with newly diagnosed myeloma, the presence of a *p53* deletion was the most significant independent parameter predicting shortened survival as compared with myeloma stage, age, β_2M and serum creatinine. The median overall survival from the start of conventional-dose chemotherapy was 16 months in newly diagnosed myeloma patients with a *p53* deletion and 39 months in patients with a *p53* deletion ($p < 0.0002$).[24]

Multiple-drug resistance (MDR) expression has been identified as an important mechanism of drug resistance in myeloma. MDR, the phenomenon of cancer cells developing cross-resistance to a variety of structurally unrelated chemotherapeutic compounds such as vinca alkaloids, anthracyclines, and epidophyllotoxins, is associated with the expression of the drug-transport-mediating protein P-glycoprotein (PgP, MDR1) and the multidrug-resistance-associated protein (MRP).

Several authors have shown that PgP is expressed at very low frequency ($<5\%$) in untreated myeloma, and has no prognostic value at that stage.[26,27] In contrast, PgP is highly expressed in VAD-refractory disease,[26] whereas

MRP is not expressed above background value in the majority of myeloma samples.[28] Another protein associated with drug resistance, the lung-resistance protein (LRP), has been identified.[29] Studies in myeloma cell lines have also related LRP expression to resistance against the alkylating agent melphalan.[30] In a series of 70 patients, LRP expression was found in 47%.[31] When newly diagnosed myeloma patients were treated with conventional-dose melphalan and prednisone, LRP expression was a significant prognostic factor affecting response and event-free and overall survival (median survival 22 months versus 40 months when LRP was not expressed; $p < 0.001$). Interestingly, dose intensification of melphalan was likely to overcome LRP-mediated resistance, and the response rates of LRP-positive patients to melphalan/prednisone and high-dose melphalan were 18% versus 81%, respectively ($p < 0.001$). LRP is considered as a predictor for response and survival after conventional-dose melphalan and prednisone.[31]

Myeloma cells are heterogeneous with regard to their phenotype, morphology, and biological character. In particular, expression of adhesion molecules such as the VLA-5 antigen clearly distinguishes immature myeloma cells (VLA-5-negative) from mature myeloma cells (VLA-5-positive). Immature myeloma cells have greater proliferation activity in vitro, whereas mature myeloma cells show almost no proliferation and secrete greater amounts of M protein.[32] It has been shown in 39 patients with conventionally treated myeloma that the percentage of immature myeloma cells present after induction therapy and maintenance therapy but not at diagnosis correlated with response.[33] No correlation with survival was available in this study.

Other adhesion molecules, such as CD56 (NCAM) and CD58 (LFA-3) are probably associated with disease activity,[23] but show no correlation with prognosis and survival in large series of patients treated with conventional-dose chemotherapy.

Cytokine activity

Interleukin-6 (IL-6) has been shown to be a major growth factor for human myeloma cells.[34,35] Anti-IL-6 monoclonal antibodies block myeloma cell proliferation in vivo, this being one piece of evidence for the in vivo role of IL-6 in myeloma pathogenesis.[36] It has been shown that IL-6 induces CRP synthesis by human hepatocytes in culture and that serum CRP level actually reflects IL-6 activity. A survival analysis carried out in 162 myeloma patients at diagnosis showed that serum CRP level was a highly significant prognostic factor, independent of serum β_2M. All 162 patients were treated with conventional chemotherapy (alternating VMCP/VBAP or melphalan and prednisone). When CRP level was greater than 6 mg/l (60 patients), the median survival was 21 months, versus 48 months in 102 patients with values less than 6 mg/l ($p < 0.001$).[37] This feature allowed stratification of patients into three groups according to CRP and β_2M serum levels: low-risk group, CRP and $\beta_2M < 6$ mg/l (50% of patients); intermediate-risk group, CRP or $\beta_2M \geq 6$ mg/l (35% of patients); high-risk group, CRP and $\beta_2M \geq 6$ mg/l (15% of patients). The median survival was 54, 27, and 6 months, respectively ($p < 0.0001$). Bataille et al[37] have proposed a new staging system based on these simple and reliable laboratory evaluations.

IL-6 also acts on hepatocytes by inhibiting albumin synthesis.[37] The serum albumin level is strongly correlated with disease activity.[10] In a series of 147 cases, Bataille et al[10] showed that the prognostic variables that correlated best with survival duration were β_2M and albumin levels. They stratified patients according to these variables into three groups and proposed a powerful prognostic system. Low-risk patients presented with both $\beta_2M < 6$ mg/l and albumin > 3 g/dl, intermediate-risk patients with $\beta_2M > 6$ mg/l but albumin > 3 g/dl, and poor-risk patients with albumin ≤ 3 g/dl. The median survival was 55, 19, and 4 months, respectively.

The action of IL-6 is dependent on an 80 kDa membrane-bound specific receptor, IL-6R, and a transmembrane signal transducer, gp130. A soluble receptor molecule (sIL-6R) can mediate the binding of IL-6 to gp130 and hence signal transduction in cells that do not produce membrane-bound IL-6R. IL-6R and membrane-bound IL-6R have a similar affinity for IL-6. Two studies have successfully correlated sIL-6R levels with disease activity and survival.[38,39] In a group of 207 newly diagnosed myeloma patients treated with melphalan and prednisone, the Finnish group found that the serum concentration of sIL-6R was raised (above the upper reference limit 185 mg/l) in 47% of patients at diagnosis. In this population of patients, the median survival was less than 30 months, compared with a 60% survival rate at 40 months in patients with sIL-6R < 185 mg/l ($p = 0.004$).[38] Of particular interest is the fact that in this trial, sIL-6R did not show linear correlation with any other parameter, including β_2M, supporting the hypothesis that β_2M and sIL-6R reflect different biological characteristics of myeloma. In 80 myeloma patients treated with VAD or melphalan–prednisone–interferon-α, Kyrtsonis et al[39] have confirmed that high sIL-6R level was strongly correlated with survival.

Combinations of factors

As mentioned previously, some authors have combined prognostic factors reflecting tumour burden or plasma cell characteristics or cytokine activity, and have proposed various staging systems (reviewed in reference 40). Three of these are commonly used: β_2M and albumin,[10] β_2M and CRP,[37] and β_2M and PCLI[19] (Table 11.2). However, none of these has superseded the 'old and simple' parameters of tumour burden such as Durie–Salmon stage and β_2M.

Prognostic factors in asymptomatic stage I myeloma

Approximately 20% of patients with myeloma are recognized by chance without significant symptoms.[41] Such patients with asymptomatic disease have been observed safely without treatment, and the temporal pattern of the development of progressive disease has been variable, ranging from a few months to several years.[42,43]

Table 11.2 Prognostic significance of β_2-microglobulin (β_2M) combined with serum albumin (SA), C-reactive protein, or plasma cell labelling index (PCLI)

Risk category	Risk parameters	No. of patients	Median survival (months)	Ref
Low	β_2M < 6 mg/l and SA > 3 g/dl	81	55	10
Intermediate	β_2M ≥ 6 mg/l and SA > 3 g/dl	46	19	
High	SA ≤ 3 g/dl	18	4	
Low	β_2M and CRP < 6 mg/l	81	54	37
Intermediate	β_2M or CRP ≥ 6 mg/l	56	27	
High	β_2M and CRP ≥ 6 mg/l	25	6	
Low	β_2M < 2.7 mg/l and PCLI < 1	9	71	19
Intermediate	β_2M ≥ 2.7 mg/l or PCLI ≥ 1	26	41	
High	β_2M ≥ 2.7 mg/l and PCLI ≥ 1	16	17	

Thus it is necessary to distinguish precisely between those asymptomatic patients who are likely to remain stable without therapy for a long period and those at high risk of serious complications who might benefit from early chemotherapy.

Several studies have defined criteria that are associated with a rapid disease progression. The group from the MD Anderson Cancer Center in Houston has shown in a series of 101 patients with asymptomatic myeloma that three factors were significantly associated with a disease progression: serum peak > 30 g/l, IgA type and Bence Jones protein > 50 mg/d.[41] Patients were then grouped into three risk categories based on these three factors: low-risk patients had no characteristic out of three, intermediate-risk patients had one characteristic, and high-risk patients had two or three characteristics. The median time to progression was 95, 39, and 17 months, respectively ($p < 0.01$), and the median survival from diagnosis was 89, 87, and 51 months, respectively ($p < 0.01$). This group also showed that magnetic resonance imaging (MRI) of the spine was an important prognostic factor among patients at intermediate risk – with an earlier disease progression (median 21 months) when MRI was abnormal compared with when it was normal (median 57 months; $p < 0.01$).

The prognostic value of vertebral lesions detected by MRI in such patients has been recently confirmed in a series of 55 consecutive newly diagnosed cases.[44] In this series, bone marrow plasmocytosis of more than 20% at diagnosis was also associated with disease progression. This latter parameter, as well as the haemoglobn level, had previously been proposed as a marker of disease activity in a series of 91 patients.[45] In this situation conflicting results have been obtained with serum β_2M level: it is not certain that this parameter has the same prognostic value as compared with stage II and III disease.[41,44–46]

AUTOLOGOUS STEM CELL TRANSPLANTATION

In the past 15 years or so, autologous stem cell transplantation (ASCT) has been widely used either as salvage therapy for patients with relapsed or refractory myeloma or as part of intial therapy in newly diagnosed patients.[47] The number of ASCTs performed per year has rapidly increased, especially after the publication of two studies – a prospective randomized trial[48] and a pair-mate analysis[49] – showing that, compared with conventional chemotherapy, high-dose therapy followed by ASCT significantly increases complete remission (CR) rate and also event-free survival (EFS) and overall survival (OS).

Three types of parameters affect the outcome of high-dose therapy: factors related to the patient, factors related to tumour burden and disease biology, and factors related to previous treatment.

Factors related to the patient

Several pilot studies suggested that greater age could be associated with shorter PFS or OS[50–53] (Table 11.3). However, in these studies, the treatments received were heterogeneous, the number of older patients was small, or patients were transplanted for refractory myeloma.[51] Other studies published in the early 1990s showed no negative impact of older age.[54–58] Retrospective analyses of large cohorts of patients also showed conflicting results. In the European Group for Blood and Marrow Transplantation (EBMT) analysis, age under 45 years was associated with both better PFS and OS.[59] In a more recent report of 259 cases from the Spanish Registry, age had no significant impact on outcome.[60] Siegel et al[61] compared 49 patients aged 65 years or more and 49 younger pair mates matched for five critical prognostic factors (β_2M cytogenetics, creatinine, albumin and CRP). All patients were prospectively entered into a tandem transplantation programme. Although the CR rate was lower in

Table 11.3 Influence of age on outcome after autologous stem cell transplantation

Study	No. of patients	Cut-off age (years)	*p*-value CR	PFS	OS
Jagannath et al (1990)[54]	55	50	NS	NS	NS
Harousseau et al (1992)[50]	97	50	NS	—	0.009
Fernand et al (1993)[55]	63	45	—	NS	NS
Vesole et al (1994)[51,a]	135	50	NS	—	0.007
Cunningham et al (1994)[56]	53	50	—	NS	NS
Harousseau et al (1995)[57]	133	50	NS	—	NS
Bensinger et al (1996)[58]	63	50	NS	NS	NS
Marit et al (1996)[52]	73	60	NS	0.001	0.0017
Björkstrand et al (1994)[59]	130	45	—	0.03	0.03
Alegre et al (1998)[60]	259	50	NS	NS	NS
Dumontet et al (1998)[53]	55	60	—	0.04	NS

CR, complete remission; PFS, progression-free survival; OS, overall survival; NS, not significant.
[a]Refractory patients.

older patients, EFS and OS duration were not significantly different. In multivariate analysis, cytogenetics, duration of prior treatment and β_2M level were the only critical prognostic parameters, whereas age was not a significant risk factor for either EFS or OS. One can conclude that when peripheral blood progenitor cells (PBPC) are used, there is no evidence that age has a significant impact on the outcome after ASCT. However, performance status plays a major role in defining patients who are candidates for high-dose therapy. Older patients in poor general condition or with concomitant diseases would probably not be included in autologous transplantation programmes.

In only one study did sex have a prognostic value, with male sex predicting for longer survival in multivariate analysis.[59]

Factors related to the disease

Factors predicting complete remission post-transplantation (Table 11.4)

In a large series of 496 consecutive patients who were transplanted in a single centre between

Table 11.4 Factors predicting complete remission after autologous transplantation

Study	No. of patients	Response to previous therapy	Duration of previous therapy	No. of lines of previous therapy	Albumin level	Isotype	Plasma cell infiltration
Harousseau et al (1995)[57]	133	+					+
Vesole et al (1996)[62]	496	+	+		+	+	
Alegre et al (1998)[60]	259	+	+				
Björkstrand et al (1994)[59]	122	+		+			

September 1989 and July 1995, Vesole et al[62] showed in multivariate analysis that factors significantly associated with higher CR rates were: disease sensitivity to standard therapy, IgA isotype, normal albumin levels, and duration of previous therapy less than 12 months.[62] In other series, response to previous therapy was also correlated with achievement of CR.[57,59,60] In one study, patients with 15% or more plasma cells in the bone marrow had significantly lower CR rates.[57] However, patients with a high percentage of plasma cells were likely to have responded poorly to previous chemotherapy.

Factors predicting longer event-free or overall survival (Table 11.5)

Two parameters that are almost invariably related to EFS and/or OS are the response to previous conventional chemotherapy and the β_2M level.

As expected, the long-term results of high-dose therapy with ASCT are better when the disease is sensitive to conventional chemotherapy. Several uncontrolled studies have suggested that ASCT is a useful salvage therapy for patients with chemosensitive relapses,[50,63] whereas it has a limited value in patients with resistant relapses.[50,54,64]

β_2M level, which is a major prognostic factor in the context of standard therapy is also critical in the context of high-dose therapy with ASCT.[51,54,55,57–59,62] However, the cut-off value is not yet clear, and varies from 2.5 mg/l to 6 mg/l, depending on the published series. Several investigators have shown that non-IgG (or IgA) isotype is associated with shorter

Table 11.5 Pretransplant characteristics negatively influencing overall survival after autologous transplantation: factors related to the disease and to previous therapy

Study	No. of patients	Response to previous therapy	β_2-microglobulin level (mg/l)	Isotype	Duration of previous therapy	Others[a]
Jagannath et al (1990)[a,54]	55	Resistant relapse	>3	Non-IgG	—	—
Fernand et al (1993)[a,55]	63	—	>2.8	—	>6 cycles	—
Björkstrand et al (1994)[59]	130	No response	>4	—	>1 line	Female sex; stage > I at diagnosis
Vesole et al (1994)[51]	135	Resistant relapse	>2.5	—	>12 months	LDH level
Harousseau et al (1995)[b,57]	133	No response	>6	IgA	—	Albumin level < 30 g/l; plasma cell infiltration > 15%
Bensinger et al (1996)[58]	63	—	>2.5	—	>8 cycles or >2 lines	Prior radiation
Marit et al (1996)[52]	73	No response after cyclophosphamide	—	Non-IgG	—	
Vesole et al (1996)[62]	496	No response	>2.5	IgA	>12 months	CRP > 4 mg/l
Alegre et al (1998)[60]	259	Progression or no response	—	—	⩾2 lines	—

[a]LDH, lactate dehydrogenase; CRP, C-reactive protein.
[b]Univariate analysis.

survival.[52,54,57,62] Other parameters have been less frequently correlated with EFS or OS: plasma cell infiltration,[57] LDH level,[56] and CRP level.[62]

Cytogenetics has been rarely evaluated in multicentric studies, mostly because of technical problems. When cytogenetics is included in the multivariate analysis, it appears to be a dominant prognostic factor. Vesole et al[62] showed that the presence of abnormalities of chromosomes 11 and 13 had a negative impact on both EFS and OS.

Factors related to previous treatment (Table 11.5)

In most studies including relapsed and refractory patients, the duration of conventional treatment prior to ASCT appeared to be a major prognostic factor, affecting not only the haematopoietic quality of the graft but also the post-transplantation outcome. Vesole et al[51] showed that when the duration of prior therapy did not exceed 12 months, the CR rate was higher and both EFS and OS were longer.

Other investigators have shown that having received two lines or more of chemotherapy prior to ASCT was also a negative prognostic factor as well.[58,60,62]

Prognostic factors in patients with previously untreated myeloma

Prognostic factors were analysed in two large prospective studies in which patients with de novo myeloma were homogeneously treated. In the IFM 94 randomized trial, 405 patients up to the age of 60 years were randomly assigned to receive either one or two ASCTs.[65] In the preliminary analysis of this trial, univariate analysis showed that the initial β_2M level, the initial CRP level, the response to conventional chemotherapy prior to ASCT, and the response obtained after ASCT were significantly related to OS. However, the initial β_2M level was the only prognostic factor in multivariate analysis.

Barlogie et al[66] have published the results of 'total therapy', a programme of intensive treatment including two cycles of high-dose therapy in 231 patients with newly diagnosed myeloma. In multivariate analysis, superior EFS and OS were observed in the absence of unfavourable karyotypes (11q breakpoints and/or partial or complete delection of chromosome 13) and with low β_2M level at diagnosis (< 4 mg/l). On combining these two factors, a subgroup of patients with a very poor prognosis was identified: patients with unfavourable cytogenetics and β_2M levels above 4 mg/l had a median survival of only 2.1 years, compared with 7 years for the remaining patients. New therapeutics are clearly needed for these patients. When taking into account treatment variables in a time-dependent covariate analysis, timely application of the second transplant increased both EFS and OS.

Selection of patients for autologous stem cell transplantation

One of the aims of defining prognostic factors is to help physicians in their therapeutic options. Therefore, it is important to have models to predict which patients are likely to benefit from high-dose therapy with ASCT as part of front-line therapy. In other cases, the risks and costs of ASCT should be avoided. Alternatively, ASCT could be postponed and used only at the time of disease progression.

Unfortunately, no clinical study can yet answer this question. In the only published randomized study, the number of patients was too small to compare the results of conventional chemotherapy and high-dose therapy in subgroups defined by their expected prognosis. However, the preliminary results of the IFM 94 study provide the beginnings of a response to this question. In patients with an unfavourable prognosis (β_2M level > 3 mg/l), there was no significant difference in overall three-year survival between one and two ASCTs (44% versus 41%; p = NS) (Figure 11.1). Conversely, in patients with a favourable prognosis (β_2M level

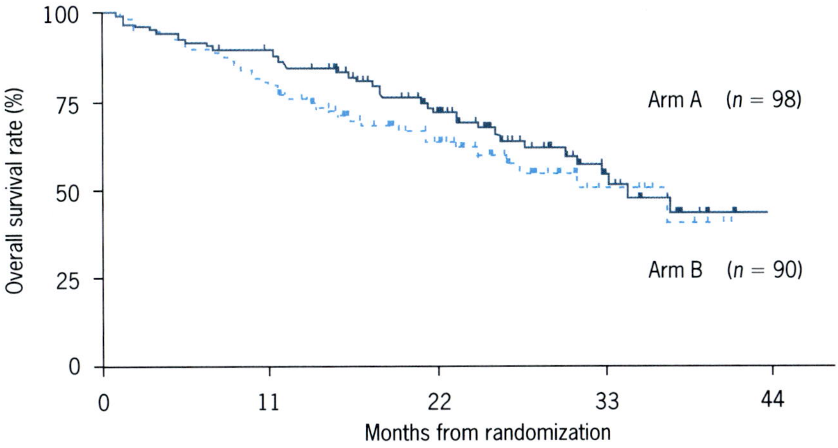

Figure 11.1 IFM 94 trial: comparison between one (Arm A) and two (Arm B) autologous transplants in patients with high β_2-microglobulin level at diagnosis (>3 mg/l).

< 3 mg/l), the three-year probability of survival was 82% after two ASCTs versus 68% after one ASCT ($p = 0.05$) (Figure 11.2). If these results are confirmed by longer follow-up, this could mean that, paradoxically, the patients who are more likely to benefit from high-dose therapy are those with the better prognosis.

ALLOGENEIC BONE MARROW TRANSPLANTATION

Few large studies are currently available to study prognostic factors in the setting of allogeneic bone marrow transplantation (alloBMT).

Gahrton et al[67] have collected data from 162 patients transplanted in European centres between 1983 and 1993. This retrospective

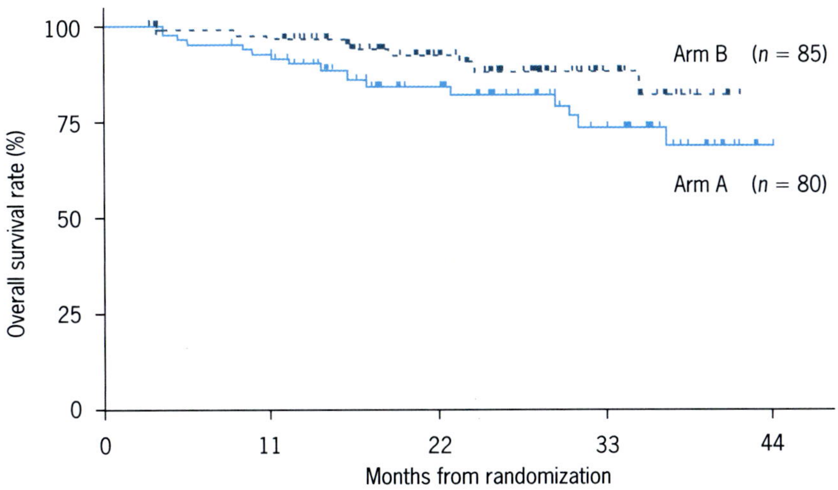

Figure 11.2 IFM 94 trial: comparison between one (Arm A) and two (Arm B) autologous transplants (Arm B) in patients with a low β_2-microglobulin level at diagnosis ($\leqslant$3 mg/l).

analysis of the EBMT Registry showed that patients with a low tumour burden who respond to chemotherapy given prior to alloBMT and are transplanted after first-line therapy have the best prognosis.

In univariate analysis, patients with stage I disease at diagnosis had a significantly better survival (52% at four years) than those in stages II and III ($p = 0.05$). Patients who had received only one line of treatment also had a better survival (42% at four years) than those who had received three or more lines of treatment ($p = 0.02$). Finally, patients in CR at the time of alloBMT survived longer (64% at three years) than other patients ($p = 0.05$). Another pretransplant favourable prognostic factor was female sex (41% survival at three years).

Post-transplant factors were also found to influence prognosis in this study. In univariate analysis, the most important one was the achievement of CR following alloBMT ($p = 0.001$). The five-year survival rate of patients who entered CR was 52%, as compared with less than 20% for these who did not. Grade III or IV acute graft-versus-host disease was the most important adverse prognostic factor in multivariate analysis.

Besinger et al[68] summarized the Seattle experience, where 80 patients were treated with high-dose busulfan and cyclophosphamide, with or without total-body irradiation. In this series with a high proportion of patients with refractory and heavily pretreated disease, transplant-related mortality was high (44%) and the actuarial probability of survival at 4.5 years was only 24%. In multivariate analysis, adverse risk factors were the following: transplantation later than one year from diagnosis, β_2M level at transplant above 2.5 mg/l, female patients transplanted from male donors, more than eight cycles of chemotherapy before transplant and stage III disease at the time of transplant.

From this limited experience, it can be concluded that patients with a low tumour burden, those who respond to conventional chemotherapy, and those who are transplanted early have the best prognosis after alloBMT.

CONCLUSIONS

The clinical impact of prognostic factors or staging systems depends on two parameters: reproducibility and practicality. A number of parameters listed above have not yet been validated by large multicentre clinical trials. Others are not easily accessible in the majority of centres. This explains why, until now, the Durie–Salmon clinical staging system has been most commonly used. This simple and reproducible system is based on easily accessible data. However, its usefulness has been demonstrated only in the context of conventional chemotherapy, and has not been confirmed in context of autologous transplantation. One of the reasons for studying prognostic factors is the identification of risk groups in order to adapt the patient treatment to the expected outcome. Therefore the initial β_2M level appears to be more accurate, since its prognostic value has been shown in a number of clinical trials with conventional chemotherapy and confirmed in studies on autologous transplantation.

Other easily accessible clinical or biological factors should be used mainly for showing the homogeneity of groups of patients enrolled in clinical trials. The prognostic impact of recently individualized parameters needs further validation.

For the future, cytogenetics appears to be an important parameter as well. The combination of β_2M level and cytogenetics could help to define therapeutic strategies. Patients with low β_2M level and without unfavourable cytogenetics could benefit from intensive strategies with autologous transplantation. New approaches are needed for patients with high β_2M level and/or unfavourable cytogenetics.

REFERENCES

1. Carbone PP, Kellerhouse LE, Gehan EA. Plasmacytic myeloma: a study of the relationship of survival to various clinical manifestations and anomalous protein type in 112 patients. *Am J Med* 1967; **42**: 937–48.

2. Bladé J, Kyle RA, Greipp PR. Presenting features and prognosis in 72 patients with multiple myeloma who were younger than 40 years. *Br J Haematol* 1996; **93**: 345–51.
3. Munshi NC. Immunoregulatory mechanisms in multiple myeloma. *Hematol Oncol Clin North Am* 1997; **11**: 51–69.
4. Kyle RA. Why better prognostic factors for multiple myeloma are needed. *Blood* 1994; **83**: 1713–16.
5. Durie BGM, Salmon SE. A clinical staging system for multiple myeloma. Correlation of measured myeloma cell mass with presenting clinical features, response to treatment and survival. *Cancer* 1975; **36**: 842–54.
6. SalmonSE,RobertCassidyJ.Plasmacellneoplasms. In: *Cancer: Principles and Practice of Oncology*, 6th edn (De Vita VT, Hellman S, Rosenberg SA, eds). Philadelphia: JB Lippincott, 2001.
7. Norfolk D, Child JA, Cooper EH et al. Serum β_2M-microglobulin in myelomatosis: potential value in stratification and monitoring. *Br J Cancer* 1980; **42**: 510–15.
8. Scarffe JH, Anderson H, Palmer MK et al. Prognostic significance of pretreatment serum β_2M-microglobulin levels in multiple myeloma. *Eur J Cancer Clin Oncol* 1983; **19**: 1361–4.
9. Bataille R, Magulo M, Grenier J et al. Serum β_2M-microglobulin in multiple myeloma: a simple reliable marker for staging. *Br J Haematol* 1983; **55**: 439–47.
10. Bataille R, Durie BGM, Grenier J et al. Prognostic factors and staging in multiple myeloma: a reappraisal. *J Clin Oncol* 1986; **4**: 80–7.
11. Cuzick J, Cooper EH, MacLennan ICM. The prognostic value of serum β_2M-microglobulin compared with other presentation features in myelomatosis. (A report to the Medical Research Council's Working Party on Leukaemia in Adults.) *Br J Cancer* 1985; **52**: 1–6.
12. Dimopoulos MA, Barlogie B, Smith TL, Alexanian R. High serum lactate dehydrogenase level as a marker for drug resistance and short survival in multiple myeloma. *Ann Intern Med* 1991; **115**: 931–5.
13. Bladé J, Rozman C, Cervantes F et al. A new prognostic system for multiple myeloma based on easily available parameters. *Br J Haematol* 1989; **72**: 507–11.
14. Rawstrom AC, Owen RC, Davies FE et al. Circulating plasma cells in multiple myeloma: characterization and correlation with disease state. *Br J Haematol* 1997; **97**: 46–55.
15. Witzig TE, Gertz MA, Lust JA et al. Peripheral blood monoclonal plasma cells as a predictor of survival of patients with multiple myeloma. *Blood* 1996; **88**: 1780–7.
16. Bayrd ED. The bone marrow on sternal aspiration in multiple myeloma. *Blood* 1948; **3**: 987.
17. Peest D, Coldewey R, Deicher H et al. Prognostic value of clinical, laboratory, and histological characteristics in multiple myeloma: Improved definition of risk groups. *Eur J Cancer* 1993; **29A:** 978–83.
18. Greipp PR, Leong T, Bennett JM et al. Plasmablastic morphology – an independent prognostic factor with clinical and laboratory correlates: Eastern Cooperative Oncology Group Myeloma Trial E9486 report by the ECOG Myeloma Laboratory Group. *Blood* 1998; **91**: 2501–7.
19. Greipp PR, Lust JA, O'Fallon WM et al. Plasma cell labelling index and β_2M-microglobulin predict survival independent of thymidine-kinase and C-reactive protein in multiple myeloma. *Blood* 1993; **81**: 3382–7.
20. San Miguel JF, Garcia-Sanz R, Gonzalez M et al. A new staging system for multiple myeloma based on the number of S-phase plasma cells. *Blood* 1995; **85**: 448–55.
21. Laï JL, Zandecki M, Mary JH et al. Improved cytogenetics in multiple myeloma: a study of 151 patients including 117 patients at diagnosis. *Blood* 1995; **85**: 2490–7.
22. Perez-Simon JA, Garcia-Sanz R, Tabernero MD et al. Prognostic value of numerical chromosome observation in multiple myeloma: a FISH analysis of 15 different chromosomes. *Blood* 1998; **91**: 3366–71.
23. Davies FE, Jack AS, Morgan GJ. The use of biological variables to predict outcome in multiple myeloma. *Br J Haematol* 1997; **99**: 719–25.
24. Preud'homme C, Facon T, Zandecki M et al. Rare occurence of P53 gene mutation in multiple myeloma. *Br J Haematol* 1992; **81**: 440–3.
25. Drach J, Ackerman J, Fritz E et al. Presence of a p53 gene deletion in patients with multiple myeloma predicts for short survival after conventional dose chemotherapy. *Blood* 1998; **92**: 802–9.
26. Grogan TM, Spier CM, Salmon SE et al. P-glycoprotein expression in human plasma cell myeloma: correlation with prior chemotherapy. *Blood* 1993; **81**: 490–5.
27. Cornelissen JJ, Sonneveld P, Schoester M et al. MDR1-expression and response to vincristine, doxorubicin and dexamethasone chemotherapy

in multiple myeloma refractory to alkylating agents. *J Clin Oncol* 1994; **12**: 115–19.
28. Burger H, Nooter K, Zaman GJR et al. Expression of the multidrug resistance associated protein (MRP) in acute and chronic leukemias. *Leukemia* 1994; **8**: 990–7.
29. Scheffer GL, Winjgaard PL, Fleus MJ et al. The drug resistance related protein LRP is the human major vault protein. *Nature Med* 1995; **1**: 578–82.
30. Scheper RJ, Broxterman HJ, Scheffer GL et al. Overexpression of a *M*(*r*) 110,000 vesicular protein in non-P-glycoprotein-mediated drug resistance. *Cancer Res* 1993; **53**: 1475–9.
31. Raaijmakers HGP, Izepmierdo MAI, Lokhorst HM et al. Lung-resistance-related protein expression is a negative predictive factor for response to conventional low but not to intensified dose alkylating chemotherapy in multiple myeloma. *Blood* 1998; **91**: 1029–36.
32. Kawano MM, Huang N, Harada H et al. Identification of immature and mature myeloma cells in the bone marrow of human myelomas. *Blood* 1993; **82**: 564–70.
33. Kawano MM, Mahmond MS, Huang N et al. High proportions of VLA-5 immature myeloma cells correlated well with poor response to treatment in multiple myeloma. *Br J Haematol* 1995; **91**: 860–4.
34. Kawano M, Hizano T, Matsuda T et al. Autocrine generation and requirement of BSF-2/IL-6 for human multiple myeloma. *Nature* 1988; **332**: 83–5.
35. Bataille R, Jourdan M, Zhang XG et al. Serum levels of interleukin 6, a potent myeloma cell growth factor, as a reflection of disease severity in plasma cell dyscrasias. *J Clin Invest* 1989; **84**: 2008–11.
36. Klein B, Wijdenes J, Zhang XG et al. Murine anti-interleukin 6 monoclonal antibody therapy in myeloma. *Blood* 1991; **78**: 1198–204.
37. Bataille R, Boccadoro M, Klein B et al. C-reactive protein and β_2 microglobulin produce a sample and powerful myeloma staging system. *Blood* 1992; **80**: 733–7.
38. Pulkki K, Pelliniemi TT, Rajamaki A et al. Soluble interleukin 6 receptor as a prognostic factor in multiple myeloma. *Br J Haematol* 1996; **92**: 370.
39. Kyrtsonis MC, Dedoussis G, Zervas C et al. Soluble interleukin-6 receptor: a new prognostic factor in multiple myeloma. *Br J Haematol* 1996; **93**: 398–400.
40. Boccadoro M, Pileri A. Diagnosis, prognosis, and standard treatment of multiple myeloma. *Hematol Oncol Clin North Am* 1997; **11**: 111–31.
41. Weber DM, Dimopoulos MA, Moulopoulos LA et al. Prognostic features of asymptomatic multiple myeloma. *Br J Haematol* 1997; **97**: 810–14.
42. Kyle RA, Greipp PR. Smoldering multiple myeloma. *N Engl J Med* 1980; **302**: 1347–9.
43. Dimopoulos MA, Moulopoulos A, Smith T et al. Risk of disease progression in asymptomatic multiple myeloma. *Am J Med* 1993; **94**: 57–61.
44. Mariette X, Zagdanski AM, Guermazi A et al. Prognostic value of vertebral lesions detected by magnetic resonance imaging in patients with stage I multiple myeloma. *Br J Haematol* 1999; **104**: 723–9.
45. Facon T, Menard JF, Michaux JL et al. Prognostic factors in low tumour mass asymptomatic multiple myeloma: a report on 91 patients. *Am J Hematol* 1995; **48**: 71–5.
46. Moulopoulos LA, Dimopoulos MA, Smith TA et al. Prognostic significance of magnetic resonance imaging in patients with asymptomatic multiple myeloma. *J Clin Oncol* 1995; **13**: 251–6.
47. Harousseau JL, Attal M. The role of autologous hematopoietic stem cell transplantation. *Semin Hematol* 1997; **34**(Suppl 1): 61–6.
48. Attal M, Harousseau JL, Stoppa AM et al. A prospective, randomized trial of autologous bone marrow transplantation and chemotherapy in multiple myeloma. *N Engl J Med* 1996; **335**: 91–7.
49. Barlogie B, Jagannath S, Vesole D et al. Superiority of tandem autologous transplantation over standard therapy for previously untreated multiple myeloma. *Blood* 1997; **89**: 789–93.
50. Harousseau JL, Milpied N, Capate JP et al. Double-intensive therapy in high-risk multiple myeloma. *Blood* 1992; **79**: 2827–33.
51. Vesole DH, Barlogie B, Jagannath S et al. High-dose therapy for refracting multiple myeloma: improved prognosis with better supportive care and double transplants. *Blood* 1994; **84**: 950–6.
52. Marit G, Faberes C, Pico JL et al. Autologous peripheral-blood progenitor-cell support following high-dose chemotherapy of chemotherapy in patients with high-risk multiple myeloma. *J Clin Oncol* 1996; **14**: 1306–13.
53. Dumontet C, Ketterrer N, Espinousse D et al. Reduced progression-free survival in elderly patients receiving intensification with autologous peripheral blood stem cell reinfusion for multiple myeloma. *Bone Marrow Transplant* 1998; **21**: 1037–41.

54. Jagannath S, Barlogie B, Dicke K et al. Autologous bone marrow transplantation in multiple myeloma: identification of prognostic factors. *Blood* 1990; **76**: 1860–6.
55. Fermand JP, Chevret S, Ravaud P et al. High-dose chemoradiotherapy and autologous blood stem cell transplantation in multiple myeloma: results of a phase II trial involving 63 patients. *Blood* 1993; **82**: 2005–9.
56. Cunningham D, Paz-Ares I, Milan S et al. High-dose melphalan and autologous bone marrow transplantation as consolidation in previously untreated myeloma. *Blood* 1994; **12**: 759–63.
57. Harousseau JL, Attal M, Divine M et al. Autologous stem cell transplantation after first remission induction treatment in multiple myeloma: a report of the French Registry on Autologous Transplantation in Multiple Myeloma. *Blood* 1995; **85**: 3077–85.
58. Bensinger WJ, Rowley SD, Demirer T et al. High-dose therapy followed by autologous hematopoietic stem-cell infusion for patients with multiple myeloma. *J Clin Oncol* 1996; **14**: 1447–56.
59. Björkstrand B, Goldstone A, Jjungman P et al. Prognostic factors in autologous stem cell transplantation for multiple myeloma: an EBMT Registry study. *Leuk Lymphoma* 1994; **15**: 265–72.
60. Alegre A, Diaz-Mediavilla J, San Miguel J et al. Autologous peripheral blood stem cell transplantation for multiple myeloma: a report of 259 cases from the Spanish Registry. *Bone Marrow Transplant* 1998; **21**: 133–40.
61. Siegel DS, Disikan KR, Mehta J et al. Age is not a prognostic variable with autotransplants for multiple myeloma. *Blood* 1999; **93**: 51–4.
62. Vesole D, Tricot G, Jagannath S et al. Autotransplantation in multiple myeloma: What have we learned? *Blood* 1996; **88**: 838–47.
63. Alexanian R, Dimopoulos MA, Hester J et al. Early myeloablative therapy for multiple myeloma. *Blood* 1994; **84**: 4278–82.
64. Alexanian R, Dimopoulos M, Smith T. Limited value of myeloablative therapy for late multiple myeloma. *Blood* 1994; **83**: 512–16.
65. Attal M, Harousseau JL, Facon T et al. Single versus double transplantation in myeloma: a prospective and randomized trial of the Intergroupe Francophone du Myélome (IFM). *Blood* 2000; **96**(Suppl 1): 557a.
66. Barlogie B, Jagannath S, Desikan KR et al. Total therapy with tandem transplants for newly diagnosed multiple myeloma. *Blood* 1999; **93**: 55–65.
67. Gahrton G, Tura S, Ljungman P et al. Prognostic factors in allogeneic bone marrow transplantation for multiple myeloma. *J Clin Oncol* 1995; **13**: 1312–22.
68. Bensinger WI, Buckner CD, Anasett C et al. Allogeneic marrow transplantation for multiple myeloma: an analysis of risk factors on outcome. *Blood* 1996; **88**: 2787–93.

12

Neuropathy in plasma cell disorders

Kenneth C Gorson, Allan H Ropper

CONTENTS • **Introduction** • **Myeloma** • **Osteosclerotic myeloma (OSM) and the POEMS syndrome** • **Waldenström's macroglobulinemia** • **Amyloidosis** • **Cryoglobulinemia** • **Monoclonal gammopathy of undertermined significance and anti-MAG antibodies** • **Anti-GM1 antibody and multifocal motor neuropathy** • **Approach to the patient with neuropathy and monoclonal gammopathy**

INTRODUCTION

A relationship between peripheral neuropathy and plasma cell dyscrasias was described early in the 20th century,[1–3] and in the last decade or so numerous studies have firmly established a link between these conditions. Monoclonal proteins are now known to be present in a sizable group of patients who were formerly thought to have idiopathic neuropathy.[4] The immunoglobulins can be detected in the serum or urine by immunoelectrophoresis or by the more sensitive immunofixation test. While the majority of patients with monoclonal gammopathy have a monoclonal protein of undetermined significance (MGUS), approximately one-third have, or ultimately develop, a malignant disorder such as myeloma or its osteosclerotic variant (POEMS syndrome, described below), Waldenström's macroglobulinemia, amyloidosis, cryoglobulinemia, or lymphoma. In certain conditions (e.g. osteosclerotic myeloma, amyloidosis, and MGUS) neuropathy may be the initial manifestation of the disease (Table 12.1).[5–10]

The prevalence of monoclonal gammopathy in the general population is 1–3%, and therefore a direct pathophysiologic relationship between the M protein and the neuropathy is often uncertain but several lines of evidence suggest that there is a causal connection. Epidemiologic data indicate that the prevalence of MGUS is higher in patients with idiopathic neuropathy than in those with a known cause,[4] and the prevalence of neuropathy is manifestly higher in patients with monoclonal gammopathy than in the general population.[11] Furthermore, under some circumstances a demyelinating neuropathy can be induced in animals by transfer of serum and by intraneural injection from patients with MGUS neuropathy.[12–14] The pivotal pieces of evidence, however, are the findings of specific anti-nerve autoantibodies in the serum of certain patients with paraproteinemic neuropathy,[15–18] the immunofluorescent staining of the responsible immunoglobulin in the endoneurium,[15–19] and improvement of the neuropathy in some cases by immunomodulating therapies, all implicating the protein as the proximate cause of nerve damage.[6,20–25]

As a prelude to understanding these conditions, a brief review of the cardinal features of peripheral nerve disease is necessary. Neuropathy may be classified into broad categories according to the clinical manifestations and the type of nerve fiber that is affected (sensory, motor, or autonomic, and large or

Table 12.1 Plasma cell disorders associated with neuropathy[a]

Disorder	Neuropathic features[b]	Systemic features[c]	Paraprotein	EMG	Nerve biopsy	Treatment[d]
Myeloma	Symmetric, distal sensory, or sensorimotor, usually mild	Bone pain, fatigue, weight loss	IgM or IgG $\kappa > 3$ g/dl	Axonal	Axonal degeneration ± amyloid deposition	None
Osteosclerotic myeloma	Symmetric, progressive proximal and distal, sensorimotor, areflexia, simulates CIDP	POEMS syndrome, Castleman's disease	IgG, IgA λ usually < 2 g/dl	Demyelinating	Demyelination + axonal degeneration ± inflammation	Resection, XRT, prednisone, melphalan, cyclophosphamide
Waldenström's macroglobulinemia	Distal, symmetric, progressive, sensory or sensorimotor, may simulate CIDP	Fatigue, oronasal bleeding, visual blurring, stroke, encephalopathy	IgM $\kappa > 3$ g/dl	Demyelinating	Demyelination; myelin separation; IgM deposition	PE, prednisone, melphalan, chlorambucil
Amyloidosis	Distal, progressive, symmetric, painful, sensory, autonomic symptoms	CHF, renal failure, HSM, macroglossia	IgG or IgA λ usually < 3 g/dl	Axonal	Axonal degeneration; amyloid deposition	Melphalan + prednisone; ? stem cell replacement
Cryoglobulinemia	Distal, painful, symmetric or multifocal, sensory or sensorimotor, mononeuritis multiplex	HSM, purpura, arthralgias, leg ulcers, Raynaud's phenomena	IgM or IgG 1–4 g/dl	Axonal	Axonal degeneration, vasculitis, inflammation	PE, prednisone, cyclophosphamide, IFN-α
IgG/IgA-MGUS	Progressive or relapsing, proximal and distal, symmetric, sensorimotor, areflexia, simulates CIDP	None	IgG or IgA $\kappa > \lambda$ < 3 g/dl	Mixed demyelinating and axonal; axonal	Demyelination; axonal degeneration	PE, prednisone, IVIG
IgM-MGUS	Progressive, symmetric, distal, sensory >> motor; areflexia	None	IgM $\kappa > \lambda$ < 3 g/dl	Demyelinating or mixed demyelinating and axonal	Demyelination; endoneural IgM deposition	PE, IVIG, chlorambucil cyclophosphamide
Anti-MAG antibody syndrome	Progressive, symmetric, distal, sensory >> motor, ataxia, tremor	None	IgM $\kappa < 3$ g/dl	Demyelinating or mixed demyelinating and axonal	Demyelination; widening of myelin lamellae; IgM deposition	PE, IVIG, cyclophosphamide, IFN-α
Anti-GM1 antibody syndrome	Progressive, asymmetric, distal, upper extremity predominant, pure motor; GBS; may simulate MND	None	IgM < 3g/dl	Demyelinating; multifocal motor conduction block or motor axonal neuropathy	degeneration of motor neurons, anterior roots; IgM deposition on myelin sheaths	IVIG, cyclophosphamide

[a] Adapted from Ropper AH, Gorson KC. Neuropathies associated with paraproteinemia. *N Engl J Med* 1998; **338**; 1601–7, with permission of the publisher.

[b] CIDP, chronic inflammatory demyelinating polyneuropathy; GBS, Guillain–Barré syndrome; MND, motor neuron disease.

[c] CHF, congestive heart failure; HSM, hepatosplenomegaly.

[d] XRT, radiation therapy; PE, plasma exchange; IFN-α, interferon-α; IVIG, intravenous immunoglobulin.

small fiber) and the pathologic nature of the process (axonal degeneration, segmental demyelination, or both). Disorders of large, myelinated sensory nerve fibers reduce joint position, touch, pressure, and vibration sensations. The typical symptoms in these disorders are numbness or 'deadness', 'pins and needles' tingling, and loss of balance. In the context of peripheral nerve disease, Romberg's sign and sensory ataxia also reflect reduced proprioceptive sense from the lower limbs. The deep tendon reflexes are diminished or absent owing to loss of large heavily myelinated Ia sensory fibers that originate in muscle spindles and constitute the afferent portion of the monosynaptic reflex arc. In contrast, spontaneous burning, stinging and stabbing pain (so-called 'neuropathic pain'), and reduced pinprick and temperature sensation indicate a disorder of small, unmyelinated and thinly myelinated sensory nerve fibers. The predominant motor symptoms and signs in all cases are muscle weakness, atrophy, cramps and fasciculations.

Peripheral nerves have a limited response to injury. The main classification separates neuropathies into disorders that affect the axon (axonal degeneration or axonopathy) and those that affect the myelin (myelinopathy), although frequently these processes coexist. Axonal degeneration is most typical of a metabolic or toxic disorder (diabetes, vitamin deficiency, hypothyroidism, medications) or a systemic illness (malignancy, connective tissue disease, vasculitis). There is a length-dependent disturbance that first affects the distal elements of the nerve fiber, and these disorders therefore manifest clinically as numbness, paresthesias, and pain beginning in the toes and feet and spreading in time in a distal-to-proximal gradient, a so-called 'glove and stocking' pattern. Most axonal sensory and sensorimotor neuropathies are symmetric polyneuropathies and have a distal predominance of signs and symptoms. As the condition advances and the symptoms approach the knee, the fingertips and hands become involved with the same symptoms. Often there is atrophy and weakness of the foot and hand muscles and absent Achilles tendon reflexes, reflecting the distal predominance in axonal diseases. In contrast, multiple mononeuropathies (mononeuritis multiplex) are characterized by a prominent asymmetry or a multifocal pattern, and are usually the result of nerve compression or ischemia (e.g., vasculitis).

Segmental demyelination signifies damage to the myelin sheaths with sparing of the axon fiber; it usually occurs in a more heterogeneous pattern throughout the nerve. The clinical features reflect the cumulative affect of multiple areas of demyelination along each nerve trunk. In distinction to most axonal neuropathies, proximal weakness and early involvement of the arms are common features, and muscle atrophy is absent. Most patients have a large-fiber type of sensory loss (position, vibration, touch senses) and generalized areflexia. Acquired demyelinating neuropathies are frequently immune-mediated and may be further classified according to the tempo of the illness. Guillain–Barré syndrome, for example, is an acute, inflammatory, demyelinating polyneuropathy characterized by rapidly progressive generalized weakness, large-fiber sensory loss, and areflexia, often with dysautonomia and ventilatory failure. Patients with similar clinical, electrodiagnostic and histopathologic features but in whom the course is more indolent or relapsing are considered to have 'chronic inflammatory demyelinating polyneuropathy' (CIDP).[23] These clinical patterns (Table 12.1) are often adequate to determine the fundamental nature of the pathologic process, but confusion easily occurs because in many cases axonal neuropathies affecting large nerve fibers cannot be distinguished from demyelinating diseases (the latter also affecting large nerve fibers), and the accumulation of multiple mononeuropathies emulates a polyneuropathy. Most importantly, as most neuropathies advance, axonal and demyelinating features become evident.

Nerve conduction studies and electromyography (EMG) are invaluable extensions of the clinical examination that allow more accurate distinctions to be made among the types of neuropathies. In particular, electrophysiologic evidence of primary demyelination, even if there is associated axonal degeneration, allows the illness to be classified within the demyelinating neuropathies, and thus limits the diagnostic possibilities. There is also a typical EMG pattern of mononeuritis multiplex. This chapter focuses primarily on the clinical manifestations and treatment of neuropathies associated with plasma cell disorders, most of which are immune-mediated.

MYELOMA

The peripheral nervous system complications of myeloma include cauda equina root compression as a result of lytic bone lesions of the spine, myelomatous infiltration of spinal roots, and a polyneuropathy.[26,27] The prevalence of neuropathy in myeloma is low, affecting 3–5% of patients in retrospective studies based on clinical criteria, but in prospective studies the frequency has been as high as 40–60%, especially if electrophysiological tests (nerve conduction studies and EMG) are used for the detection of peripheral nerve disease.[28–30] Neuropathy is a late complication in most myeloma patients; however, it may rarely be the presenting feature, and in both cases represents a remote effect of the malignancy.[3]

There are several types of myeloma neuropathy. The most common is a mild, distal sensorimotor polyneuropathy that reflects the severity and duration of the myeloma. These patients usually have advanced disease, with weight loss, bone pain, fatigue, anemia, renal insufficiency, or hypercalcemia. Acral pain and paresthesias are prominent, and distal, symmetric sensory loss, absent Achilles tendon reflexes, and minimal weakness are characteristic. Nerve conduction studies indicate an axonal process with reduced or absent sural nerve sensory action potentials, reduced motor amplitudes, mild slowing of conduction velocities, and denervation in distal muscles. Sural nerve biopsy specimens show axonal degeneration with secondary segmental demyelination, and a minority of patients have superimposed amyloid deposits.[3,31,32] The mechanism of the neuropathy is unknown, and may be related to the paraprotein, weight loss, or other metabolic or toxic factors associated with the malignancy.[27,31] The polyneuropathy is static or slowly progressive, and usually does not respond to chemotherapy for myeloma.

Rarely, myeloma produces mononeuritis multiplex or a pure sensory neuropathy or ganglionopathy, the latter with substantial sensory loss and ataxia. Other infrequent cases have displayed a predominantly motor, demyelinating polyneuropathy that is indistinguishable from Guillain–Barré syndrome or from CIDP.[27,32] The course of the pure sensory neuropathy and motor demyelinating neuropathy are independent of the malignancy, and may improve with the standard therapies for immune-mediated neuropathies that are discussed further on.

OSTEOSCLEROTIC MYELOMA (OSM) AND THE POEMS SYNDROME

This is a rare plasma cell disorder characterized by a plasmacytoma, usually in one or more sclerotic bone lesions, polyneuropathy, and monoclonal protein. Although OSM comprises only 3–5% of myeloma cases, its importance lies with the high frequency of polyneuropathy (85%) as the presenting feature.[33] These patients tend to be younger than others with myeloma, and have a more indolent course. OSM causes a chronic, slowly progressive, sensorimotor demyelinating polyneuropathy sharing many features with CIDP, except that spontaneous remissions do not occur.[34] Paresthesias in the legs are often the initial symptoms, followed by sensory loss and then weakness that usually begins distally and gradually spreads to involve proximal muscles. Severe weakness occurs in more than one-half of cases and patients may become bed- or wheelchair-bound. Autonomic symptoms and pain are uncommon. There is symmetric proximal and distal weakness, atrophy, areflexia, and prominent large-fiber sensory loss (touch, vibration, and joint position). Temperature and pain sensation are reduced to a lesser degree. The cranial nerves are rarely affected, except for the occasional finding of papilledema, which is unexplained.

Electrodiagnostic studies show moderate or marked slowing of conduction velocities, temporal dispersion of the compound muscle action potential (CMAP) waveform, and prolonged distal latencies, denoting a demyelinating neuropathy. Axonal loss is also common, and most patients have reduced CMAP amplitudes and fibrillation potentials in distal muscles, indicating denervation. A neuropathy with purely axonal features occurs rarely.[35] One helpful distinguishing feature of this neuropathy is an almost invariable elevation of the cerebrospinal fluid protein concentration, often to greater than 0.1 g/dl. The sural nerve sampled by a biopsy typically shows features of mixed axonal degeneration and demyelination, with little or no inflammatory infiltration.[34,36,37] Electron microscopy demonstrates numerous axons wrapped in spirals of Schwann cell cytoplasm with increased myelin periodicity, so-called 'uncompacted' myelin.[19,37] This finding, even in the absence of a circulating paraprotein, strongly suggests OSM, and is found in over half of cases.[37] Immunolabeling techniques have shown deposition of the monoclonal protein in the endoneurium and on the myelin sheath, indicating that the paraprotein probably has a direct role in generating the neuropathy.[19, 38–39]

The M protein, usually an IgA or IgG, is found in the serum in 75–90% of cases and rarely in the urine. In contrast to ordinary myeloma, however, the concentration of the paraprotein is small (usually <2 g/dl) and may not be detected unless immunofixation is performed. The light chain is virtually always of the λ subtype.[34]

Plasmacytomas, sclerotic in over two-thirds of cases and mixed lytic and sclerotic in the remainder, occur in the pelvis, ribs, proximal long bones or axial skeleton, usually sparing the skull and distal extremities, and are multiple in 50%.[33,36,40] A skeletal bone survey is more sensitive than radionuclide bone scanning in detecting these bone lesions, and a biopsy of the bone lesion demonstrating monoclonal plasma cells establishes the diagnosis of OSM.[7,9,34] The sclerotic lesions can simulate the radiographic changes of degenerative joint disease in the elderly, especially when found in the lumbar spine, and thus a low threshold for bone biopsy is appropriate in elderly patients with monoclonal gammopathy and a chronic, progressive demyelinating polyneuropathy.

Patients with OSM have a variable constellation of systemic features that has been referred to as the POEMS syndrome (polyneuropathy, organomegaly, endocrinopathy, M spike, skin changes).[2,40–42] Although considered a distinct entity, it has been indicated that the differences between POEMS and OSM are largely artificial.[42] It is also noteworthy that adenopathy from angiofollicular lymph node hyperplasia (Castleman's disease) occurs in 60% of cases (Figure 12.1).[33,36] Furthermore, few patients with OSM and neuropathy have all the features of the POEMS syndrome; approximately 50% have hepatosplenomegaly or lymphadenopathy, and 80% have thrombocytosis.[33,36,40,42] The endocrine abnormalities may include diabetes, gynecomastia, and hypogonadism, and occur in approximately one-half of cases. Patients frequently have distal limb edema, hypertrichosis, hyperpigmentation, hemangiomas, or diffuse thickening of the skin.

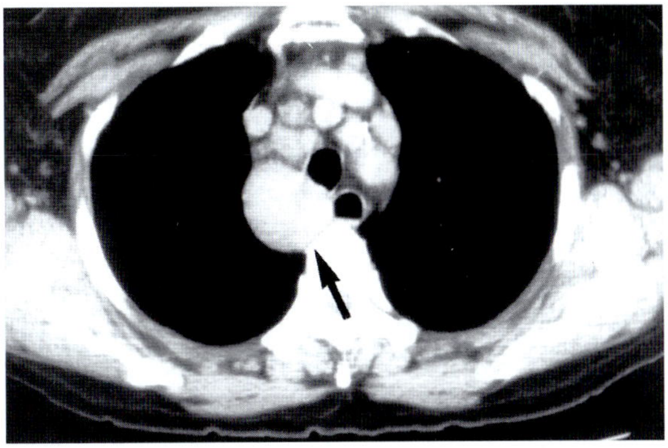

Figure 12.1 A 49-year-old patient with 2.2 g/dl of IgGλ monoclonal protein and progressive generalized weakness, areflexia, and ataxia. EMG showed a demyelinating sensorimotor polyneuropathy. Chest computed tomography scan demonstrated mediastinal adenopathy (arrow). Lymph node biopsy showed angiofollicular lymph node hyperplasia (Castleman's disease).

The cause of the neuropathy and the other systemic features of OSM are unknown. It may be that the circulating paraprotein contains a substance that is toxic to peripheral nerves and produces the widespread systemic abnormalities in some patients.[27] For example, it has been postulated that the neuropathy is a remote effect of circulating proinflammatory cytokines, such as tumor necrosis factor and interleukin-6, which are greatly elevated in some of these patients.[43,44]

Therapy for OSM includes surgical resection of an isolated plasmacytoma and radiation therapy for multiple lesions located in a limited region, thus emphasizing the need to obtain tissue samples from single bone lesions.[27,34] Patients with widespread sclerotic lesions require chemotherapy, usually prednisone and melphalan administered in six-week cycles.[45] Combining modalities may be beneficial in some patients.[46] Half the patients show substantial improvement of the neuropathy, but the response may not be evident for six months or more.[27,34] Prednisone alone, azathioprine, and plasma exchange are relatively ineffective.[41,42,47,48] Interferon (IFN-α2a, 3 MIU daily) has been beneficial in a few patients with neuropathy who were refractory to other therapies.[49,50]

WALDENSTRÖM'S MACROGLOBULINEMIA

Peripheral neuropathy occurs in up to 40% of patients with Waldenström's macroglobulinemia (WM).[51,52] It is chronic, slowly progressive, and symmetric, and shares many of the clinical features of the neuropathy in patients with IgM-MGUS neuropathy (see below).[53] Most patients have large-fiber sensory loss, primarily in the lower limbs, paresthesias, ataxia, mild or moderate distal weakness, and generalized hypo- or areflexia. Other patients have a pure sensory or pure motor neuropathy, typical amyloid neuropathy (see below) or mononeuritis multiplex associated with cryoglobulinemia and vasculitis.[54,55] The EMG shows a demyelinating polyneuropathy with varying degrees of axonal loss. Immunofluorescence studies of sural nerve biopsies demonstrate immunoglobulin deposition on myelin sheaths, and indicate that the monoclonal protein probably has a central role in the pathogenesis of the neuropathy.[19,56–58]

Improvement in the neuropathy has been reported following treatment with plasma exchange, chlorambucil, or prednisone.[56,59] Remission was reported in one patient who was treated with high-dose melphalan followed by autologous stem cell transplant.[60]

AMYLOIDOSIS

Amyloid is an amorphous, hyaline-like fibrillary protein with a β-sheet structure composed of non-branching filaments, and is characterized by pink staining with routine hematoxylin and eosin and apple-green birefringence when stained with Congo red and viewed under polarized light.

A neuropathy occurs in approximately 15–20% of patients with primary systemic amyloidosis and is the presenting feature in 15% of these cases.[61–63] There is an M spike in the serum or urine in 90% of patients, usually IgG, IgA, or a λ light chain alone, and the disorder may complicate multiple myeloma or Waldenström's macroglobulinemia. Amyloidosis afflicts older individuals (median age > 60 years) and is twice as common in men than women. Burning, aching, and lancinating pain over the soles of the feet are prominent symptoms, with relative sparing of large-fiber proprioceptive sensation and strength, at least early in the course. The small-diameter sensory fibers are most affected, typically causing loss of pain and temperature sensation in the acral extremities. Sensory loss tends to be distal, greater in the legs than the arms, and symmetric.[64] Paresthesias and numbness frequently accompany painful sensory symptoms, and weakness develops as the disease progresses. Carpal tunnel syndrome is common due to amyloid infiltration of the flexor retinaculum, and is the initial feature of the neuropathy in 25% of patients. Autonomic symptoms occur in 65% and can dominate the clinical picture, particularly postural hypotension with recurrent syncope, diarrhea, impotence, and bladder dysfunction, and any of these may eclipse the sensory manifestations.[64,65] The neuropathy also may be overshadowed by symptoms of amyloid deposition in other organs, most commonly congestive heart failure with cardiac conduction abnormalities and renal insufficiency with nephrotic syndrome. Occasionally, amyloid deposits occur in proximal muscles and cause a myopathy.[66]

EMG studies demonstrate a symmetric, distal sensory or sensorimotor axonal neuropathy. CMAP amplitudes are low or absent, but conduction velocities and distal latencies are normal or near-normal. Sensory nerve action potentials are usually absent. Needle EMG shows acute and chronic denervation in distal muscles.[64,65] Autonomic tests demonstrate severe adrenergic, sudomotor, and cardiovagal impairment. Nerve biopsy shows axonal degeneration, with predominant involvement of small myelinated and unmyelinated fibers; in advanced cases, the large-fiber population is also depleted. Amyloid deposition occurs in the epineurium, perineurium, and endoneurium and around blood vessel walls (Figure 12.2). Nerve biopsy and immunostaining with antisera to κ and λ light chains is crucial in establishing the diagnosis in the minority of patients (approximately 10%) without a detectable paraprotein in whom clinical suspicion for amyloid neuropathy is high.[19] The diagnosis is established by demonstrating amyloid in bone marrow (50%), abdominal fat pad (70%), rectal biopsy (80%), or sural nerve biopsy (85%).[61,62,64,67]

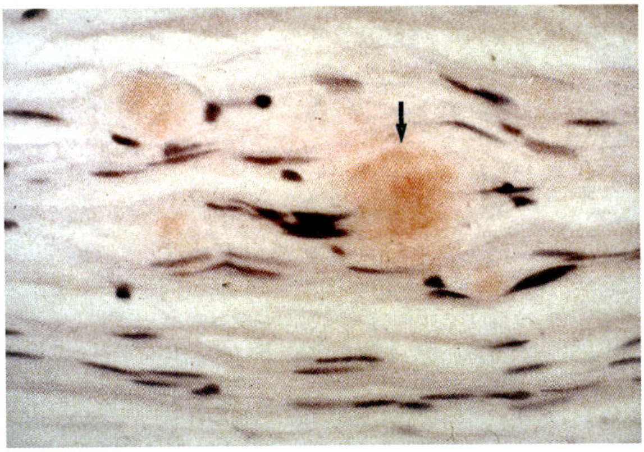

Figure 12.2 Sural nerve biopsy of a 62-year-old man who complained of burning feet and acral sensory loss and had a monoclonal λ light chain. The pink-staining material (arrow) is amyloid deposited in the endoneurium. (H & E stain, 10×.)

The prognosis for these patients is poor, with death occurring generally one to three years after the diagnosis. A recent review of 26 patients in whom neuropathy was the dominant manifestation indicated that the median survival was only 25 months from the time of diagnosis. However, their survival was still better than that of patients who had renal involvement (median 17 months) or cardiac involvement (median 10 months).[65] A serum albumin level of less than 3 g/dl was a negative prognostic factor in neuropathy patients. Melphalan combined with prednisone administered daily for seven days every six weeks prolonged survival in a small proportion of patients, but there was little effect on the neuropathy.[65,68] Pulse dexamethasone for three to six cycles followed by IFN-α showed promise in a small study.[69] A few reports have documented short-term remission in several patients treated with high-dose intravenous melphalan followed by autologous blood stem cell rescue or bone marrow transplant. The durability of remission remains uncertain, but a few patients have survived for considerable periods.[70–72] The effect on the neuropathy with these therapies is unknown.

CRYOGLOBULINEMIA

Neuropathy has a prevalence ranging from 8% to 82% in patients with cryoglobulinemia, and rarely may be the sole manifestation of the disorder.[73–74] In mixed essential cryoglobulinemia, neuropathy is the presenting feature of the disease in 12–19% of patients.[73–74] The neuropathy is almost always painful, and may be generalized, focal, or multifocal. Approximately one-third of cases have mononeuritis multiplex, but more commonly there is a pattern of a subacute or chronic, generalized and symmetric, distal sensorimotor polyneuropathy that cannot be easily appreciated as the confluence of multiple mononeuropathies caused by vasculitic nerve infarction. In patients with the generalized sensorimotor pattern, the legs are more affected than the arms, and there is sensory loss, moderate distal leg weakness with atrophy, and absent ankle jerks. Pure or predominantly sensory neuropathies and a CIDP-like illness also have been described.[73,75–77] Cranial nerve involvement and autonomic dysfunction are rare. There is no evident relationship between the amount of the cryoglobulin and the severity of the neuropathy. Hepatitis C antibodies are found in the majority of patients with cryoglobulinemic neuropathy.[78]

The EMG typically shows an axonal pattern, which may be symmetric or multifocal, with absent sensory potentials, low motor amplitudes, and normal conduction velocities. A minority of cases have demyelinating features.[73,75,76] Nerve biopsy shows necrotizing vasculitis in epineurial vessels, perivascular inflammatory cells, or micro-occlusion of the vasa nervorum by intravascular deposits of cryoglobulins.[19,75,77,79–80] Axonal loss is usually evident, often with selective depletion of large myelinated fibers in a multifocal pattern, a finding indicative of vasculitis even in the absence of vessel wall changes. The different histopathologic findings may reflect various stages of the disease process rather than distinct pathological processes.[78]

Plasma exchange, corticosteroids, and cytotoxic agents have been used with some success in stabilizing or reversing the neuropathy. IFN-α may be beneficial for cryoglobulinemic neuropathy associated with hepatitis C.[75,77,78,81]

MONOCLONAL GAMMOPATHY OF UNDETERMINED SIGNIFICANCE AND ANTI-MAG ANTIBODIES

In approximately two-thirds of patients with a monoclonal protein there is no associated systemic disorder. Although a monoclonal IgG is the most frequent immunoglobulin in patients with MGUS, IgM is more common in those with neuropathy (60%), followed by IgG (30%) and IgA (10%), and the light chain is predominantly a κ type.[6,82,83]

The neuropathy associated with MGUS occurs predominantly in men. The onset is insidious, and symptoms advance slowly after months or years. Approximately 20% have a relapsing course. Sensory features dominate, and include distal leg numbness, paresthesias, imbalance, and gait ataxia.[6–10,23,82–85] Wasting and weakness of leg muscles occurs as the disorder progresses, although these are not prominent or obligate findings, but patients rarely have a pure motor disorder simulating motor neuron disease.[86,87] The majority have generalized areflexia, but reflex abnormalities may be restricted to the legs. The arms are seldom if ever affected in isolation, and the cranial nerves are usually spared. Upper-extremity tremor occurs in 10% of cases, typically in the variety associated with anti-myelin-associated glycoprotein antibodies (see below).[23,82–85]

Electrodiagnostic studies demonstrate mixed features of demyelination and axonal degeneration. Many patients with MGUS also fulfill the EMG criteria for CIDP, with slowed motor nerve conduction velocities (approximately 40% of patients) and prolonged motor distal latencies and F responses, although conduction block, the electrophysiologic hallmark of CIDP, is less commonly observed.[7,9–10,23,82–85] Sensory potentials are reduced or absent. The needle-electrode examination shows fibrillation potentials in distal limb muscles. A few patients have a predominantly axonal neuropathy.[24,88] The spinal fluid protein concentration is mildly elevated in most cases, but a wide range of cerebrospinal fluid protein occurs. Pathologic studies show demyelinating changes that are especially prominent in patients with IgM-MGUS, active axonal degeneration, and loss of large myelinated fibers. Inflammatory cell infiltrates composed of lymphocytes and macrophages are common. Immunofluorescence staining shows deposits of immunoglobulin on myelin sheaths or axons in approximately one-third of nerve biopsies in patients with IgG/IgA-MGUS and up to 80% of patients with IgM-MGUS.[17,19,83,89,90]

The relationship between the neuropathy that is associated with MGUS and the condition known as idiopathic CIDP is controversial, and in some patients the clinical and electrophysiological abnormalities are indistinguishable. Indeed, as many as one-quarter of CIDP cases occur in the context of a paraproteinemia.[6,23,84,85] Several studies have compared patients with idiopathic CIDP with patients with CIDP–MGUS and have demonstrated subtle differences.[23,84,85] For example, CIDP–MGUS patients tend to be older, with a more indolent, progressive course, have less severe weakness and functional impairment but greater sensory loss, more often have abnormal sensory conduction studies, and may be less responsive to immunotherapy.[23,84,85]

Several studies have indicated a relationship between the class of the monoclonal protein (IgM, IgG, or IgA) and the clinical and EMG characteristics of the neuropathy.[24,82,91] It can be said that IgM neuropathy produces greater sensory loss, ataxia, and tremor, more severe demyelinating findings on EMG, and is less responsive to immune therapy,[24,25,82,91,92] but none of these attributes has been entirely dependable, and some studies have failed to demonstrate such differences.[25,83,84]

Approximately one-half of patients with IgM neuropathy have an illness that is associated with antibodies against a specific myelin-associated glycoprotein (anti-MAG) or one of its sulfated glycolipid derivatives (SGPG, SGLPG) that are found in the periaxonal membrane of the Schwann cell (Figure 12.3).[5,15,17,18,25,82,93–95] The neuropathy is slowly progressive, and is

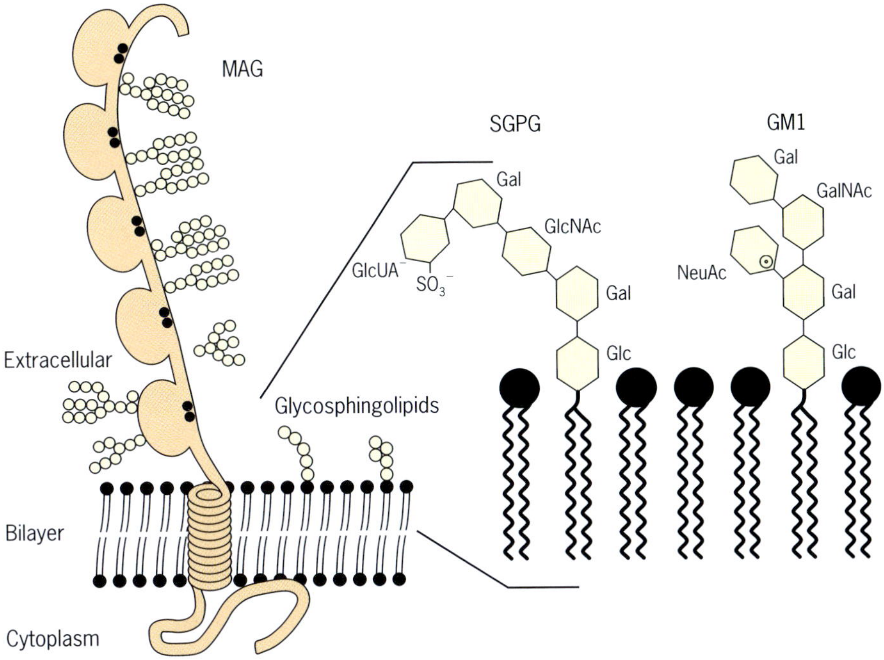

Figure 12.3 Structure of myelin-associated glycoprotein (MAG), sulfated glycolipids (SGPG), and ganglioside antigens (GM1) on peripheral nerves that have been implicated in certain neuropathies associated with monoclonal gammopathy. MAG is shown with its five extracellular immunoglobulin domains, a transmembrane domain, and a cytoplasmic component. Gal, galactose; GlcNAc, *N*-acetylglucosamine; Glc, glucose; GlcUA, glucuronic acid; GalNAc, *N*-acetylgalactosamine; NeuAc, *N*-acetylneuraminic acid. Adapted from Ropper AH, Gorson KC. Neuropathies associated with paraproteinemia. *N Engl J Med* 1998; **338**: 1601–7, with permission of the publisher. Copyright © 1998 Massachusetts Medical Society. All rights reserved.

characterized by distal numbness, paresthesias, impaired joint position, and Romberg sign.[9,15–17,93–95] Gait ataxia, generalized areflexia, and tremor are also frequent findings. The cranial nerves are spared and autonomic involvement is rare. Distal limb weakness occurs in the majority of cases (65%), and seldom surpasses the sensory features.[15,17,94] The neuropathy usually occurs in the context of IgM-MGUS; however, one quarter of patients with anti-MAG antibodies have Waldenström's macroglobulinemia, and a few have lymphoma, chronic lymphocytic leukemia, or cryoglobulinemia.[15] The monoclonal protein is an IgMκ in the majority of the cases. Rarely there may be high anti-MAG antibodies in the absence of a monoclonal gammopathy or the M spike is detected later.[96,97] Electrodiagnostic studies show demyelinating features in approximately 75% of patients, frequently accompanied by axonal degeneration.[15,17,25,82,83,91] Disproportionately prolonged distal motor latencies are a characteristic electrodiagnostic feature, and, in contrast to CIDP, conduction block occurs infrequently.[98,99] Nerve biopsy shows demyelination with widely spaced myelin, a distinctive finding that results from a lack of apposition of the outer layers of the Schwann cell membrane (Figure 12.4).[83, 89] Immunocytochemical staining shows deposition of IgM and complement on myelin sheaths in periaxonal regions of nerve fibers. Despite these observations, several studies have indicated that patients with anti-MAG antibodies cannot be reliably distinguished from those with IgM-MGUS lacking these antibodies.[25,82,84,91]

The EMG demonstrates features of an axonal neuropathy in a minority of patients, usually with IgG-MGUS.[24,88,100] In this group, the relationship between the paraprotein and the neuropathy is not clear and may be coincidental, particularly in an older patient with an 'idiopathic' neuropathy.[24,100] However, in a few cases, there are IgM or IgG antibodies directed against antigens on the nerve axon, such as sulfatide or chondroitin sulfate C, and some improve with immunotherapy.[24,101–106]

The optimal therapy for the neuropathy associated with MGUS has not been established. One-third or more of patients with IgG and IgA-MGUS respond to intravenous immuno globulin (IVIG) (2 g/kg administered over two to five days), plasma exchange, (200 ml/kg in four or five exchanges), corticosteroids or cytotoxic agents.[5,9,22–24,82,84–85,88,107,108] The efficacy of plasma exchange has been confirmed in a randomized, controlled study.[92] It must be recognized that these treatments usually provide only temporary stability or improvement and need to be repeated periodically.

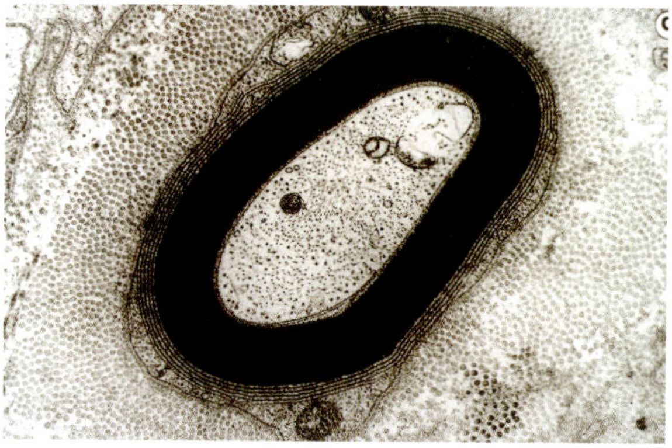

Figure 12.4 Electron micrograph of a sural nerve biopsy specimen from a patient with a demyelinating neuropathy, IgM-MGUS, and raised anti-MAG antibodies. There is separation of the outer myelin layer due to deposition of IgM immunoglobulin (× 25 000). Reproduced from Ropper AH, Gorson KC. Neuropathies associated with paraproteinemia. *N Engl J Med* 1998; **338**: 1601–7, with permission of the publisher. Copyright © 1998 Massachusetts Medical Society. All rights reserved.

The IgM neuropathies are frequently refractory to immunomodulatory therapy. Plasma exchange and pulse corticosteroids combined with cyclophosphamide or chlorambucil have been effective in some patients.[20–22,109] IVIG is beneficial in only a small minority of cases.[110] Patients with neuropathy associated with IgM-MGUS and anti-MAG antibodies also tend to be resistant to treatment.[111] Therapeutic reduction of antibody concentrations has been associated with clinical improvement in some, but there is no consistent relationship between the antibody titer and the severity of the neuropathy.[111] A number of immunosuppressive regimens have been advocated, but large, well-controlled trials have not been performed.

Monthly plasma exchanges followed by pulse intravenous cyclophosphamide have reversed the deficits in some, and may delay progression.[5,22,25,111,112] Corticosteroids alone are not effective.

ANTI-GM1 ANTIBODY AND MULTIFOCAL MOTOR NEUROPATHY

Multifocal motor neuropathy (MMN) manifests as slowly progressive, painless, asymmetric weakness, usually beginning in the arms, minimal or no atrophy early in the course, and normal or reduced reflexes, all without sensory findings. This condition may mimic amyotrophic lateral sclerosis, and can be distinguished clinically by the lack of upper motor neuron signs (Babinski signs, hyperreflexia, spasticity), oropharyngeal weakness and progressive ventilatory failure. This condition is frequently associated with high titers of antibodies directed at a particular ganglioside epitope (GM1) on the axonal membrane (see Figure 12.3). In 20% of patients, the anti-GM1 antibody is contained in an IgM monoclonal protein.[113–115] The presence of focal areas of electrical conduction block of the motor nerves is the distinctive finding on EMG studies, and additional electrophysiologic features of a demyelinating motor neuropathy also are common.[116,117] In contrast to other demyelinating neuropathies that have been linked to MGUS, the sensory nerve action potentials are invariably normal. The anti-GM1 antibody has been detected in as many as 70% of patients, but its role in producing multifocal motor neuropathy is still somewhat uncertain. Pathologic studies have demonstrated antibody binding at nodes of Ranvier, and this observation may partially explain the electrophysiologic abnormalities.[118–120] IVIG is an effective treatment in as many as 90% of patients, but most relapse, and repeated infusions are necessary.[121–123] Cyclophosphamide is beneficial in patients who relapse or fail to improve with IVIG.[113,114,116,124]

APPROACH TO THE PATIENT WITH NEUROPATHY AND MONOCLONAL GAMMOPATHY (Figure 12.5)

The diagnostic evaluation of a patient with idiopathic neuropathy should include both serum and urine immunoelectrophoresis and immunofixation. The detection of a monoclonal protein warrants investigation for a malignant plasma cell dyscrasia before concluding that the M spike is related to MGUS; an M protein greater than 3 g/dl is usually associated with a plasma cell disorder, whereas a level less than 1.5 g/dl is more often observed in patients who have MGUS. The serum should be evaluated for the presence of cryoglobulins and β_2-microglobulin, and serum viscosity should be measured when over 3 g/dl of IgM monoclonal protein is detected. A bone scan and bone marrow biopsy are necessary in patients who have over 3 g/l of monoclonal protein and systemic features suggesting myeloma. A skeletal bone survey is required in most cases to exclude bone lesions associated with osteosclerotic myeloma and the POEMS syndrome, especially if there is an IgG or IgA monoclonal protein, λ light chain and demyelinating neuropathy. Suspicious sclerotic lesions should be biopsied. Chest and abdominal CT scanning is useful in patients suspected of having lymphoma or the POEMS syndrome associated with Castleman's disease.

Electrodiagnostic testing is essential to classify the neuropathy. Axonal neuropathies are most commonly encountered in patients with myeloma, amyloidosis, IgG-MGUS, and cryoglobulinemic neuropathy. In contrast, a demyelinating neuropathy is most often associated with osteosclerotic myeloma, Waldenström's macroglobulinemia, IgM and IgG/A-MGUS, and Castleman's disease. Patients who have IgM paraproteinemia and a demyelinating neuropathy should be tested for anti-MAG antibodies. A sural nerve biopsy is generally advisable when vasculitis, amyloid, or neoplastic infiltration is considered or when immunofluorescence studies are indicated.

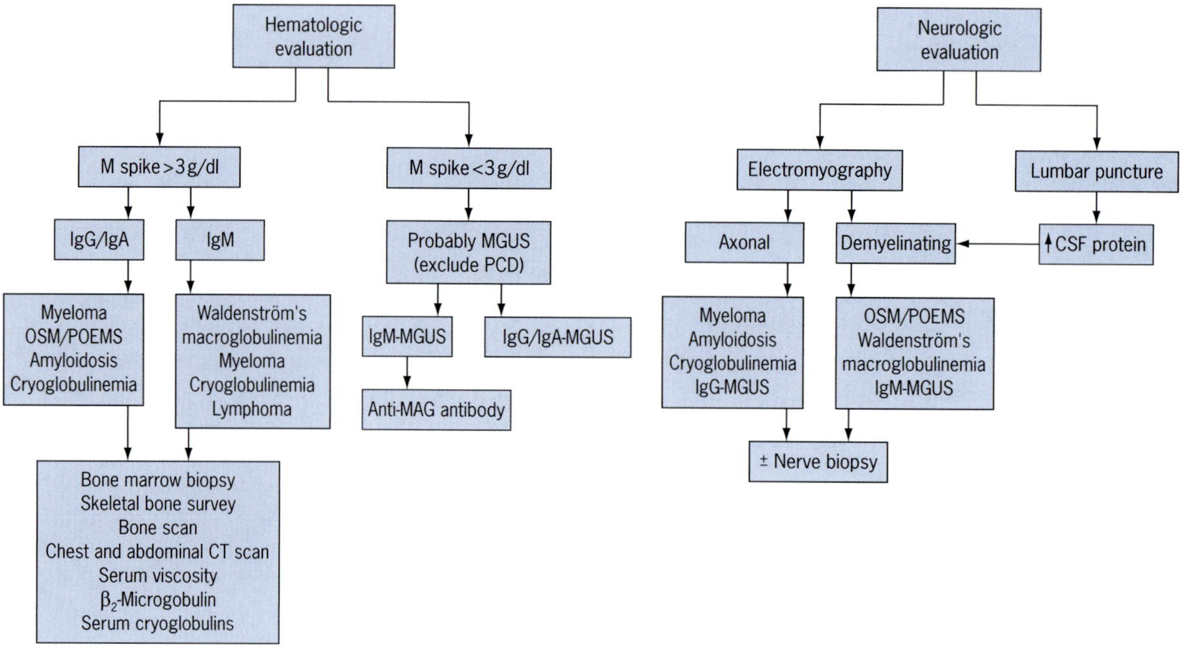

Figure 12.5 Diagnostic approach to a patient with a plasma cell disorder and neuropathy. MGUS, monoclonal gammopathy of undetermined significance; PCD, plasma cell dyscrasia; OSM, osteosclerotic myeloma; CSF, cerebrospinal fluid.

ACKNOWLEDGEMENTS

We thank Dr Jean M Jacobs, Senior Lecturer in Neuropathology, National Hospital, Queen Square, England for Figure 12.3, and Richard H Quarles of the Laboratory of Molecular and Cellular Neurobiology, National Institute of Neurological Disorders and Stroke, for assistance with Figure 12.4.

REFERENCES

1. Davison C, Balser BH. Myeloma and its neural complications. *Arch Surg* 1937; **35**: 913–36.
2. Crow RS. Peripheral neuritis in myelomatosis. *BMJ* 1956: **ii**: 802–4.
3. Victor M, Banker BQ, Adams RD. The neuropathy of multiple myeloma. *J Neurol Neurosurg Psychiatry* 1958; **21**: 73–88.
4. Kelly JJ Jr, Kyle RA, O'Brien PC, Dyck PJ. Prevalence of monoclonal protein in peripheral neuropathy. *Neurology* 1981; **31**: 1480–3.
5. Ropper AH, Gorson KC. Neuropathies associated with paraproteinemia. *N Engl J Med* 1998; **338**: 1601–7.
6. Kyle RA. Dyck PJ. Neuropathy associated with monoclonal gammopathies. In: *Peripheral Neuropathy*, 3rd edn (Dyck PJ, Thomas PK, Griffin JW et al, eds). Philadelphia: WB Saunders, 1993: 1275–87.
7. Kelly JJ Jr. Peripheral neuropathies associated with monoclonal proteins: a clinical review. *Muscle Nerve* 1985; **8**: 138–50.
8. Bosch EP, Smith BE. Peripheral neuropathies associated with monoclonal proteins. *Med Clin North Am* 1993; **77**: 125–39.
9. Kissel JT, Mendell JR. Neuropathies associated with monoclonal gammopathies. *Neuromusc Disord* 1995; **6**: 3–18.
10. Kyle RA. Monoclonal proteins in neuropathy. *Neurol Clin* 1992; **10**: 713–34.
11. Vrethem M, Cruz M, Wen-Xin Huang et al. Clinical, neurophysiological, and immunological evidence of polyneuropathy in patients with monoclonal gammopathies. *J Neurol Sci* 1993; **114**: 193–9.

12. Hays AP, Latov N, Takatsu M, Sherman WH. Experimental demyelination of nerve induced by serum of patients with neuropathy and an anti-MAG IgM M-protein. *Neurology* 1987; **37**: 242–56.
13. Tatum AH. Experimental paraprotein neuropathy; demyelination by passive transfer of human IgM anti-myelin-associated glycoprotein. *Ann Neurol* 1993; **33**: 502–6.
14. Trojaborg W, Gallassi G, Hays AP et al. Electrophysiologic study of experimental demyelination induced by serum of patients with IgM M protein and neuropathy. *Neurology* 1989; **39**: 1581–6.
15. Latov N, Hays AP, Sherman WH. Peripheral neuropathy and anti-MAG antibodies. *CRC Crit Rev Neurobiol* 1988; **3**: 301–32.
16. Nobile-Orazio E, Manfredini E, Carpo M et al. Frequency and clinical correlates of anti-neural IgM antibodies in neuropathy associated with IgM monoclonal gammopathy. *Ann Neurol* 1994; **36**: 416–24.
17. Ellie E, Vital A, Steck A et al. Neuropathy associated with 'benign' anti-myelin-associated glycoprotein IgM gammopathy: clinical, immunological, neurophysiological, pathological findings and response to treatment in 33 cases. *J Neurol* 1996; **243**: 34–43.
18. Monaco S, Bonetti B, Ferrari S et al. Complement-mediated demyelination in patients with IgM monoclonal gammopathy and polyneuropathy. *N Engl J Med* 1990; **322**: 649–52.
19. Midroni G, Bilbao JM (eds). *Biopsy Diagnosis of Peripheral Neuropathy*. Boston: Butterworth-Heinemann, 1995.
20. Oksenhendler E, Chrevet S, Leger JM et al. Plasma exchange and chlorambucil in polyneuropathy associated with monoclonal IgM gammopathy. *J Neurol Neurosurg Psychiatry* 1995; **59**: 243–7.
21. Sherman WH, Olarte MR, McKiernan G et al. Plasma exchange treatment of peripheral neuropathy associated with plasma cell dyscrasia. *J Neurol Neurosurg Psychiatry* 1984; **47**: 813–19.
22. Notermans NC, Lokhorst HM, Franssen H et al. Intermittent cyclophosphamide and prednisone treatment of polyneuropathy associated with monoclonal gammopathy of undetermined significance. *Neurology* 1996; **47**: 1227–33.
23. Gorson KC, Allam G, Ropper AH. Chronic inflammatory demyelinating polyneuropathy: Clinical features and response to treatment in 67 consecutive patients with and without monoclonal gammopathy. *Neurology* 1997; **48**: 321–8.
24. Gorson KC, Ropper AH. Axonal neuropathies associated with monoclonal gammopathy of uncertain significance. *J Neurol Neurosurg Psychiatry* 1997; **63**: 163–8.
25. Simovic D, Gorson KC, Ropper AH. Comparison of IgM-MGUS and IgG-MGUS neuropathy. *Acta Neurol Scand* 1998; **97**: 194–200.
26. Barron KD, Rowland LP, Zimmerman HM. Neuropathy with malignant tumor metastasis. *J Nervous Ment Dis* 1960; **131**: 10–31.
27. Kelly JJ Jr. Polyneuropathies associated with myeloma, POEMS, and non-malignant IgG and IgA monoclonal gammopathies. In: *Immunological and Infectious Diseases of the Peripheral Nerves* (Latov N, Wokke JHJ, Kelly JJ Jr, eds). Cambridge: Cambridge University Press, 1998: 225–37.
28. Silverstein A, Doniger DE. Neurologic complications of myelomatosis. *Arch Neurol* 1963; **9**: 534–44.
29. Hesselvik M. Neuropathological studies on myelomatosis. *Acta Neurol* Scand 1969; **45**: 95–108.
30. Walsh JC. The neuropathy of multiple myeloma. *Arch Neurol* 1971; **25**: 404–14.
31. Ohi T, Kyle RA, Dyck PJ. Axonal attenuation and secondary segmental demyelination in myeloma neuropathies. *Ann Neurol* 1985; **17**: 255–61.
32. Kelly JJ, Kyle RA, Miles JM et al. The spectrum of peripheral neuropathy in myeloma. *Neurology* 1981; **31**: 24–31.
33. Soubrier MJ, Dubost JJ, Sauvezie BJM et al. POEMS syndrome: a study of 25 cases and a review of the literature. *Am J Med* 1994; **97**: 543–53.
34. Kelly JJ, Kyle RA, Miles JM, Dyck PJ. Osteosclerotic myeloma and peripheral neuropathy. *Neurology (NY)* 1983; **33**: 202–210.
35. Ropper AH, McKee AC. Case Records of the Massachusetts General Hospital: Case 21-1993. *N Engl J Med* 1993; **328**: 1550–8.
36. Nakanishi T, Sobue I, Toyokura Y et al. The Crow–Fukase syndrome: a study of 102 cases in Japan. *Neurology (Cleveland)* 1984; **34**: 712–20.
37. Vital C, Gherardi R, Vital A et al. Uncompacted myelin lamellae in polyneuropathy, organomegaly, endocrinopathy, M-protein and skin changes syndrome. Ultrastructural study of peripheral nerve biopsy from 22 patients. *Acta Neuropathol* 1994; **87**: 302–7.
38. Lavenstein B, Dalakas M, Engel WK. Polyneuropathy in nonsecretory osteosclerotic

multiple myeloma with immunoglobulin deposition in peripheral nerve tissue. *Neurology* 1979; **29**: 611 (abst).
39. Adams D, Said G. Ultrastructural characterisation of the M protein in nerve biopsy of patients with POEMS syndrome. *J Neurol Neurosurg Psychiatry* 1998; **64**: 809–12.
40. Iwashita H, Ohnishi A, Asada M et al. Polyneuropathy, skin hyperpigmentation, edema, and hypertrichosis in localized osteosclerotic myeloma. *Neurology* 1977; **27**: 675–81.
41. Bardwick PA, Zvaifler NJ, Gill GN et al. Plasma cell dyscrasia with polyneuropathy, organomegaly, endocrinopathy, M protein and skin changes: the POEMS syndrome. *Medicine (Baltimore)* 1980; **59**: 311–22.
42. Miralles GD, O' Fallon JR, Taller NJ. Plasma-cell dyscrasia with polyneuropathy. The spectrum of the POEMS syndrome. *N Engl J Med* 1992; **327**: 1919–23.
43. Gherardi R, Belec L, Soubrier M et al. Overproduction of proinflammatory cytokines imbalanced by their antagonists in POEMS syndrome. *Blood* 1996; **87**: 1458–65.
44. Mandler RN, Kerrigan DP, Smart J et al. Castleman's disease in the POEMS syndrome with elevated interleukin 6. *Cancer* 1992; **69**: 2697–703.
45. Kuwabara S, Hattori T, Shimoe Y, Kamitsukasa I. Long term melphalan-prednisolone chemotherapy for POEMS syndrome. *J Neurol Neurosurg Psychiatry* 1997; **63**: 385–7.
46. Rotta FT, Bradley WG. Marked improvement of severe polyneuropathy associated with multifocal myeloma following surgery, radiation, and chemotherapy. *Muscle Nerve* 1997; **20**: 1035–7.
47. Silberstein LE, Duggan D, Berkman EM. Therapeutic trial of plasma exchange in osteosclerotic myeloma associated with the POEMS syndrome. *J Clin Apheresis* 1985; **2**: 253–7.
48. Delauche MC, Clauvel JP, Seligmann M. Peripheral neuropathy and plasma cell neoplasias: a report of 10 cases. *Br J Haematol* 1981; **48**: 383–92.
49. Coto V, Auletta M, Cocozza M et al. POEMS syndrome: an Italian case with diagnostic and therapeutic implications. *Ann Ital Med Int* 1991; **6**: 416–19.
50. Saida K, Kawakami H, Ohta M, Iwamura K. Coagulation and vascular abnormalities in Crow–Fukase syndrome. *Muscle Nerve* 1997; **20**: 486–92.
51. Baldini L, Nobile-Orazio E, Guffanti A et al. Peripheral neuropathy in IgM monoclonal gammopathy and Waldenström's macroglobulinemia: a frequent complication in elderly males with low MAG-reactive serum monoclonal component. *Am J Hematol* 1994; **45**: 25–31.
52. Nobile-Orazio E, Baldini L, Barbieri S et al. Treatment of patients with neuropathy and anti-MAG IgM M-proteins. *Ann Neurol* 1988; **24**: 83–97.
53. Pollard JD, Young GAR. Neurology and the bone marrow. *J Neurol Neurosurg Psychiatry* 1997; **63**: 706–18.
54. Dellagi K, Dupouey P, Brouet JC et al. Waldenström's macroglobulinemia and peripheral neuropathy: a clinical and immunologic study of 25 patients. *Blood* 1983; **62**: 280–5.
55. Julien J, Vital L, Vallat JM et al. Polyneuropathy in Waldenström's macroglobulinemia. *Arch Neurol* 1978; **35**: 423–5.
56. Meier C, Roberts K, Steck AJ et al. Polyneuropathy in Waldenström's macroglobulinemia: reduction in endoneurial IgM deposits after treatment with chlorambucil and plasmapheresis. *Acta Neuropathol* 1984: **64**: 297–307.
57. Vital C, Deminiere C, Bourgouin B et al. Waldenström's macroglobulinemia and peripheral neuropathy: deposition of M-component and kappa light chain in the endoneurium. *Neurology* 1985; **35**: 603–6.
58. Vital C, Vital A, Deminiere C et al. Myelin modifications in 8 cases of peripheral neuropathy with Waldenström's macroglobulinemia and anti-MAG activity. *Ultrastruct Pathol* 1997; **21**: 509–16.
59. Dalakas M, Flaum MA, Rick M et al. Treatment of polyneuropathy in Waldenström's macroglobulinemia: role of paraproteinemia and immunologic studies. *Neurology* 1983; **33**: 1406–10.
60. Rudnicki SA, Harik SI, Dhodapkar M et al. Nervous system dysfunction in Waldenström's macroglobulinemia: response to treatment. *Neurology* 1998; **51**: 1210–13.
61. Kyle RA, Bayrd ED. Amyloidosis: review of 236 cases. *Medicine (Baltimore)* 1975; **54**: 271–99.
62. Kyle RA, Greipp PR. Amyloidosis (AL). Clinical and laboratory features in 229 cases. *Mayo Clin Proc* 1983; **58**: 665–83.
63. Duston MA, Skinner M, Anderson J et al. Peripheral neuropathy as an early marker of AL amyloidosis. *Arch Intern Med* 1989; **149**: 358–60.
64. Kelly JJ, Kyle RA, O Brien PC, Dyck PJ. The natural history of peripheral neuropathy in

primary systemic amyloidosis. *Ann Neurol* 1979; **6**: 1–7.
65. Rajkumar SV, Gertz MA, Kyle RA. Prognosis of patients with primary systemic amyloidosis who present with dominant neuropathy. *Am J Med* 1998; **104**: 232–7.
66. Spuler S, Emslie-Smith A, Engel AG. Amyloid myopathy: an underdiagnosed entity. *Ann Neurol* 1998; **43**: 719–28.
67. Kyle RA. 'Benign' monoclonal gammopathy after 20 to 30 years of followup. *Mayo Clin Proc* 1993; **68**: 26–36.
68. Kyle RA, Gertz MA, Greipp PR. A trial of three regimens for primary amyloidosis: colchicine alone, melphalan and prednisone, and melphalan, prednisone and colchicine. *N Engl J Med* 1997; **336**: 1202–7.
69. Dhodapkar MV, Jagannath S, Vesole D et al. Treatment of AL-amyloidosis with dexamethasone plus alpha interferon. *Leuk Lymphoma* 1997; **27**: 351–6.
70. Comenzo RL, Vosburgh E, Simms RW et al. Dose-intensive melphalan with blood stem cell support for the treatment of AL amyloidosis: one year followup in five patients. *Blood* 1996; **88**: 2801–6.
71. van Buren M, Hene RJ, Verdonck LF et al. Clinical remission after syngeneic bone marrow transplantation in a patient with AL amyloidosis. *Ann Intern Med* 1995; **122**: 508–10.
72. Gilmore JD, Davies J, Iqbal A et al. Allogeneic bone marrow transplantation for systemic AL amyloidosis. *Br J Haematol* 1998; **100**: 226–8.
73. Gemignani F, Pavesi G, Fiocchi A et al. Peripheral neuropathy in essential mixed cryoglobulinaemia. *J Neurol Neurosurg Psychiatry* 1992; **55**: 116–20.
74. Gorevic PD, Kassab HJ, Levo Y et al. Mixed cryoglobulinemia: clinical aspects and long term follow-up of 40 patients. *Am J Med* 1980; **69**: 287–308.
75. Garcia-Bragado F, Fernandez JM, Navarro C et al. Peripheral neuropathy in essential mixed cryoglobulinemia. *Arch Neurol* 1988; **45**: 1210–14.
76. Ferri C, La Civita L, Cirafisi C et al. Peripheral neuropathy in mixed essential cryoglobulinemia: clinical and electrophysiological investigations. *J Rheumatol* 1992; **19**: 889–95.
77. Lippa CF, Chad DA, Smith TW et al. Neuropathy associated with cryoglobulinemia. *Muscle Nerve* 1986; **9**: 626–31.
78. Apartis E, Leger JM, Musset L et al. Peripheral neuropathy associated with essential mixed cryoglobulinemia: a role for hepatitis C virus infection? *J Neurol Neurosurg Psychiatry* 1996; **60**: 661–6.
79. Vallat JM, Desproges-Gotteron R, Leboutet MJ et al. Cryoglobulinemic neuropathy: a pathological study. *Ann Neurol* 1980; **8**: 179–85.
80. Vital C, Deminiere C, Lagueny A et al. Peripheral neuropathy with essential mixed cryoglobulinemia: biopsies from 5 cases. *Acta Neuropathol* 1988; **75**: 605–10.
81. Khella SL, Frost S, Hermann GA et al. Hepatitis C infection, cryoglobulinemia, and vasculitic neuropathy. Treatment with interferon alpha: case report and literature review. *Neurology* 1995; **45**: 407–11.
82. Gosselin S, Kyle RA, Dyck PJ. Neuropathy associated with monoclonal gammopathies of undetermined significance. *Ann Neurol* 1991; 30: 54–61.
83. Yeung KB, Thomas PK, King RHM et al. The clinical spectrum of peripheral neuropathies associated with benign monoclonal IgM, IgG and IgA paraproteinemia. *J Neurol* 1991; **238**: 383–391.
84. Simmons Z, Albers JW, Bromberg MB et al. Presentation and initial clinical course in patients with chronic inflammatory demyelinating polyradiculoneuropathy. Comparison of patients with and without monoclonal gammopathy. *Neurology* 1993; **43**: 2202–9.
85. Simmons Z, Albers JW, Bromberg MB, Feldman EL. Long-term followup of patients with chronic inflammatory demyelinating polyneuropathy, without and with monoclonal gammopathy. *Brain* 1995; **118**: 359–68.
86. Gordon PH, Rowland LP, Younger DS et al. Lymphoproliferative disorders and motor neuron disease: an update. *Neurology* 1997; **48**: 1671–8.
87. Younger DS, Rowland LP, Latov N et al. Motor neuron disease and amyotrophic lateral sclerosis: relation of high CSF protein content to paraproteinemia and clinical syndromes *Neurology* 1990; **40**: 595–99.
88. Notermans NC, Wokke JHJ, Lokhorst HM et al. Polyneuropathy associated with monoclonal gammopathy of undetermined significance. A prospective study of the prognostic value of clinical and laboratory abnormalities. *Brain* 1994; **117**: 1385–93.
89. Vital A, Vital C, Julien J et al. Polyneuropathy associated with IgM monoclonal gammopathy: immunological and pathological study in 31 patients. *Acta Neuropathol* 1989; **79**: 160–7.
90. Bleasel AF, Hawke SH, Pollard JD, McLeod JG. IgG monoclonal paraproteinemia and peripheral

neuropathy. *J Neurol Neurosurg Psychiatry* 1993; **56**: 52–7.
91. Suarez GA, Kelly JJ Jr. Polyneuropathy associated with monoclonal gammopathy of undetermined significance: further evidence that IgM-MGUS neuropathies are different than IgG-MGUS. *Neurology* 1993; 43: 1304–8.
92. Dyck PJ, Low PA, Windebank AJ. Plasma exchange in polyneuropathy associated with monoclonal gammopathy of undetermined significance. *N Engl J Med* 1991; **325**: 1482–6.
93. Mendell JR, Sahenk Z, Whitaker JN et al. Polyneuropathy and IgM monoclonal gammopathy: studies of the pathogenic role of anti-myelin associated glycoprotein antibody. *Ann Neurol* 1985; 17: 243–54.
94. van den Berg LH, Hays AP, Nobile-Orazio E et al. Anti-MAG and anti-SGPG antibodies in neuropathy. *Muscle Nerve* 1996; **19**: 637–43.
95. Pestronk A, Li F, Griffin J et al. Polyneuropathy syndromes associated with serum antibodies to sulfatide and myelin-associated glycoprotein. *Neurology* 1991; **41**: 357–62.
96. Nobile-Orazio E, Latov N, Hays AP et al. Neuropathy and anti-MAG antibodies without detectable serum M-protein. *Neurology* 1984; **34**: 218–21.
97. Gabriel JM, Erne B, Bernasconi I et al. Confocal microscopic localization of anti-myelin-associated glycoprotein autoantibodies in a patient with peripheral neuropathy initially lacking a detectable IgM gammopathy. *Acta Neuropathol (Berl)* 1998; **95**: 540–6.
98. Kaku DA, England JD, Sumner AJ. Distal accentuation of conduction slowing in polyneuropathy associated with antibodies to myelin associated glycoprotein and sulfated glucuronyl paragloboside. *Brain* 1994; **117**: 941–7.
99. Trojaborg W, Hays AP, Van den berg L et al. Motor conduction parameters in neuropathies associated with anti-MAG antibodies and other types of demyelinating and axonal neuropathies. *Muscle Nerve* 1995; **18**: 730–5.
100. Notermans NC, Wokke JHJ, van der Berg LH et al. Chronic idiopathic axonal polyneuropathy. Comparison of patients with and without monoclonal gammopathy. *Brain* 1996; **119**: 421–7.
101. Sherman WH, Latov N, Hays AP et al. Monoclonal IgMk antibody precipitating with chondroitin sulfate C from patients with axonal polyneuropathy and epidermolysis. *Neurology* 1983; **33**: 192–201.
102. Nemni R, Fazio R, Quattrini A et al. Antibodies to sulfatide and to chondroitin sulfate C in patients with chronic sensory neuropathy. *J Neuroimmunol* 1993; **43**: 79–86.
103. Lopate G, Parks BJ, Goldstein JM et al. A. Polyneuropathies associated with high titre anti-sulfatide antibodies: characteristics of patients with and without serum monoclonal proteins. *J Neurol Neurosurg Psychiatry* 1997; **62**: 581–5.
104. van den Berg LH, Lankamp CL, de Jager AE et al. Anti-sulfatide antibodies in peripheral neuropathy. *J Neurol Neurosurg Psychiatry* 1993; **56**: 1164–8.
105. Freddo L, Hays AP, Sherman WH, Latov N. Axonal neuropathy in a patient with IgM M-protein reactive with nerve endoneurium. *Neurology* 1985; **35**: 1321–5.
106. Yee WC, Hahn AF, Hearn SA, Rupar AR. Neuropathy in IgM lambda paraproteinemia. Immunoreactivity to neural proteins and chrondroitin sulfate. *Acta Neuropathol* 1989; **78**: 57–64.
107. Fineman SM, McKendall RR. Plasma exchange: a treatment for neuropathy associated with IgG-kappa gammopathy. *J Neurol* 1990; **237**: 85–7.
108. Cook D, Dalakas M, Galdi A et al. High dose intravenous immunoglobulin in the treatment of demyelinating neuropathy associated monoclonal gammopathy. *Neurology* 1990; 40: 212–14.
109. Ernerudh J, Brodtkorb E, Olsson T et al. Peripheral neuropathy and monoclonal IgM with antibody activity against peripheral nerve myelin; effect of plasma exchange. *J Neuroimmunol* 1986; **11**: 171–8.
110. Dalakas, MC, Quarles RH, Farrer RG et al. A controlled study of intravenous gammaglobulin in demyelinating neuropathy with IgM gammopathy. *Ann Neurol* 1996; **40**: 792–5.
111. Gorson KC, Ropper AH, Weinberg DH, Weinstein R. Treatment experience in patients with anti-MAG neuropathy. *Muscle Nerve* 2001; **24**: 778–86.
112. Blume G, Pestronk A, Goodnough LT. Anti-MAG antibody associated polyneuropathies: improvement following immunotherapy with monthly plasma exchange and IV cyclophosphamide. *Neurology* 1995; **45**: 1577–80.
113. Pestronk A Cornblath DR, Ilyas AA et al. A treatable multifocal motor neuropathy with antibodies to GM1 ganglioside. *Ann Neurol* 1988; **24**: 73–8.
114. Nobile-Orazio E. Multifocal motor neuropathy. *J Neurol Neurosurg Psychiatry* 1996; **60**: 599–603.
115. Parry GJ. Motor neuropathy with multifocal motor conduction block. In: *Peripheral Neuropathy,*

3rd edn (Dyck PJ, Thomas PK, Griffin JW et al, eds). Philadelphia: WB Saunders, 1993: 1518–24.

116. Chaudhry V. Multifocal motor neuropathy. *Semin Neurol* 1998; **18**: 73–81.

117. Katz JS, Wolfe GI, Bryan WW et al. Electrophysiological findings in multifocal motor neuropathy. *Neurology* 1997; **48**: 700– 7.

118. Santoro M, Thomas FP, Fink ME. IgM deposits at nodes of Ranvier in a patient with amyotrophic lateral sclerosis, anti-GM1 antibodies, and multifocal motor conduction block. *Ann Neurol* 1990; **28**: 373–7.

119. Thomas FP, Adapon PH, Goldberg GP et al. Localization of neural epitopes that bind to IgM monoclonal antibodies (M-proteins) from two patients with motor neuron disease. *J Neuroimmunol* 1989; **23**: 167–74.

120. Adams D, Kuntzer T, Steck A et al. Motor conduction block and high titers of anti-GM1 ganglioside antibodies: pathological evidence of a motor neuropathy in a patient with a lower motor neuron syndrome. *J Neurol Neurosurg Psychiatry* 1993; **56**: 982–7.

121. van der Berg LH, Kerkhoff H, Oey PL et al. Treatment of multifocal motor neuropathy with high-dose intravenous immunoglobulins: a double-blind, placebo controlled study. *J Neurol Neurosurg Psychiatry* 1995; **59**: 248–52.

122. Bouche P, Moulonguet A, Younes-Chennoufi AB et al. Multifocal motor neuropathy with conduction block: a study of 24 patients. *J Neurol Neurosurg Psychiatry* 1995; **59**: 38–44.

123. Azulay JP, Blin O, Puget J et al. Intravenous gammaglobulin treatment in patients with motor neuron syndromes associated with GM1 antibodies: a double-blind, placebo-controlled trial. *Neurology* 1994; **44**: 429–32.

124. Krarup C, Stewart JD, Sumner AJ et al. A syndrome of asymmetric limb weakness with motor conduction block. *Neurology* 1990; **40**: 118–27.

13

The kidney in plasma cell disorders

Mary Jo Shaver-Lewis, Sudhir V Shah

CONTENTS • **Introduction** • **Spectrum of renal diseases** • **Cast nephropathy** • **Light-chain deposition disease** • **Amyloidosis** • **Fanconi syndrome** • **Pathophysiology of paraproteins and nephrotoxicity** • **Acute renal failure** • **Treatment** • **Renal disorders in hematopoietic stem cell transplant recipients** • **Conclusions**

INTRODUCTION

The spectrum of disorders that involve the kidney in patients with plasma cell dyscrasias includes asymptomatic proteinuria, nephrotic syndrome, and both acute and chronic renal insufficiency.

In addition, we have come to recognize several kidney-related syndromes (Table 13.1) in patients who have undergone hematopoietic stem cell transplantation (HSCT); a widely employed therapeutic measure in myeloma.

Impairment of renal function is a common feature of myeloma.[1–5] In early studies describing the management of myeloma, renal insufficiency was associated with a worse prognosis. With the advent of modern and intensive supportive therapy, it has been shown that survival is not dramatically changed by the presence of renal failure, and the overall prognosis is determined by the response of the underlying disease to chemotherapy rather than renal function.[6–8]

Table 13.1 Kidney and plasma cell disorders

- Renal disease due to plasma cell disorders
  - Myeloma kidney or cast nephropathy
  - Light-chain deposition disease
  - Amyloidosis
  - Fanconi syndrome
- Acute renal failure
- Renal disorders associated with hematopoietic stem cell transplantation

SPECTRUM OF RENAL DISEASES

Patients with plasma cell dyscrasias who have renal involvement present primarily with proteinuria and/or an elevation in serum creatinine and blood urea nitrogen. The urinary dipstick for protein may be the first clue to a renal process. However, it detects albumin and may be negative if Bence Jones proteinuria is present without albuminuria.[9] Immunofixation electrophoresis or immunoelectrophoresis, which are antibody detection assays that can be performed on both serum and urine, are the tests of choice for the detection of paraprotein or light chains.

The most common histological diagnosis, found in 80% of patients with myeloma, is cast nephropathy or myeloma kidney. Light-chain deposition disease (LCDD), occurring in 5–10%, and amyloidosis, in 10%, can present as nephrotic syndrome, which is present in up to 25% of cases.[10] A much rarer cause of chronic renal impairment is plasma cell infiltration of the kidney.

Renal failure develops in approximately half of patients with myeloma at some point in the course of the disease,[1,2,11–13] and renal damage is more frequent in patients with light-chain and IgD disease.[14, 15]

CAST NEPHROPATHY

Patients with cast nephropathy usually present with proteinuria and renal insufficiency. Renal failure can evolve rapidly despite stable paraprotein production and excretion. Although the renal insufficiency is progressive in nature, whenever an unexpected deterioration in renal function occurs, every attempt should be made to elucidate precipitating factors such as dehydration, hypercalcemia, and exposure to nephrotoxic agents.[16]

Aggressive treatment with alkaline diuresis, chemotherapy, elimination of nephrotoxic agents, and avoidance of unnecessary investigations (exposure to radiographic contrast material), offer some potential for reversibility.[7,16–18]

The typical light-microscopic findings include large refractile tubular casts[19,20] surrounded by multinucleated giant cells located in the distal and collecting tubules (Figure 13.1). These casts have a multilamellar solid appearance, with multiple areas of fracture. They are composed of light chains (LC; see the section below on pathophysiology of paraproteins), Tamm–Horsfall protein (THP), fibrinogen, and albumin, and are strongly eosinophilic, non-argyrophilic, and periodic acid–Schiff-positive.[19,20] Figure 13.1 shows the findings on immunofluorescence studies as well as the characteristic light-microscopic picture of cast nephropathy.

There may be evidence of tubulointerstitial disease, particularly in patients who have renal impairment. The tubular cells are flattened, and show varying degrees of degeneration with necrosis and denudation of the tubular basement membrane,[21] leading to tubuloepithelial cell atrophy and interstitial fibrosis.[22] It has been suggested that tubulointerstitial damage correlates best with the lack of recovery of renal function.[23,24] In addition, severe cast formation has also been suggested to predict lack of recovery of renal function.[18,25]

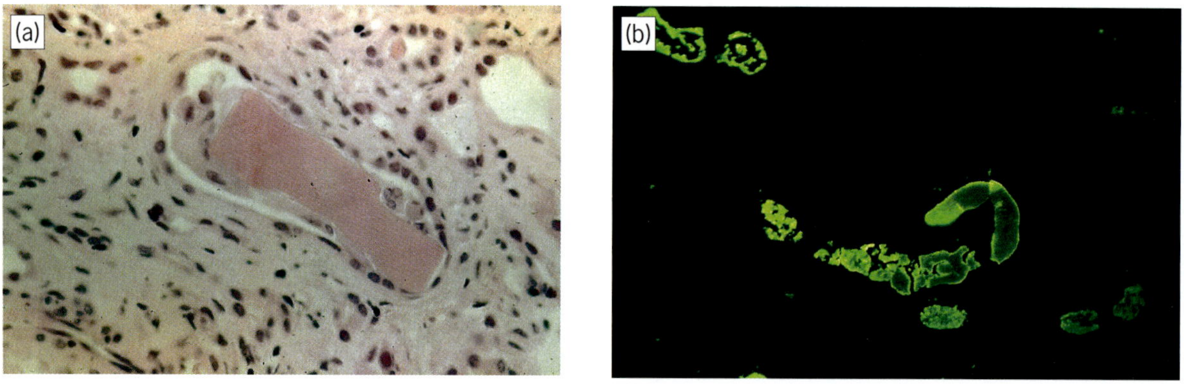

Figure 13.1 (a) Light-microscopic findings for myeloma cast nephropathy include large refractile tubular casts surrounded by multinucleated giant cells located in the distal and collecting tubules. These casts have a multilamellar appearance, with multiple areas of fracture. (b) On immunofluorescence, the casts are strongly positive for their selected light chain. In this case, the cast is strongly positive for κ light-chain deposition. (Provided by Dr Patrick Walker and Dr Stephen Bonsib from the Department of Pathology, University of Arkansas for Medical Sciences, Little Rock, Arkansas.)

In addition to the degree of tubulointerstitial damage and fibrosis[26] on renal biopsy, several other factors such as hypercalcemia and early infection have been associated with a poor prognosis. Sex, tumor load, the severity of renal failure, and light-chain isoelectric point have not been shown to correlate with prognosis.[27] Response to chemotherapy, disease stage, and creatinine at one month have also been suggested to be important predictors of survival.[17]

LIGHT-CHAIN DEPOSITION DISEASE

Light-chain deposition disease (LCDD) is a monoclonal gammopathy characterized by the deposition of light chains in the kidney and other vital organs (liver, heart, peripheral nerves)[28,29–33] (see Chapter 29 for details). The primary renal presentation is with elevated serum creatinine and proteinuria, the latter being in the nephrotic range in 25%.[10]

Figure 13.2 shows the typical light-microscopic and immunofluorescence findings of LCDD. The characteristic light-microscopic findings range from normal glomeruli to varying degrees of mesangial expansion along with thickened tubular basement membranes outlined by continuous deposits. One-third of biopsy cases have a pattern of nodular glomerulosclerosis similar to Kimmelstiel–Wilson glomerulopathy seen with diabetic nephropathy.[21] The biopsy may also show varying degrees of tubulointerstitial fibrosis. Immunofluorescence shows diffuse precipitates along the basement membrane of renal tubules, glomeruli, blood vessels, and the mesangium, and/or nodular deposits composed of monoclonal light chains, usually κ type. Electron microscopy shows discrete punctate and granular deposits in the same pattern detected by immunohistochemical techniques.[19,20] The deposits of LCDD are non-amyloidotic (non-fibrillar) and Congo-red-negative.[19, 20]

The median survival of patients surviving beyond three months is not drastically different from that of myeloma patients without renal impairment.[10] Symptomatic management of these patients with correction of volume depletion and hypercalcemia, and chemotherapy for control of the underlying malignancy may improve renal function in up to 50%.[10]

AMYLOIDOSIS

Tissue infiltration with immunoglobulin light chains results in primary (AL) amyloidosis, in

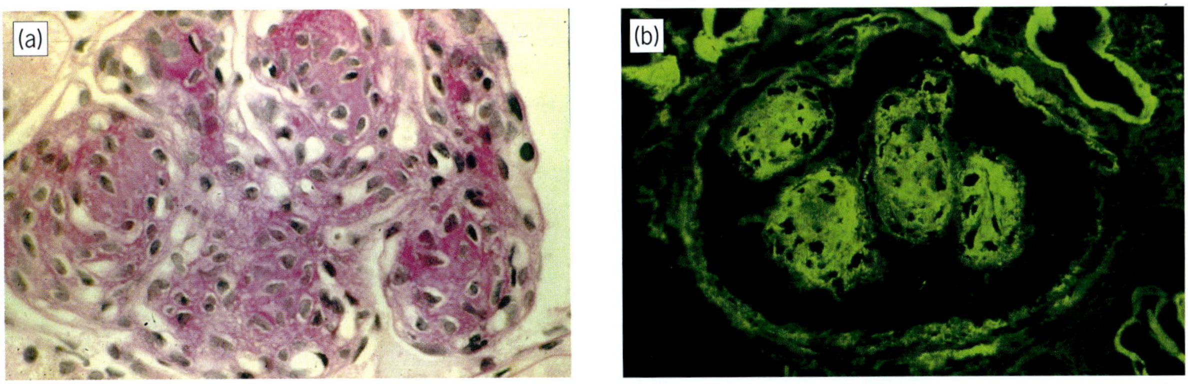

Figure 13.2 (a) One of the classic patterns of light-chain deposition disease found on light microscopy. This is typical of nodular glomerulosclerosis similar to Kimmelstiel–Wilson glomerulopathy seen with diabetic nephropathy. (b) Immunofluorescence shows these deposits to be composed of monoclonal light chains usually κ type, as nodular deposits or diffuse precipitates along the basement membrane of renal tubules, glomeruli, blood vessels and the mesangium. (Provided by Dr Patrick Walker and Dr Stephen Bonsib from the Department of Pathology, University of Arkansas for Medical Sciences, Little Rock, Arkansas.)

contrast to secondary amyloidosis (AA protein), which is commonly associated with chronic infectious, inflammatory, immune, genetic, and neoplastic disorders. β_2-Microglobulin amyloidosis occurs in patients on long-term hemodialysis, and presents as carpal tunnel syndrome or destructive arthropathy. AL amyloidosis is most commonly associated with IgD myeloma[34] and light-chain disease.[35]

Patients with AL amyloidosis present with renal impairment and proteinuria, often in the nephrotic range (>3.5 g/24 h).[1,11,12,22] In a review of 236 cases of amyloidosis published by Kyle and Bayrol[12] in 1975, renal insufficiency was present in approximately 50% at diagnosis and proteinuria was detected in over 90%.

On ultrasonography, the kidneys are normal in size or enlarged. Deposits are found in the glomerular basement membrane, the interstitium and in the blood vessels, and derive mainly from fragments of λ monoclonal light chains,[10,22] frequently of the λ VI subgroup.[36] On light microscopy, the deposits are extracellular, eosinophilic, and metachromatic. These deposits eventually replace the normal glomerular architecture, with loss of cellularity. When the tubules and interstitium are involved, tubular atrophy and interstitial fibrosis ensues. The amyloid deposits are Congo-red-positive and show apple-green birefringence under polarized light and are fibrillar on electron microscopy. Figure 13.3 shows the typical Congo red staining and electron-microscopic findings of AL amyloidosis.

FANCONI SYNDROME

Light-chain deposition in the proximal tubules of the kidney can cause tubular dysfunction with an acquired Fanconi syndrome. Fanconi syndrome is a generalized disorder of proximal tubular transport dysfunction, leading to urinary excretion of amino acids, glucose, bicarbonate, uric acid, phosphate, potassium, and low-molecular-weight proteins. The presence of hypokalemia, hypophosphatemia, hypouricemia, and a normal anion gap metabolic acidosis point to the possibility of Fanconi syndrome. An additional clue is glycosuria in a patient with normal serum glucose.

Maldonado et al[37] reviewed 17 cases of Fanconi syndrome associated with Bence Jones proteinuria or amyloidosis. Features of Fanconi syndrome preceded the diagnosis of myeloma or amyloidosis in 11 patients.[38–44] Of interest was the detection of crystalline cytoplasmic inclusion bodies in the lymphoplasmacytic elements of the bone marrow and renal tubular cells in 9 cases. The inclusion bodies were rectangular, rhomboid or rounded, with slight basophilic staining. More recent case reports have revealed similar findings.[45–47]

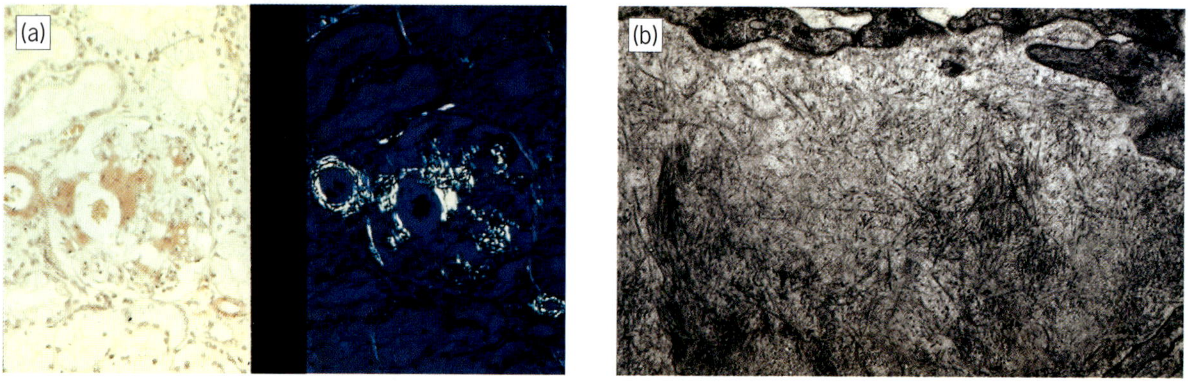

Figure 13.3 (a) Typical Congo red appearance of amyloid in the kidney. (b) Electron-microscopic findings of amyloidosis, showing the typical fibrillar appearance. (Provided by Dr Patrick Walker and Dr Stephen Bonsib from the Department of Pathology, University of Arkansas for Medical Sciences, Little Rock, Arkansas).

PATHOPHYSIOLOGY OF PARAPROTEINS AND NEPHROTOXICITY

An abnormal urinary protein, later to be called Bence Jones protein (BJP), was characterized by Dr Henry Bence Jones in 1847. These proteins were found to be immunoglobulin light chains. Light chains are low-molecular-weight proteins (approximately 22 kDa) and may be of two types: kappa (κ) and lambda (λ). Plasma cells synthesize light chains independently of heavy chains and combine them in the endoplasmic reticulum to form immunoglobulin molecules.[48] When excess light chains are synthesized, they escape as free light chains into the circulation,[49,50] and appear in the urine as BJP.[51]

Light chains are readily filtered by the glomerulus,[52, 53] and are reabsorbed by the proximal tubule. The proteins are subsequently handled by endocytosis, and then they are hydrolyzed by lysosomal enzymes, with amino acids being returned to the circulation.[54] Reabsorption in the proximal tubule is a saturable process. Therefore, any excess protein will be delivered to the distal nephron and will appear in the urine.[55] Proximal tubular damage may be due to overload of the endolysosomal system with release of toxic lysosomal enzymes or to the diversion of cell metabolism away from essential functions.[22] Ultimately, light chains precipitate as intratubular casts or are deposited in tubular, glomerular, or vascular basement membranes and the mesangium.

Koss et al[56] were the first to report that the intraperitoneal injection of nephrotoxic human BJP into mice resulted in cast deposition in the distal tubules, while other proteins failed to cause such deposition. Subsequent studies have shown that the injection of BJP from patients with myeloma or amyloidosis into mouse models produces a pathologic process similar to that seen in the human patients from whom the protein is derived, i.e. tubular cast, basement membrane precipitates, crystals, or amyloid fibrils.[57]

Exactly what makes some paraproteins nephrotoxic and others not is not well known. Several factors may contribute to the aggregation of THP with BJP to form obstructive distal tubular casts. An acidic urinary environment, high calcium concentration, and furosemide have been shown to enhance the binding rates and aggregation rates of THP and BJP.[58] Infusion of urinary proteins obtained from patients with cast nephropathy has been shown to result in intraluminal obstruction in the kidney.[59] The addition of furosemide aggravated the obstruction by two mechanisms: increase in the sodium chloride concentration in the distal nephron, which facilitated the coprecipitation of BJP with THP in vitro,[60] and direct binding to THP.[59]

The isoelectric point (pI) of the light chain may also play a role in renal toxicity. There are several studies showing that light chains with a high isoelectric point ($pI > 6$) are more likely to precipitate in the acidic urinary environment of the distal tubules, thus forming casts and causing renal damage.[61] It has been suggested that light chains with $pI > 5.5$, being positively charged in the presence of an acidic urine, may be more avidly absorbed by the anionic brush border of the tubular cells and would co-precipitate with THP in the distal tubule.[62–64] Other investigators have reported that BJP with $pI < 5.5$ may be more likely to lead to cast formation and thus be more nephrotoxic.[65] Most investigators have found no correlation between the pI of light chains or the amount of protein excreted and renal insufficiency.[61,65,66] Acute reversible renal failure seems to be associated with low-pI light chains and chronic irreversible renal failure with high-pI light chains.[66] Table 13.2 is a summary of the factors that can potentiate cast formation.

THP is rich in carbohydrate, which accounts for 30% of its molecular weight.[58] Physical properties of light chains such as the extent of glycosylation and polymerization have been implicated in the pathogenesis of renal toxicity.[67, 68] Complete deglycosylation of THP has been shown to abolish co-aggregation.[59] In both animal and human studies, treatment with colchicine has been shown to decrease the carbohydrate content of THP, specifically the sialic acid moiety, thus preventing co-aggregation with BJP.[59] These data suggest that the binding

Table 13.2 Factors that can potentiate cast formation

- Loop diuretics such as furosemide
- Concentration of Bence Jones protein and Tamm–Horsfall protein in the early distal tubule
- Distal nephron pH
- Ion concentration in the distal nephron
- Hypercalcemia
- Extracellular fluid volume depletion
- Amino acid sequence of the variable region of light chains
- Extent of light-chain glycosylation or polymerization
- Light-chain isoelectric point (pI)

site on THP for cast-forming BJP is the carbohydrate moiety.[59] It is also hypothesized that the amino acid sequence of the variable region of the monoclonal light chain may contribute to its toxicity and to the binding to a particular segment of THP.[69] This may also be the mechanism for the formation of amyloid fibrils.[22]

The co-aggregation of BJP and THP in the lumen of the distal nephron appears to be the main pathogenic factor in cast nephropathy in the rat.[10] Thus, with adequate control of plasma cell proliferation with chemotherapy, tissue deposition and injury may be prevented.

ACUTE RENAL FAILURE

Acute renal failure (ARF) is a common feature of myeloma. More than 50% of patients have impaired renal function at presentation or during the course of the disease.[1,2,5] In up to half of the patients with ARF, there are potentially reversible causes that contribute to renal failure. These include dehydration, hypercalcemia, infection, intravenous contrast agents, hyperuricemia, and drugs such as non-steroidal anti-inflammatory agents, angiotensin-converting enzyme inhibitors, amphotericin B, and aminoglycosides (Table 13.3). Thus, every patient with a plasma cell disorder that presents with or develops renal failure must be carefully evaluated for potentially reversible factors.

Table 13.3 Factors associated with acute renal failure

- Volume depletion
- Hypercalcemia
- Hyperuricemia and tumor lysis syndrome
- Infection
- Drug Toxicity
  - NSAIDs
  - Intravenous contrast
  - Amphotericin B
  - Aminoglycosides
  - Acyclovir
  - Angiotensin-converting enzyme inhibitors
- Heart failure
- Liver failure
- Chronic renal disorders unrelated to myeloma

Dehydration and hypercalcemia

One of the commonest reasons for reversible renal failure is volume depletion, which leads to decreased renal perfusion, resulting in prerenal azotemia. In addition, enhanced reabsorption of fluids in response to volume depletion results in an increased concentration of paraproteins in the distal tubules, promoting aggregation and cast formation.

Compounding this is the presence of hypercalcemia, which is not uncommonly seen with progressive myeloma. Hypercalcemia can cause dehydration due to an osmotic diuresis induced by the high serum calcium level, hypercalcemia-induced emesis, and nephrogenic diabetes insipidus. Hypercalcemia and dehydration have accounted for up to 58% of the causes of ARF in myeloma.[18]

In addition to the effect of hypercalcemia in causing volume depletion, several studies have shown other potentially detrimental effects. Hypercalcemia can cause a decrease in the glomerular filtration rate secondary to renal vasoconstriction[70] and an alteration in the glomerular permeability coefficient.[71] Hypercalcemia may have an effect on glomerular filtration even in the absence of vasoconstriction. Smolens et al[72] studied rats injected with non-toxic BJP in the presence of hypercalcemia. In this group of rats, the inulin clearance was decreased by 46% without a significant difference in the urine flow rate, mean arterial blood pressure, renal blood flow, or histology on renal biopsy compared with controls. The mechanism by which calcium causes increased toxicity of BJP is somewhat unclear. However, hypercalcemia itself has been shown to enhance the direct toxic effect of light chains by increasing the aggregability of THP and BJP.[65,72,73]

Infection

Infection is a common problem in myeloma patients as a result of hypogammaglobulinemia and compromised cell-mediated immunity. Bacteremia without hemodynamic compromise or full-blown sepsis can decrease renal perfusion, with resultant acute tubular necrosis (ATN).

Nephrotoxic antibiotics, not uncommonly needed to treat patients with myeloma, also contribute to ARF. These include aminoglycosides and amphotericin B, both of which can cause ATN,[74] and acyclovir which can cause acute interstitial nephritis,[75] acute tubular necrosis,[76] and obstruction secondary to tubular deposition of crystals.

Aminoglycoside nephrotoxicity, occurring in 15–20% of therapeutic courses,[77,78] is typically noticed five to seven days after therapy has been initiated. Changes in proximal tubular function may occur, as well as hypokalemia and hypomagnesemia. Risk factors for aminoglycoside toxicity include advanced age, renal hypoperfusion, and sepsis.[77,79]

Nephrotoxicity during early therapy with amphotericin B is vascular in origin, secondary to vasoconstriction with a fall in glomerular filtration rate.[80] The early signs include hypokalemia and a decreased urinary concentrating ability. Patients who receive a higher average daily dose of the medication develop nephrotoxicity more frequently.[81] As the total dose exceeds 5 g, both the incidence of nephrotoxicity[74] and the potential for permanent renal damage increase.[82] Salt loading is probably the most nephroprotective intervention that can be used with amphotericin B therapy.[82] With the introduction of lipid preparations of amphotericin B, such as amphotericin B lipid complex (ABLC), in the treatment of fungal infections, there appears to be a decrease in the incidence of nephrotoxicity.[83]

Non-steroidal anti-inflammatory drugs

The non-steroidal anti-inflammatory drugs (NSAIDs) are frequently used to relieve bone pain in myeloma patients with lytic bone lesions. NSAIDs exert their effect by inhibition of prostaglandin production via inhibition of cyclo-oxygenase. By blocking production of vasodilatory prostaglandins, NSAIDs cause a reduction in renal blood flow and GFR, leading to ARF. Sodium and water retention occur, which contribute further to cast precipitation. The risk of acute renal failure due to NSAID administration in patients with myeloma is well documented,[84–86] and the use of these agents should be avoided.

Radiographic contrast

The most important risk factor for contrast-induced ARF is prior renal insufficiency. The additional risk factors in patients with plasma cell dyscrasias include hypercalcemia and dehydration.[5] Earlier studies, in the 1950s and 1960s, reported a high incidence of contrast-induced ARF. Contrast agents in use during that period were characterized by high protein binding,[87] which predisposed them to precipitate and obstruct tubular fluid flow.[88] The incidence of contrast-induced ARF in myeloma patients is between 0.6% and 1.26%,[87] as compared with 0.15% in the general population. In a myeloma patient with normal renal function, the risk of contrast-induced ARF is thought to be low when there is no hypercalcemia and volume depletion. The lesser degree of protein binding by non-ionic contrast agents suggests that these agents may have a greater role in patients with myeloma although there are no studies addressing this issue.

Urate nephropathy

Acute uric acid nephropathy refers to the development of ARF due to renal tubular obstruction by urate or uric acid crystals. Uric acid precipitation primarily occurs in the distal tubule and collecting duct. Hyperuricemia is a common complication of active myeloma due to rapid cell turnover; especially after chemotherapy or HSCT secondary to tumor lysis syndrome. The classic metabolic presentation of tumor lysis syndrome is hyperuricemia, hyperkalemia, and hyperphosphatemia, with subsequent hypocalcemia, and elevated blood urea nitrogen and creatinine.

A useful test to help differentiate uric acid nephropathy from other forms of ARF is a urinary uric acid to creatinine ratio. A ratio of greater than 1 is consistent with uric acid nephropathy.[89] The urine sediment examination may be normal or may contain rhomboidal crystals composed of urates.[90] Treatment consists of aggressive hydration, alkalinization of the urine, and allopurinol.[91] Urinary alkalinization enhances uric acid excretion. A patient with severe hyperuricemia who becomes oliguric is a candidate for hemodialysis to reduce the uric acid level rapidly.

TREATMENT

Therapeutic intervention in patients with acute renal impairment

Plasma exchange

As light chains have been shown to play a dominant role in renal damage in myeloma, one of the primary goals of therapy is a rapid reduction in the paraprotein level. Several studies have examined plasma exchange as a means of rapidly lowering paraprotein concentrations and improving or reversing acute renal failure.[92,93] Plasma exchange may have a role, in combination with hydration, forced alkaline diuresis, dialysis, and chemotherapy in the treatment of myeloma.[92–94]

Zucchelli et al[95] explored the role of plasmapheresis in myeloma with ARF in a controlled study. In 11 of 13 patients treated with plasma exchange in addition to conventional measures, there was an improvement in renal function in 9–34 days. In contrast, only 2 of 11 patients who did not undergo plasma exchange experienced improved renal function. Patients receiving plasma exchange also had a better one–year survival rate (66% versus 28%). The majority of the deaths in the study were secondary to infection.

Pozzi et al[18] retrospectively reviewed 50 cases of myeloma with ARF. Thirty-two patients received a mean of 4.7 plasma exchange treatments (range 2–18), with renal function improvement in 61% versus 27% of those who did not receive plasma exchange. The biopsy data in this study showed a good correlation between the severity of the histological picture and the gravity of prognosis, as has been shown in other studies.[23–25] The most frequent causes of death in the first six months were infection and cancer cachexia.[18]

Johnson et al[25] performed the most recent study of plasmapheresis in myeloma patients with ARF. Twenty-one patients were randomized to receive either forced diuresis and chemotherapy (10 patients) or forced diuresis, chemotherapy, and plasmapheresis (11 patients). Of the 12 patients who required renal replacement therapy, the only ones to recover renal function were 3 patients treated with plasmapheresis. The primary factor predicting irreversibility of renal failure was severity of the renal lesion on biopsy.[25] Overall, it appears that plasma exchange plays a beneficial role in the treatment of patients with myeloma who have high paraprotein levels and renal impairment. Renal biopsy may be important in predicting those expected to recover renal function with this mode of therapy.

Therapeutic intervention in patients with chronic renal impairment

Renal replacement therapy

Approximately 3–12% of patients with myeloma require long-term renal replacement therapy (RRT), either peritoneal dialysis (PD) or hemodialysis (HD), for end-stage renal disease.[96] Advantages of PD include minimal blood loss and elimination of systemic heparinization, both of which increase the risk in a patient with anemia and thrombocytopenia. PD has been shown to enhance the removal of paraproteins.[97–99] While continuous ambulatory PD (CAPD) clears light chains better than HD, this has not been shown to influence recovery of renal function,[95] and further loss of immunoglobulin may be a disadvantage. Although some have questioned the safety of CAPD,[100] others have found no difference in survival between HD and CAPD.[8] The rate of peritonitis is similar to that in patients without myeloma.[101] When considering the high rates of infection-related morbidity and mortality in myeloma patients, it may be best to hold CAPD until after the first two months of therapy when most infections can be brought under control.

There is no contraindication to HD in patients with myeloma. When a patient presents with significant renal impairment, the need for permanent vascular access must be borne in mind. Patients receiving chemotherapy for myeloma almost invariably require a central venous catheter. When placing central venous lines in this population of patients, thought must be given to the future need of a permanent arm access, an arteriovenous fistula, or graft, because preservation of arm and central neck veins is critical to securing permanent access. Early creation of an arteriovenous fistula can obviate the need for large-diameter central venous hemodialysis catheters in the acute setting.

The response rate to chemotherapy of patients who survive beyond the first two months from initiation of dialysis seems to be similar to that of patients with normal renal function.[102] The overall survival of patients accepted into dialysis programs is comparable to that of other myeloma patients.[6]

Renal transplantation

There are 11 reported cases of renal transplantation in patients who either had myeloma prior to the allograft or developed it shortly thereafter.[6,103–112] This limited experience suggests that prolonged survival with excellent graft function can be achieved following renal transplantation in these patients. In the majority, antitumor chemotherapy has seemed to provide adequate immunosuppression.[103]

There are no established criteria for selection of patients for transplantation, but it is suggested that they have chemotherapy-induced disease remission of at least one year's duration in the absence of extrarenal disease prior to consideration of transplantation. Legitimate concerns about renal transplantation in myeloma patients include the relatively limited life expectancy, reduced rehabilitation potential, relative shortage of cadaveric kidneys, and the possibility that post-transplant immunosuppression given to prevent rejection may promote tumor growth.

Monoclonal gammopathies are not infrequent after solid organ transplantation.[113–118] The frequency varies depending on the organ transplanted, the intensity of the immunosuppressive treatment, age, the interval post transplant[119] and the sensitivity of the method used to detect clonality.[120] The pathologic clonal expansion is felt to be secondary to the impaired control of B cell clones by suppressor T cells due to immunosuppression.[121] However, myeloma has been rarely reported after renal transplantation.[113]

RENAL DISORDERS IN HEMATOPOIETIC STEM CELL TRANSPLANT RECIPIENTS

ARF or renal insufficiency develops in approximately 40% of patients after HSCT, with 10–50% of those with renal dysfunction requiring dialysis.[122,123] Renal complications are far more common after allogeneic transplantation compared with autologous.[122,123]

A number of factors predispose to the development of ARF requiring dialysis after HSCT.[124] The strongest risk factor is use of amphotericin B prior to the doubling of serum creatinine. It is hard to gauge what contributes most to renal dysfunction during therapy for sepsis – sepsis *per se* on the amphotericin B. Other risk factors include weight gain (reflecting renal sodium avidity, which is commonly seen in hepatorenal syndrome/veno-occlusive disease, HRS/VOD) and clinically detectable jaundice. At the time of the doubling of serum creatinine, 84% of patients who eventually went on to require dialysis had a bilirubin of 2 mg/dl or more.[124]

Renal impairment can be classified according to the time of occurrence after HSCT (Figure 13.4). Problems that can occur shortly after HSCT include the tumor lysis syndrome (TLS) and stem cell infusion toxicity; occurring within a week. VOD usually occurs between days 10 and 28 post transplantation. Late renal complications occurring after the first month include the hemolytic–uremic syndrome (HUS) and chronic cyclosporine nephrotoxicity.

Tumor lysis syndrome

ARF after TLS is most typically observed after cytoreductive radiochemotherapy in patients with active disease and a high tumor burden.[125,126] TLS is uncommon in myeloma, but may be seen with anaplastic, rapidly proliferative disease. The common metabolic abnormalities associated with cell death of this degree are hyperuricemia, hyperkalemia, hyperphosphatemia, secondary hypocalcemia, metabolic acidosis, and azotemia. The etiology of ARF is felt to be

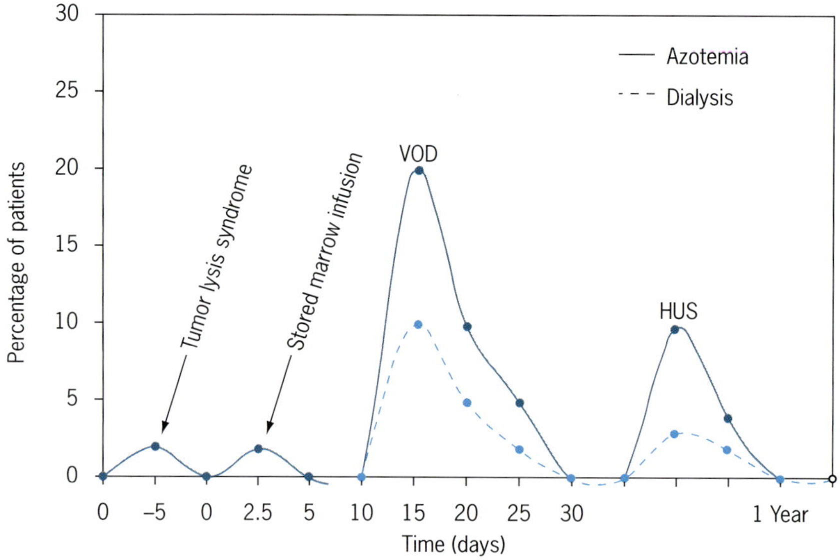

Figure 13.4 Time distribution and frequency of renal syndromes in the setting of bone marrow transplantation. The solid line depicts the approximate frequency of renal insufficiency, as defined by at least doubling of the baseline serum creatinine concentration (azotemia); the dashed line represents the frequency of dialysis-requiring ARF. During the period of conditioning, tumor lysis syndrome and stored marrow-infusion toxicity are most common; between 10 and 28 days, the peak incidence of ARF is observed, most notably due to a veno-occlusive–disease (VOD) associated hepatorenal-like syndrome. Beyond one month, the hemolytic–uremic syndrome (HUS), and less commonly chronic cyclosporine toxicity, can be observed. Reprinted with permission from Zager RA. Acute renal failure syndromes after bone marrow transplantation. *Advances in Nephrology*. Vol 27; 1997. St Louis, MO: Mosby-Year Book: 263–79.

secondary to the deposition of both phosphate and uric acid within the renal tubules.[127–129] Typically, uric acid levels will be greater than 15 mg/dl, but lesser degrees of elevation can also precipitate ARF. A urinary uric acid to creatinine ratio of greater than 1 is consistent with a diagnosis of acute uric acid nephropathy associated with TLS.[89]

Preventive measures for the development of acute uric acid nephropathy include allopurinol, forced saline diuresis, and urinary alkalinization to increase the solubility of xanthine and uric acid. Urinary alkalinization can be achieved with 100 mmol/m^2/day of sodium bicarbonate and 1 g/m^2/day of acetazolamide. Potassium supplementation may be needed to prevent hypokalemia.[91] If TLS does develop, intensive treatment with allopurinol, volume expansion, and urinary alkalinization (urinary pH $>$ 7) should be initiated promptly. Dialysis may be indicated for critical hyperkalemia as well as for marked elevations of phosphorus and uric acid. Other proteins derived from the intracellular milieu may cause ARF secondary to ATN and tubular obstruction.[130]

Nephrotoxicity related to stem cell infusion

The second early cause of ARF after HSCT is nephrotoxicity of the cryopreserved hematopoietic stem cells. This is secondary to the release of free hemoglobin during stem cell storage and thawing. Although hemoglobinuria occurs in 75–100% of HSCT patients,[131–133] ARF is rare. Clinically, these patients present with nausea, vomiting, abdominal pain, shortness of breath, or headache, and may have flushing, fever, chills, hypertension or hypotension, on physical examination.[131,134] The hemoglobin release appears to be due to red blood cell disruption secondary to the cryopreservation process as well as in vivo hemolysis from dimethylsulfoxide (DMSO).[135]

Several mechanisms exist for the induction of ARF due to heme proteins. Proximal tubular cell injury leading to tubular cell death or necrosis can be secondary to a cascade of events triggered by intracellular free-iron release.[123] Precipitation of heme proteins into tubular cast can occur both proximally and distally, leading to tubular obstruction and tubular cell damage. This occurs most frequently in an acidic urinary environment,[124,136] making urinary alkalinization an important step in therapy. Renal vasoconstriction may result secondary to scavenging of nitric oxide[137] and endothelin generation.[138] Prophylaxis both with volume expansion and with urinary alkalinization is usually adequate to prevent infusion nephrotoxicity. Studies are needed to evaluate alternative therapeutic interventions, including iron-chelation therapy, endothelin antagonist, and nitric oxide supplementation using L-arginine in pre-emptive treatment of this group of patients.[123,139–142]

Veno-occlusive disease (VOD)

Hepatic VOD closely resembles the hepatorenal syndrome (HRS),[122] and is the most common form of post-HSCT ARF occurring in the first month after transplantation. Mortality rates are as high as 40% and 90% in patients experiencing doubling of serum creatinine and requiring dialysis, respectively.[124]

VOD is usually diagnosed clinically.[143,144] Jones et al[143] define VOD as the onset of jaundice before day 21 (bilirubin $>$ 34 mmol/l) as well as two of the following: (i) hepatomegaly, (ii) ascites, and (iii) weight gain. The Jones criteria identify patients with more severe VOD and predict early mortality.[145]

Urine studies can assist with the diagnosis and evaluation of VOD: over 80% of these patients have a urine sodium concentration of less than 20–40 mmol/l, despite diuretic use.[122] This sodium retentive state is probably the earliest sign of hepatic VOD.[122,146] Supportive of a pre-renal state is a high blood urea nitrogen to creatinine ratio of more than 30 : 1 (both in mg/dl). Despite this pre-renal state, approximately 50% of patients are not oliguric at the initiation of dialysis. The urine sediment is often unremarkable, with no cellular elements or cast formation.[124,136]

The most widely accepted cause of VOD is cytoreductive chemoradiotherapy leading to fibrous narrowing of small hepatic venules and sinusoids with subendothelial edema and thrombosis with sinusoidal congestion and portal hypertension.[143,144,147,148] The risk factors associated with the development of VOD include prior liver disease, HLA-mismatched donor, age over 25 years, and selected medications.[146] Table 13.4 summarizes the risk factors for VOD/HRS and ARF.

Increased production of vasoconstrictor substances such as endothelin-1 and vasodilator substances such as nitrous oxide (NO) have been found in VOD. Renal vasoconstriction secondary to circulating endothelin-1 has been suggested as an important mediator of ARF in HRS.[149] Preliminary data in animal studies lends support to the use of endothelin antagonist and nitric oxide supplementation using L-arginine in the treatment of these patients.[140–142] Dopamine has been used in the hope of increasing renal blood flow, but any clinical benefit obtained is usually transient.[150] Preliminary data show promising results with atrial natriuretic peptide (ANP) in acute renal failure,[151] but studies in ARF patients with HRS have shown elevated levels of plasma ANP suggesting a renal insensitivity to this product.[152,153]

Table 13.4 Risk factors predisposing transplant recipients to veno-occlusive disease

- Hepatitis B or C
- Liver disease
- Vancomycin during cytoreductive therapy
- High-dose chemoradiotherapy regimen
- Acyclovir therapy before transplantation
- Mismatched graft
- Previous radiation therapy to the abdomen
- Age >25 years
- Medications
  - Estrogen/progesterone
  - Methotrexate
  - Amphotericin B
- Sepsis

Heparin plus thrombolytic therapy has been used with some success in VOD.[154] Prophylactic use of low-dose intravenous heparin, at 100 U/kg/day, in the prevention of VOD after bone marrow transplantation has resulted in significant improvement without added risk of bleeding.[155] Supportive therapy, comprising meticulous management of fluids and electrolytes, aggressive drug dosage adjustment, and dialysis, is crucial.

There are potential risks incurred by the initiation of hemodialysis in a hemodynamically unstable patient. We have conducted sustained low-efficiency dialysis (SLED) in hemodynamically unstable patients with renal failure requiring renal replacement therapy with encouraging results.[156,157]

Hemolytic–uremic syndrome

Beyond the first month after HSCT, the most common cause of ARF, with an incidence of 6%, is HUS.[158] The classic presentation of HUS includes microangiopathic hemolytic anaemia, thrombocytopenia, and end-organ damage primarily involving the kidneys and the central nervous system, beginning anywhere from a few weeks to 12 months after HSCT.[158]

The common pathophysiologic events include vascular endothelial damage, platelet aggregation, activation of the coagulation system, and red blood cell fragmentation due to the microangiopathic process.[158]

The hallmark laboratory findings are microangiopathic hemolytic anaemia with schistocytes and thrombocytopenia. Other parameters of hemolysis including elevated lactate dehydrogenase, increased indirect bilirubin, and low haptoglobin, are seen. Table 13.5 shows factors associated with the development of post-transplant HUS.[159–161]

Light-microscopic findings include microthrombi in arterioles and capillaries, thickening of capillary walls, endothelial cell swelling, and subsequent arteriolar and capillary occlusion.[162,163] HUS is poorly responsive to most interventions, and these patients usually progress to end-stage

Table 13.5 Factors associated with the development of hemolytic–uremic syndrome after transplantation

- Radiation nephritis (TBI) with increased susceptibility in children
- Conditioning chemotherapy
  - Cyclophosphamide
  - Cisplatin
- Cyclosporine
- Graft-versus-host disease
- Type of graft
  - Allograft
  - HLA-mismatch
- Bacterial infections
- Cytomegalovirus infection

renal disease if they develop ARF or require dialysis. Plasma exchange and modification of immunosuppression (cyclosporine to tacrolimus and vice versa) may be of some benefit.[159]

The current evidence appears to suggest that HUS is a result of the conditioning regimen. Endothelial cell injury is present in both HUS and radiation nephritis, and they have similar histological features.[164,165] Supporting evidence for this is that shielding of the kidney during total-body irradiation (TBI) decreases the incidence of post-HSCT HUS,[166] and the fact that HUS is seen in HSCT recipients not receiving cyclosporine.[160]

Late renal dysfunction

Late renal dysfunction after HSCT has been reported to occur in up to 17% of patients,[167] with the single most important etiology being TBI.[168] Various chemotherapeutic agents may potentiate radiation-induced nephrotoxicity. Radiation nephritis is felt to be the result of direct endothelial damage with a long latent period secondary to the slow turnover of the endothelium.[169]

It is difficult to say if acute radiation nephritis with subsequent HUS predisposes to chronic renal failure or if 'chronic radiation nephritis' develops independently of HUS.[123] TBI may lead to a 20% reduction in the glomerular filtration rate.[170] Shielding of the kidneys during TBI significantly decreases the incidence of late renal dysfunction.[166]

Chronic renal insufficiency can also develop as a result of chronic cyclosporine nephrotoxicity. Chronic cyclosporine nephrotoxicity is rare, because most allogeneic HSCT recipients take the drug for a relatively short period time (under a year). However, prolonged therapy may result in irreversible renal changes.[171] A third potential etiology of late renal dysfunction is membranous nephropathy.[172,173] There have been reports in both humans and animals suggesting that membranous nephropathy may develop in the setting of graft-versus-host disease.[174]

CONCLUSIONS

It is evident that patients with plasma cell dyscrasias can present with a whole spectrum of renal syndromes, including proteinuria, progressive renal failure, ARF, and various acid–base and electrolyte disorders. Determining the etiology may present a challenge that requires consideration of not only the underlying plasma cell dyscrasia but also complicating illnesses, medications, and procedures. Development of renal failure is not necessarily associated with a poor prognosis. Nonetheless, further improvements will require a better understanding of the pathogenic mechanisms of renal injury. Such an understanding may permit early therapeutic intervention to prevent progression of renal failure and improve prognosis.

REFERENCES

1. Kyle RA. Multiple myeloma: review of 869 cases. *Mayo Clin Proc* 1975; **50**: 29–40.
2. Martinez-Maldonado M, Yium J, Suki WN, Eknoyan G, Renal complications in multiple myeloma: pathophysiology and some aspects of clinical management. *J Chron Dis* 1971; **24**: 221–37.

3. Alexanian R, Barlogie B, Dixon D. Renal failure in multiple myeloma. *Arch Intern Med* 1990; **150**: 1693–5.
4. Knudsen LM, Hippe E, Hjorth M et al. Renal function in newly diagnosed multiple myleoma – a demographic study of 1353 patients. *Eur J Haematol* 1994; **53**: 207–12.
5. Defronzo RA, Humphrey RL, Wright JR, Cooke CR. Acute renal failure in multiple myeloma. *Medicine (Baltimore)* 1975; **543**: 209–23.
6. Cosio FG, Pence TV, Shapiro FL, Kjellstrand CM. Severe renal failure in multiple myeloma. *Clin Nephrol*. 1981; **15**: 206–10.
7. Misiani R, Tiraboschi G, Mingardi G, Mecca G. Management of myeloma kidney: an anti-light-chain approach. *Am J Kidney Dis* 1987; **10**: 28–33.
8. Iggo N, Palmer ABD, Severn A et al. Chronic dialysis in patients with multiple myeloma and renal failure: a worthwhile treatment. *QJM* 1989; **73**: 903–10.
9. Ganeval D, Cathomen M, Noel L-H, Grunfeld J-P. Kidney involvement in multiple myeloma and related disorders. *Contr Nephrol* 1982; **33**: 210–22.
10. Choukroun G, Varet B, Grunfeld J-P. Multiple myeloma. Part I: Renal involvement. *Clin Issues Nephrol* 1995; **70**: 11–17.
11. Kyle RA, Jowsey J, Kelly PJ, Taves DR. Multiple-myeloma bone disease. The comparative effect of sodium fluoride and calcium carbonate or placebo. *N Engl J Med* 1975; **293**: 1334–8.
12. Kyle RA, Bayrd ED. Amyloidosis: review of 236 cases. *Medicine* 1975; **54**: 271–99.
13. Cohen HJ, Rundles RW. Managing the complications of plasma cell myeloma. *Arch Intern Med* 1975; **135**: 177–84.
14. Fibbe WE, Jansen J. Prognostic factors in IgD myeloma: a study of 21 cases. *Scand J Haematol* 1984; **33**: 471–5.
15. Bergesio F, Salvadori M, Lombardi M et al. Renal involvement in IgD myeloma. *Scand J Urol Nephrol* 1988; **22**: 309–12.
16. Iggo N, Winearls CG, Davies DR. The development of cast nephropathy in multiple myeloma. *QJM* 1997; **90**: 653–6.
17. Ganeval D, Rabian C, Guerin V et al. Treatment of multiple myeloma with renal involvement. *Adv Nephrol* 1992; **21**: 347–70.
18. Pozzi C, Pasquali S, Donini U et al. Prognostic factors and effectiveness of treatment in acute renal failure due to multiple myeloma: a review of 50 cases. *Clin Nephrol* 1987; **28**: 1–9.
19. Sanders PW, Herrera GA, Kirk KA et al. Spectrum of glomerular and tubulointerstitial renal lesions associated with monotypical immunoglobulin light chain deposition. *Lab Invest* 1991; **64**: 527–37.
20. Pirani CL, Silva F, D'Agati V et al. Renal lesions in plasma cell dyscrasias: ultrastructural observations. *Am J Kidney Dis* 1987; **10**: 208–21.
21. Picken MM, Shen S. Immunoglobulin light chain and the kidney: an overview. *Ultrastruct Pathol* 1994; **18**: 105–12.
22. Iggo N, Parsons V. Renal disease in multiple myeloma: current perspectives. *Nephron* 1990; **56**: 229–33.
23. Levi DF, Williams RC, Lindstrom FD. Immunofluorescent studies of the myeloma kidney with special reference to light chain disease. *Am J Med* 1968; **44**: 922–33.
24. DeFronzo RA, Cooke CR, Wright JR, Humphrey RL. Renal function in patients with multiple myeloma. *Medicine (Baltimore)* 1978; **57**: 151–66.
25. Johnson WJ, Kyle RA, Pineda AA et al. Treatment of renal failure associated with multiple myeloma: plasmapheresis, hemodialysis, and chemotherapy. *Arch Intern Med* 1990; **150**: 863–9.
26. Pasquali S, Zucchelli P, Casanova S et al. Renal histological lesions and clinical syndromes in multiple myeloma. *Clin Nephrol* 1987; **27**: 222–8.
27. Pasquali S, Casanova S, Zucchelli A, Zucchelli P. Long-term survival patients with acute and severe renal failure due to multiple myeloma. *Clin Nephrol* 1990; **34**: 247–54.
28. Pozzi C, Fogazzi GB, Banfi G et al. Renal disease and patient survival in light chain deposition disease. *Clin Nephrol* 1995; **43**: 281–7.
29. Droz D, Noel LH, Carnot F et al. Liver involvement in nonamyloid light chain deposits disease. *Lab Invest* 1984; **50**: 683–9.
30. Staros E, Katz SM. Myocardial necrosis in light chain deposition. *Am Heart J* 1985; **110**: 1295–6.
31. Vital C, Pautrizel B, Lagueny A et al. Hypermyelination in a case of peripheral neuropathy with benign IgM monoclonal gammopathy. *Rev Neurol (Paris)* 1985; **141**: 729–34.
32. Bedossa P, Fabre M, Paraf F et al. Light chain deposition disease with liver dysfunction. *Hum Pathol* 1988; **19**: 1008–14.
33. McAllister HA, Seger J, Bossart M, Ferrans VJ. Restrictive cardiomyopathy with kappa light chains deposits in myocardium as a complication of multiple myeloma. Histochemical and electron microscopic observations. *Arch Pathol Lab Med* 1988; **112**: 1151–4.

34. Jancelewicz Z, Takatsuki K, Sugai S, Pruzanski W. IgD multiple myeloma. *Arch Intern Med* 1975; **135**: 87–93.
35. Stone MJ, Frendel EP. The clinical spectrum of light chain myeloma. A study of 35 patients with special reference to the occurrence of amyloidosis. *Am J Med* 1975; **58**: 601–19.
36. Solomon A, Frangione B, Franklin EC. Bence Jones proteins and light chains of immunoglobulins. *J Clin Invest* 1982; **70**: 453–60.
37. Maldonado JE, Velosa JA, Kyle RA et al. Fanconi syndrome in adults, a manifestation of a latent form of myeloma. *Am J Med* 1975; **58**: 354–64.
38. Dragsted PJ, Hjorth N. The association of the Fanconi syndrome with malignant disease. *Danish Med Bull* 1956; **3**: 177–9.
39. Horn ME, Knapp MS, Page FT, Walker WH. Adult Fanconi syndrome and multiple myelomatosis. *J Clin Pathol* 1969; **22**: 414–16.
40. Headley RN, King JS, Cooper MR, Felts JH. Multiple myeloma presenting as adult Fanconi syndrome. *Clin Chem* 1972; **18**: 293–5.
41. Lee DB, Drinkard JP, Rosen VJ, Gonick HC. The adult Fanconi syndrome: observations on etiology, morphology, renal function and mineral metabolism in three patients. *Medicine (Baltimore)* 1972; **51**: 107–38.
42. Finkel PN, Kronenberg K, Pesce AJ et al. Adult Fanconi syndrome, amyloidosis and marked kappa-light chain proteinuria. *Nephron* 1973; **10**: 1–24.
43. Sirota JH, Hamerman D. Renal function studies in an adult subject with the Fanconi syndrome. *Am J Med* 1954; **16**: 138–52.
44. Dedmon RE, West JH, Schwartz TB. The adult Fanconi syndrome: report of two cases, one with multiple myeloma. *Med Clin North Am* 1963; **47**: 191–206.
45. Aucouturier P, Bauwens M, Khamlichi AA et al. Monoclonal Ig L chain and L chain V domain fragment crystallization in myeloma-associated Fanconi's syndrome. *J Immunol* 1993; **150**: 3561–8.
46. Orfila C, Lepert JC, Modesto A et al. Fanconi's syndrome, kappa light-chain myeloma, non-amyloid fibrils and cytoplasmic crystals in renal tubular epithelium. *Am J Nephrol* 1991; **11**: 345–9.
47. Troung LD, Mawad J, Cagle P, Mattioli C. Cytoplasmic crystals in multiple myeloma-associated Fanconi's syndrome. A morphological study including immunoelectron microscopy. *Arch Pathol Lab Med* 1989; **113**: 781–5.
48. Bergman LW, Kuehl WM. Co-translational modification of nascent immunoglobulin heavy and light chains. *J Supramol Struct* 1979; **11**: 9–24.
49. Baumal R, Scharff MD. Synthesis, assembly and secretion of mouse immunoglobulin. *Transplant Rev* 1973; **14**: 163–83.
50. Shapiro AL, Scharff MD, Maizel JV, Uhr JW. Synthesis of excess light chains of gamma globulin by rabbit lymph node cells. *Nature* 1966; **211**: 243–5.
51. Edelman GM, Gally JA. The nature of Bence-Jones proteins' chemical similarities to polypeptide chains of myeloma globulins and normal gamma-globulins. *J Exp Med* 1962; **116**: 207–27.
52. Baylis C, Folconer-Smith J, Ross B. Glomerular and tubular handling of differently charged human immunoglobulin light chains by the rat kidney. *Clin Sci* 1988; **74**: 639–44.
53. Pesce AJ, Clyne DH, Pollak VE et al. Renal tubular interactions of proteins. *Clin Biochem* 1980; **13**: 209–15.
54. Maack T, Johnson V, Kau ST, Figueiredo J, Sigulem D. Renal filtration, transport, and metabolism of low-molecular-weight proteins: a review. *Kidney Int* 1979; **16**: 251–70.
55. Sanders PW, Herrera GA. Monoclonal immunoglobulin light chain-related renal diseases. *Semin Nephrol* 1993; **13**: 324–41.
56. Koss MN, Pirani CL, Osserman EF. Experimental Bence Jones cast nephropathy. *Lab Invest* 1976; **34**: 579–91.
57. Solomon A, Weiss DT, Kattine AA. Nephrotoxic potential of Bence Jones proteins. *N Engl J Med* 1991; **324**: 1845–51.
58. Huang ZQ, Sanders PW. Biochemical interaction between Tamm–Horsfall glycoprotein and Ig light chains in the pathogenesis of cast nephropathy. *Lab Invest* 1995; **73**: 810–17.
59. Sanders PW, Booker BB. Pathobiology of cast nephropathy from human Bence Jones proteins. *J Clin Invest* 1992; **89**: 630–9.
60. Sanders PW, Booker BB, Bishop JB, Cheung HC. Mechanisms of intranephronal proteinaceous cast formation by low molecular weight proteins. *J Clin Invest* 1990; **85**: 570–6.
61. Coward RA, Delamore IW, Mallick NP, Robinson EL. The importance of urinary immunoglobulin light chain isoelectric point (pI) in nephrotoxicity in multiple myeloma. *Clin Sci* 1984; **66**: 229–32.
62. Clyne DH, Pesce AJ, Thompson RE. Nephrotoxicity of Bence Jones proteins in the rat:

importance of protein isoelectric point. *Kidney Int* 1979; **16**: 345–52.
63. Clyne DH, Kant KS, Pesce AJ, Pollak VE. Nephrotoxicity of low molecular weight serum proteins: physicochemical interactions between myoglobulin, hemoglobulin, Bence-Jones proteins and Tamm–Horsfall mucoprotein. *Curr Probl Clin Biochem* 1979; **9**: 299–308.
64. Weiss JH, Williams RH, Galla JH et al. Pathophysiology of acute Bence-Jones protein nephrotoxicity in the rat. *Kidney Int* 1981; **20**: 198–210.
65. Smolens P, Barnes JL, Stein JH. Effect of chronic administration of different Bence Jones proteins on rat kidney. *Kidney Int* 1986; **30**: 874–82.
66. Melcion C, Mougenot B, Baudouin B et al. Renal failure in myeloma: relationship with isoelectric point of immunoglobulin light chains. *Clin Nephrol* 1984; **22**: 138–43.
67. Johns EA, Turner R, Cooper EH, MacLennan ICM. Isoelectric points of urinary light chains in myelomatosis: analysis in relation to nephrotoxicity. *J Clin Pathol* 1986; **39**: 833–7.
68. Solling K, Solling J, Nielsen JL. Polymeric Bence Jones proteins in serum in myeloma patients with renal insufficiency. *Acta Med Scand* 1984; **216**: 495–502.
69. Sanders PW. Pathogenesis and treatment of myeloma kidney. *J Lab Clin Med* 1994; **124**: 484–8.
70. Chomdeg B, Bell PD, Navar LG. Renal hemodynamic and autoregulatory responses to acute hypercalcemia. *Am J Physiol* 1977; **232**: F490–6.
71. Humes HD, Ichikawa I, Troy JL, Brenner BM. Evidence for a parathyroid hormone-dependent influence of calcium on the glomerular ultrafiltration coefficient. *J Clin Invest* 1978; **61**: 32–40.
72. Smolens P, Barnes JL, Kreisberg R. Hypercalcemia can potentiate the nephrotoxicity of Bence Jones proteins. *J Lab Clin Med* 1987; **110**: 460–5.
73. Stevenson FK, Cleave AJ, Kent PW. The effect of ions on the viscometric and ultracentrifugal behaviour of Tamm–Horsfall glycoprotein. *Biochim Biophys Acta* 1971; **236**: 59–66.
74. Hoitsma AJ, Wetzels JF, Koene RA. Drug-induced nephrotoxicity. Aetiology, clinical features and management. *Drug Saf* 1991; **6**: 131–47.
75. Rashed A, Azadeh B, Abu Romeh SH. Acyclovir-induced acute tubulo-interstitial nephritis. *Nephron* 1990; **56**: 436–8.
76. Becker BN, Fall P, Hall C et al. Rapidly progressive acute renal failure due to acyclovir: case report and review of the literature. *Am J Kidney Dis* 1993; **22**: 611–15.
77. Fabrizzi V, Thalhammer F, Horl WH. Aminoglycoside-induced nephrotoxicity. *Wien Klin Wochenschr* 1997; **109**: 830–5.
78. Swan SK. Aminoglycoside nephrotoxicity. *Semin Nephrol* 1997; **17**: 27–33.
79. Whelton A. Therapeutic initiatives for the avoidance of aminoglycoside toxicity. *J Clin Pharmacol* 1985; **25**: 67–81.
80. Sawaya BP, Weihprecht H, Campbell WR et al. Direct vasoconstriction as a possible cause for amphotericin B-induced nephrotoxicity in rats. *J Clin Invest* 1991; **87**: 2097–107.
81. Fisher MA, Talbot GH, Maislin G et al. Risk factors for amphotericin B-associated nephrotoxicity. *Am J Med* 1989; **87**: 547–52.
82. Sabra R, Takahashi K, Branch RA, Badr KF. Mechanisms of amphotericin B-induced reduction in the glomerular filtration rate: a micropuncture study. *J Pharmacol Exp Ther* 1990; **253**: 34–7.
83. Mehta J, Kelsey SM, Chu P et al. Amphotericin B lipid complex (ABLC) for the treatment of confirmed or presumed fungal infections in immunocompromised patients with hematologic malignancies. *Bone Marrow Transplant* 1997; **20**: 39–43.
84. Yussim E, Schwartz E, Sidi Y, Ehrenfeld M. Acute renal failure precipitated by non-steroidal anti-inflammatory drugs (NSAIDs) in multiple myeloma. *Am J Hematol* 1998; **58**: 142–4.
85. Shpilberg O, Douer D, Ehrenfeld M et al. Naproxen-associated fatal acute renal failure in multiple myeloma. *Nephron* 1990; **55**: 448–9.
86. Wu MJ, Kumar KS, Kulkarni G, Kaiser H. Multiple myeloma in naproxen-induced acute renal failure. *N Engl J Med* 1987; **317**: 170–1.
87. McCarthy CS, Becker JA. Multiple myeloma and contract media. *Radiology*.1992; **183**: 519–21.
88. Winearls CG. Acute myeloma kidney. *Kidney Int* 1995; **48**: 1347–61.
89. Kelton J, Kelley WN, Holmes EW. A rapid method for the diagnosis of acute uric acid nephropathy. *Arch Intern Med* 1978; **138**: 612–15.
90. Crittenden DR, Ackerman GL. Hyperuricemic acute renal failure in disseminated carcinoma. *Arch Intern Med* 1977; **137**: 97–9.
91. Barri YM, Shah SV. Prevention and nondialytic management of acute renal failure. In: *Current Therapy in Nephrology and Hypertension*, 4th edn

(Glassock RJ, ed). St Louis, MO: Mosby, 1998: 240–8.
92. Feest TG, Burge PS, Cohen SL. Successful treatment of myeloma kidney by diuresis and plasmaphoresis. *BMJ* 1976; **i**: 503–7.
93. Misiani R, Remuzzi G, Bertani T et al. Plasmapheresis in the treatment of acute renal failure in multiple myeloma. *Am J Med* 1979; **66**: 684–8.
94. Locatelli F, Pozzi C, Pedrini L et al. Steroid pulses and plasmapheresis in the treatment of acute renal failure in multiple myeloma. *Proc EDTA* 1980; **17**: 690–4.
95. Zucchelli P, Pasquali S, Cagnoli L, Ferrari G. Controlled plasma exchange trial in acute renal failure due to multiple myeloma. *Kidney Int* 1988; **33**: 1175–80.
96. Torra R, Blade J, Cases A et al. Patients with multiple myeloma requiring long-term dialysis: presenting features, response to therapy, and outcome in a series of 20 cases. *Br J Haematol* 1995; **91**: 854–9.
97. Rosansky SJ, Richards FW. Use of peritoneal dialysis in the treatment of patients with renal failure and paraproteinemia. *Am J Nephrol* 1985; **5**: 361–5.
98. Nolph KD, Ghods AJ, Brown PA, Twardowski ZJ. Effects of intraperitoneal nitroprusside on peritoneal clearances in man with variations of dose, frequency of administration and dwell times. *Nephron* 1979; **24**: 114–20.
99. Solling K, Solling J. Clearances of Bence-Jones proteins during peritoneal dialysis or plasmapheresis in myelomatosis associated with renal failure. *Contrib Nephrol* 1988; **68**: 259–62.
100. Tapson JS, Mansy H, Wilkinson R. End-stage renal failure due to multiple myeloma – poor survival on peritoneal dialysis. *Int J Artif Organs* 1988; **11**: 39–42.
101. Shetty A, Oreopoulos DG. Myeloma patients do well on CAPD too! *Br J Haematol* 1997; **96**: 654–7.
102. Bergsagel DE. The role of chemotherapy in the treatment of multiple myeloma. *Baillière's Clin Haematol* 1995; **8**: 783–94.
103. Walker F, Bear RA. Renal transplantation in light-chain multiple myeloma. *Am J Nephrol* 1983; **3**: 34–7.
104. Humphrey RL, Wright JR, Zachary JB et al. Renal transplantation in multiple myeloma. *Ann Int Med* 1975; **83**: 651–3.
105. Martin DW, Siegel RC, Smith LH. The kidney in multiple myeloma. *Western J Med* 1978; **129**: 41–8.
106. Spence RK, Hill GS, Goldwein MI et al. Renal transplantation for end-stage myeloma kidney. *Arch Surg* 1979; **114**: 950–2.
107. De Lima JJG, Kourilsky O, Meyrier A, Sraer J-D. Kidney transplant in multiple myeloma. *Transplantation* 1981; **31**: 223–4.
108. Scully RE, Galdabini JJ, McNeely BU. Case records of the Massachusetts General Hospital: Case 1–1981. *N Engl J Med* 1981; **304**: 33–43.
109. Briefel GR, Spees EK, Humphrey RL et al. Renal transplantation in a patient with multiple myeloma and light chain nephropathy. *Surgery* 1983; **93**: 579–84.
110. Gerlag PGG, Koene RAP, Berden JHM. Renal transplantation in light chain nephropathy: case report and review of the literature. *Clin Nephrol* 1986; **25**: 101–4.
111. Passweg J, Bock HA, Tichelli A, Thiel G. Transient multiple myeloma after intense immunosuppression in a renal transplant patient. *Nephrol Dial Transplant* 1993; **8**: 1393–4.
112. Sammett D, Dagher F, Abbi R et al. Renal transplantation in multiple myeloma. *Transplantation* 1996; **62**: 1577–80.
113. Howard AD, Moore J, Tomaszewski M-M. Occurrence of multiple myeloma three years after successful renal transplantation. *Am J Kidney Dis* 1987; **10**: 147–50.
114. Brown JH, Newstead CG, Jos V et al. Multiple myeloma in a renal transplant recipient. *Nephrol Dial Transplant* 1992; **7**: 447–9.
115. Aparicio M, de Precigout V, Reiffers J et al. Multiple myeloma and AL amyloidosis in a renal transplant recipient. *Nephron* 1989; **53**: 373–5.
116. Radl J, Valentijn RM, Haaijman JJ, Paul LC. Monoclonal gammapathies in patients undergoing immunosuppressive treatment after renal transplantation. *Clin Immunol Immunopathol* 1985; **37**: 98–102.
117. Renoult E, Bertrand F, Kessler M. Monoclonal gammopathies in HBsAg-positive patients with renal transplants. *N Engl J Med* 1988; **318**: 1205.
118. Penn I. Multiple myeloma in a renal transplant recipient. *Am J Kidney Dis* 1988; **11**: 201.
119. Peest D, Burkardt S, Bjorn N et al. High incidence of monoclonal immunoglobulins in patients after liver or heart transplantation. *Transplantation* 1988; **46**: 389–93.
120. Kyle RA, Greipp PR. The laboratory investigation of monoclonal gammopathies. *Mayo Clin Proc* 1978; **53**: 719–39.

121. Stanko CK, Jeffery JR, Rush DN. Monoclonal and multiclonal gammopathies after renal transplantation. *Transplant Proc* 1989; **21**: 3330–2.
122. Zager RA. Acute renal failure in the setting of bone marrow transplantation. *Kidney Int* 1994; **46**: 1443–1458.
123. Zager RA. Acute renal failure syndromes after bone marrow transplantation. *Adv Nephrol* 1998; **27**: :263–79.
124. Zager RA, O'Quigley J, Zager BK et al. Acute renal failure following bone marrow transplantation: a retrospective study of 272 patients. *Am J Kidney Dis* 1989; **13**: 210–16.
125. Nomdedeu J, Martino R, Sureda A H et al. Acute tumor lysis syndrome complicating conditioning therapy for bone marrow transplantation in a patient with chronic lymphocytic leukemia. *Bone Marrow Transplant* 1994; **13**: 659–60.
126. Fleming DR, Henslee-Downey PJ, Coffey CW. Radiation induced acute tumor lysis syndrome in the bone marrow transplant setting. *Bone Marrow Transplant* 1991; **8**: 235–6.
127. Conger JD. Acute uric acid nephropathy. *Med Clin North Am* 1990; **74**: 859–71.
128. Jones DP, Mahmound H, Chesney RW. Tumor lysis syndrome: pathogenesis and management. *Pediatr Nephrol* 1995; **9**: 206–12.
129. Kjellstrand CM, Cambell DC, von Hartitzsch B, Buselmeier TJ. Hyperuricemic acute renal failure. *Arch Intern Med* 1974; **133**: 349–59.
130. Zager RA. Precipitable tissue proteins can cause experimental acute renal failure. *Lab Invest* 1988; **59**: 798–808.
131. Okamoto Y, Takaue Y, Saito S et al. Toxicities associated with cryopreserved and thawed peripheral blood stem cell autografts in children with active cancer. *Transfusion* 1993; **33**: 578–81.
132. Kessinger A, Schmit-Pokorny D, Smith D, Armitage J. Cryopreservation and infusion of autologous peripheral blood stem cells. *Bone Marrow Transplant* 1990; **5**(Suppl 1): 25–7.
133. Smith DM, Weisenburger DD, Bierman P et al.. Acute renal failure associated with autologous bone marrow transplantation. *Bone Marrow Transplant* 1987; **2**: 195–210.
134. Davis JM, Rowley SC, Braine HG et al. Clinical toxicity of cryopreserved bone marrow graft infusion. *Blood* 1990; **75**: 781–6.
135. Yellowlees P, Greenfield C, McIntyre N. Dimethylsulphoxide-induced toxicity. *Lancet* 1980; **ii:** 1004–6.
136. Zager RA. Studies of mechanisms and protective maneuvers in myoglobinuric acute renal injury. *Lab Invest* 1989; **60**: 619–29.
137. Maree A, Peer G, Schwartz D et al. Role of nitric oxide in glycerol-induced acute renal failure in rats. *Nephrol Dial Transplant* 1994; **9**(Suppl 4): 78–81.
138. Karam H, Bruneval P, Clozel J-P et al. Role of endothelin in acute renal failure due to rhabdomyolysis in rats. *J Pharmacol Exp Ther* 1995; **274**: 481–6.
139. Zager RA. Rhabdomyolysis and myohemoglobinuric acute renal failure. *Kidney Int* 1996; **49**: 314–26.
140. Krause SM, Walsh TF, Greenlee WJ et al. Renal protection by a dual ETA/ETB endothelin antagonist, L-754,142, after aortic cross-clamping in the dog. *J Am Soc Nephrol* 1997; **8**: 1061–71.
141. Schramm L, Heidbreder E, Lopau K et al. Influence of nitric oxide on renal function in toxic acute renal failure in the rat. *Miner Electrolyte Metab* 1996; **22**: 168–77.
142. Ito S, Carretero OA, Abe K. Nitric oxide in the regulation of renal blood flow. *New Horiz* 1995; **3**: 615–23.
143. Jones RJ, Lee KSK, Beschorner WE et al. Venoocclusive disease of the liver following bone marrow transplantation. *Transplantation* 1987; **44**: 778–83.
144. McDonald GB, Sharma P, Matthews DE et al. Venoocclusive disease of the liver after bone marrow transplantation: diagnosis, incidence, and predisposing factors. *Hepatology* 1984; **4**: 116–22.
145. Blostein MD, Paltiel OB, Thibault A, Rybka WB. A comparison of clinical criteria for the diagnosis of veno-occlusive disease of the liver after bone marrow transplantation. *Bone Marrow Transplant* 1992; **10**: 439–43.
146. McDonald GB, Hinds MS, Fisher LD et al. Veno-occlusive disease of the liver and multiorgan failure after bone marrow transplantation: a cohort study of 355 patients. *Ann Intern Med* 1993; **118**: 255–67.
147. Ganem G, Saint-Marc Girardin MF, Kuentz M et al. Venoocclusive disease of the liver after allogeneic bone marrow transplantation in man. *Int J Radiat Oncol Biol Phys* 1988; **14**: 879–84.
148. Rollins BJ. Hepatic veno-occlusive disease. *Am J Med* 1986; **81:** 297–306.
149. Moore K, Wendon J, Frazer M et al. Plasma endothelin immunoreactivity in liver disease and

the hepatorenal syndrome. *N Engl J Med* 1992; **327**: 1774–8.
150. Graziani G, Casati S, Cantaluppi A et al. Dopamine-frusemide therapy in acute renal failure. *Proc Eur Dial Transplant Assoc* 1983; **19**: 319–24.
151. Rahman SN, Kim GE, Mathew AS et al. Effects of atrial natriuretic peptide in clinical acute renal failure. *Kidney Int* 1994; **45**: 1731–8.
152. Pasqualetti P, Casale R. The atrial natriuretic peptide–renin–aldosterone system in hepatorenal syndrome. *Riv Eur Sci Med Farmacol* 1996; **18**: 137–41.
153. Morgan TR, Imada T, Hollister AS, Inagami T. Plasma human atrial natriuretic factor in cirrhosis and ascites with and without functional renal failure. *Gastroenterology* 1988; **95**: 1641–7.
154. Bearman SI, Shuhart MC, Hinds MS, McDonald GB. Recombinant human tissue plasminogen activator for the treatment of established severe venoocclusive disease of the liver after bone marrow transplantation. *Blood* 1992; **80**: 2458–62.
155. Attal M, Huguet F, Rubie H et al. Prevention of hepatic veno-occlusive disease after bone marrow transplantation by continuous infusion of low-dose heparin: a prospective, randomized trial. *Blood* 1992; **79**: 2834–40.
156. Chatoth DK, Shaver MJ, Marshall MR, Golper TA. Daily 12-hour sustained low-efficiency hemodialysis (SLED) for the treatment of critically ill patients with acute renal failure (ARF): initial experience. *Blood Purification* 1999; **17**: 29 (abst).
157. Shaver MJ, Marshall MR, Chatoth DK et al. Adequacy, solute and acid-base control with daily sustained low-efficiency hemodialysis (SLED) for acute renal failure. *Blood Purification* 1999; **17**: 36. (abst).
158. Pettitt AR, Clark RE. Thrombotic microangiopathy following bone marrow transplantation. *Bone Marrow Transplant* 1994; **14**: 495–504.
159. Juckett M, Perry EH, Daniels BS, Weisdorf DJ. Hemolytic uremic syndrome following bone marrow transplantation. *Bone Marrow Transplant* 1991; **7**: 405–9.
160. Rabinowe SN, Soiffer RJ, Tarbell NJ et al. Hemolytic–uremic syndrome following bone marrow transplantation in adults for hematologic malignancies. *Blood* 1991; **77**: 1837–44.
161. Van Why SK, Friedman AL, Wei LJ, Hong R. Renal insufficiency after bone marrow transplantation in children. *Bone Marrow Transplant* 1991; **7**: 383–8.
162. Antignac C, Gubler M-C, Leverger G et al. Delayed renal failure with extensive mesangiolysis following bone marrow transplantation. *Kidney Int* 1989; **35**: 1336–44.
163. Iskandar SS, Browning MC, Lorentz WB. Mesangiolytic glomerulopathy in a bone marrow allograft recipient. *Hum Pathol* 1989; **20**: 290–2.
164. Down JD, Berman AJ, Wahrol M et al. Late complications following total body irradiation and bone marrow rescue in mice: Predominance of glomerular nephropathy and hemolytic anemia. *Int J Radiat Biol Phys* 1990; **57**: 551–65.
165. Moulder JE, Fish BL. Late toxicity of total body irradiation with bone marrow transplantation in a rat model. *Int J Radiat Oncol Biol Phys* 1989; **16**: 1501–9.
166. Lawton CA, Barber-Derus SW, Murray KJ et al. Influence of renal shielding on the incidence of late renal dysfunction associated with T-lymphocyte deplete bone marrow transplantation in adult patients. *Int J Radiat Oncol Biol Phys* 1992; **23**: 681–6.
167. Lonnerholm G, Carlson K, Bratteby LE et al. Renal function after autologous bone marrow transplantation. *Bone Marrow Transplant* 1991; **8**: 129–34.
168. Kamil ES, Latta H, Johnston WH et al. Radiation nephritis following bone marrow transplantation. *Kidney Int* 1978; **14**: 713.
169. Krochak RJ, Baker DG. Radiation nephritis. Clinical manifestations and pathophysiologic mechanisms. *Urology* 1986; **27**: 389–93.
170. Leblond V, Sutton L, Jacquiaud C et al. Evaluation of renal function in 60 long term survivors of bone marrow transplantation. *J Am Soc Nephrol* 1995; **6**: 1661–5.
171. Dieterle A, Gratwohl A, Nizze H et al. Chronic cyclosporine-associated nephrotoxicity in bone marrow transplant patients. *Transplantation* 1990; **49**: 1093–100.
172. Hiesse C, Goldschmidt E, Santelli G et al. Membranous nephropathy in a bone narrow transplant recipient. *Am J Kidney Dis* 1988; **11**: 188–91.
173. Muller GA, Muller CA, Markovic-Lipkowski J et al. Membranous nephropathy after bone marrow transplantation in ciclosporin treatment. *Nephron* 1989; **51**: 555–6.
174. Barbara JAJ, Thomas AC, Smith PS et al. Membranous nephropathy with graft-versus-host disease in a bone marow transplant recipient. *Clin Nephrol* 1992; **37**: 115–18.

14

Infections: Principles of prevention and therapy

Peter Kelleher, Helen Chapel

INTRODUCTION

Infections play an important role in the morbidity and mortality associated with myeloma. The predominant pathogens isolated from patients with myeloma are bacterial, which reflects the defect in humoral immunity seen in this condition. The principal immune deficits associated with infection are a reduction in polyclonal immunoglobulin synthesis and a failure to make appropriate antibody responses post immunization. The timing of serious infection varies with the phase of disease. Preliminary studies show that antimicrobial prophylaxis significantly reduces the rate of serious infection in the initial phase of disease. Immunoglobulin replacement therapy is effective as primary infection prophylaxis in the stable phase of disease.

In addition to discussing infectious complications in myeloma, this chapter will briefly review the possible role of infection in the pathogenesis of the disease.

CONTRIBUTION OF INFECTION TO THE PATHOGENESIS OF MYELOMA

The detection of human herpesvirus-8 (HHV-8; also known as Kaposi sarcoma-associated herpesvirus, KSHV) DNA in bone marrow dendritic cells obtained from patients with myeloma raised the intriguing possibility that this virus may be implicated in the pathogenesis of myeloma (Figure 14.1).[1] This virus encodes for a protein similar to interleukin-6 (IL-6), which is an important growth factor for myeloma cells.[2–5] Conflicting results have been reported by several groups on whether this virus is present in bone marrow dendritic cells of patients with myeloma[6–17] (Chapter 3). It has been suggested that differences in methods used to detect this virus or the presence of different strains of HHV-8 (in Kaposi sarcoma compared with myeloma) may explain the contrasting results of viral DNA studies to date. It is not yet known if biologically active HHV-8 gene products are present in myeloma. At the moment, the jury is still out on the possible pathogenic relationship between HHV-8 and myeloma, but, if confirmed, this finding would have important implications for the prevention and treatment of plasma cell disorders.

INCIDENCE OF INFECTION

A number of studies published between 1953 and 1963 showed that infections occurred often

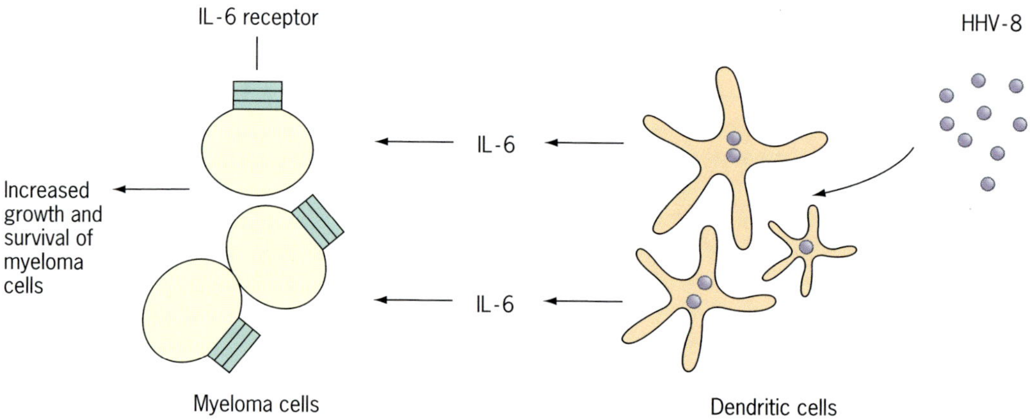

Figure 14.1 Paracrine effects of human herpesvirus-8 (HHV-8)-infected dendritic cells in the pathogenesis of myeloma.

as a complication of myeloma.[18–21] In these studies, the increased incidence of bacterial pneumonia was emphasized, and the risk of recurrent bacterial infection highlighted. Most of these studies were unable to estimate the risk of infection in myeloma, since they lacked both normal and other disease-related controls. More systematic reports estimated the risk of infection in patients with myeloma. Twomey[22] demonstrated that patients with myeloma have 15 times more infections per year than hospitalized control patients with ischaemic heart disease.[22] In this study, the majority of infections were confirmed either microbiologically or at autopsy, and included bacteria, viruses, and fungi. In another study, the annual rate of cultured bacterial infection in patients with myeloma was seven times greater than that of hospital inpatients and three times the rate of patients with Waldenström's macroglobinaemia.[21]

The overall incidence of infection in myeloma ranges from 0.8 to 2.2 infections per patient-year.[23] The reasons for the variation in incidence probably reflect differences in the definition and classification of infection, patient characteristics, and the duration of patient follow-up. A study of 102 patients with myeloma who were monitored prospectively for one year confirmed the high incidence and risk of recurrent infection in this disorder.[24] In this study, 56 patients (55%) suffered one infection, and 22 patients (22%) experienced more than one infection. Most infections in this report were not microbiologically confirmed, depending on clinical, radiological, and laboratory findings (Table 14.1).

TYPES OF INFECTION

The principal sites of infection are the respiratory tract, the urinary tract, and the skin.[19,21,24] Septicaemia occurs less frequently but it does cause significant morbidity and mortality in this patient group (Table 14.1).

Table 14.1 The distribution of serious infections (n = 78) in patients with myeloma[24]

Respiratory tract	40
Blood	11
Urinary tract	10
Skin	8
Other sites	6
Pyrexia of unknown origin	5

Serious infections were defined as septicaemia, meningitis, pneumonia (radiological evidence), fever of unknown origin (cullture-negative), bronchitis, urinary tract infection, skin abscess/cellulitis, localized herpes zoster, and an upper respiratory tract infection complicated by secondary bactgerial infection.

Streptococcus pneumoniae is the commonest organism isolated in respiratory tract infection in myeloma.[19–21] *Haemophilus influenzae*[22,25] and Gram-negative organisms[26,27] have also been implicated in respiratory tract infections.

Gram-negative organisms such as *Escherichia coli, Pseudomonas, Klebsiella* and *Enterobacter* spp. and *Proteus mirabilis* are commonly found in urinary tract infections.[21,26,27] The commonest organisms that are associated with septicaemia are *S. pneumoniae*, *Staphylococcus aureus*, *E. coli* and *Pseudomonas* spp.[25,26,28] *S. aureus* infection is the most common isolate in skin infections.[25]

The only viral infection that has been consistently reported in studies of patients with myeloma is herpes zoster.[22,24,25,27] This infection, however, is common in aged-matched controls and in those treated with chemotherapy: it is therefore unlikely that herpes zoster is specifically associated with myeloma. Systemic, fungal, protozoal, and mycobacterial infections are uncommon in patients with myeloma.[23]

TIMING OF INFECTION

There is a clear relationship between the length of time after the initial diagnosis of myeloma and susceptibility to infections (Figure 14.2). Infections are also more frequent when chemotherapy is used. The risk of infection has been correlated with disease progression using criteria devised by the UK Medical Research Council to define plateau phase in myeloma.[29] All newly diagnosed patients are designated as being in induction phase. Plateau phase is defined as minimal disease symptoms or asymptomatic patients with stable paraprotein and β_2-microglobulin measurements over three months. Patients receiving chemotherapy for recurrence of symptoms are categorized as having relapsed or progressive disease.

A small proportion of patients with myeloma (5–14%) present initially with infection.[9,26] The risk of infection is high in the induction phase[24,28] when patients receive induction chemotherapy; it then declines in plateau-phase disease and in those who respond to chemotherapy. Finally, relapsed disease or progressive disease is associated with a rising incidence of infection.[24,26,28] In one study, there were 1.58 serious infections per patient-year in the induction phase, compared with 0.49 in the plateau phase and 1.90 during relapsed/progressive disease.[24]

The spectrum of bacterial infection varies with the phase of the illness. Although pneumococcal pneumonia was the commonest infection described in early studies of patients with myeloma,[17–21] more recent data indicate that there has been an increase in the overall incidence of infection and in the proportion of Gram-negative bacteria.[23,25]

Infections with *S. pneumoniae* and *H. influenzae* have been noted in patients who present with myeloma and in the first six months post diagnosis.[20,26] The same organisms are responsible for the majoirity of infections that occur in patients responding to chemotherapy and in the plateau phase of disease.[24,26] Episodes of infection with Gram-negative organisms have been described in the initial phase of disease, particularly in individuals who are on induction chemotherapy[28] and in patients who experience relapse.[26]

SEVERITY OF INFECTION

Infection is a major contributor to morbidity and mortality in myeloma. Rayner and colleagues[25] estimated that infection in myeloma was associated with a 2.75-fold increased risk of death, independent of other risk factors. In two studies, infection was a significant factor in the cause of death in one-third of patients with myeloma.[19,28] In a prospective study of 102 individuals with myeloma, bacterial infection was the primary cause of death in 11 patients.[24] Recurrent infection is a feature of myeloma occurring in approximately 20% of patients.[24,25]

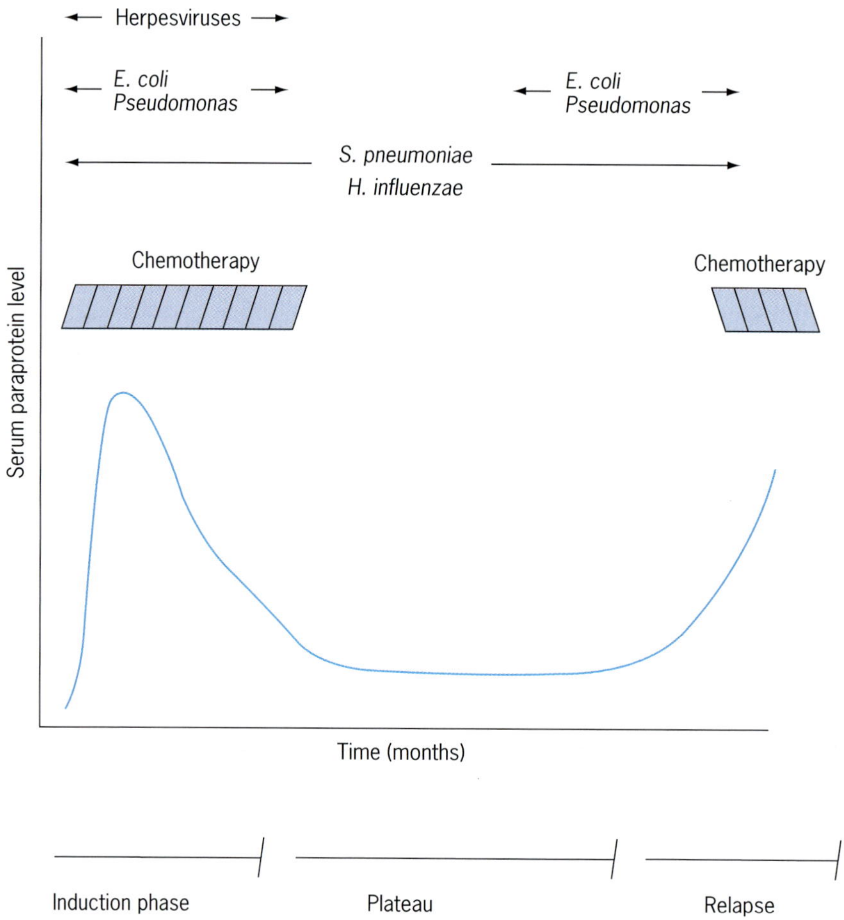

Figure 14.2 Relationship of infections to the phase of disease in myeloma.

IMMUNE DEFECTS IN MYELOMA

The principal factors determining susceptibility to infection in myeloma are polyclonal humoral immunosuppression, low levels of circulating CD19+ B cells, and the inability to respond to immunization[24,28,30] (Table 14.2). In addition, renal impairment, progressive disease, and, in some studies, the use of chemotherapy significantly increase the risk of infection.[25,26,28] The immunological deficits have been best defined for patients with plateau-phase disease. The mechanisms responsible for immunosuppression are not clear. Currently, the contribution of distinct CD8+ T cells and CD19+ B cells to the immune deficits in myeloma are the focus of research.[31,32] Table 14.3 shows the various immune defects in myeloma patients at various stages of the disease and therapy, and Table 14.4 shows the various organisms to which patients are susceptible during those time periods.

HUMORAL IMMUNITY

Non-paraprotein immunoglobulins and B cells

The majority of patients with myeloma have depressed levels of polyclonal (non-paraprotein) immunoglobulin in serum.[21,24,26 28,33] This is due to defective antibody synthesis, which manifests

Table 14.2 Immune deficits in myeloma that are associated with an increased risk of infection

- Decreased polyclonal immunoglobulin synthesis
- Decreased specific antibody levels
- Impaired antibody responses post immunization
- $CD19^+$ B cells $< 0.125 \times 10^9$/l at initial diagnosis
- Impaired binding of C3b to *Streptococcus pneumoniae*

in two ways: functionally, by a decreased ability to form specific antibodies, and clinically, by an increased susceptibility to bacterial infection.

Decreased antibody synthesis rather than accelerated catabolism is primarily responsible for the low serum polyclonal immunoglobulin concentration.[34,35] This deficiency in humoral immunity is not related to the presence or absence of a paraprotein,[21] nor is it correlated with the extent of disease.[24,28]

Table 14.3 Host defence mechanisms at various stages of the disease and therapy in myeloma

Impaired host defence mechanism	Untreated disease	Initial therapy	High-dose chemotherapy	Plateau phase or remission (maintenance: none or interferon)	Plateau phase or remission (corticosteroid maintenance)	Recurrent disease
Humoral immunity	+++	+++	+++	++	+++	+++
Cell-mediated immunity	+/−	++	+++	+/−	++	++
Neutropenia	−	+	++	−	−	+

Table 14.4 Susceptibility to infections during various disease stages and therapy in myeloma

Type of infection	Untreated disease	Initial therapy	High-dose chemotherapy	Plateau phase or remission (maintenance: none or interferon)	Plateau phase or remission (corticosteroid maintenance)	Recurrent disease
Viruses	+	++	+++	+/−	++	++
Varicella zoster	+	++	+++	+/−	++	++
Cytomegalovirus	+/−	+/−	+	−	+/−	+/−
Other	+/−	+/−	+	−	+/−	+/−
Fungi	+/−	+	++	−	++	+
Candida	−	+	++	−	++	+
Aspergillus	−	+	++	−	++	+
Bacteria	+	+	++	+	+	+
Encapsulated organisms	+	+	++	++	++	++
Gram-negative	+/−	+/−	++	+/−	+/−	+
Pneumocystis carinii	+/−	++	++	−	++	+

Decreased polyclonal imunoglobulin levels are a risk factor for the development of infection in patients undergoing induction chemotherapy.[28] Low serum non-paraprotein IgG and IgA concentrations predicted the risk of serious infection in two prospective studies of patients with myeloma.[24, 28]

In patients who do achieve complete remission, polyclonal serum immunglobulin levels tend to return to normal.[36]

Analyses of circulating B cells in myeloma have generated conflicting data on the exact level of these cells, and whether they may represent circulating polyclonal cells or clonal tumour cells.[30] It is now accepted that expanded clonal B-cell populations can be found in peripheral blood.[37] There is no relationship between the numbers of circulating $CD19^+$ B cells and the number of clonal cells in blood.[30] A recent multicentre study has shown that, in comparison with healthy controls, patients with myeloma exhibit marked heterogeneity in the numbers of circulating $CD19^+$ B cells.[30] Low B-cell numbers are associated with disease stage, and there is a strong inverse association between the level of $CD19^+$ cells at diagnosis and infections within the first two months of diagnosis. Thus, 35% of patients with $CD19^+$ cell counts of less than $0.125 \times 10^9/l$ experienced at least one documented infection during the first two months, compared with 24% of patients with $CD19^+$ cell counts above $0.125 \times 10^9/l$. The number of deaths due to infection in the induction phase of disease was significantly greater in individuals with low $CD19^+$ cell counts compared with those with high $CD19^+$ cell numbers (5.6% versus 1.7%; $p = 0.02$).

Specific antibodies

A number of studies published in the 1950s showed that the patients with myeloma had depressed levels of circulating antibodies to a number of recall antigens.[38–40] Marks[39] showed the titres of specific antibodies to proteins of both *Streptococcus pyogenes* and *Staphylococcus aureus* were low in patients with myeloma compared with healthy controls. In addition, American investigators also demonstrated that specific antibodies to several Gram-negative organisms were either absent or significantly reduced in patients who had myeloma.[40] The study by Hargreaves et al[24] also confirmed that levels of IgG specific to both protein and carbohydrate antigens were reduced when compared with an age-matched control population, although the difference was not significant for anti-*E. coli* lipopolysaccharide antibodies.

It has been shown that there is a correlation between increased infection risk and reduced titres of both anti-pneumococcal and anti-*E. coli* lipopolysaccharide antibodies.[24,41]

RESPONSE TO IMMUNIZATION

Antibody levels after test immunization are used to assess the functional integrity of the humoral immune system. Several studies have shown that patients with myeloma have impaired IgG responses to pneumococcal vaccination when compared with healthy controls.[19,24,38,41–44] Suboptimal immune responses to other carbohydrate, protein, and viral antigens have been noted.[19,21,24,45] In one study, primary antibody responses were depressed more than secondary antibody responses.[33] In general, most studies have found a correlation between the amount of specific antibody measured to the test antigen before immunization and its concentration post immunization.[21,24,38,41–45]

Fahey and colleagues[21] reported an association between impaired antibody responses post immunization and susceptibility to infection. This finding was confirmed by Chapel and colleagues,[24] who demonstrated an association between poor response to Pneumovax II immunization and the occurrence of septicaemia.[24] In this study, a poor response to Pneumonvax II was not associated with a poor response to protein antigens or to disease stage. In addition, the heterogeneity of patients' responses to pneumococcal vaccination was demonstrated: 38% of patients made no antibodies to Pneumovax II, whereas 44% of patients mounted a good response to immunization; in the remaining patients, responses to Pneumovax II were suboptimal.

CELL-MEDIATED IMMUNITY

Depressed numbers of circulating lymphocytes have been noted in myeloma.[46–47] CD4+ T cells are reduced in myeloma, particularly in treated patients and in those with advanced disease.[47–49] In addition, abnormalities of lymphocytes within the CD4+ T-cell compartment have been described in myeloma, although the relevance of these changes to the pathogenesis or the complications of the disease is unclear.[49] Delayed-type hypersensitivity responses to previously encountered antigens are normal in patients with myeloma; however, the development of primary delayed-type hypersensitivity is impaired.[33] There is no correlation between the number of CD4+ T cells and the presence or absence of infection in myeloma.[49]

CD8+ cell counts are also reduced in patients with myeloma.[49] Within the CD8+ compartment, the numbers of cells expressing CD11b is increased.[31] This abnormality has been correlated with disease stage and impaired non-paraprotein immunoglobulin synthesis. Finally, oligoclonal expansions of both CD4+ and CD8+ T cells have been described in myeloma, but the significance of these findings to the pathogenesis or complications of this disease are unclear.[50] In conclusion, although abnormalities in cell-mediated immunity have been described in patients with myeloma, these defects are subtle and do not usually predispose individuals to infection with fungi, protozoa, and viruses.

OTHER IMMUNE DEFECTS

Neutropenia is an important risk factor for infection during periods of high-dose chemotherapy. Some studies, however, have shown no relationship between neutrophil counts and risk of infection.[24,26] Several studies have shown that there are functional neutrophil defects in myeloma, but there is no clear relationship between the abnormalities that have been described and either the risk of infection or the use of chemotherapy.[51–54]

Reduced serum concentrations of complement components and defects in the activation in of the classical and alternative complement pathways have also been described.[55–57] Apart from one study, there was no association between the abnormalities noted in the function of complement and the risk of infection.[57]

Renal impairment is an important risk factor for infection in myeloma.[25, 28] This may in part be associated with defects in macrophage function. Antigen uptake by antigen-presenting cells in myeloma is normal.[58] However, the more pronounced defects in primary as opposed to secondary immunization responses suggests that more systematic studies of dendritic cell function may be warranted in this disease. This may be of relevance in light of the recent studies implicating infection of this cell type by HHV-8 in the pathogenesis of this condition. With the renewed interest in the role of Fc (IgG) receptors in antibody production and catabolism, this may also be a fruitful area for study again.

TREATMENT OF INFECTIONS IN MYELOMA

Antimicrobial prophylaxis and therapy for standard myeloma treatment

The conventional therapy for myeloma is a combination of melphalan and prednisone, with a resulting median survival of three years.[5] The initial first two months of standard induction chemotherapy has been identified as a high-risk period for infection for patients with myeloma.[28]

In a small study, trimethoprim–sulfamethoxazole (co-trimoxazole) at 960 mg/day significantly reduced the number of patients who experienced a serious infection during induction chemotherapy.[59] The number of patients enrolled (57) was too small to ascertain whether this approach reduced the number of infection-related deaths. One point to note, however, was the relatively poor tolerability of this drug; a problem that has been noted in other groups of immunocompromised patients. Up to 25% of individuals discontinued co-trimoxazole: skin rashes, nausea and vomiting were the commonest reasons for stopping therapy. Larger studies are needed to confirm the result of this trial.

In addition the use of alternative antibiotics that are better tolerated, and the selection of patients who should be offered chemoprophylaxis (such as those individuals with laboratory parameters suggesting an increase rate of infection), remain to be determined. Finally, it is not known whether a similar approach will be beneficial in individuals with disease relapse.

There are no data on the role of antimicrobial prophylaxis in the prevention of infection in the plateau phase of disease. Given the reduced rate of infection in this patient group, it seems reasonable to consider prophylactic antimicrobial therapy against encapsulated bacteria for those at increased risk of serious infection as defined by laboratory parameters. The efficacy of this approach needs to be assessed in double-blind randomized trials.

Treatment of infection in early disease needs to cover both encapsulated bacteria and Gram-negative organisms, and will be influenced by the local pattern of antibiotic resistance.

ANTIMICROBIAL PROPHYLAXIS AND THERAPY DURING INTENSIVE TREATMENT

Recent clinical trials have shown that more intensive chemotherapeutic regimens combined with haematopoietic stem cell transplantation extends both event-free and overall survival in patients with myeloma compared with standard treatment.[60] High-dose therapy can be administered to patients aged up to 76 years[61] and to those with renal failure,[62] thereby significantly increasing the number of patients eligible for this form of therapy. The intensification of chemotherapy regimens means that patients with myeloma experience infections associated with defects in T-cell and neutrophil function, similar to those seen in recipients of organ transplants. This is in addition to the defects in humoral immunity seen in myeloma.

General approaches to limit mortality and morbidity, including infection, in patients treated with high-dose therapy have been transplantation at an earlier stage of disease, less toxic conditioning regimens, the use of peripheral blood stem cells and haematopoietic growth factors, and improved therapy of graft-versus-host disease.[63–65] Although there is little evidence as yet supporting the use of prophylactic antimicrobials, the principles of prophylaxis used in other transplant settings may be applicable.[66] These depend on the pattern of infection varying with time post transplant, the association of specific immune deficits with an increased risk of particular microbial pathogens (Figure 14.3) and the effectiveness of prophylactic antibiotics against clinically significant infections.

The best example of antimicrobial prophylaxis in transplant recipients is the use of co-trimoxazole in organ transplantation.[66] Co-trimoxazole reduces the incidence of bacterial infections and *Toxoplasma gondii* in recipients of organ tranplants. It would also provide effective prophylaxis against *Listeria monocytogenes* and. *Nocardia asteroides*.[67–70] Other antimicrobial propylactic strategies include quinolones to prevent Gram-negative sepsis and acyclovir to prevent herpesvirus infections (Table 14.5). Fluconazole has been used to prevent systemic fungal infection; however, in some studies, its use has been associated with the emergence of infection with drug-resistant *Candida* spp. in bone marrow transplant recipients.[71,72] Furthermore, fluconazole offers little protection against *Aspergillus* infections.

Despite the availability of antimicrobial prophylaxis, infection remains a common complication of organ transplantation and is a common cause of death in allogeneic bone marrow transplantation. Systemic fungal infection in particular is associated with a poor prognosis.[73] In myeloma, infections are much more common in patients who receive allografts compared with autograft recipients.[74] In some studies transplantation with either T-cell-depleted bone marrow or $CD34^+$-selected haematopoietic progenitor

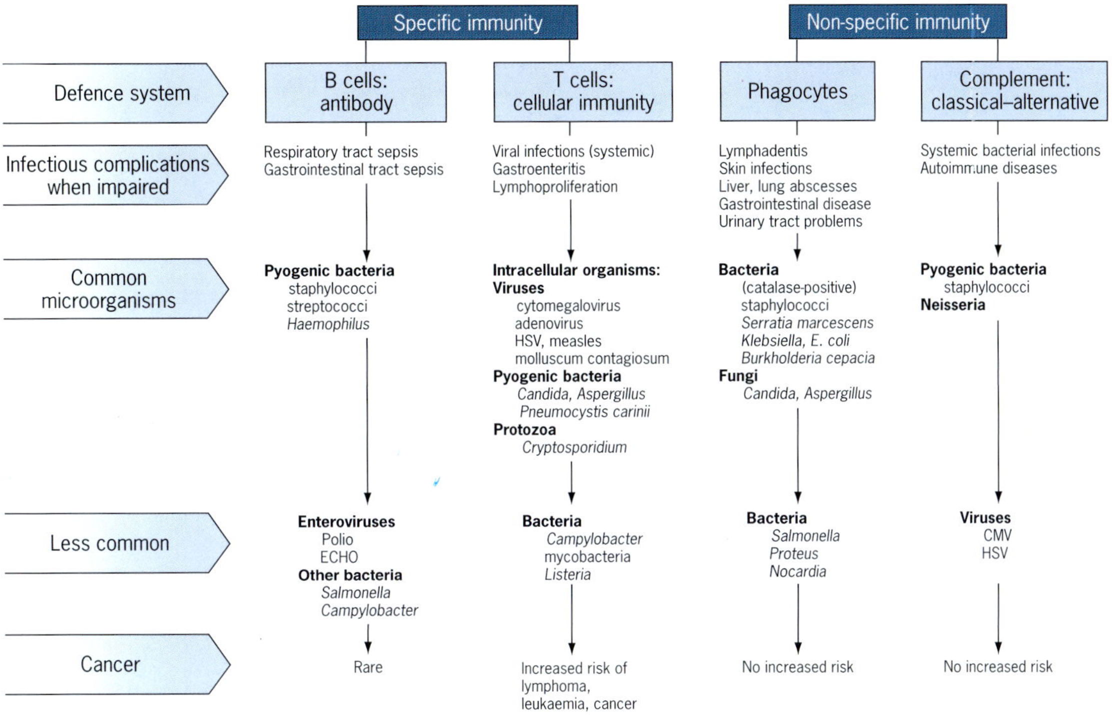

Figure 14.3 Relationship between type of immune deficiency and infective organisms. From Chapel H, Haeney M. *Essentials of Clinical Immunology*, 3rd edn. Oxford: Blackwell Science, 1993.

cells is associated with an increased risk of infections.[75–77] Effective immune reconstitution may be associated with an infused dose of at least 2×10^6 $CD34^+$ cells/kg.[78] The risk of infection is also increased in patients who receive corticosteroids for prophylaxis of graft-versus-host disease. Finally, HLA-matched sibling allograft recipients are less immunosuppressed than unrelated donor and mismatched donor transplant recipients, and therefore at less risk of infection.

There are a number of issues that need to be clarified in order to limit the risks of infection associated with more intensive chemotherapeutic regimens for myeloma. First, the details of antimicrobial prophylaxis and types of infection in such patients need to be documented. Secondly, the limitations of current anti-mycotic regimens imply that antimicrobial research in transplantation should concentrate on the need to develop agents to both prevent and treat systemic fungal infections. Thirdly, more research is required to identify patients at high risk of infection defined on epidemiological, clinical, or laboratory criteria. The application of highly specific assays to detect, for example, cytomegalovirus viraemia[79,80] or *Aspergillus* respiratory colonization[81] could form the basis of appropriate preemptive antimicrobial therapy. Fourthly, for patients in complete remission the kinetics of immune reconstitution could be studied to determine whether parameters of immune function could be used as a guide to discontinue antimicrobial chemoprophylaxis.

For B cells, the levels of immunoglobulins, specific antibodies, and antibody levels to test immunizations with protein or carbohydrate antigens may be useful measures of immune function. The study of T-cell regeneration is likely to be more complex, since the markers of naive T-cells are limited in humans; however, there is hope that the development of antigen-specific T-cell assays for various pathogens will allow one to monitor for the risks of infections

Table 14.5 Suggested antimicrobial prophylaxis in myeloma patients based upon specific impaired defence mechanisms

Prophylaxis	Untreated disease	Initial therapy	High-dose chemotherapy	Plateau phase or remission (maintenance: none or interferon)	Plateau phase or remission (corticosteroid maintenance)	Recurrent disease
Acyclovir (famciclovir, valaciclovir)	+	++	+++	+/−	++	++
Co-trimoxazole for prevention of *Pneumocystis carinii* infections (pentamidine, atovaquone)	−	++	+	+/−	++	+/−
Co-trimoxazole as an antibacterial agent[a]	+/−	++[a]	+[a]	+[a]	+[a]	+
Clarithromycin (azithromycin, erythromycin, penicillin V)	+/−	++	++	+/−	++	++
Quinolones (levofloxacin, Ciprofloxacin)	+/−	++	++	+/−	++	++
Intravenous immunoglobulin in selected patients not responding to immunization[a]	+/−	+	+	++[a]	++	+

−, no utility; +/−, doubtful utility; +, ++, +++, definite utility (increasing magnitude).
[a]Approaches for which there is published evidence in myeloma.

with these organisms in the transplant setting.[82,83] It will be important to correlate T-cell numbers with T-cell function (T-cell proliferation, cytokine production, cytolytic activity) if these tests are to be clinically meaningful.

IMMUNOGLOBULIN REPLACEMENT THERAPY

Administration of replacement immunoglobulin therapy to individuals with myeloma was proposed as a logical approach to the treatment of this disorder, since many of these patients are hypogammaglobulinaemic Figure 14.4.

In an early study, administration of intramuscular immunoglobulin failed to reduce the incidence of severe infections,[84] implying that much higher doses of immunoglobulin may be required. In a preliminary randomized crossover study of 94 patients, Schedel et al[85] showed that intravenous immunoglobulin (IVIG) reduced the incidence of infection. The dose of IVIG was lower than that used in patients with primary antibody deficiency.

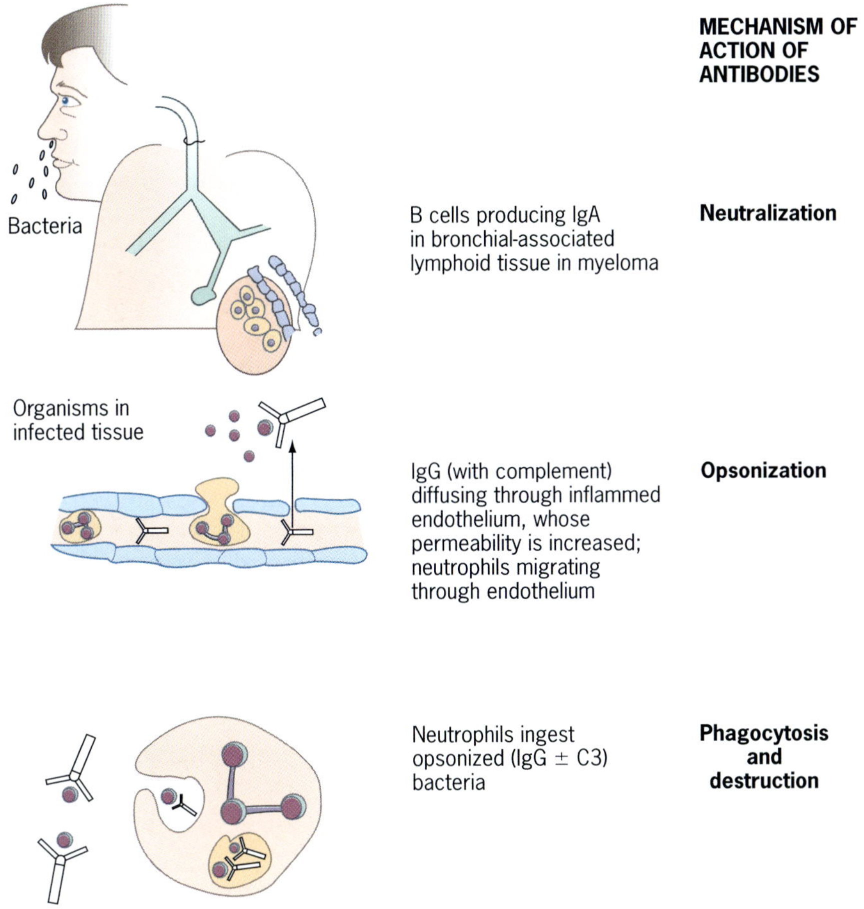

Figure 14.4 Presumed mechanism of action of intravenous immunoglobulin (IVIG) in the prevention of infections.

A randomized, placebo-controlled trial showed that monthly IVIG at a dose of 400 mg/kg significantly reduced the rate of serious as well as recurrent infections in patients with myeloma.[86] The majoirity of patients had stable disease and received either no or low-dose chemotherapy during the trial period. There were no episodes of pneumonia or septicaemia in patients who received IVIG, although the numbers of urinary tract or skin infections were not significantly different from those in patients who received placabo (0.4% albumin). Immunoglobulin therapy was safe and well tolerated. Adverse reactions were generally minor and occurred in 12.5% of patients receiving IVIG, compared with 6% in the patients receiving placebo.

A poor IgG antibody response to Pneumovax II was a characteristic of those who benefited most from this treatment. The conclusions of this study were that IVIG protected patients with stable myeloma against life-threatening infections and significantly reduced the rate of recurrent infections.

There are a number of issues to be resolved before prophylactic immunoglobulin therapy can be used in the routine management of patients with myeloma. In the placebo-controlled trial, the number of clinically significant infections was small: only 10 episodes of pneumonia and septicaemia were reported in this study, and the total number of serious bacterial infections was 15 in the IVIG group compared with 29 in the placebo group. The small patient numbers and short duration of follow-up (one year) meant that no conclusions could be drawn on the efficacy of immunoglobulin therapy in preventing infection-related mortality. The incidence of serious infection (1 case every 12.4 months in the placebo arm and 1 case every 26.2 months in the IVIG group) was higher than previously described for patients in the plateau phase.[87] The wider applicability of this treatment to patients with myeloma remains uncertain since patients with poor bone marrow reserve and those who had received multi-agent chemotherapy did not appear to benefit from prophylactic IVIG. There is no reason to think that immunoglobulin prophylaxis would be effective in patients being treated for newly diagnosed or relapsed disease.

One potential approach to the use of IVIG as prophylaxis against infection in patients in the plateau phase is shown in Figure 14.5. A randomized control trial needs to be undertaken to compare the efficacy of immunoglobulin therapy with antimicrobial prophylaxis in patients with stable disease post induction therapy.

ACTIVE IMMUNIZATION

In general, patients with myeloma mount impaired antibody responses to vaccination. Pneumococcal vaccination of myeloma patients did not appear to prevent either pneumococcal bacteraemia or meningitis.[88] This is probably due to the poor IgG responses to such immunization, since only 45% of patients have an appropriate response to pneumococcal vaccination.[24] Immune response to influenza vaccine is also impaired in myeloma patients,[40] as are responses to other proteins,[24] suggesting that these patients may not benefit from conjugate vaccines either.

The increasing use of transplantation in the treatment of myeloma raises issues about the need to reimmunize long-term survivors. The response to vaccination depends upon the type of transplant, the immune status of the patient, and the vaccine used.[89] It is recommended that all autologous and allogeneic stem cell recipients should receive tetanus, diphtheria, and inactivated poliovirus vaccines 6–12 months post transplantation.[90] Vaccination against *Haemophilus* and

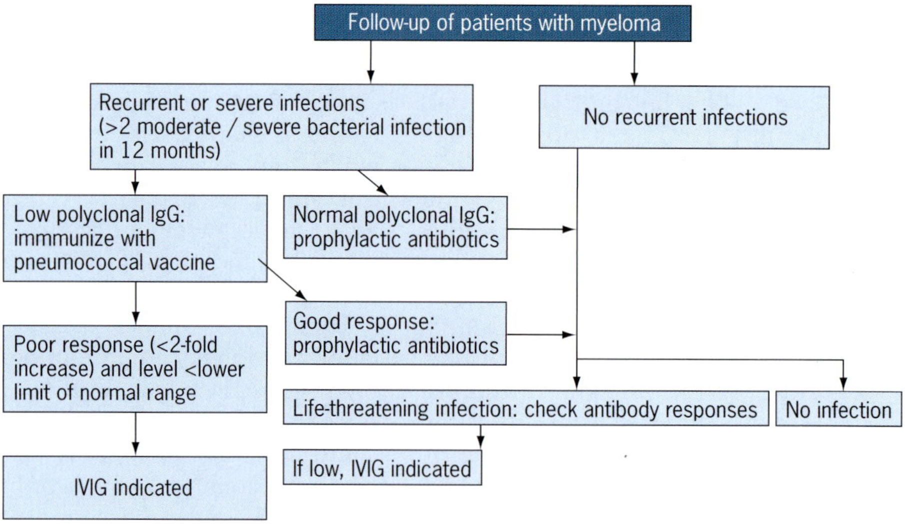

Figure 14.5 An approach to the use of IVIG in patients with myeloma.

Pneumococcus would also appear indicated for post-transplant myeloma patients. Further studies are required to study the optimal timing, dose, and type of vaccine (conjugated pneumococcal vaccines) to prevent pneumococcal and *Haemophilus* infections. In addition, there is little data to date on the relationship between immune reconstitution and the extent of response to immunization.

FUTURE DIRECTIONS

Infection is one of several variables that influence morbidity and mortality in this disease. Although the results of treating this tumour are disappointing, there is an association between complete remission and restoration of humoral immune function as determined by serum immunoglobulin levels in a relatively small number of patients.[36] The numbers and types of infection that occur in patients with more intensive regimens for myeloma are under current study.[91] The ability of patients to respond to immunization and the measures that may be needed to prevent infection if it occurs in these patients remain to be determined. Ultimately the prevention of infection in myeloma will depend on improved therapy for the disease itself.

In the interim, clinical trials are needed to confirm the efficacy of antimicrobial chemoprophylaxis in the prevention of infection in the initial phase of the disease. In addition, the feasibility of replacement immunoglobulin therapy needs to be compared with antimicrobial prophylaxis in preventing significant bacterial sepsis in patients with stable myeloma. If the link between HHV8 and myeloma is confirmed, the development of more potent antiviral agents against HHV8 might prevent both the progression and hence the infectious complications of myeloma.

REFERENCES

1. Rettig MB, Ma HJ, Vescio RA et al. Kaposi's sacoma-associated herpes virus infection of bone marrow dendritic cells from multiple myeloma patients. *Science* 1997; **276**: 1851–4.
2. Kawano M, Hirano T, Matsuda T, et al. Autocrine generation and requirement of BSF-2/Il-6 for human multiple myelomas. *Nature* 1988; **332**: 83–5.
3. Klein B, Zhang X-G, Jourdan, M et al. Paracrine rather autocrine regulation of myeloma-cell growth and differentiation by interleukin-6. *Blood* 1989; **73**: 517–26.
4. Hardin J, McLeod S, Grigorieva I et al. Interleukin-6 prevents dexamethasone-induced myeloma cell death. *Blood* 1994; **84**: 3063–70.
5. Bataille R, Harousseau J-L. Multiple myeloma. *N Engl J Med* 1997; **336**: 1657–65.
6. O'Leary JJ, Silva, I, Uhlmann V et al. HHV-8 in multiple myeloma; is this the first paracrine model of human tumorogenesis and do Koch's postulates apply? *J Clin Pathol Mol Pathol* 1998; **51**: 201–3.
7. Parravicini C, Lauri E, Baldini L et al. Kaposi's sarcoma-associated herpes virus infection and multiple myeloma. *Science* 1997; **278**: 1969–70.
8. Whitby D, Boshoff C, Lupp, M, Torelli G. Kaposi's sarcoma-associated herpes virus infection and multiple myeloma. *Science* 1997; **278**: 1971–2.
9. Marcelin A-G, Dupin N, Bouscary D et al. HHV-8 and multiple myeloma in France. *Lancet* 1997; **350**: 1144.
10. MacKenzie J, Sheldon J, Morgan G et al. HHV-8 and multiple myeloma in the UK. *Lancet* 1997; **350**: 1144–5.
11. Santarelli R, Angeloni A, Farina A et al. Lack of serological association between human herpesvirus-8 and multiple myeloma and monoclonal gammopathies of undetermined significance. *J Natl Cancer Inst* 1998; **80**: 781–2.
12. Masood R, Zheng T, Tulpule A et al. Kaposi sarcoma's associated herpes virus infection and multiple myeloma. *Science* 1997; **278**: 1970–1.
13. Rabkin CS, Schultz TF, Whitby D et al. Interassay correlation of human herpesvirus 8 serologic tests. *J Infect Dis* 1998; **178**: 304–9.

14. Brousset P, Meggetto F, Attal M, Delsol G. Kaposi's sarcoma and herpes virus infection in multiple myeloma. *Science* 1997; **287**: 1972–3.
15. Gao S-J, Alsina M, Deng J-H et al. Antibodies to Kaposi's sarcoma herpesvirus (human herpesvirus 8) in patients with multiple myeloma. *J Infect Dis* 1998; **178**: 846–9.
16. Chauhan D, Bharti A, Raje N et al. Detection of Kaposi's sarcoma herpesvirus DNA sequences in multiple myeloma bone marrow stromal cells. *Blood* 1999; **93**: 1483–6.
17. Tisdale JF, Stewart AK, Dickenstein B et al. Molecular and serological examination of the relationship of human herpesvirus 8 to multiple myeloma: orf 26 sequences in bone marrow stroma are not restricted to myeloma patients and other regions of the genome are not detected. *Blood* 1998; **92**: 2681–7.
18. Snapper I, Turner LB, Moscovitz HL. *Multiple Myeloma*. New York: Grune and Stratton, 1953.
19. Zinnemann HH, Hall WD. Recurrent pneumonia in multiple myeloma and some observations on the immune response. *Ann Intern Med* 1954; **41**: 1152–63.
20. Glenchur H, Zinnemann HH, Hall WH. A review of fifty-one cases of multiple myeloma. *Arch Intern Med* 1959; **103**: 173–83.
21. Fahey JL, Scoggins R, Utz JP, Szewed CF. Infection, antibody response and gamma globulin components in multiple myeloma and macroglobulinaemia. *Am J Med* 1963; **35**: 698–707.
22. Twomey JJ. Infections complicating multiple myeloma and chronic lymphocytic leukaemia. *Arch Intern Med* 1973; **132**: 562–5.
23. Jacobson DR, Zolla-Palmer S. Immunosuppression and infection in multiple myeloma. *Semin Oncol* 1986; **13**: 282–90.
24. Hargreaves RM, Lea JR, Griffiths H et al. Immunological factors and risk of infection in plateau phase myeloma. *J Clin Pathol* 1995; **48**: 260–6.
25. Rayner HC, Haynes AP, Thompson JR et al. Perspectives in multiple myeloma: survival, prognostic factors and disease complications in a single centre between 1975 and 1988. *QJM* 1991; **79**: 517–25.
26. Savage DG, Lindenbaum J, Garrettt TJ. Biphasic pattern of infection in multiple myeloma. *Ann Intern Med* 1982; **96**: 47–50.
27. Meyers BR, Hirschmann SZ, Axelford JA. Current patterns of infection in multiple myeloma. *Am J Med* 1972; **52**: 87–92.
28. Perri RT, Hebbel RP, Oken MM. Influence of treatment and response status on infection in multiple myeloma. *Am J Med* 1981; **71**: 935–40.
29. Cuzick J, DeStavola BL, Cooper EH et al. Long term prognostic value of serum beta 2 microglobulin in myelomatosis. *Br J Haematol* 1990; **75**: 506–10.
30. Kay NE, Leong T, Kyle RA et al. Circulating blood B cells in multiple myeloma: analysis and relationship to circulating clonal cells and clinical parameters in a cohort of patients entered on the Eastern Cooperative Oncology Group phase III E9486 clinical trial. *Blood* 1997; **80**: 340–5.
31. Walchner M, Wick M. Elevation of $CD8^+$ $CD11b^+$ Leu8-T cells is associated with the humoral immunodeficiency in myeloma patients. *Clin Exp Immunol* 1997; **109**: 310–16.
32. Paglieroni T, Caggiano V, McKenzie M. Abnormalities in immune regulation precede the development of multiple myeloma. *Am J Hematol* 1992; **40**: 51–5.
33. Cone L, Uh, J. Immunological deficiency disorders associated with chronic lymphocytic leukaemia and multiple myeloma. *J Clin Invest* 1964; **43**: 2241–8.
34. Waldmann T, Strober W. Metabolism of immunoglobulins. *Prog Allergy* 1969; **13**: 1–110.
35. Broder S, Humphrey R, Durm M et al. Impaired synthesis of polyclonal (non-paraprotein) immunoglobulins by circulating lymphocytes from patients with multiple myeloma. Role of suppressor cells. *N Engl J Med* 1975; **293**: 887–92.
36. Gore ME, Viner C, Meldru, M et al. Intensive treatment of multiple myeloma and criteria for complete remission. *Lancet* 1989; **ii**: 879–82.
37. van Reit I, Heirman C, Lacor P et al. Detection of monoclonal B lymphocytes in bone marrow and peripheral blood of multiple myeloma by immunoglobulin gene rearrangement studies. *Br J Haematol* 1989; **73**: 289–98.
38. Larson DL, Tomlinson LJ. Quantitative antibody studies in man. II. The relationship of the level of serum proteins to antibody production. *J Lab Clin Med* 1952; **39**: 129–33.
39. Marks J. Antibody formation in myelomatosis. *J Clin Pathol* 1953; **6**: 62–3.
40. Lawson HA, Stuart CA, Paull AM et al. Observations on the antibody content of the

blood in patients with multiple myeloma. *N Engl J Med* 1955; **252**: 13–18.
41. Stoll C, Schedel I, Peest D et al. Serum antibodies against common antigens of bacterial lipopolysaccharides in healthy adults and patients with multiple myeloma. *Infection* 1985; **13**: 115–19.
42. Lazarus HM, Lederman M, Lubin A et al. Pneumococcal vaccination: the response of patients with multiple myeloma. *Am J Med* 1980; **69**: 419–23.
43. Schmid GP, Smith RP, Baltch AL et al. Antibody response to pneumococcal vaccine in patients with multiple myeloma. *J Infect Dis* 1981; **143**: 590–7.
44. Birgens HS, Espersen F, Hertz JB et al. Antibody response to pneumococcal vaccination in patients with myelomatosis. *Scand J Haematol* 1983; **30**: 324–30.
45. Heath RB, Hamilton Fairley G, Malpas JS. Production of antibodies against viruses in leukaemia and related diseases. *Br J Haematol* 1962; **10**: 365–70.
46. Sewell RL. Lymphocyte abnormalities in myeloma. *Br J Haematol* 1977; **36**: 545–51.
47. Bergmann L, Mitriou PS, Kelker W, Weber KC. T-cell subsets in malignant lymphomas and monoclonal gammopathies. *Scand J Haematol* 1985; **34**: 170–6.
48. Mills KHG, Cawley JC. Abnormal monoclonal antibody defined helper/suppressor T-cell subpopulations in multiple myeloma: relationship to treatment and clinical stage. *Br J Haematol* 1983; **53**: 271–5.
49. Kay NE, Leong T, Bone N et al. T-helper phenotypes in the blood of myeloma patients on ECOG phase III trials E9486/E3A93. *Br J Haematol* 1998; **100**: 459–63.
50. Moss P, Gillespie G, Frodsham P, Reyburn H. Clonal populations of CD41 and CD81 T cells in patients with multiple myeloma and paraproteinaemia. *Blood* 1996; **87**: 3297–306.
51. Penny R, Galton DAG. Studies on neutrophil functions. II Pathological aspects. *Br J Haematol* 1966; **12**: 633–45.
52. Spitler LE, Spath P, Petz L et al. Phagocytes and C4 in paraproteinaemia. *Br J Haematol* 1975; **29**: 279–92.
53. MacGregor RR, Negendank WG, Schreiber, AD. Impaired granulocyte adherence in multiple myeloma: relationship to complement system, granulocyte delivery, and infection. *Blood* 1978; **51**: 591–9.
54. Hopen G, Glette J, Halstensen A et al. Granulocyte function in malignant monoclonal gammopathy. *Scand J Haematol* 1983; **31**: 133–43.
55. Cheson BD, Plass RR, Rothstein G. Defective opsonisation in multiple myeloma. *Blood* 1980; **55**: 602–6.
56. Krauf EH, Sagone AL. Alternative pathway of complement in multiple myeloma. *Am J Hematol* 1981; **11**: 335–45.
57. Cheson BD, Walker HS, Heath ME et al. Defective binding of the third component of complement (C3) to *Streptococcus pneumoniae* in multiple myeloma. *Blood* 1984; **63**: 949–57.
58. Paglieroni T, MacKenzie MR. Studies on the pathogenesis of an immune defect in multiple myeloma. *J Clin Invest* 1977; **59**: 1120–33.
59. Oken MM, Pomeroy C, Weisdorf D, Bennett JM. Prophylactic antibiotics for the prevention of early infection in multiple myeloma. *Am J Med* 1996; **100**: 624–8.
60. Attal M, Harousseau JL, Stoppa AM et al. A prospective randomised trial of autologous bone marrow transplantation and chemotherapy in multiple myeloma. *N Engl J Med* 1996; **335**; 91–7
61. Siegel DS, Desikan KR, Mehta J et al. Age is not a prognostic variable with autotransplants for multiple myeloma. *Blood* 1999; **93**: 51–4.
62. Barlogie B, Jagannath S, Desikan KR et al. Total therapy with tandem transplants for newly diagnosed multiple myeloma. *Blood* 1999; **93**: 55–65.
63. Vesole DH, Barlogie B, Jagannath S et al. High dose therapy for refractory myeloma: improved prognosis with better supportive care and double transplants. *Blood* 1994; **84**: 950–6.
64. Besinger WI, Buckner CD, Anasetti C et al. Allogeneic marrow transplantation for multiple myeloma: an analysis of risk factors on outcome. *Blood* 1996; **88**: 2787–93.
65. Russell NH, Milfin G, Sainer C et al. Allogeneic bone marrow transplant for multiple myeloma. *Blood* 1997: **89**: 2610–11.
66. Fishmann JA, Rubin RH. Medical progress: infection in organ-transplant recipients. *N Engl J Med* 1998; **338**: 1741–51.
67. Fox BC, Sollinger HW, Belzer FO, Maki DG. A prospective, randomised, double-blind study of trimethoprim-sulfamethoxazole for prophylaxis in renal transplantation: clinical efficacy, absorption of trimethoprim–sulfamethoxazole, effects

on the microflora, and cost-benefit of prophylaxis. *Am J Med* 1990: **89**: 255–74.

68. Orr KE, Gould FK, Short G et al. Outcome of *Toxoplasma gondii* mismatches in heart transplant recipients over a period of 8 years. *J Infect* 1994; **29**: 249–53.
69. Merle-Melet M, Dossou-Gbete L, Maurer P et al. Is amoxicillin–cotrimoxazole the most appropriate antibiotic regimen for listeria meningoencephalitis? Review of 22 cases and the literature. *J Infect* 1996; **33**: 79–85.
70. Chapman SW, Wilson JP. Nocardiosis in transplant recipients *Semin Resp Infect* 1990; **5**: 74–9.
71. Wingard JR, Merz WG, Rinaldi MG et al. Increase in *Candida krusei* infection among patients with bone marrow transplantation and neutropenia treated prophylactically with fluconazole. *N Engl J Med* 1991; **325**: 1274–7.
72. Castagnola E, Buccci B, Montinaro E, Viscoli C. Fungal infections in patients undergoing bone marrow transplantation: an approach to rational management protocol. *Bone Marrow Transplant* 1996; **18**(Suppl 2): 97–106.
73. Kruger W, Russmann B, Kroger N et al. Early infections in patients undergoing bone marrow or blood stem cell transplantation – a 7 year single centre investigation of 409 cases. *Bone Marrow Transplant* 1999; **23**: 589–97.
74. Mehta J, Ayers D, Mattox S et al. Allogeneic bone marrow transplantation in multiple myeloma patients; single-centre experience of 97 patients. *Blood*. 1997; **90**(Suppl 1): 225a.
75. Siegel D, Mehta J, Anaissie E et al. Prolonged immunosuppression after $CD34^+$ or $CD34^+$/Thy-1^+/Lin- selected autologous peripheral blood stem cells (PBSC) transplants (Tx) for multiple myeloma. *Blood* 1997; **90**(Suppl 1): 112a.
76. Rossi JF, Legouffe E, Fegeux N et al. Autologous transplantation (AT) of $CD34^+$ peripheral blood progenitor cells (PBDC) after double (D) high dose chemotherapy (HDC) in multiple myeloma (MM) is followed by severe immunodeficiency (ID) and high production of interleukin-6 (IL-6) related-C reactive protein (CRP) requiring additive immunotherapy (IT). *Blood* 1996; **88**(Suppl 1): 132a.
77. Tricot G, Gazzit Y, Leemhuis T et al. Collection, tumour contamination and engraftment kinetics of highly purified hematopoietic progenitor cells to support high dose therapy in multiple myeloma. *Blood* 1998; **91**: 4489–95.
78. Vescio R, Schiller G, Stewart K et al. Multicentre trial to evaluate $CD34^+$ selected versus unselected autologous peripheral blood progenitor cell transplantation in multiple myeloma. *Blood* 1999; **93**: 1858–68.
79. Zaia JA, Gallez-Hawkins GM, Tegtmeier BR et al. Late cytomegalovirus disease in marrow transplantation is predicted by viral load in plasma. *J Infect Dis* 1997; **176**: 782–5.
80. Herbart H, Schroder A, Loffler J et al. Cytomegalovirus monitoring by polymerase chain reaction of whole blood samples from patients undergoing autologous bone marrow or peripheral blood progenitor cell transplantation. *J Infect Dis* 1997; **175**: 1490–3.
81. Horvath JA, Dummer S. The use of respiratory-tract cultures in the diagnosis of invasive pulmonary aspergillosis. *Am J Med* 1996; **100**: 171–8.
82. Schwartz RS. Direct visualisation of antigen-specific cytotoxic T cells – a new insight into immune defences. *N Engl J Med* 1998; **339**: 1076–8.
83. Komanduri KV, Viswanathan MN, Wieder ED et al Restoration of cytomegalovirus-specific $CD4^+$ T-lymphocyte responses after ganciclovir and highly active antiretroviral therapy in individuals infected with HIV-1. *Nature Med* 1998; **4**: 953–6.
84. Salmon SE, Samal BA, Hayes DM et al. Role of gamma globulin for immunoprophylaxis in multiple myeloma. *N Engl J Med* 1967; **277**: 1336–40.
85. Schedel I. Application of Ig preparations in multiple myeloma. In: *Clinical Uses of Intravenous Immunoglobulins* (Morell A, Nydegger U, eds). London: Academic Press, 1986: 123–30.
86. Chapel H, Lee M, Hargreaves R et al, for the UK Group for Immunoglobulin Replacement Therapy in Multiple Myeloma. Randomised trial of intravenous immunoglobulin as prophylaxis against infection in plateau-phase multiple myeloma. *Lancet* 1994; **343**: 1059–63.
87. Snowdon L, Gibson J, Joshua DE. Frequency of infection in plateau-phase multiple myeloma. *Lancet* 1994; **344**: 262.
88. Butler JC, Breiman RF, Campbell JF et al. Pneumococcal polysaccharide vaccine efficacy. An evaluation of current recommendations. *JAMA* 1993: **270**: 1826–31.

89. Singhal S, Mehta J. Reimmunisation after blood or marrow stem cell transplantion. *Bone Marrow Transplant* 1999; **23**: 637–46.
90. Ljungman P. Immunisation of transplant recipients. *Bone Marrow Transplant* 1999; **23**: 635–6.
91. Reich G, Mapara M, Reichardt P et al. Infectious complications after high dose chemotherapy and autologous stem cell transplantation: comparison between patients with lymphoma or multiple myeloma and patients with solid tumours. *Bone Marrow Transplant* 2001; **27**: 52–9.

Part 3

Investigations

15

Laboratory investigations

Jesus F San Miguel, Julia Almeida, Alberto Orfao

INTRODUCTION

Laboratory investigations in patients with suspected plasma cell disorders serve to confirm a diagnosis, differentiate between the various monoclonal gammopathies, help determine prognosis, decide on the best therapeutic approach, and monitor the course of the disease and the therapy.

In this chapter, we have grouped the different laboratory investigations according to the biological factor analysed into 10 different areas: plasma cell morphology, monoclonal protein studies (including immunoglobulin levels), haematological parameters, biochemical parameters, immunophenotyping, cytogenetics, DNA ploidy, molecular studies, plasma cell labelling index, and multidrug resistance (MDR). Table 15.1 gives the relative values of these broad groups of investigations at various stages of the disease and its therapy.

MORPHOLOGY

Morphological assessment of the bone marrow, based on the evaluation of aspirates as well as biopsies, is one of the three major criteria for the diagnosis of myeloma. The number of plasma cells in the marrow is also an important criterion for differentiating myeloma from monoclonal gammopathy of undetermined significance (MGUS) and solitary plasmacytoma; more than 10% plasmacytosis is usually indicative of myeloma.

However, the extent of marrow plasmacytosis does not appear to influence the prognosis; probably owing to the heterogeneous distribution of plasma cells in the marrow. The percentage of plasma cells detected may vary significantly from one place to another (areas with bone tenderness or lytic lesions usually show more plasma cells), and is therefore not a reliable marker of the tumour mass.

Marrow plasmacytosis is not a criterion for monitoring response to treatment, although the detection of less than 5% plasma cells is necessary to define complete remission (CR).

All too often, when a marrow sample from a patient with a monoclonal gammopathy is evaluated, only the extent of plasmacytosis is taken into account and little attention is paid to the morphological characteristics of these cells. In fact, morphology plays a very important role in determining the biological nature of the disease, and can yield information of great prognostic

Table 15.1 Investigations in patients with plasma cell disorders

	Diagnosis and differential diagnosis	Prognosis	Monitoring therapy
Bone marrow morphology	High	Intermediate	High
Monoclonal protein studies	High	Low	High
Haematological parameters[a]	Intermediate	Intermediate	Intermediate
Biochemical parameters	Low	High[b]	Intermediate[c]
Immunophenotyping	Intermediate	Low	High
Cytogenetics	Intermediate	High	Intermediate
DNA ploidy	Low	Intermediate	Intermediate
Molecular studies	Low	High	High
Labelling index	Intermediate	High	Low
Multidrug resistance (MDR) assessment	Low	Intermediate	Low

[a] Haemoglobin.
[b] β_2-Microglobulin, C-reactive protein, creatinine, lactate dehydrogenase.
[c] β_2-Microglobulin, C-reactive protein.

value. Chapter 16 discusses bone marrow morphology in myeloma in depth.

The morphology of plasma cells in myeloma is quite heterogeneous. Greipp et al[1] described four morphological subtypes of plasma cells:

- *Mature*: Small eccentric nucleus with a prominent hof and dense chromatin clumping, and well-developed cytoplasm.
- *Intermediate*: Do not fulfil criteria for other subtypes.
- *Immature*: Large eccentric nucleus with a hof and diffuse chromatin; with or without a nucleolus, and abundant cytoplasm.
- *Plasmablast*: Very high nuclear/cytoplasmic ratio, with scanty cytoplasm and a central, immature, large nucleus with a reticular chromatin pattern, prominent nucleolus, and little or no hof.

Based upon plasma cell morphology, myeloma can be divided into four subtypes:

- *Mature myeloma*: More than 10% mature plasma cells, less than 2% plasmablasts, and less than 13% immature plasma cells.
- *Immature myeloma*: More than 12% immature plasma cells, less than 10% mature plasma cells, and less than 2% plasmablasts.
- *Plasmablastic myeloma*: More than 2% plasmablasts.
- *Intermediate myeloma*: Does not fulfil criteria for other subtypes

Bartl et al[2,3] have focused on morphological analysis of marrow histology. They established six morphological subgroups according to the predominant type of plasma cells: Marschalko, small cell, cleaved, polymorphous, asynchronous, and blastic. The first two types are classified as low-grade disease, and have a median survival of 51 months. Intermediate-grade myeloma consists of the cleaved, polymorphous, and asynchronous cell types, and has a median survival of 20 months. High-grade myeloma is represented by the plasmablastic cells, and has a median survival of 9 months. Additionally, six architectural patterns were also recognized: interstitial, interstitial with paratrabecular sheets, interstitial/nodular, nodular, packed marrow, and sarcomatous.

Although the prognostic value of plasma cell morphology had been recognized by Bayrd[4] in 1948 – with a median survival of less than one year for the 10 patients with poorly-differentiated morphology compared with more than five years for the seven patients with well-differentiated cells – the prognostic influence of plasma cell morphology on disease outcome was evaluated comprehensively only in 1980. Several groups have now shown that plasmablastic morphology is associated with poor outcome and has independent prognostic significance.[1–3,5–8]

Little attention has been paid to the immunocytochemical characteristics of plasma cells, although some reports suggest that acid phosphatase score can be of value in the diagnosis of plasma cell disorders and may even have prognostic impact. However, neither acid phosphatase nor α-naphthyl acetate esterase can consistently differentiate between myeloma and MGUS, because stage I myeloma in particular displays low values similar to those found in MGUS.[9]

ANALYSIS OF MONOCLONAL PROTEIN

The detection of a monoclonal protein ('M protein') in the serum or urine is the most characteristic biological marker of myeloma. Although the quantity of the M protein has frequently been used to differentiate between myeloma and MGUS (the latter usually shows less than 3 g/dl), it is not a reliable parameter, because many myeloma patients show less than 3 g/dl.

M protein is the most widely used marker for monitoring the course of the disease. Serum as well as urine M protein should be monitored, since there could be a divergence between the two.[10] Serum protein studies also provide information about the levels of polyclonal (uninvolved) immunoglobulins, which are usually depressed in myeloma, and the level of albumin, where a decline is associated with an adverse prognosis.

Detection and identification of monoclonal protein

Screening serum and urine for M protein requires a rapid and sensitive assay.[11–17] Electrophoresis on agarose or cellulose acetate membrane is the method of choice for detection of serum M protein. This is seen as a dense, discrete band on the cellulose membrane or as a narrow peak in the densitometer tracing. Monoclonal light chains are rarely detected on cellulose acetate electrophoresis, and IgD paraprotein may be difficult to see. For the latter, a more sensitive technique such as high-resolution agarose gel electrophoresis is more useful.[11–14]

IgD, non-secretory, or light-chain disease should be suspected in the absence of serum M protein if there is a severe hypogammaglobulinaemia and marrow plasmocytosis. On serum electrophoresis, the sharp monoclonal band is frequently accompanied by a corresponding decrease in the intensity of staining for the remaining proteins of the gamma region, reflecting a decrease in polyclonal immunoglobulins.

Once a monoclonal protein has been detected, the heavy- and light-chain isotypes must be identified by using immunoelectrophoresis or immunofixation. The former shows a localized distortion (thickening or bowing) in the precipitin arc of the monoclonal heavy chain and, significantly, a corresponding thickening in either the κ or the λ arcs, since monoclonality is defined by the presence of only one type of light chain in the abnormal protein. If there is bowing in the light chain arc without the corresponding abnormality in the IgG, IgA, or IgM arcs, the possibility of an IgD or IgE paraprotein should be investigated.[13]

Immunofixation is more sensitive than immunoelectrophoresis, and therefore is particularly useful for the assessment of small residual M components following treatment. However, it requires experienced and skilled personnel for the interpretation of the results.[11–14] Appropriate sample dilution may be critical if there is antigenic excess in order to distinguish a sharp monoclonal component from a dense polyclonal band. Antigenic excess is seen most frequently in IgAλ myeloma. It is also important to apply the cellulose acetate strip containing the antibody to the appropriate part of the gel, because urine M protein may migrate close to the albumin and may be missed once immunofixation techniques are used.[13]

Immunoisoelectric focusing is probably the most sensitive method for the detection of monoclonal proteins, but it requires technically skilled personnel and is not used in routine screening. Nephelometry has frequently been used to detect the light-chain type of a monoclonal gammopathy based on the existence of a marked imbalance in the κ/λ ratio. However, cases with small monoclonal proteins may display a normal κ/λ ratio and be overlooked with the rate nephelometer.[14]

Several groups[11,12] have studied different protocols for cost-effective detection of monoclonal gammopathies. One of the best alternatives is the combination of electrophoresis followed by immunofixation, which is rapid and avoids the need for immunoelectrophoresis.

Quantitation of immunoglobulins and paraprotein

Quantitation of immunoglobulins was performed in the past by radial immunodiffusion. However, this technique is time-consuming and somewhat imprecise for IgA and IgM paraproteins. The method of choice for immunoglobulin quantitation is rate nephelometry.[11–17] This measures the amount of monoclonal protein as well as the individual polyclonal immunoglobulins. The amount of M protein can also be assessed with the densitometer tracing of serum protein electrophoresis.

The two methods frequently give discrepant results, with higher values usually being obtained by nephelometry.[13] When evaluating response to treatment, it is important to recognize that in responding patients, polyclonal immunoglobulins may increase as the M protein decreases. In these instances, quantitation of the M protein by electrophoresis is more accurate. In any case, for the evaluation of changes in the M protein, it is important to select one technique, either electrophoresis or nephelometry, and to always use the same method for comparison throughout the course of the disease.

Analysis of urine

Most laboratories use sulfosalicylic acid precipitation as the screening test for urinary protein, since dipsticks are not reliable for the identification of Bence Jones proteinuria. However, if the sulfosalicylic acid test is negative in a patient with a suspected monoclonal gammopathy, other tests such electrophoresis or immunofixation should be performed on the urine.[11–14]

For the analysis of urinary monoclonal protein, a 24-hour collection of urine is mandatory for the determination of the total amount of protein excreted per day. An aliquot of the 24-hour sample must be concentrated 150- to 200-fold for electrophoresis, which will show a dense band on cellulose acetate or a peak on the densitometer tracing. To define the type of light chain, immunoelectrophoresis of concentrated urine using monospecific antisera to κ and λ light chains (that recognize both free and combined light chains) should be performed. As previously mentioned, immunofixation is more sensitive than immunoelectrophoresis, and may be of value in cases of small amounts of proteinuria.[11–13]

HAEMATOLOGICAL PARAMETERS

Moderate normochromic, normocytic anaemia (haemoglobin, Hb > 9 g/dl) is present in 50% of myeloma patients at diagnosis. A further 20% present with severe anaemia (Hb < 8 g/dl). The origin of anaemia in myeloma is multifactorial, and includes displacement of erythroid cells by the infiltrating plasma cells, renal failure, iron deficiency, mild shortening of red cell survival, expanded plasma volume, and insufficient erythropoietin production.[14–16]

Thrombocytopenia is uncommon at diagnosis, with only 10–15% of patients showing a platelet count below 100×10^9/l secondary to marked marrow infiltration. Leukopenia only occurs in very advanced disease or after chemotherapy.[14–16]

The peripheral blood smear frequently shows an increase in the intensity of blue staining ('background staining') due to the high immunoglobulin level, as well as rouleaux formation.[15,16] The blood film may occasionally show circulating plasma cells,[16] usually in association with advanced disease. Only in 2% of the cases does the proportion of plasma cells exceed 5%.[16] If more sensitive techniques such as immunophenotyping or polymerase chain reaction are used, circulating plasma cells can be detected in 80% of patients.[18,19]

Increased erythrocyte sedimentation rate (ESR) (usually greater than 50 mm in 1 hour) as well as rouleaux formation, due to hypergammaglobulinaemia, are present in about two-thirds of patients.[15,16] Ten percent of myeloma patients, mainly those with light-chain disease, have ESR values of less than 20 mm. The detection of an ESR value of more than 100 mm should point to a possible diagnosis of myeloma.

BIOCHEMICAL MARKERS AND CYTOKINES

Evaluation of renal function, either by serum blood urea nitrogen (BUN) or creatinine levels, is most important because it has an influence on disease outcome.[20] Around 25–30% of myeloma patients have creatinine values above 2 mg/dl at diagnosis, and the proportion of patients with renal impairment doubles during disease evolution.[15,16,20] Hypercalcaemia is detected in a similar proportion of patients. Severe hyperuricaemia is less frequent in our experience (15%), although others have seen it in almost one-third of patients.[16]

Lactate dehydrogenase (LDH) activity, reflecting cell turnover, is increased in very aggressive forms of myeloma, usually associated with tumour masses and short survival. In our experience, only 20% of myeloma patients display high LDH levels at diagnosis.[20]

False hyperphosphataemia due to interference of the M protein with the molybdate reagent used in the phosphate assay has been reported.[21] Severe hypoglycaemia, secondary to hyperinsulinaemia, may also occur.[15] Hyperamylasaemia has been described secondary to the secretion of amylase by malignant plasma cells.[22]

β_2-Microglobulin

β_2-Microglobulin (β_2M) is a low-molecular-weight protein found on the surface of all nucleated cells, representing the light chain of the HLA class I histocompatibility antigen complex. β_2M can be measured by radioimmunoassay (RIA) or enzyme-linked immunosorbant assay (ELISA).

In myeloma patients, β_2M levels may increase owing to renal impairment or advanced stage.[23–28] The increases seen in renal insufficiency result from decreased glomerular filtration of this molecule, which, in fact, is a very sensitive indicator of glomerular filtration. Initially, it was suggested that β_2M should be corrected according to serum creatinine. However, further studies showed that it was better to use the uncorrected value, because it could provide prognostic information on tumour burden as well as renal function.[23–30] At the time of diagnosis, most myeloma patients have increased serum β_2M levels. In general, β_2M levels cannot discriminate early-stage and smouldering myeloma from MGUS.[24,28] Nevertheless, a serum β_2M level of more than 3 µg/dl in a patient with a monoclonal protein and normal renal function strongly suggests a diagnosis of myeloma.[28]

The most important application of serum β_2M is as a prognostic factor. In all reported studies,[23–30] it has proven to be one of the most, if not *the* most, relevant prognostic factor in myeloma: β_2M levels above 5 µg/ml identify a subgroup of patients with a median survival of only two years.[30] In contrast, β_2M is not helpful for monitoring the course of the disease, because there are patients who relapse without a preceding increase in β_2M level whereas others have levels in the upper normal limit without any evidence of disease progression.[10] Additionally, β_2M levels are elevated in patients on interferon, even if the disease is in remission.

Serum thymidine kinase

Thymidine kinase (TK) catalyses the phosphorylation of deoxythymidine in the DNA salvage pathway. The thymidine kinase 1 isoenzyme is present in high concentrations in proliferating cells.[31] Serum TK activity can be determined by radioenzyme assay. About 25% of all myeloma patients display high TK levels, and this feature confers an adverse prognosis.[31] However, determination of serum TK does not give diagnostic or prognostic information in patients with MGUS, because only stage III disease is associated with significantly increased activity compared with MGUS.[32]

Interleukin-6 and soluble IL-6 receptor

The availability of RIA and ELISA has facilitated laboratory evaluation of serum cytokine and cytokine receptor levels in myeloma. Of these, interleukin (IL)-6 and its soluble receptor (sIL-6R) have been the most widely explored.

IL-6 is a pleiotropic cytokine that induces differentiation of B lymphocytes into Ig-secreting cells and proliferation of plasma cells, playing a key role in the pathogenesis of myeloma.[33] Although it has been suggested that IL-6 may be produced directly by plasma cells (autocrine secretion), there is stronger evidence that this cytokine is produced by other cells from the marrow microenvironment (paracrine secretion).[34] Stimulation of cells by IL-6 requires binding to the IL-6 receptor (IL-6R). This receptor is composed of two subunits: an 80 kDa glycoprotein (CD126) to which IL-6 binds, and a signal-transducing glycoprotein of 130 kDa (gp130 or CD130).[35] Soluble IL-6R is generated through the shedding of the receptor from the cell membrane or by alternative RNA splicing.[36]

Serum IL-6 and sIL-6R may be measured by ELISA or RIA.[29,37] Recently, immunoassay kits for IL-6 have become available that have a sensitivity of a few femtograms and are not influenced by the presence of soluble receptor in the assay mixture.[21]

An attractive alternative for investigation of in situ production of IL-6 can be the use of double-staining methods (one antibody for the identification of plasma cells and another anti-IL-6) analysed by multiparameter flow cytometry.

Serum IL-6 levels are increased in 30–50% of myeloma patients.[37–42] Although the levels in myeloma are higher than in MGUS, the serum IL-6 level does not have a significant predictive value for the differential diagnosis between myeloma and MGUS, because the levels in early-stage myeloma and MGUS overlap.[37] In myeloma, high serum IL-6 levels reflect active disease and a poor prognosis.[37–42]

Although sIL-6R levels do not show a linear correlation with serum IL-6 levels,[42] sIL-6R levels are also elevated in 25–50% of myeloma patients.[8,42,43] sIL-6R is also not a reliable marker for differentiating between myeloma and MGUS.[43] It has been reported that serial measurements of serum sIL-6R levels could be useful for monitoring disease activity.[43] However, its prognostic value has not been established well. Some groups have found that increased s-IL6R levels are associated with a shorter survival,[8,42] although others have not been able to confirm this.[43]

Several other cytokines, such as IL-2, IL-4, and IL-10, have also been analysed in myeloma, but do not appear to have any clear diagnostic or prognostic value. Blade et al[44] have suggested that the measurement of tumour necrosis factor α (TNF-α) by ELISA could contribute to predicting the risk of transformation of MGUS into myeloma. TNF-α levels were elevated in 55% of myeloma patients and 22% of MGUS patients, and MGUS patients with high TNF-α levels had a higher probability of transformation into myeloma.

Acute-phase reactants

C-reactive protein (CRP) is an acute-phase reactant protein whose synthesis by human hepatocytes is induced by IL-6. Actually, serum CRP levels reflect IL-6 activity, and they represent a surrogate for IL-6 concentration, and infusion of anti-IL-6 monoclonal antibodies in myeloma decreases CRP levels to undetectable values.[27] Serum CRP levels can be measured by commercially available ELISA kits or nephelometry. Both methods give very similar results.[27]

Forty percent of myeloma patients have increased serum CRP values (>6 mg/l), while this only occurs in 8% of MGUS patients. Moreover, myeloma patients who remain in remission have significantly lower CRP values than those who relapse, suggesting that this marker may be of help in disease monitoring. However, CRP is not a specific marker of disease activity in myeloma, and increases because of several different factors. Evaluation of CRP is important in myeloma at diagnosis, since it is an independent prognostic factor that can substitute for serum IL-6 levels (its determination is more rapid, simpler, and cheaper), and together with β_2M it constitutes an excellent combination for the prognostic stratification of myeloma patients.[27]

IL-6 also influences the hepatic synthesis of other acute-reactant-phase proteins, such as α_1-antitrypsin and orosomucoid, which can also be measured by nephelometric assays. α_1-Antitrypsin offers very similar information to CRP, since it is also raised in 40% of myeloma patients, correlates with IL-6 values, and together with β_2M, constitutes an excellent combination of prognostic factors.[29] Orosomucoid is increased in 20% of myeloma patients, but its correlation with prognosis is less clear.[29,45]

Laboratory markers of bone disease

Radiographic techniques do not provide information on bone metabolism. Several biochemical markers are available for the specific evaluation of bone resorption.[46–48] The pyridinium crosslinks of collagen have been established as specific urinary markers of bone resorption. Pyridinoline (PYD) and deoxypyridinoline (DPD) are mature, covalent crosslinks of collagen, and contribute to the stability of the extracellular matrix of bone. In healthy adults, about 40% of the urinary crosslinks are excreted in a free form; the remaining 60% are bound to fragments of collagen peptides.[46] The standard method for determining urinary pyridinium crosslinks is ion-paired high-performance liquid chromatography (HPLC), which may be used to measure both total and free pyridinium crosslink levels in urine.[48] An enzyme immunoassay that is highly specific for free urinary DPD has been developed, and results obtained with this immunoassay are reported to correlate well with HPLC measurements of total DPD.[48] A possible shortcoming of these studies is that they require specific conditions of urine sample collection: at least 12 hours fasting or collection of the sample in mid-morning in order to avoid diurnal variations, and collection of the second void urine.

Patients with advanced myeloma (clinical stage III) show significantly higher levels of urinary excretion of PYD and DPD than healthy individuals and patients with MGUS.[46] However, these parameters are not useful for discriminating MGUS from early-stage myeloma. Although the urinary levels of DPD are increased in myeloma with advanced clinical stages and progressive disease, and are associated with CRP, creatinine, and albumin serum levels, the correlation with survival is only marginal.[46] An attractive possibility would be to use pyridinium crosslinks to monitor bisphosphonate therapy.[47]

The crosslinked carboxy-terminal telopeptide of collagen I (ICTP) is a stable fragment of collagen that can be used as a marker of bone resorption.[49,50] It can be measured by RIA or ELISA, which represents an important advantage over pyridinium crosslinks. Its main disadvantage is its renal elimination: levels increase when the glomerular filtration rate is less than 50 ml/min. Determination of ICTP provides prognostic information, since an inverse correlation with survival has been shown.[49,50] The crosslinked amino-terminal telopeptide of collagen I (Ntx), assessed by ELISA in urine, has recently been introduced as a marker of bone resorption. Ntx, as well as ICTP, should be useful in monitoring treatment with bisphosphonates.

Serum bone sialoprotein is another biochemical marker of bone turnover that affords similar results to DPD. It is significantly increased in stage III disease, but it does not discriminate between MGUS and stage I myeloma. Serum osteocalcin (elevated in myeloma) and bone-specific alkaline phosphatase (decreased in myeloma) have been used for a long time as markers of bone formation, but they are less specific than pyridinium crosslinks for the evaluation of bone disease.[48]

IMMUNOPHENOTYPING

Immunophenotyping studies on myeloma plasma cells over 15 years have shown some variability of results.[51–64] Heterogeneous or even discrepant results reported are related, at least to some extent, to methodological problems and the lack of standardization of the techniques used. For example, monoclonal antibodies of the same cluster of differentiation (CD) may detect different epitopes and therefore give discrepant reactivities.[65] The fluorochrome used for conjugation of the antibody may modify the positivity threshold by its effect on the intensity of the signal, and, as a result, change the number of reactive cells detected. Furthermore, very few previous studies have included multiple staining techniques with markers for antigens specifically expressed on plasma cells.[59]

In terms of technique, flow cytometry has many advantages over fluorescence microscopy and APAAP (immuno-alkaline phosphatase): higher number of cells analysed, simultaneous multiple marker analysis, assessment of fluorescence intensity (crucial for CD38; see below), and higher sensitivity.

It is well established that CD38 and CD138 (B-B4) are the two best markers for identifying plasma cells. Although the CD38 antigen is widely distributed in the haematopoietic system, flow cytometry has shown that the intensity at which it is expressed on plasma cells is clearly higher than on any other cell type. This strong reactivity for CD38 ('CD38^{+++}') has converted it into a 'specific' plasma cell marker, ideal for multiple-staining studies in which plasma cells must be identified.[57,59,64,66,67] Anti-CD138 antibodies, which recognize syndecan-1,[68] have been shown to be highly specific for the detection of both benign and malignant plasma cells.

In the bone marrow, anti-CD138 antibodies stain the CD38^{+++} fraction of cells that exclusively contains plasma cells[68] and vice versa.[69,70] Several other monoclonal antibodies recognizing antigens on plasma cells, such as R1–3, 62B1, 8A, PCA-1, and PCA-2, have been produced.[51,52,71] However, they are not specific to plasma cells.

Thus, at present, CD38^{+++} and CD138^{+} are the best markers for the identification of plasma cells (Figure 15.1).[59] In addition, plasma cells display singular light-scattering characteristics, which also contribute to their unequivocal identification by flow cytometry (Figure 15.1).[59]

Although early studies showed that myeloma plasma cells usually displayed very low or no expression of antigens classically considered pan-B-lymphoid-associated,[72] later studies in larger series of patients, in which more sensitive techniques were used, showed that plasma cells express some B-cell antigens in a variable proportion of patients. Pellat-Deceunynck et al[69] found CD19-positivity in 35% of myeloma patients, although in the experience of other groups (including ours), positivity is seen in a much lower proportion of patients.[16,56,64] While some groups have reported that myelomatous plasma cells show no expression of either CD20[16] or CD22,[64] other groups[73] have found reactivity for these markers in around 15% of patients. Likewise, the presence of sIg has been reported in up to one-third of all myeloma patients.[61,74] Several groups have also detected CD10 (frequently present in B-lymphoid malignancies) on plasma cells with a highly variable frequency (10–60%).[54,58,59,73]

The heterogeneity of the expression of B-cell-associated antigens could reflect different stages of maturation. This is consistent with the fact that the neoplastic clone may be able to undergo a certain degree of differentiation. In line with this hypothesis, it has been reported that two plasma cell populations exist in myeloma: CD45^{+} and CD45^{-}, with CD45^{+} plasma cell population corresponding to more immature cells.[75]

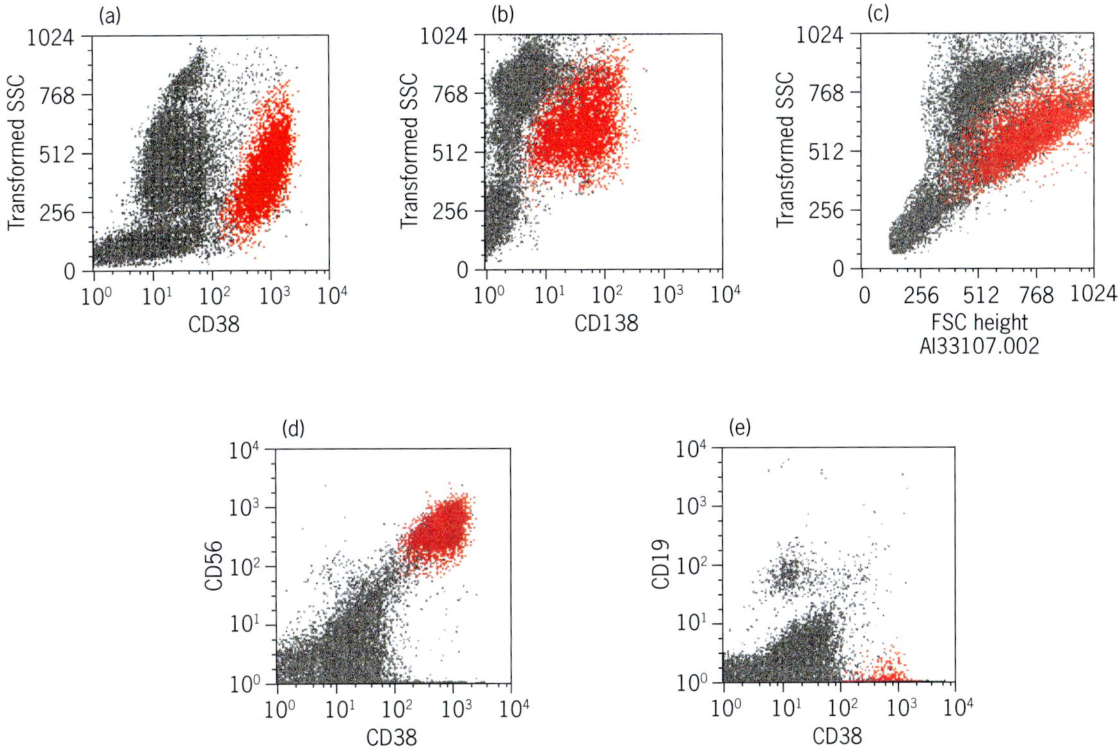

Figure 15.1 Immunophenotypic identification of bone marrow plasma cells in myeloma on the basis of their strong reactivity for CD38 (a), positivity for CD138 (b), and their light-scattering characteristics (c). Malignant plasma cells usually display a strong positivity for CD56 (d) in the absence of reactivity for CD19 (e).

Malignant plasma cells strongly express the CD56 adhesion molecule in two-thirds of the patients[55,56,76] (Figure 15.1). The other cell surface adhesion molecules expressed by myeloma cells include β_1-integrins (VLA-1, -4, and -5) and a β_2-integrin (LFA-1), and other adhesion molecules of the immunoglobulin superfamily, such as CD54 (ICAM-1), CD102 (ICAM-2), and CD50 (ICAM-3); also, plasma cells display reactivity for proteoglycans such as syndecan-1 and CD44.[33,56,62,63,67,70,77]

Other surface antigens are found on myelomatous plasma cells in a variable proportion of patients: CD117 (in one-third of the patients[60]), the granulomonocytic antigens CD13 and CD33 (in one-quarter of patients[64]), and co-stimulatory molecules involved in the activation of B and T lymphocytes, such as CD40 and CD28 (positive in 70% and 40%, respectively[69]).

Several groups[59,65,69,70,74] have analysed the prognostic implication of the immunophenotypic characteristics of plasma cells. Markers associated with immature cells (CD20 and sIg) have been associated with a poor outcome.[65,74] Downregulation of CD11a and CD56, and a greater expression of CD44, has been associated with extramedullary spread.[69,70] CD28 expression has been related to disease activity – mainly the highly proliferative accelerated phase of the disease.[69] The presence of myelomonocytic antigens has been associated with a poor outcome.[65] Nevertheless, none of these markers has been clearly shown to have an independent prognostic value on multivariate analysis.

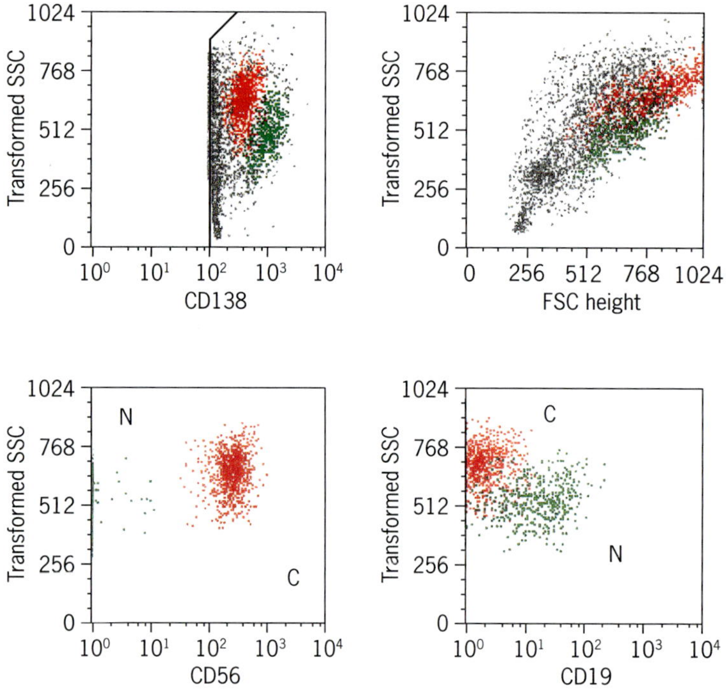

Figure 15.2 Immunophenotypic identification of bone marrow plasma cell populations in MGUS after acquisition of CD38^{+++} - gated cells: the N population (green) displays a phenotypic profile similar to that of normal bone marrow plasma cells, representing the normal residual plasma cells, while the C population (red) represents the clonal plasma cell subset, which displays a phenotype identical to that of myelomatous plasma cells.

Immunophenotypic studies for the differential diagnosis of myeloma and MGUS

Immunophenotypic characteristics of myeloma plasma cells differ from those of normal plasma cells in terms of CD19 and CD56 expression.[16,56,78] Malignant plasma cells display strong reactivity for CD56, usually associated with CD19-negativity (CD19^{-}/CD56^{++}). This phenotype is never seen in plasma cells from healthy individuals. Additionally, we have reported that malignant plasma cells express lower levels of CD38 and higher flow-cytometry light-scattering values compared with normal plasma cells.[78]

In MGUS patients, the coexistence of both normal and clonal plasma cell populations has been reported[56,78] (Figure 15.2). Interestingly, we have found that the presence of residual polyclonal (normal) plasma cells is a constant finding in MGUS patients but it is rare in myeloma (22% of the patients), and, when present, the amount of normal cells is significantly lower than that observed in MGUS.[78] Multivariate analysis showed that the proportion of normal residual plasma cells (> or <3% of the total number of plasma cells) was the most powerful single parameter for discriminating between MGUS and myeloma patients at diagnosis, even when only stage I disease was considered.[78]

Immunophenotypic studies for the investigation of residual disease

In our experience, most myeloma patients have abnormal immunophenotypic characteristics on their malignant cells that allow their unequivocal distinction from normal plasma cells, which is useful for monitoring therapy. These abnormalities can be easily identified using four triple combinations of monoclonal antibodies (CD38/CD56/CD19, CD20/CD28/CD38, CD117/CD33/CD38, and κ/λ/CD38) which makes this approach cost-effective.

Using a two-step acquisition procedure with a specific live gate for plasma cells (gate drawn on the CD38^{+++} fraction) to increase the number of plasma cells analysed, we have shown that it is possible to reach a detection limit of 10^{-4} to 10^{-5} (1 aberrant plasma cell among 10 000 to 100 000 normal haematopoietic cells).[79] Using this technique, we have detected residual malignant plasma cells in 44% of autologous blood stem cell collections and in 61% of marrow samples obtained three months post transplant. Follow-up studies are necessary to see whether this is useful in predicting relapse early.

Immunophenotypic studies for assessment of immunoregulatory cells

The immune status of the patient may play an important role in tumour growth control. The laboratory analysis of immunoregulatory cells in myeloma patients has focused mainly on the distribution of peripheral blood T-cell and natural killer (NK)-cell subsets.

Several studies have shown that myeloma patients have decreased $CD4^+$ cells, with significantly decreased $CD4^+/CD8^+$ ratio.[80,81] The decline of $CD4^+$ cells mainly involves naive cells ($CD4^+/CD45RA^+$), while the memory $CD4^+$ T cells are almost totally preserved.[82] A correlation has been reported between lower peripheral blood $CD4^+$ cell numbers and lower survival[81] and greater disease progression.[83] However, in our experience, this is not an independent prognostic factor.[81] An increase in the absolute number of $CD8^+$ cells has not been consistently seen.[84] The reduced $CD4^+/CD8^+$ ratio is seen in myeloma and not in MGUS. This could represent a useful parameter for differentiating between the two.[84]

The number of NK cells in the blood and marrow of myeloma patients has been studied using flow cytometry for the CD56, CD57, and CD16 antigens.[85] Österborg et al[86] reported a reduction in the number of cells expressing CD56, CD57, and CD16 in myeloma, particularly with advanced stage, as compared with MGUS and healthy donors. However, in this study, dual monoclonal antibody staining was not used to specifically identify NK cells. This is important, since these antigens can be expressed by other cells too. We have found, in fact, a significant increase in the number of NK cells in myeloma patients.[85] In our experience, the number of mature NK cells increases in early stages of the disease, probably reflecting an attempt by the immune system to control tumour growth. In advanced disease stages, the number of mature NK cells in the blood decreases, while the relative number of immature NK cells increases.[85] Since NK cells may affect tumour growth through immunoregulation, it is possible that their numbers could vary according to the clinical stage of the disease. This, and the existence of functionally different subpopulations of NK cells, may also explain the discrepant results reported in the literature.

CYTOGENETIC STUDIES

Chromosomal abnormalities have become one of the most important prognostic factors in myeloma, and karyotyping should be mandatory in all patients with newly diagnosed disease.

Conventional cytogenetics (G-banding) has evolved in recent years into so-called molecular cytogenetics with the introduction of fluorescence in situ hybridization (FISH) techniques that allow direct analysis of specific DNA sequences, not only in metaphase chromosomes but also in interphase nuclei. Nevertheless, conventional cytogenetic analysis continues to be the first step for screening.[87–96]

The major shortcoming of G-banding is the difficulty in obtaining good-quality mitoses owing to the low proliferative rate of plasma cells. To avoid this problem, several modifications of the culture conditions have been explored. At present, a 72-hour culture without mitogen or a five-day culture with the addition of IL-6 and granulocyte–macrophage colony-stimulating factor (GM-CSF) appear to be the best culture conditions, since they yield the highest percentage of clonal mitosis.[97–99] We have also described a five-day culture system with IL-4 that yields excellent results in terms of the number of clonally abnormal metaphases obtained.[100]

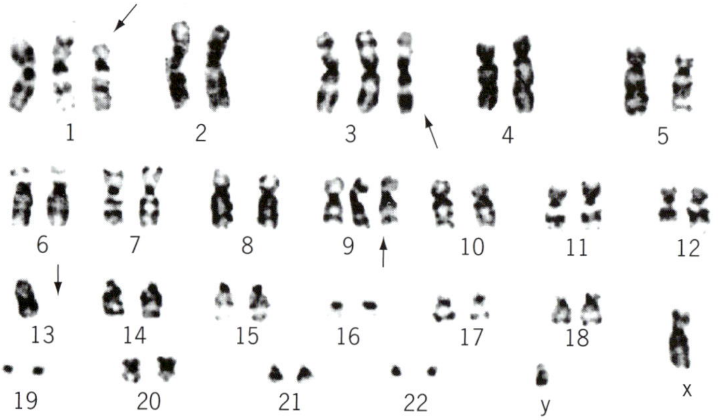

Figure 15.3 Representative karyotype in a patient with myeloma, showing several numerical changes, including trisomy 1, 3, and 9, and monosomy 13.

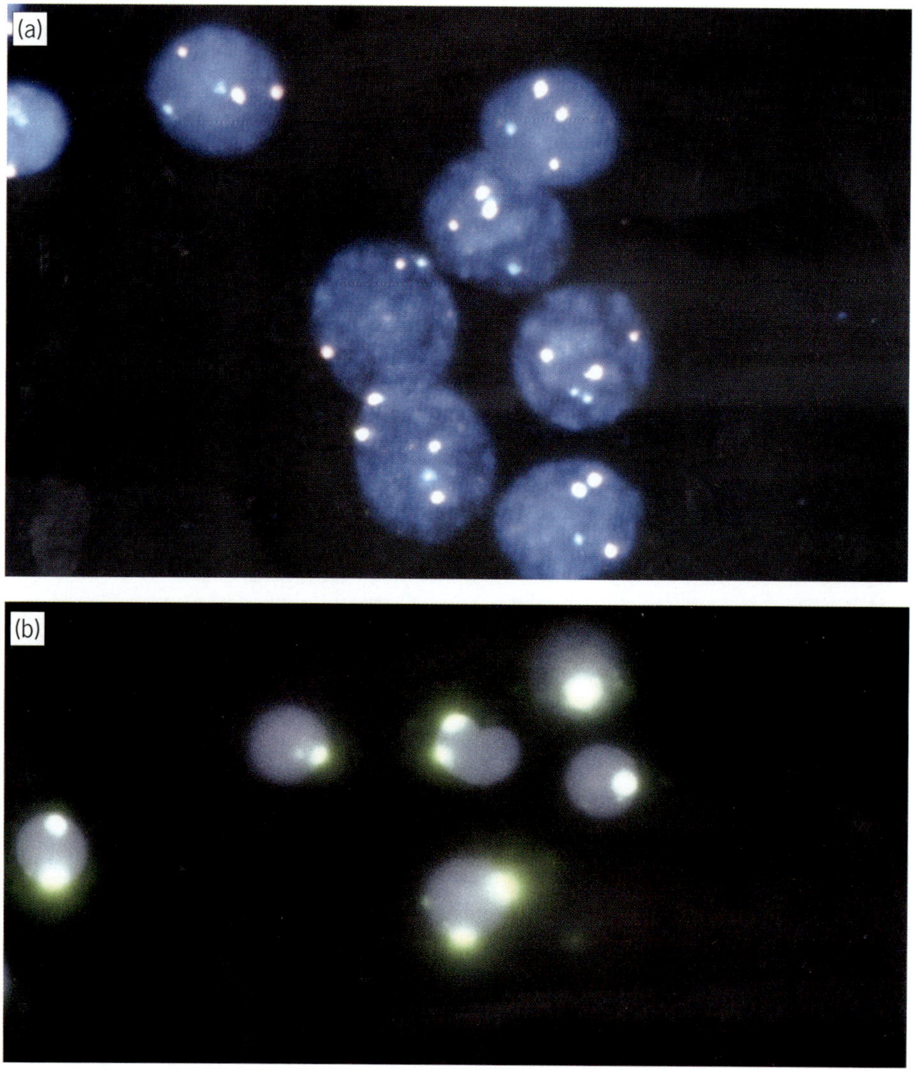

Figure 15.4 (a) Fluorescence in situ hybridization (FISH) signals for chromosomes 7 (green spots) and 9 (red spots). (b) FISH signals for chromosome 13 (green spots). Normal cells show two fluorescence spots for chromosomes 7 and 9 (a) and 13 (b), while malignant cells show trisomy 9 (three red spots per cell) in (a) and monosomy 13 (one spot per cell) in (b).

Overall, the percentage of myeloma cases with clonal cytogenetic changes ranges from 25% to 60%, depending upon the clinical status of the patient.[87–89,98–100] Figure 15.3 shows a karyotype from a myeloma patient, displaying several numerical changes.

FISH is an optimal method for the detection of numerical chromosomal changes, since it can be used on interphase cells, it does not require cell mitosis, and centromeric probes are available for almost all chromosomes.[101–103] FISH techniques are useful for the study of cryptic chromosomal abnormalities, and for the investigation of specific chromosomal regions[104] (Figure 15.4a,b).

In recent years, several techniques based on FISH, such as comparative genomic hybridization (CGH) and multicolour FISH, have been developed.[105–106] These techniques can be used to analyse complex karyotypes with large numbers of rearrangements involving different chromosomes.[107]

Not only do cytogenetic studies contribute to the knowledge of the pathogenesis of myeloma, but they also provide important prognostic information: the presence of a monosomy 13, abnormalities of 11q, or a complex karyotype are associated with poor prognosis.[108,109] Cytogenetic aspects of plasma cell disorders are discussed in depth in Chapter 5.

DNA PLOIDY STUDIES

Flow-cytometric measurement of cell DNA contents provides rapid and objective information on the presence of clonal quantitative abnormalities in the total DNA content per cell (DNA aneuploidy). This type of measurement has now been used for over 20 years. However, significant variations exist in sample preparation techniques, staining, instrumentation, and even data interpretation.

The DNA content of a given cell should be compared with that of a diploid cell population in the same cell cycle phase from a normal sex-matched individual. Accordingly, the DNA content of a cell population as assessed by flow cytometry is usually expressed as its DNA index, which is obtained by dividing the modal fluorescence channel of the G_0/G_1 peak of the tumour cells by the modal fluorescence channel of the residual G_0/G_1 normal cells present in the sample. If this DNA index is 1, the tumour cells are considered to be DNA-diploid, whereas if it is not 1, the cells are considered to be DNA-aneuploid (<1 is hypodiploid and >1 is hyperdiploid).

Reports of cell DNA content in myeloma show considerable variability in the frequency of DNA aneuploidy, and its clinical and prognostic implications. The overall incidence of DNA aneuploidy in myeloma has been reported to range between 28% and 80%.[110–112] The reasons for such discrepancies were evaluated in a DNA Cytometry Consensus Conference held in October 1992.[113] At the conference, it was stated that the discrepancies can be largely attributed to poorly designed studies involving small numbers of patients and lacking sufficient follow-up, and to technical artefacts.

The use of samples containing too few tumour cells or samples stored under inappropriate

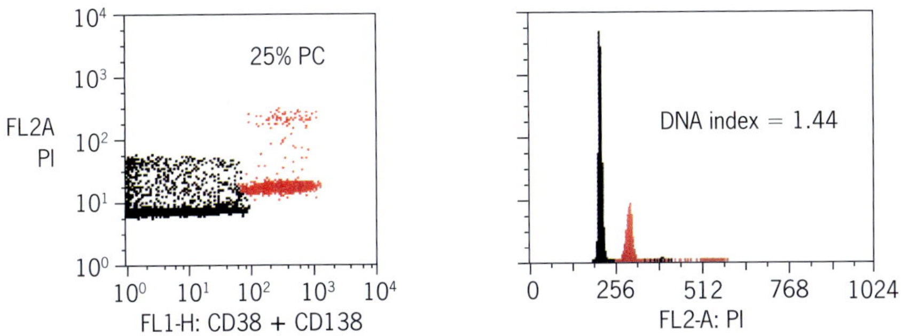

Figure 15.5 Simultaneous staining for plasma cell markers (with a combination of monoclonal antibodies directed against CD38 and CD138 antigens) and DNA (with propidium iodide, PI). Malignant plasma cells from a myeloma patient show hyperdiploid DNA content (DNA index 1.44).

conditions, the lack of specific stainings for the identification of neoplastic cells, and the use of preparation procedures in which tumour cells can be selectively lost or destroyed are some of the technical pitfalls that may interfere with results.

Using a highly sensitive method in which simultaneous staining for plasma cells ($CD38^{+++}/CD138^{+}$) and DNA was performed, we have analysed more than 300 untreated myeloma patients. DNA aneuploidy was present in 62% of cases, the overwhelming majority being hyperdiploid.[78,114] Figure 15.5 shows a representative aneuploid myeloma sample.

It has been suggested that DNA hypoploidy may be associated with a poor response to treatment and short survival.[115] However, the incidence of DNA hypodiploidy is very low in the majority of series. A high incidence of DNA hypoploidy has been reported for plasma cell leukaemia,[111] which supports the hypothesis of a worse prognosis for DNA hypodiploid myeloma.

Although some studies have suggested that DNA hyperploidy may be associated with a worse prognosis (especially when the DNA index is higher than 1.15),[116] in our experience patients with DNA hyperdiploidy have a significantly better outcome than diploid cases.[114,117]

The incidence of DNA aneuploidy in MGUS patients has been reported to range from 0% to 61%.[110,118,119] None of these reports describes a method in which the analysis of cell DNA content was specifically performed on plasma cells. In addition, the variation found in the relative distribution of normal and clonal plasma cells in MGUS patients may also help explain the variation.

We have analysed the plasma cell DNA-ploidy status in a series of 76 MGUS cases using simultaneous staining for plasma cells and

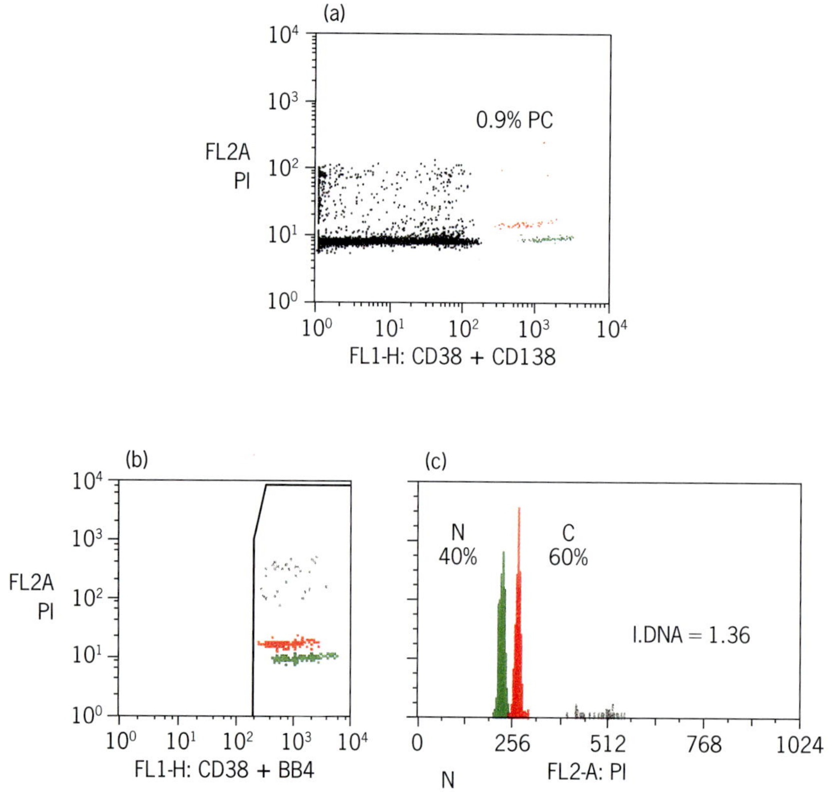

Figure 15.6 Plasma cell DNA-ploidy analysis in a MGUS patient. Using simultaneous staining for plasma cells and DNA, two clearly distinct plasma cell subsets can be distinguished based on their differing DNA content (a). These two subpopulations can be more clearly distinguished upon acquiring plasma cells through a live gate drawn on the $CD38^{+++}/CD138^{+}$ fraction (b): 60% of plasma cells display hyperdiploidy (clonal population, red), while the remaining plasma cells display diploid DNA content (normal population, green) (c).

DNA. Based on this methodological approach, two clearly different plasma cell subsets could be detected in 73% of the cases[78] – one showing normal DNA content (corresponding to polyclonal plasma cells) and the other displaying DNA aneuploidy (corresponding to the malignant clone) (Figure 15.6).

The aneuploid subpopulation found in MGUS marrow samples always showed a DNA index greater than 1.[78] These results are in line with the fact that the presence of DNA hyperdiploidy in myeloma patients is associated with a better prognosis, since most MGUS patients do not develop myeloma. The presence of two plasma cell subpopulations with different DNA content would be useful in differentiating between myeloma and MGUS, because there is usually only one plasma cell population in myeloma – either aneuploid or diploid.

DNA aneuploidy constitutes a specific tumour marker that is present in a high proportion of myeloma patients at diagnosis, and could be used for monitoring these patients for the presence of residual tumour cells following high-dose chemotherapy. Using dilutional experiments, we have shown that aneuploid plasma cells can be detected even when present at frequencies lower than 10^{-4}.[79]

MOLECULAR GENETIC TECHNIQUES

Molecular laboratory investigations in myeloma patients have focused on two main objectives: the analysis of monoclonal immunoglobulin gene rearrangements and the study of the oncogenes and tumour suppressor genes involved in the pathogenesis of the disease.

Monoclonal immunoglobulin gene rearrangements

Myeloma cells show a specific heavy chain *VDJ* gene rearrangement (a molecular hallmark of a B-cell malignancy). Although these genes have been reported to be in germinal configuration in 10–20% of cases, this is probably due to technical pitfalls, since, by definition, all myeloma patients must have a *VDJ* gene rearrangement.[120]

Molecular techniques identify tumour-related DNA sequences based on the unique CDR3 region that is generated during the rearrangement of the immunoglobulin heavy-chain (*IgH*) genes. Somatic mutations, but not intraclonal variations, frequently occur, reflecting the mature post-germinal-centre origin of the neoplastic cells.[121] The main applicability of laboratory investigations of the *VDJ* gene rearrangements is for monitoring minimal residual disease; either employing a polymerase chain reaction (PCR)-based strategy (clone-specific sequences derived from the *IgH* gene rearrangement) or using an *IgH* fingerprinting technique. These studies show that although some myeloma patients achieve molecular remission following allografting or double autografting,[122] clonal cells persist in most cases.[123] Moreover, most leukapheresis products and marrow harvests from myeloma patients undergoing autotransplantation contain residual myeloma cells.[123]

Investigation of the CDR3 sequence has also been used to demonstrate clonal involvement of circulating B cells in myeloma, with a small subset of marrow and peripheral blood B lymphocytes displaying the same rearrangement pattern as myelomatous plasma cells in 50% and 25% of myeloma patients, respectively.[124] The number of clonal peripheral blood B cells may help identify MGUS patients at a higher risk of transformation to myeloma.[125] Fifty-three percent of MGUS cases displaying an excess of peripheral blood clonal B lymphocytes transformed into myeloma, compared with 17% of cases who did not show an excess of clonal B cells.[125]

Oncogenes and tumour suppressor genes

Dysregulation of oncogenes and tumour suppressor genes contributes to the pathogenesis of myeloma. Some of these genetic abnormalities may have an impact on prognosis. The value of most of these studies for discriminating myeloma from MGUS is relatively low, since many of the genetic abnormalities are also present in a variable proportion of MGUS patients.

c-myc

The t(8;14) translocation occurs in less that 5% of patients with myeloma.[33,126] However, DNA rearrangements involving *c-myc* or the *MLVI-4* locus (located 20 kb downstream of *c-myc*) are seen in up to 20% of patients. Increased expression of *c-myc* and a selective expression of one of the *c-myc* alleles frequently occurs in myeloma, and expression of c-Myc protein is commonly increased in myeloma cells and myeloma-derived cell lines.[33] A significant correlation has been found between c-Myc expression and the histologic grade, the isotype of the M protein and tumour burden.[126]

bcl-1 / cyclin D1

The t(11;14) translocation is present in 25–40% of myeloma patients. Interestingly, the breakpoint in myeloma is different from that observed in mantle cell lymphoma (*MTC* region). The breakpoint in myeloma is 120 kb upstream from the *cyclin D1* gene. Thus, there is a close association between t(11;14) and enhanced expression of *cyclin D1*, although it is possible that other genes may also be involved.[127] Cyclin D1, together with CDK4, phosphorylates Rb (the retinoblastoma tumour suppressor gene product), inactivating it, and allows progression through G_1 to S phase of the cell cycle. The presence of t(11;14) (q13;q32) in myeloma is associated with a lymphoplasmacytic cell morphology as well as with aggressive disease forms and a poor prognosis.[128]

FGFR3

The fibroblast growth factor (FGF) receptor 3 gene has been found to be dysregulated by t(4;14)(p16;q32) in approximately 25% of newly diagnosed myeloma patients and myeloma cell lines.[129] This translocation has not been described before, and may be unique to myeloma. Hallek et al[33] have suggested that, as a result of t(4;14), myeloma cells receive an FGFR3–mediated signal from FGF produced by marrow stromal cells, and this continuous signal interferes with their terminal differentiation and ability to undergo apoptosis.

bcl-2

Overexpression of Bcl-2 protein, as assessed by immunohistochemistry, has been reported in the majority of myeloma patients and in myeloma cell lines, in spite of the fact that t(14;18) is rarely detected (0–15%).[130] It should be noted that high levels of Bcl-2 protein have also been detected in normal marrow plasma cells. The prognostic implication of *bcl-2* overexpression by myelomatous plasma cells remains controversial.

Other evidence of oncogenic dysregulation related to disease progression

According to the multistep pathogenetic model suggested by Hallek et al,[33] tumour progression requires the accumulation of sequential additional mutations/deletions. These molecular changes are usually not seen in MGUS, but are associated with aggressive disease and refractoriness to treatment in myeloma. A number of oncogenic events are involved in the 'escape' of plasma cells, and are discussed in depth in Chapter 2.

Mutations of N- and K-*ras* are not present in MGUS, but are seen in 9–30% of myeloma cases. The incidence increases (up to 70%) with progressive disease and plasma cell leukaemia.[131] Myeloma patients with K-*ras* mutations have a shorter survival than those who do not.[132]

p53 tumour suppressor gene mutations occur in only around 5% of inactive myeloma, but the incidence increases with disease progression, and reaches up to 40% in plasma cell leukaemia.[133]

The retinoblastoma (*Rb*) tumour suppressor gene is located on chromosome 13. Monosomy of chromosome 13 have been identified in approximately 30% of abnormal myeloma karyotypes. By Southern blot or interphase FISH analysis, monoallelic deletion of *Rb* has been reported in about 30–60% of myeloma cases and cell lines, independent of disease stage. By contrast, bi-allelic loss of the *Rb* gene is

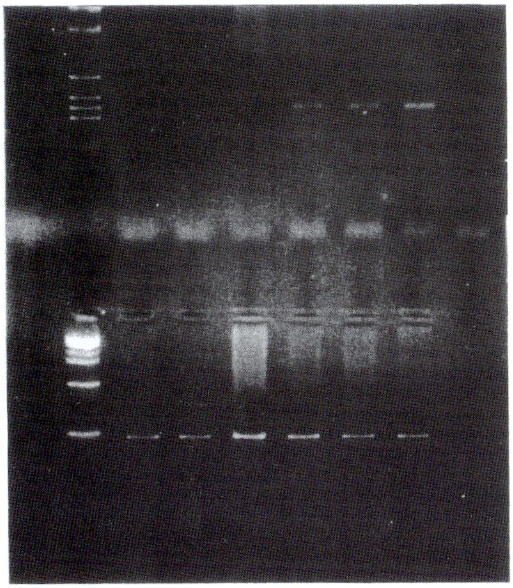

Figure 15.7 Methylation pattern of exon E1 of the *p16* gene in myeloma patients analysed by PCR. Products of exons E1 and E2 are shown at the top and the bottom respectively. The amplification of exon E1 after digestion with *Eag*I, a methylation-sensitive restriction enzyme, indicates that this restriction site was methylated and the amplification of exon E2 of the *p16* gene indicates a good PCR. Lane 1: Marker and DNA digested with *Hin*dIII. Lane 2: DNA from a healthy donor, digested with *Eag*I. Lane 7: Undigested DNA from the same healthy donor. Lane 8: Distilled water. The presence of a band corresponding to exon 1 of the *p16* gene in lanes 6 and 7 represents methylated samples.

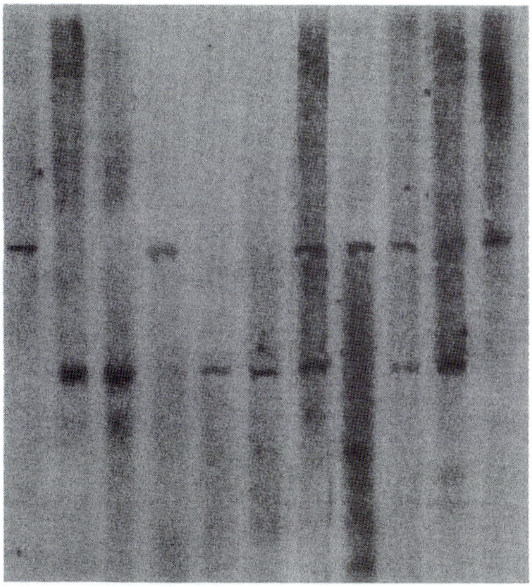

Figure 15.8 Methylation status at the 5′CpG island of the *p16* gene by Southern blot. Sizes of the fragments (Kb) are specified on the left. Cases were digested using *Hin*dIII, a methylation-non-sensitive restriction enzyme, and *Sac*II, a methylation-sensitive restriction enzyme, and hybridized with the exon E1 probe. Lane 1: DNA sample from a healthy donor digested only with *Hin*dIII, which originates a 6 kb fragment. Lane 2: The same DNA sample digested with both enzymes, originating a 3.9 kb fragment (unmethylated sample). Lanes 3–11: DNA from myeloma cases digested with the *Hin*dIII and *Sac*II restriction enzymes. Lanes 3, 5, and 6 show only the 3.9 kb band, indicating that they are unmethylated cases. Lanes 4, 8, and 11 show the presence of the 6 kb band alone, indicating that they are methylated cases with high plasma cell infiltration. Lanes 7, 9, and 10 show the presence of both 6 and 3.9 kb bands, indicating the presence of methylated cells accompanied by residual normal cells. In these cases, the 6 kb band originates from methylated neoplastic plasma cells, while the 3.9 kb band is derived from the unmethylated normal cells.

infrequent in myeloma, and thus the majority of myeloma patients (with monoallelic lesions) do not manifest changes in Rb expression.[33]

Deletion of *Rb* has been associated with an adverse prognosis.[109] No evidence exists so far showing the presence of this abnormality in MGUS patients. By contrast, we have shown that monoallelic deletion of *Rb* occurs in 85% of plasma cell leukaemia cases.[134]

Other cell-cycle regulatory genes, such as inhibitors of cyclin-dependent kinases (*p16*, *p21*^{Waf1} and *MDM2*), have also been thought to be involved in myeloma progression, but the information is still too limited to allow firm conclusions to be drawn. Figures 15.7 and 15.8 show the methylation status of the *p16* gene in myeloma patients analysed by PCR and Southern-blot, respectively.

PLASMA CELL LABELLING INDEX

Plasma cell labelling index (PCLI) usually refers to the percentage of plasma cells in S phase of the cell cycle, and therefore it reflects the cell kinetics of the myeloma cell clone. Joshua et al[135] have shown recently that proliferative activity is almost entirely attributable to increased labelling index of immature plasma cells.

Initially, PCLI was assessed by the incorporation of [^{3}H]thymidine, and proved to be an excellent independent prognostic factor in myeloma. Patients with a high tumour cell mass and over 3% of myeloma cells incorporating [^{3}H]thymidine (PCLI > 3%) had a median survival of only five months.[136] However, this technique uses in vitro radioactive labelling and is difficult for routine use. Because of this limitation, non-radioactive approaches such as the in vitro or in vivo incorporation of bromodeoxyuridine (BRDU), another thymidine analogue, have been developed, and have been shown to have a similar prognostic impact.[137]

An alternative technique is to analyse the expression of the Ki-67 nuclear antigen. However, correlation between Ki-67-positivity and PCLI measured by other techniques is relatively poor.[10]

Propidium iodide (PI) staining and flow-cytometric analysis permits the identification of cellular distribution along the different cell cycle phases. PI analysis is based on the assumption that S-phase cells have a DNA content that is between that of the G_0/G_1-phase and the G_2/M-phase populations. The use of appropriate mathematical models would then allow an accurate estimation of the distribution of a tumour population along the different cell cycle phases.[59] However, bone marrow contains many other cells apart from plasma cells. It is therefore critical to simultaneously identify the neoplastic cells present in the sample, so that their cell cycle distribution can be analysed separately from that of the normal haematopoietic cells. We have reported that the combined use of plasma-cell-related antigens ($CD38^{+++}/CD138^{+}$) and PI on flow cytometry can permit the assessment of the cell cycle distribution of myeloma plasma cells separately from that of normal haematopoietic cells.[138] With this method, we have found a clear correlation between a high percentage of S-phase plasma cells (>3%) and poor outcome.[114] With the same technique, additional information about the regenerative activity of normal haematopoietic cells can also be obtained.

PCLI may also help to differentiate between myeloma, MGUS, and smouldering myeloma.[28] In patients with a monoclonal gammopathy, elevated PCLI assessed by BRDU incorporation is a strong indication that myeloma is already present or that symptomatic myeloma will develop soon. However, more than one-third of patients with symptomatic myeloma have a normal PCLI,[139] which undermines its diagnostic specificity.

MULTIDRUG RESISTANCE (MDR)

Myeloma cells develop resistance to therapy through various mechanisms. These are inactivation or elimination of drugs by the cell,[140–142] increased activity of mechanisms involved in repairing drug-induced cell damage,[143] and anti-apoptotic mechanisms that prevent tumour cells affected by chemotherapy from undergoing apoptosis.[144]

The expression of the multidrug-resistance protein (MDR1 or P-glycoprotein, PgP) has been one of the most extensively explored mechanisms of drug resistance, and is associated with a poor response to chemotherapy.[140] MDR1 is a member of the ABC (ATP-binding cassette) membrane transporters,[145] which is coded on chromosome 7 at q21–31.

MDR1 expression can be measured by using molecular techniques, monoclonal antibodies, or functional assays. A consensus meeting held in 1994[146] concluded that more than one technique must be employed to assess MDR1 in order to avoid the great variability of results seen in different reports.

Western blot, Northern blot, and reverse-transcriptase (RT)-PCR are molecular techniques for MDR1 assessment, but do not allow discrimination between plasma cells and normal bone marrow cells (which also express MDR1), and may show false-positive results.[147]

A number of monoclonal antibodies are available to detect MDR1 expression by flow cytometry. However, many of these antibodies detect intracellular epitopes (JSB1, C219), making the technique cumbersome.[146,148,149] The ideal monoclonal antibody for MDR1 assessment should detect an external epitope, should have a high affinity for the MDR1 protein, and should be conjugated with phycoerythrin. Preliminary results indicate that the UIC2, 4E3, and 15D3 monoclonal antibodies possess these characteristics, but only 15D3 is available commercially in a phycoerythrin-conjugated format.[150] It should be noted that flow-cytometric studies must include multiple labelling to simultaneously identify the malignant clone and MDR1.

The expression of the MDR1 phenotype does not mean that the protein is functionally active. Several approaches have been developed to determine activity in which rhodamine 123 (rh123) and doxorubicin are employed.[151–153] Cells are incubated with rh123/doxorubicin for a short period of time (15 minutes) in order to incorporate high levels of the substrates into the cells. After that, cells are incubated for an hour at 37°C without rh123/doxorubicin. Cells expressing MDR1 eliminate more substrate than MDR1–negative cells. Simultaneous incubation with an MDR1–blocking agent such as verapamil or cyclosporine serves as a control. As with immunophenotyping, it is important to perform simultaneous antigenic labelling for plasma cells to ensure specificity of the analysis (substrate efflux from malignant cells as opposed to normal cells).

The reported incidence of MDR1 overexpression in myeloma varies greatly.[142,146,153] This is related, at least in part, to methodological issues since most reports have employed a single technique.

MDR1 expression has been related to previous chemotherapy.[154] Although some studies have suggested the existence of a relationship between the MDR1 phenotype and low response rates to VAD (vincristine–doxorubicin–dexamethasone),[155] other groups have not found this to be the case.[153] Similarly, conflicting results have been reported on the independent prognostic value of MDR1 expression.[155,156]

Expression of the multidrug-resistance-associated protein (MRP) has not been detected in myeloma. Recently, the expression of lung resistance protein (LRP), a cytoplasmic transporter protein, has been shown to be associated with a poor response to conventional doses of chemotherapy in myeloma.[140] Its adverse influence disappeared with the use of high-dose chemotherapy.

Information on other cellular mechanisms of multidrug resistance in myeloma is scanty or controversial. Linsenmeyer et al[157] have shown the presence of increased levels of the glutathione-*S*-transferase enzymes in myeloma. Potential anti-apoptotic mechanisms such as Bcl-2 overexpression[130] and *p53* gene mutations[133] have also been reported in myeloma. However, the clinical impact of these findings largely remains unclear.

REFERENCES

1. Greipp PR, Raymond NM, Kyle RA, O'Fallon M. Multiple myeloma: significance of plasmablastic subtype in morphological classification. *Blood* 1985; **65:** 305–10.

2. Bartl R, Frisch B, Burkhardt R et al. Bone marrow histology in myeloma: its importance in diagnosis, prognosis, classification and staging. *Br J Haematol* 1982; **51:** 361–75.
3. Bartl R, Frisch B, Fateh-Moghadam A et al. Histologic classification and staging of multiple myeloma. A retrospective and prospective study of 674 cases. *Am J Clin Pathol* 1987; **87:** 342–55.
4. Bayrd ED. The bone marrow on sternal aspiration in multiple myeloma. *Blood* 1948; **3:** 987–1018.
5. Fritz E, Ludwig H, Kundi M. Prognostic relevance of cellular morphology in multiple myeloma. *Blood* 1984; **63:** 1072–9.
6. Wutke K, Varbiro M, Rudiger KD, Kelenyi G. Cytological and histological classification of multiple myeloma. *Haematologia (Budap)* 1981; **14:** 315–29.
7. Schambeck CM, Bartl R, Hochtlen-Vollmar W et al. Characterization of myeloma cells by means of labeling index, bone marrow histology, and serum beta 2-microglobulin. *Am J Clin Pathol* 1996; **106:** 64–8.
8. Greipp PR, Leong T, Bennett JM et al. Plasmablastic morphology – an independent prognostic factor with clinical and laboratory correlates: Eastern Cooperative Oncology Group (ECOG) myeloma trial E9486 report by the ECOG Myeloma Laboratory Group. *Blood* 1998; **91:** 2501–7.
9. Portero JA, Martin S, Gonzalez M, San Miguel JF. Cytochemistry in the differential diagnosis of monoclonal gammopathies. *Br J Haematol* 1985; **60:** 768–9.
10. Greipp PR. Monoclonal gammopathies: new approaches to clinical problems in diagnosis and prognosis. *Blood Rev* 1989; **3:** 222–36.
11. Keren DF, Warren JS, Lowe JB. Strategy to diagnose monoclonal gammopathies in serum: high-resolution electrophoresis, immunofixation, and kappa/lambda quantification. *Clin Chem* 1988; **34:** 2196–201.
12. Normansell DE. Cost-effective detection of anomalous immunoglobulins in serum. *Clin Chem* 1988; **34:** 2193.
13. Kyle RA, Garton JP. Immunoglobulins and laboratory recognition of monoclonal proteins. In: *Neoplastic Diseases of the Blood* (Wiernik PH, Canellas GP, Kyle RA, Schiffer CA, eds). New York: Churchill Livingstone, 1991: 373–92.
14. Kyle RA. Diagnostic criteria of multiple myeloma. *Hematol Oncol Clin North Am* 1992; **6:** 347–58.
15. McIntyre OR. Laboratory investigation of myeloma. In: *Myeloma: Biology and Management* (Malpas JS, Bergsagel DE, Kyle RA, Anderson KC, eds). Oxford: Oxford University Press, 1998: 210–34.
16. Kyle RA, Bayrd ED. *The Monoclonal Gammopathies: Multiple Myeloma and Related Plasma-Cell Disorders*. Springfield: Charles C Thomas, 1976.
17. Boccadoro M, Pileri A. Plasma cell dyscrasias: classification, clinical and laboratory characteristics, and differential diagnosis. *Baillière's Clin Haematol* 1995; **8:** 705–19.
18. Witzig TE, Gertz MA, Lust JA et al. Peripheral blood monoclonal plasma cells as predictor of survival in patients with multiple myeloma. *Blood* 1996; **88:** 1780–7.
19. Rawstron AC, Owen RG, Davies FE. Circulating plasma cells in multiple myeloma: characterization and correlation with disease stage. *Br J Haematol* 1997; **97:** 46–55.
20. San Miguel JF, Sanchez Y, Gonzalez M. Prognostic factors and classification in multiple myeloma. *Br J Cancer* 1989; **59:** 113–18.
21. Oren S, Feldman A, Turkot S, Lugassy G. Hyperphosphatemia in multiple myeloma. *Ann Hematol* 1994; **69:** 41–3.
22. Delannoy A, Hamels J, Mecucci C et al. Amylase-producing IgD-type myeloma. *J Intern Med* 1992; **232:** 457–60.
23. Bataille R, Grenier J, Sany J. Beta-2-microglobulin in myeloma: optimal use for staging, prognosis and treatment: a prospective study of 160 patients. *Blood* 1984; **63:** 468–76.
24. Garewal H, Durie BGM, Kyle RA, Finley P, Bower B, Serokman R. Serum beta 2-microglobulin in the initial staging and subsequent monitoring of monoclonal plasma cell disorders. *J Clin Oncol* 1984; **2:** 51–7.
25. Boccadoro M, Omede D, Frieri R et al. Multiple myeloma: beta-2-microglobulin is not a useful follow-up parameter. *Acta Haematol* 1989; **82:** 122–5.
26. Cuzick J, De Stavola BL, Cooper EH et al. Long-term prognostic value of serum beta-2–microglobulin in myelomatosis. *Br J Haematol* 1990; **75:** 506–10.
27. Bataille R, Boccadoro M, Klein B et al. C-reactive protein and beta-2-microglobulin produce a simple and powerful myeloma staging system. *Blood* 1992; **80:** 733–7.
28. Kyle RA. Monoclonal gammopathy of undetermined significance and solitary plasmacytoma:

implications for progression to overt multiple myeloma. *Hematol Oncol Clin North Am* 1997; **11:** 71–88.
29. Pelliniemi TT, Irjala K, Mattila K et al. Immunoreactive interleukin-6 and acute phase proteins as prognostic factors in multiple myeloma. Finnish Leukemia Group. *Blood* 1995; **85:** 765–71.
30. San Miguel JF, Garcia-Sanz R, Gonzalez M et al. A new staging system for multiple myeloma based on the number of S-phase plasma cells. *Blood* 1995; **85:** 448–55.
31. Brown RD, Joshua DE, Nelson M et al. Serum thymidine kinase as a prognositc indicator for patient with multiple myeloma: results from the MRC (UK) V trial. *Br J Haematol* 1993; **84:** 238–44.
32. Back H, Jagenburg R, Rodjer S, Westin J. Serum deoxythymidine kinease: no help in the diagnosis and prognosis of monoclonal gammopathy. *Br J Haematol* 1993; **84:** 746–8.
33. Hallek M, Bergsagel PL, Anderson KC. Multiple myeloma: increasing evidence for a multistep transformation process. *Blood* 1998; **91:** 3–21.
34. Klein B. Cytokine, cytokine receptors, transduction signals and oncogenes in multiple myeloma. *Semin Hematol* 1995; **32:** 4–19.
35. Murakami M, Hibi M, Nakagawa N et al. IL-6 induced homodimerization of gp 130 and associated activation of a tyrosine kinase. *Science* 1993; **260:** 1808–10.
36. Lust JA, Donovan KA, Kline MP et al. Isolation of an mRNA encoding a soluble form of the human interleukin-6 receptor. *Cytokine* 1992; **4:** 96–100.
37. Du Villard L, Guiguet M, Casanovas RO et al. Diagnostic value of serum IL-6 level in monoclonal gammopathies. *Br J Haematol* 1995; **89:** 243–9.
38. Gaillard JP, Bataille R, Brailly H et al. Increased and highly stable levels of functional soluble interleukin-6 receptor in sera of patients with monoclonal gammopathy. *Eur J Immunol* 1993; **23:** 820–4.
39. Filella X, Blade J, Guillermo AL et al. Cytokines (IL-6, TNF-alpha, IL-1 alpha) and soluble interleukin-2 receptor as serum tumor markers in multiple myeloma. *Cancer Detect Prev* 1996; **20:** 52–6.
40. Papadaki H, Kyriakou D, Foudoulakis A et al. Serum levels of soluble IL-6 receptor in multiple myeloma as indicator of disease activity. *Acta Haematol* 1997; **97:** 191–5.
41. Bataille R, Jourdan M, Zhang XG, Klein B. Serum levels of interleukin 6, a potent myeloma cell growth factor, as a reflection of disease severity in plasma cell dyscrasias. *J Clin Invest* 1989; **84:** 2008–11.
42. Pulkki K, Pelliniemi RT, Rajamaki A et al. Soluble interleukin-6 receptor as a prognostic factor in multiple myeloma. *Br J Haematol* 1996; **92:** 370–4.
43. Ohtani K, Ninomiya H, Hasegawa Y et al. Clinical significance of elevated soluble interleukin-6 receptor levels in the sera of patients with plasma cell dyscrasias. *Br J Haematol* 1995; **91:** 116–20.
44. Filella X, Blade J, Montoto S et al. Impaired production of interleukin 6 and tumour necrosis factor alpha in whole blood cell cultures of patients with multiple myeloma. *Cytokine* 1998; **12:** 993–6.
45. Merlini G, Perfetti V, Gobbi PG et al. Acute phase proteins and prognosis in multiple myeloma. *Br J Haematol* 1993; **83:** 595–601.
46. Pecherstorfer M, Seibel MJ, Woitge HW et al. Bone resorption in multiple myeloma and in monoclonal gammopathy of undetermined significance: quantification by urinary pyridinium cross-links of collagen. *Blood* 1997; **90:** 3743–50.
47. Peest D, Deicher H, Feet W et al. Pyridinium cross-links in multiple myeloma: correlation with clinical parameters and use for monitoring of intravenous clodronate therapy: a pilot study of the German Myeloma Treatment Group (GMTG). *Eur J Cancer* 1996; **32:** 2053–7.
48. Woitge HW, Horn E, Keck AV et al. Biochemical markers of bone formation in patients with plasma cell dyscrasias and benign osteoporosis. *Clin Chem* 2001; **47:** 686–93.
49. Carlson K, Larsson A, Simonsson B et al. Evaluation of bone disease in multiple myeloma: a comparison between the resorption markers urinary deoxypyridinoline/creatinine (DPD) and serum ICTP, and an evaluation of the DPD/osteocalcin and ICTP/osteocalcin ratios. *Eur J Haematol* 1999; **62:** 300–6.
50. Elomaa I, Virkkunen P, Risteli L, Risteli J. Serum concentration of the cross-linked carboxyterminal telopeptide of type I collagen (ICTP) is a useful prognostic indicator in multiple myeloma. *Br J Cancer* 1992; **66:** 337–41.
51. Anderson KC, Park EK, Bates PM et al. Antigens on human plasma cells identified by monoclonal antibodies. *J Immunol* 1983; **130:** 1132–8.
52. Gonchoroff NJ, Katzmann JA, Garton JP et al. A monoclonal antibody reactive with a subset of human plasma cells. *Br J Haematol* 1986; **62:** 619–30.

53. Jackson N, Ling NR, Ball J et al. An analysis of myeloma plasma cell phenotype using antibodies defined at the IIIrd International Workshop on Human Leucocyte Differentiation Antigens. *Clin Exp Immunol* 1988; **72:** 351–6.
54. Epstein J, Xiao HQ, He XY. Markers of multiple hematopoietic-cell lineages in multiple myeloma. *N Engl J Med* 1990; **322:** 664–8.
55. Barker HF, Hamilton MS, Ball J et al. Expression of adhesion molecules LFA-3 and N-CAM on normal and malignant human plasma cells. *Br J Haematol* 1992; **81:** 331–5.
56. Harada H, Kawano MM, Huang N et al. Phenotypic difference of normal plasma cells from mature myeloma cells. *Blood* 1993; **81:** 2658–63.
57. Kawano MM, Huang N, Harada H et al. Identification of immature and mature myeloma cells in the bone marrow of human myelomas. *Blood* 1993; **82:** 564–70.
58. Ruiz-Argüelles GJ, San Miguel JF. Cell surface markers in multiple myeloma. *Mayo Clin Proc* 1994; **69:** 684–90.
59. San Miguel JF, Garcia-Sanz R, Gonzalez M, Orfao A. Immunophenotype and DNA cell content in multiple myeloma. *Baillière's Clin Haematol* 1995; **8:** 735–59.
60. Ocqueteau M, Orfao A, Garcia-Sanz R et al. Expression of the CD117 antigen (c-kit) on normal and myelomatous plasma cells. *Br J Haematol* 1996; **95:** 489–93.
61. Ocqueteau M, San Miguel JF, Gonzalez M et al. Do myelomatous plasma cells really express surface immunoglobulins? *Haematologica* 1996; **81:** 460–3.
62. Drew M, Barker HF, Ball J et al. Very late antigens (VLA) expression by normal and neoplastic human plasma cells; including an assessment of antibodies submitted to the Vth International Workshop on Leukocyte Differentiation Antigens using human myeloma cell lines. *Leuk Res* 1996; **20:** 619–24.
63. Helfrich MH, Livingston E, Franklin IM, Soutar RL. Expression of adhesion molecules in malignant plasma cells in multiple myeloma: comparison with normal plasma cells and functional significance. *Blood Rev* 1997; **11:** 28–38.
64. Almeida J, Orfao A, Mateo G et al. Immunophenotypic and DNA content characteristics of plasma cells in multiple myeloma and monoclonal gammopathy of undetermined significance. *Pathol Biol* 1999; **47:** 119–27.
65. San Miguel JF, González M, Gascón A et al. Immunophenotype heterogeneity of multiple myeloma: influence on the biology and clinical course of the disease. *Br J Haematol* 1991; **77:** 185–90.
66. Harada Y, Kawano MM, Huang N et al. Identification of early plasma cells in peripheral blood and their clinical significance. *Br J Haematol* 1996; **92:** 184–91.
67. Leo R, Boeker M, Peest D et al. Multiparameter analyses of normal and malignant human plasma cells: CD3811, CD561, CD541, cIg1 is the common phenotype of myeloma cells. *Ann Hematol* 1992; **64:** 132–9.
68. Wijdenes J, Vooijs WC, Clement C et al. A plasmocyte selective monoclonal antibody (B-B4) recognizes syndecan-1. *Br J Haematol* 1996; **94:** 318–23.
69. Pellat-Deceunynck C, Bataille R, Robillard N et al. Expression of CD28 and CD40 in human myeloma cells: a comparative study with normal plasma cells. *Blood* 1994; **84:** 2597–603.
70. Pellat-Deceunynck C, Barille S, Puthier D et al. Adhesion molecules on human myeloma cells: significant changes in expression related to malignancy, tumour spreading and immortalization. *Cancer Res* 1995; **55:** 3647–53.
71. Tazzari PL, Gobbi M, Dinota A. Normal and neoplastic plasma cell membrane phenotype: studies with new monoclonal antibodies. *Clin Exp Immunol* 1987; **70:** 192–200.
72. Tominaga N, Katahiri S, Ohnishi M. Analysis of surface antigen expression of human immunoglobulin-secreting cells: phenotype heterogeneity in normal counterparts of myeloma cells. *Br J Haematol* 1989; **73:** 302–8.
73. Zandecki M, Obein V, Bernardi F et al. Monoclonal gammopathy of undetermined significance: chromosome changes are a common finding within bone marrow plasma cells. *Br J Haematol* 1995; **90:** 693–6.
74. Omede P, Boccadoro M, Fusaro A et al. Multiple myeloma: 'early' plasma cell phenotype identifies patients with aggressive biological and clinical characteristics. *Br J Haematol* 1993; **85:** 504–13.
75. Schneider U, Lessen AV, Huhn D, Serke S. Two subsets of peripheral blood plasma cells defined by differential expression of CD45 antigen. *Br J Haematol* 1997; **97:** 56–64.
76. Van Camp B, Durie BGM, Spier C et al. Plasma cells in multiple myeloma express a natural killer cell-associated antigen: CD56 (NKH-1; Leu-19). *Blood* 1990; **76:** 377–82.

77. Teoh G, Anderson KC. Interaction of tumor and host cells with adhesion and extracellular matrix molecules in the development of multiple myeloma. *Hematol Oncol Clin North Am* 1997; **11:** 27–40.
78. Ocqueteau M, Orfao A, Almeida J et al. Immunophenotypic characterization of plasma cells from monoclonal gammopathy of undetermined significance (MGUS) patients. Implications for the differential diagnosis between MGUS and multiple myeloma. *Am J Pathol* 1998; **152:** 1655–65.
79. Almeida J, Orfao A, Ocqueteau M et al. High-sensitivity immunophenotyping and DNA ploidy studies for the investigation of minimal residual disease in multiple myeloma. *Br J Haematol* 1999; **107:** 121–31.
80. Mills KH, Cawley JC. Abnormal monoclonal antibody-defined helper/supressor T-cell subpopulations in multiple myeloma: relationship to treatment and clinical stage. *Br J Haematol* 1983; **53:** 271–5.
81. San Miguel JF, González M, Gascón A. Lymphoid subsets and prognostic factors in multiple myeloma. *Br J Haematol* 1992; **80:** 305–9.
82. Serra HM, Mant MJ, Ruether BA et al. Selective loss of CD41CD45R1 T cells in peripheral blood of multiple myeloma patients. *J Clin Immunol* 1988; **8:** 259–65.
83. Tienhaara A, Pelliniemi TT. Peripheral blood lymphocyte subsets in multiple myeloma and monoclonal gammopathy of undetermined significance. *Clin Lab Haematol* 1994; **16:** 213–23.
84. Munshi NC. Immunoregulatory mechanisms in multiple myeloma. *Hematol Oncol Clin North Am* 1997; **11:** 51–68.
85. García-Sanz R, González M, Orfao A et al. Analysis of natural killer-associated antigens in peripheral blood and bone marrow of multiple myeloma patients and prognostic implications. *Br J Haematol* 1996; **93:** 81–8.
86. Österborg A, Nilsson B, Björkholm M et al. Natural killer cell activity in monoclonal gammopathies: relation to disease activity. *Eur J Haematol* 1990; **45:** 153–7.
87. Dewald GW, Kyle RA, Hicks GA, Greipp PR. The clinical significance of cytogenetic studies in 100 patients with multiple myeloma, plasma cell leukemia, or amyloidosis. *Blood* 1985; **66:** 380–90.
88. Gould J, Alexanian R, Goodacre A et al. Plasma cell karyotype in multiple myeloma. *Blood* 1988; **71:** 453–6.
89. Van den Berghe H. Chromosomes in plasma-cell malignancies. *Eur J Haematol* 1989; **43**(Suppl 51): 47–51.
90. Weh HJ, Gutensohn K, Selbach J et al. Karyotype in multiple myeloma and plasma cell leukaemia. *Eur J Cancer* 1993; **29A:** 1269–73.
91. Sawyer JR, Waldron JA, Jagannath S, Barlogie B. Cytogenetic findings in 200 patients with multiple myeloma. *Cancer Genet Cytogenet* 1995; **82:** 41–9.
92. Laï JL, Zandecki M, Mary JY et al. Improved cytogenetics in multiple myeloma: a study of 151 patients including 117 patients at diagnosis. *Blood* 1995; **85:** 2490–7.
93. Weh HJ, Bartl R, Seeger D et al. Correlations between karyotype and cytologic findings in multiple myeloma. *Leukemia* 1995; **9:** 2119–22.
94. Zandecki M, Laï JL, Facon T. Multiple myeloma: almost all patients are cytogenetically abnormal. *Br J Haematol* 1996; **94:** 217–27.
95. Calasanz MJ, Cigudosa JC, Odero MD et al. Cytogenetic analysis of 280 patients with multiple myeloma and related disorders: primary breakpoints and clinical correlations. *Genes Chromosomes Cancer* 1997; **18:** 84–93.
96. Seong C, Delasalle K, Hayes K et al. Prognostic value of cytogenetics in multiple myeloma. *Br J Haematol* 1998; **101:** 189–94.
97. Facon T, Laï JL, Nataf E et al. Improved cytogenetic analysis of bone marrow plasma cells after cytokine stimulation in multiple myeloma: a report on 46 patients. *Br J Haematol* 1993; **84:** 743–5.
98. Smadja NV, Louvet C, Isnard F et al. Cytogenetic study in multiple myeloma at diagnosis: comparison of two techniques. *Br J Haematol* 1995; **90:** 619–24.
99. Brigaudeau C, Trimoreau F, Gachard N et al. Cytogenetic study of 30 patients with multiple myeloma: comparison of 3 and 6 days bone marrow cultures stimulated or not with cytokines by using a miniaturized karyotypic method. *Br J Haematol* 1997; **96:** 594–600.
100. Hernández JM, Gutiérrez NC, Almeida J et al. IL-4 improves the detection of cytogenetic abnormalities in multiple myeloma and increases the proportion of clonally abnormal metaphases. *Br J Haematol* 1998; **103:** 163–7.
101. Drach J, Schuster J, Nowotny H et al. Multiple myeloma: high incidence chromosomal aneuploidy as detected by interphase fluorescence in situ hybridization. *Cancer Res* 1995; **55:** 3854–9.

102. Lee W, Han K, Drut RM et al. Use of fluorescence in situ hybridizatiion for retrospective detection of anueploidy in multiple myeloma. *Genes Chromosomes Cancer* 1993; **7:** 137–43.
103. Tabernero D, San Miguel JF, García-Sanz R et al. Incidence of chromosome numerical changes in multiple myeloma. Fluorescence in situ hybridization analysis using 15 chromosome-specific probes. *Am J Pathol* 1996; **149:** 153–61.
104. Taniwaki M, Nishida K, Takashima T et al. Nonrandom chromosomal rearrangements of 14q32 and 19p13.3 and preferential deletion of 1p in 21 patients with multiple myeloma and plasma cell leukemias. *Blood* 1994; **84:** 2283–90.
105. Avet-Loiseau H, Andree-Ashley LE, Moore D et al. Molecular cytogenetic abnormalities in multiple myeloma and plasma cell leukemia measured using comparative genomic hybridization. *Genes Chromosomes Cancer* 1997; **19:** 124–33.
106. Cigudosa JC, Rao PH, Calasanz MJ et al. Characterization of nonrandom chromosomal gains and losses in multiple myeloma by comparative genomic hybridization. *Blood* 1998; **91:** 3007–10.
107. Rao PH, Cigudosa JC, Ning Y et al. Multicolor spectral karyotyping identifies new recurring breakpoints and translocations in multiple myeloma. *Blood* 1998; **92:** 1743–8.
108. Tricot G, Sawyer JR, Jagannath S et al. Unique role of cytogenetics in the prognosis of patients with myeloma receiving high-dose therapy and autotransplants. *J Clin Oncol* 1997; **15:** 2659–66.
109. Pérez-Simón JA, García-Sanz R, Tabernero MD et al. Prognostic value of numerical chromosome aberrations in multiple myeloma: a FISH analysis of 15 different chromosomes. *Blood* 1998; **91:** 3366–71.
110. Danova M, Riccardi A, Ucci G et al. *Ras* oncogene expression and DNA content in plasma cell dyscrasias: a flow cytofluorimetric study. *Br J Cancer* 1990; **62:** 781–5.
111. Shimazaki C, Gotoh H, Ashihara E et al. Immunophenotype and DNA content of myeloma cells in primary plasma cell leukemia. *Am J Hematol* 1992; **39:** 159–62.
112. Tienhaara A, Pelliniemi TT. Flow cytometric DNA analysis and clinical correlations in multiple myeloma. *Am J Clin Pathol* 1991; **97:** 322–30.
113. Duque RE, Andreef M, Braylan RC et al. Consensus review of the clinical utility of DNA flow cytometry in neoplastic hematopathology. *Cytometry* 1993; **14:** 492–6.
114. Garcia-Sanz R, Orfao A, Gonzalez M et al. Prognostic implications of DNA aneuploidy in 156 untreated multiple myeloma patients. *Br J Haematol* 1995; **90:** 106–12.
115. Morgan RJ, Gonchoroff NJ, Katzmann JA et al. Detection of hypodiploidy using multi-parameter flow cytometric analysis: a prognostic indicator in multiple myeloma. *Am J Hematol* 1989; **30:** 195–200.
116. Tafuri A, Meyers J, Lee BJ, Andreeff M. DNA and RNA flow cytometric study in multiple myeloma. Clinical correlations. *Cancer* 1991; **67:** 449–54.
117. San Miguel JF, García-Sanz R, González M, Orfao A. DNA cell content studies in multiple myeloma. *Leuk Lymphoma* 1996; **23:** 33–41.
118. Leo E, Kropff M, Lindemann A et al. DNA aneuploidy, increased proliferation and nuclear area of plasma cells in monoclonal gammopathy of undetermined significance and multiple myeloma. *Anal Quant Cytol Histol* 1995; **17:** 113–20.
119. Zandecki M, Facon T, Bernardi F et al. CD19 and immunophenotype of bone marrow plasma cells in monoclonal gammopathy of undetermined significance. *J Clin Pathol* 1995; **48:** 548–52.
120. Zaccaria A, Tassinari A, Saglio G et al. Immunoglobulin gene rearrangements in human multiple myeloma. *Br J Haematol* 1989; **73:** 425–32.
121. Vescio RA, Cao J, Hong CH et al. Myeloma Ig heavy chain V region sequences reveal prior antigenic selection and marked somatic mutation but not intraclonal diversity. *J Immunol* 1995; **155:** 2487–93.
122. Bird JM, Russell NH, Samson D. Minimal residual disease after bone marrow transplantation for multiple myeloma: evidence for cure in long-term survivors. *Bone Marrow Transplant* 1993; **12:** 651–4.
123. Corradini P, Voena C, Astolfi M et al. High-dose sequential chemoradiotherapy in multiple myeloma: residual tumor cells are detectable in bone marrow and peripheral blood cell harvests and after autografting. *Blood* 1995; **85:** 1596–602.
124. Van Riet Y, Heirman C, Lacor P et al. Detection of monoclonal B lymphocytes in bone marrow and peripheral blood of multiple myeloma patients by immunoglobulin gene rearrangement studies. *Br J Haematol* 1989; **73:** 289–95.
125. Isaksson E, Björkholm M, Holm G et al. Blood clonal B-cell excess in patients with monoclonal gammopathy of undetermined significance (MGUS): association with malignant transformation. *Br J Haematol* 1996; **92:** 71–6.

126. Skopelitou A, Hadjiyannakis M, Tsenga A et al. Expression of c-myc p62 oncoprotein in multiple myeloma: an immunohistochemical study of 180 cases. *Anticancer Res* 1993; **13:** 1091–5.
127. Akiyama N, Tsuruta H, Sasaki H et al. Messenger RNA levels of five genes located at chromosome 11q13 in B-cell tumors with chromosome translocation t(11;14)(q13;q32). *Cancer Res* 1994; **54:** 377–9.
128. Tricot G, Barlogie B, Jagannath S et al. Poor prognosis in multiple myeloma is associated with partial or complete deletions of chromosome 13 or abnormalities involving 11q and not with other karyotype abnormalities. *Blood* 1995; **86:** 4250–6.
129. Chesi M, Nardini E, Brents LA et al. Frequent translocation t(4;14)(p16.3;q32.3) in multiple myeloma: association with increased expression and activating mutations of fibroblastic growth factor receptor 3. *Nature Genet* 1997; **16:** 260–5.
130. Ong F, Nieuwkoop JA, De Groot-Swings GMJS et al. Bcl-2 protein expression is not related to short survival in multiple myeloma. *Leukemia* 1995; **9:** 1282–4.
131. Corradini P, Ladetto M, Voena C et al. Mutational activation of N- and K-*ras* oncogenes in plasma cell dyscrasias. *Blood* 1993; **81:** 2699–707.
132. Liu P, Leong T, Quam L et al. Activating mutations of N- and K-*ras* in multiple myeloma show different clinical associations: analysis of the Eastern Cooperative Oncology Group phase III trial. *Blood* 1996; **88:** 2699–706.
133. Corradini P, Inghirami G, Astolfi M et al. Inactivation of tumor suppressor genes, p53 and Rb1 in plasma cell dyscrasias. *Leukemia* 1994; **8:** 758–66.
134. Garcia-Sanz R, Orfao A, Gonzalez M et al. Primary plasma cell leukemia: clinical, immunophenotypic, DNA ploidy, and cytogenetic characteristics. *Blood* 1999; **93:** 1032–7.
135. Joshua D, Petersen A, Brown R et al. The labelling index of primitive plasma cells determines the clinical behaviour of patients with myelomatosis. *Br J Haematol* 1996; **94:** 76–81.
136. Durie BGM, Salmon SE, Moon TE. Pretreatment tumor mass, cell kinetics and prognosis in multiple myeloma. *Blood* 1980; **55:** 364–9.
137. Greipp PR, Lust JA, O´Fallon M et al. Plasma cell labeling index and beta2-microglobulin predict survival independent of thymidine kinase and C-reactive protein in multiple myeloma. *Blood* 1993; **81:** 3382–7.
138. Orfao A, García-Sanz R, López-Berges MC et al. A new method for the analysis of plasma cell DNA content in multiple myeloma samples using a CD38/propidium iodide double staining technique. *Cytometry* 1994; **17:** 332–9.
139. Kyle RA. Monoclonal gammopathy of undetermined significance (MGUS). *Baillières Clin Haematol* 1995; **8:** 761–81.
140. Raaijmakers HGP, Izquierdo MAI, Lokhorst HM et al. Lung resistance related protein expression is a negative predictive factor for response to conventional low but not to intensified dose alkylating chemotherapy in multiple myeloma. *Blood* 1998; **91:** 1029–36.
141. Shen H, Paul S, Breuninger LM et al. Cellular and in vitro transport of glutathione conjugates by MRP. *Biochemistry* 1996; **35:** 5719–25.
142. Sonneveld P, Lokhorst H, Vossebeld P. Drug resistance in multiple myeloma. *Semin Hematol* 1997; **34**(Suppl 5): 34–8.
143. D'Arpa P, Liu LF. Topoisomerase-targeting antitumor drugs. *Biochim Biophys Acta* 1989; **989:** 163–77.
144. Reed JC. Bcl-2 family proteins: regulators of apoptosis and chemoresistance in hematologic malignancies. *Semin Hematol* 1997; **34**(Suppl 5): 9–19.
145. Juliano RL, Ling V. A surface glycoprotein modulating drug permeability in Chinese hamster ovary cell mutants. *Biochim Biophys Acta* 1976; **455:** 152–62.
146. Beck WT, Grogan T, Willman CL et al. Methods to detect P-glycoprotein-associated multidrug resistance in patients' tumors: consensus recommendations. *Cancer Res* 1996; **56:** 3010–20.
147. Drach D, Zhao S, Drach J et al. Subpopulations of normal peripheral blood and bone marrow cells express a functional multidrug resistant phenotype. *Blood* 1992; **80:** 2729–34.
148. Beck WT, Grogan TM. Methods to detect P-glycoprotein and implications for other drug resistance-associated proteins. *Leukemia* 1997; **11:** 1107–9.
149. Okochi E, Iwahashi T, Tsuruo T. Monoclonal antibodies specific for P-glycoprotein. *Leukemia* 1997; **11:** 1119–23.
150. Krishan LA, Sauerteig A, Andritsch I, Wellham L. Flow cytometric analysis of the multiple drug resistance phenotype. *Leukemia* 1997; **11:** 1138–46.
151. Lamy T, Drenou B, Grulois I et al. Multi-drug resistance (MDR) activity in acute leukemia determined by rhodamine 123 efflux assay. *Leukemia* 1995; **9:** 1549–55.

152. Bailly JD, Muller C, Jaffrezou JP et al. Lack of correlation between expression and function of P-glycoprotein in acute myeloid leukemia cell lines. *Leukemia* 1995; **9:** 799–807.
153. Ludescher C, Gattringer C, Drach J et al. Rapid functional assay for the detection of multidrug-resistant cells using the fluorescent dye rhodamine 123. *Blood* 1991; **78:** 1385–7.
154. Grogan TM, Spier CM, Salmon SE et al. P-glycoprotein expression in human plasma cell myeloma: correlation with prior chemotherapy. *Blood* 1993; **81:** 490–5.
155. Sonneveld P, Marie JP, Huisman C et al. Reversal of multidrug resistance by SDZ PSC 833, combined with VAD (vincristine, doxorubicin, dexamethasone) in refractory multiple myeloma. A phase I study. *Leukemia* 1996; **10:** 1741–50.
156. Gieseler F, Nuessler V. Cellular resistance mechanisms with impact on the therapy of multiple myeloma. *Leukemia* 1998; **12:** 1009–12.
157. Linsenmeyer ME, Jefferson S, Wolf M. Levels of expression of the MDR1 gene and glutathione-S-transferase genes 2 and 3 and response to chemotherapy in multiple myeloma. *Br J Cancer* 1992; **65:** 471–5.

16

Clinical significance of bone marrow and bone morphology in myeloma

Reiner Bartl, Bertha Frisch

CONTENTS • Bone marrow biopsy and aspiration • Normal plasma cells • The role of morphology in the diagnosis of myeloma • Growth patterns in myeloma • Haematopoiesis, stroma, and bone in myeloma • Morphologic classification of myeloma • Morphology in staging of myeloma • Morphologic features of myeloma variants • Monitoring the course of the disease with morphology

BONE MARROW BIOPSY AND ASPIRATION

Biopsy and aspiration sites (Figure 16.1)

Multiple myeloma is a systemic disorder of the bone marrow,[1,2] and consequently, specimens obtained from any skeletal site containing red, haematopoietic marrow are useful for investigation.

Three main considerations determine the choice of the skeletal site for biopsy in a patient with myeloma:

- easy accessibility with minimum risk to the patient;
- access to representative haematopoietic marrow;
- ability to obtain sequential biopsies and aspirates with minimal variability.

The os ilium comes nearest to fulfilling these criteria, and the posterior iliac crest is the preferred site from which the biopsies and aspirates are taken.[3]

Biopsy and aspiration instruments

The majority of bone marrow biopsies are obtained under local anaesthesia with a manual trephine needle (Jamshidi or other).[4] An adequate biopsy should be at least 15 mm long with a diameter of 2–3 mm.[3] The length varies greatly – up to 70 mm.

Aspiration is performed immediately *after* the biopsy, using a separate aspiration needle and selecting another spot within the anaesthesized area. This needle technique is less traumatic, can be performed easily, and is particularly suitable for outpatients.

Biopsy and aspirate processing (Figure 16.2)

The biopsy is fixed, dehydrated, and embedded in methyl methacrylate without decalcification, and semithin sections are cut at 3 µm. This procedure requires only 48 hours.

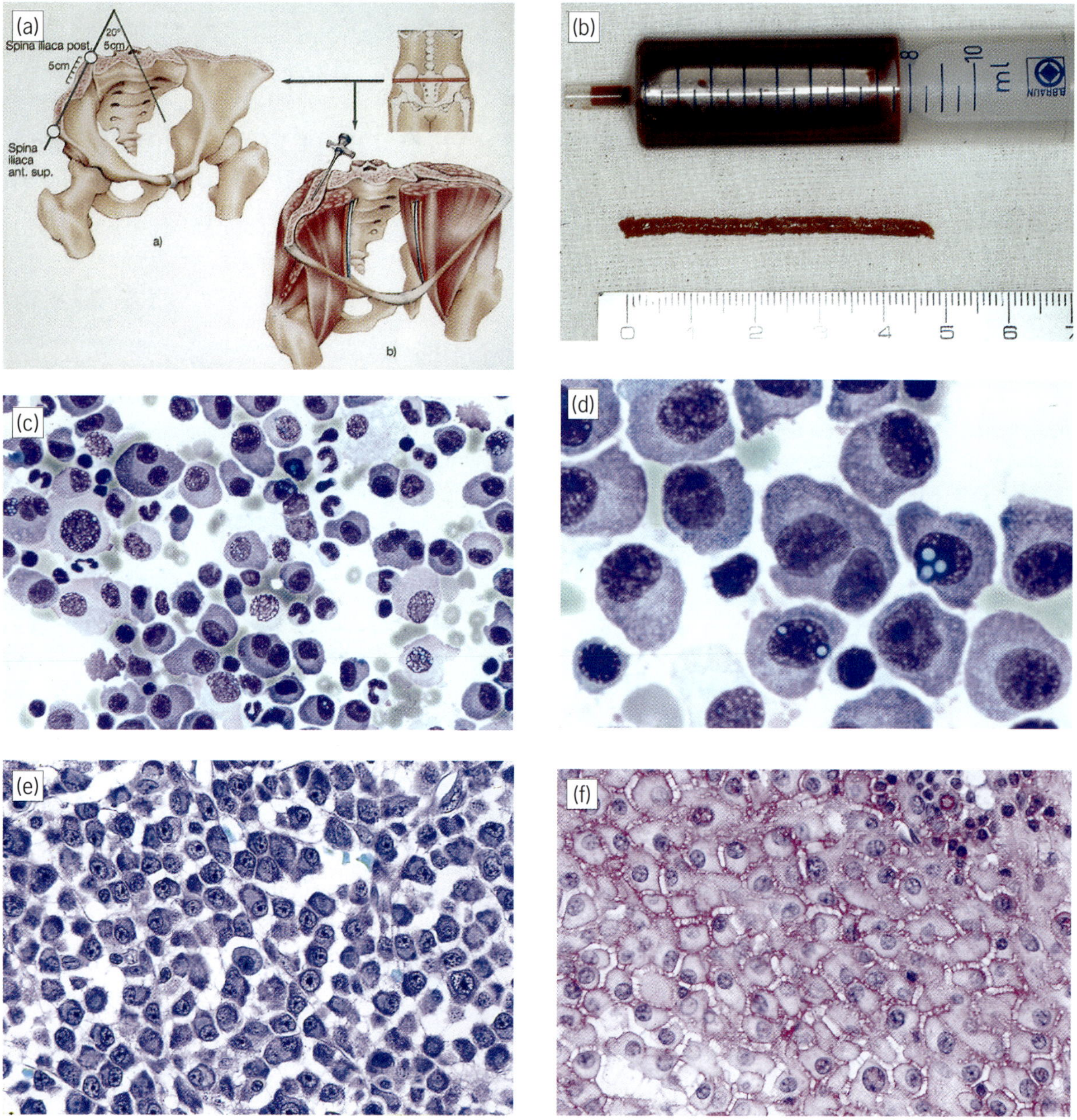

Figure 16.1 (a) Sketches of horizontal section of the anterior superior spinous process of the ilium. Note that the posterior ilium is broader than the anterior, and long biopsies can safely been taken from the posterior ilium. In addition, both external and internal surfaces of the ilium are protected by muscles. (b) Posterior iliac crest biopsy taken with an 8-gauge manual trephine and an aspirate taken after the biopsy from another spot within the anaesthesized area. (c) Smear of bone marrow aspirate, with intensive infiltration by polymorphic plasma cells. (d) At higher magnification, polymorphous plasma cells, partly nucleolated and with intranuclear inclusions ('Dutcher bodies'). (e) Large, asynchronous myeloma cells in the centre of a nodule, with prominent nucleoli (Giemsa, ×400). (f) Dense infiltration of monoclonal plasma cells, Marschalko type, κ light chain.

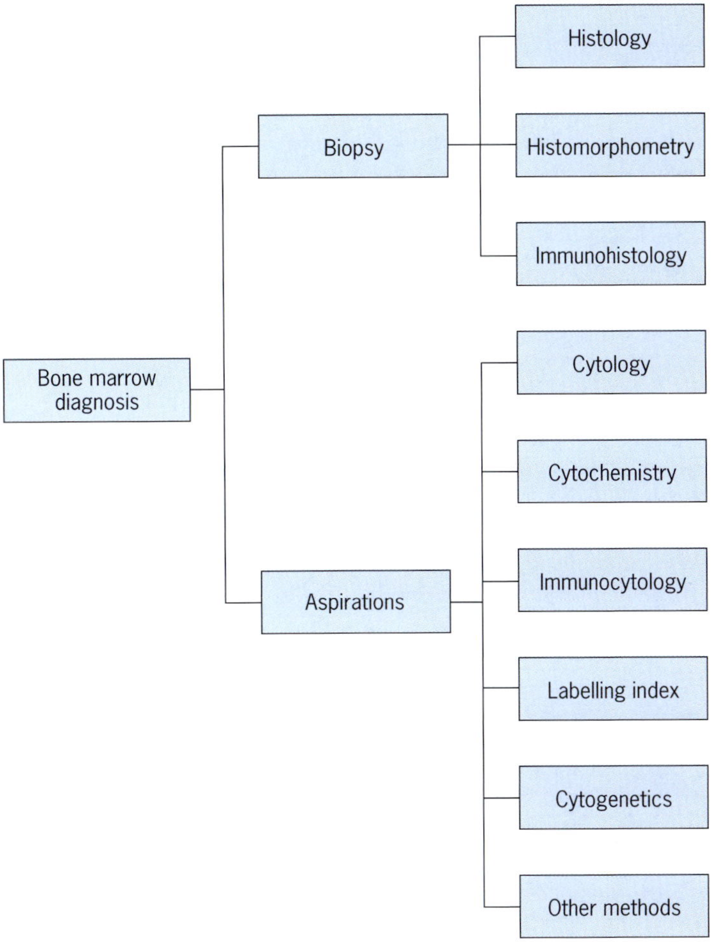

Figure 16.2 Work-up of bone marrow biopsy and aspirates in myeloma patients.

The following histologic stains are routinely employed:

- gallamin-blue–Giemsa for cytologic details;
- Gomori for bone structures and fibres;
- PAS for glycoprotein;
- Ladewig for osteoid;
- Berlin blue for iron;[5]
- immunohistology utilizing appropriate combinations of the following antibodies: CD10, CD19, CD20, CD40, Cd45, CD56, Ki67, BCL2, P53, κ, λ, IgG, IgA, IgD, IgE;
- histomorphometry: quantitative estimation of plasma cells, fatty tissue, haematopoiesis, bone structure and bone cells, using the grid technique.

Bone marrow aspirates are used for the following studies:

- smears, which are stained with May–Gruenwald–Giemsa and for acid phosphatase activity;
- plasma cell labelling index (PCLI);[6]
- immunophenotyping using flow cytometry (FACS);
- cytogenetic and other specialized studies.

Diagnostic evaluation of smears and sections

Bone marrow diagnosis is made on the basis of cytologic and histologic findings (smears and sections).[7] The smears are examined first, and the differential count including the percentage of plasma cells is made on a minimum of 300 nucleated cells. The histologic and histomorphometric findings are then correlated with the cytologic features, and a preliminary report is made. The final bone and marrow report also includes PCLI, immunophenotyping of the plasma cells, and cytogenetic findings. This report provides important information on the tumour itself and on the alterations of haematopoiesis, bone marrow stroma, and bone[8] (Figure 16.3).

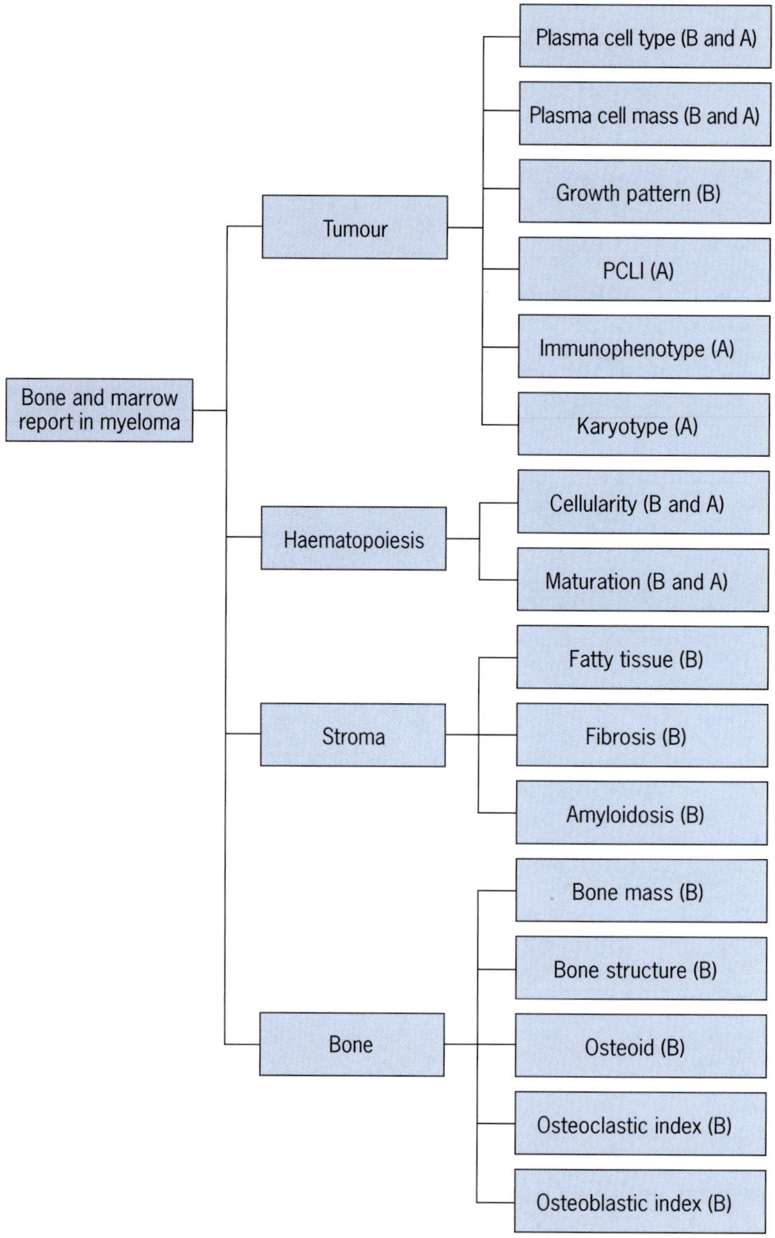

Figure 16.3 Bone and bone marrow report in myeloma, using biopsy (B) and aspirates (A).

NORMAL PLASMA CELLS

These are normally seen in the bone marrow,[4,5,9] and represent the final developmental stage of the B-cell lineage.[10,11] They constitute about 1% of the nucleated cells from a normal bone marrow aspirate of an adult, with a range of up to 4%. Plasma cells are equally distributed throughout the red marrow, with no significant differences between the various skeletal sites, but are almost absent from the yellow marrow.[3] There are more than 100 million plasma cells in the red marrow, producing more than 90% of the serum immunoglobulins. Plasma cells have low proliferative activity, and they survive in the bone marrow for about 30 days.

The mature 'Marschalko' plasma cell is the predominant plasma cell (80%) in the normal marrow and in reactive plasmacytosis. In aspirate smears, these plasma cells are usually oval, 8–25 mm in diameter, with abundant basophilic cytoplasm, a paranuclear 'hof', and, in sections more than smears, a 'spoke-wheel' nuclear pattern. Nucleoli are rare.[12]

Plasma cells exhibit acid phosphatase, β-glucuronidase, and non-specific esterase activity. Plasma cells are found in close apposition to capillaries and small blood vessels, as well as singly and in clusters of two or three within the bone marrow.[4,9,13] Less frequent are the lymphoplasmacytoid cells, with less cytoplasm and less characteristic nuclei.

THE ROLE OF MORPHOLOGY IN THE DIAGNOSIS OF MYELOMA (Figure 16.1)

Clinical, laboratory and radiologic findings are considered together with bone marrow morphology, utilizing both aspirates and biopsies.[7] The majority of cases can be diagnosed on morphology alone. The few equivocal cases can be elucidated by checking for monoclonality utilizing antibodies to κ and λ light chains. This can be done on sections, smears, and imprints of biopsies.

Quantity of plasma cells

In many centres, the diagnosis of myeloma is still based on the percentage of plasma cells in an aspirated marrow sample, ranging from 5–10% to 30%, although equal or higher numbers of plasma cells may be present in other non-neoplastic conditions.[14,15]

Reactive plasmacytosis is common in association with chronic inflammatory diseases, infections, and other conditions such as hepatic cirrhosis, Hodgkin's disease (especially after therapy), and diabetes mellitus.[16–20]

Occasionally, discrepancies may occur between numbers of plasma cells in aspirate smears and biopsy sections. This is due to fibrosis or nodular bone marrow infiltration preventing aspiration of plasma cells, resulting in low numbers in the smears.[21] Conversely, aspirates of patients with reactive plasmacytosis and/or monoclonal gammopathy of undetermined significance (MGUS) may contain over 30% plasma cells, and in many of these cases the biopsy sections reveal a hypocellular bone marrow.[16] The volume percentage of plasma cells on biopsy is estimated from overall cellularity and percentage of plasma cells (% cellularity × % plasma cells/100).

Qualitative abnormalities of plasma cells

These may be as important as the quantity of plasma cells. Although there are no characteristics pathognomonic for myeloma, many are suggestive:[22–31]

- variations in cell size;
- variations in nuclear size and shape;
- multinuclearity and hypersegmentation;
- presence of Dutcher, Russell, and other inclusion bodies;
- grape cells;
- Mott cells;
- flaming cells;
- tadpole-like cells;
- thesaurocytes;
- cytoplasmic heterogeneity in staining and in enzyme reactions.

Conversely, plasmacytic satellitosis (histiocyte surrounded by plasma cells), and increased eosinophils, mast cells, and megakaryocytes are typical of reactive plasmacytosis.[18]

Nuclear–cytoplasmic asynchrony of plasma cells

Instead of the typical spoke-wheel pattern seen in normal and reactive plasmacytoses, the nuclear chromatin in myeloma is often finely dispersed like that of a blast, and contains a large, sharply demarcated nucleolus.[32,33] The nuclei in myeloma plasma cells are often variably shaped: notched, cleaved, multilobulated, convoluted, or cerebriform, sometimes with multiple nucleoli or inclusion bodies (Figure 16.4).

No differences were found in plasma cell morphology when patients were grouped according to the type of M component. Histochemically, there are considerable variations in reactivity between plasma cells and between myeloma, MGUS, and reactive plasmacytosis.[34,35] Therefore, these reactions cannot be used to differentiate between them.

In summary, the presence of three cytologic features enables a morphologic diagnosis of myeloma despite a low number of plasma cells (<5%) in aspirate smears:[16,36,37]

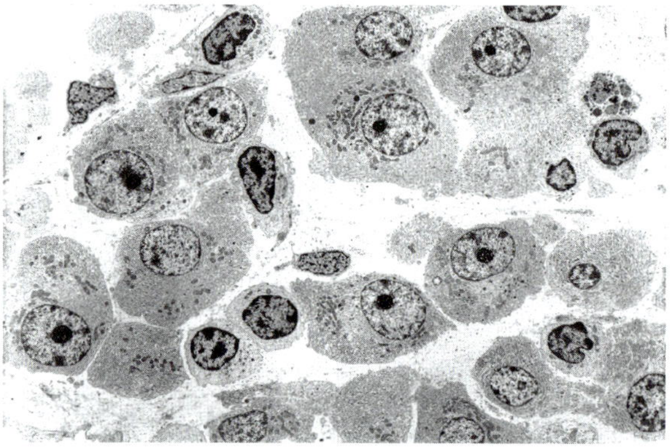

Figure 16.4 Electron micrograph of myeloma cells in the bone marrow, showing different degrees of nuclear–cytoplasmic asynchrony (×5000).

- nuclear–cytoplasmic asynchrony with large nucleoli;
- irregularities of nuclear configuration;
- variations in cell size and cytoplasmic staining.

Plasma cell labelling index (PCLI)

As myeloma is a slowly growing tumour, only about 1–2% of plasma cells are in the S-phase of the cell cycle as shown by the PCLI, which is useful for distinguishing myeloma from MGUS.[38,39] BU-1, Ki-67, other monoclonal antibodies, and flow cytometry may be used for this purpose.[6,39–41]

Histotopography of plasma cells

This is also useful for distinguishing reactive from neoplastic plasmacytosis.[13,17,42–45] In the former, many typical reticular plasma cells are located around the small blood vessels. In the latter, there is also a random interstitial infiltration among fat and haematopoietic cells initially; subsequently denser aggregates of myeloma cells accumulate along endosteal surfaces and around ectatic sinusoids and arteries, eventually forming nodules or sheets that replace the haematopoietic and fat tissues (Figure 16.5).

Patients with endosteal sheets of myeloma cells respond well to bisphosphonates, with a marked decline in the M protein level as well as a lower incidence of skeletal events during the course of disease. Patients without endosteal accumulation of plasma cells have lower osteoclastic activity and do not show osteolytic lesions on skeletal X rays.

GROWTH PATTERNS IN MYELOMA (Figure 16.6)

Six architectural patterns have been observed in the biopsy sections: their frequencies, radiographic appearances, and median survivals are

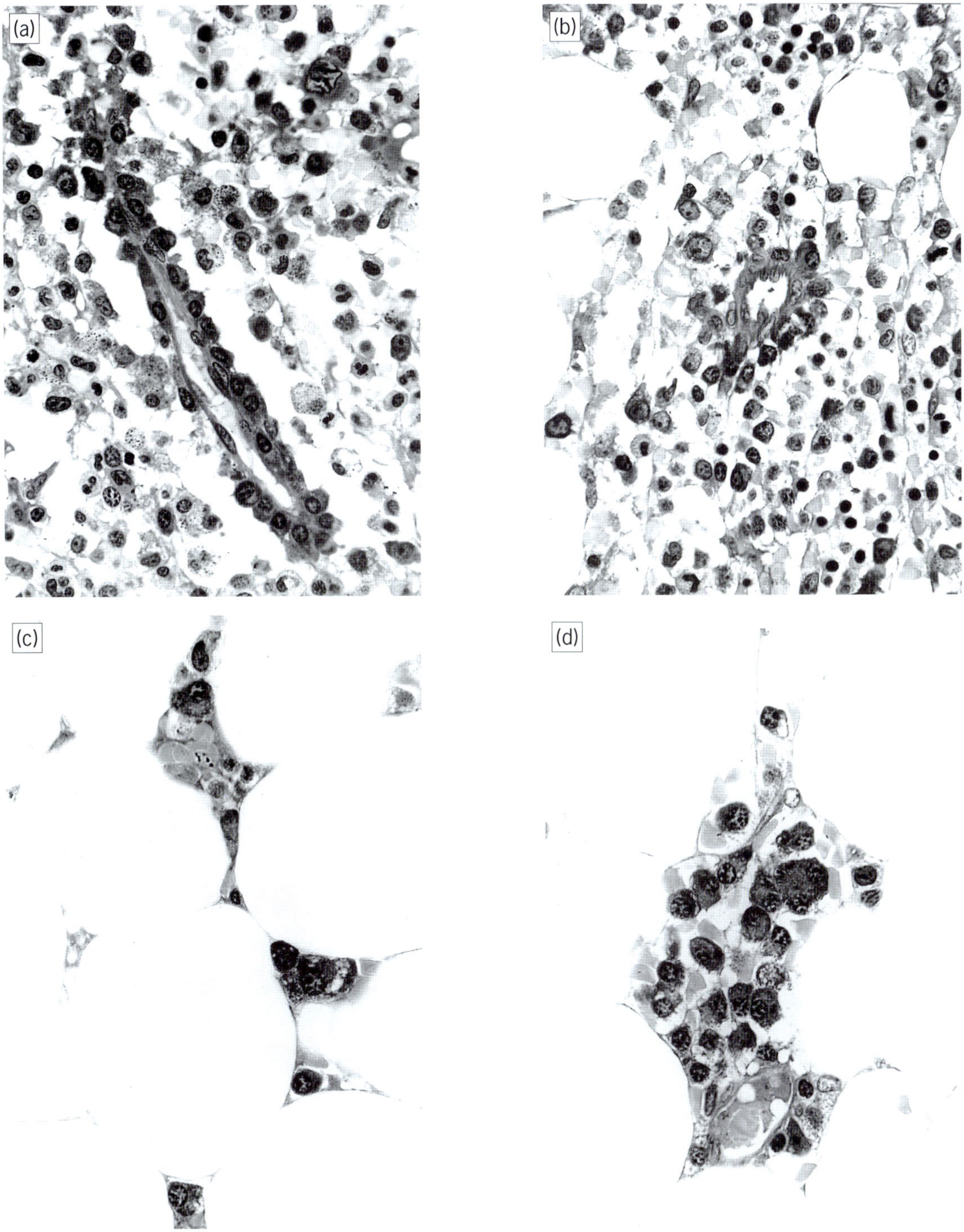

Figure 16.5 Histotopography for differential diagnosis of reactive plasmacytosis and early myeloma. (a, b) Reactive plasmacytosis, with mature plasma cells located around capillaries, together with granulocytes and eosinophils (Giemsa, ×400). (c, d) Early myeloma, with plasma cells loosely distributed between fat cells. There is no definite topographic orientation to capillaries. Some plasma cells are nucleolated and of variable size (Giemsa, ×400).

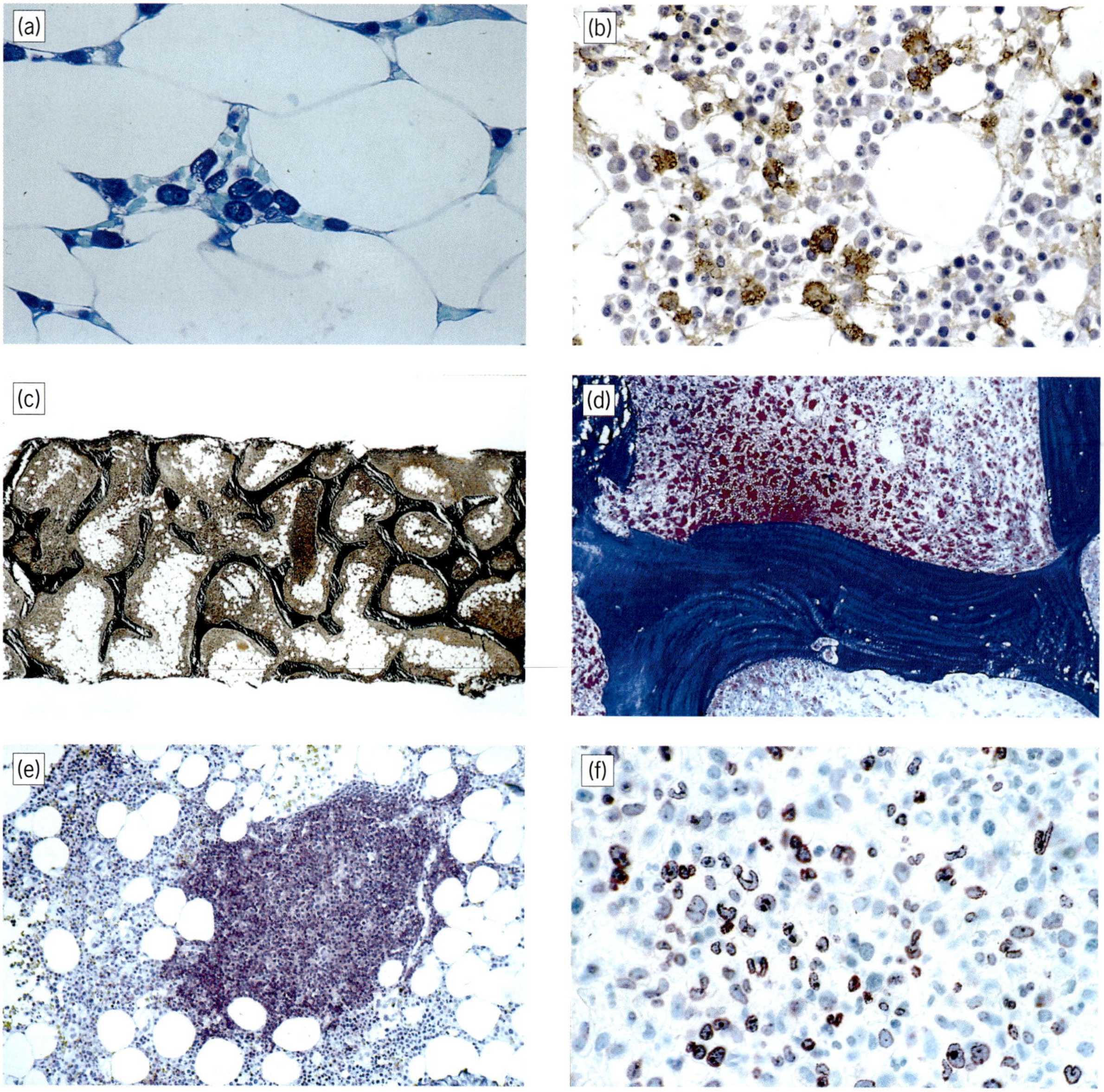

Figure 16.6 (a) Some atypical, mature plasma cells distributed between fat cells, without any topographic orientation to capillaries, in a patient with smouldering myeloma (Giemsa, ×400). (b) Monoclonal Marschalko-type plasma cells (anti-λ, ×400), loosely interspersed with normal haematopoiesis in an interstitial growth pattern in a patient with stage I myeloma. (c) Bone marrow biopsy, showing an interstitial pattern with endosteal seams of plasma cells ('paratrabecular pattern') and marrow atrophy in the centres of the marrow spaces (Gomori, ×15). (d) Myeloma cell aggregate radiating from the surface of an ossicle. Note the deep resorption cavity (left) and the intratrabecular bone resorption by osteoclasts (below) (Ladewig, ×100). (e) Myeloma nodule, too small to be detected by magnetic resonance imaging (anti-κ, ×100). (f) At higher magnification, high proliferative activity in the centre of the nodule is demonstrated by dense positivity of Ki-67.

given in Figures 16.7 and 16.8.[36,37,46] An exclusively nodular infiltration is rare. It characterizes the multifocal variant of myeloma and may be the reason for negative aspirate/biopsy at initial presentation.

Immunohistology using the Ki-67 antibody shows that plasma cells in the S phase were predominantly located in the centre of the myeloma nodules, explaining the unfavourable significance of the nodular pattern. In contrast, chronic lymphocytic leukaemia (CLL) patients with nodular pattern in the bone marrow have very low proliferative activity (Ki-67) in the centres of the lymphocytic nodules. An increase in coarse fibrosis or in lymphocytic infiltration within dense myelomatous infiltrates also correlates with an unfavourable prognosis.

Magnetic resonance imaging (MRI) can detect nodules and foci of disease not observed on conventional radiographs. MRI of the whole spine was performed in 108 patients with myeloma (Data kindly supplied by Professor M Reiser and Dr Andrea Baur, Department of Radiologic Diagnosis, Klinikum Großhadern, University of Munich). The five different types of growth patterns and their frequencies were as follows: normal 21% (0%), 'salt and pepper' 5% (0%), nodular 33% (40%), nodular/diffuse 22% (45%), and diffuse 19% (41%). The figures in parentheses represent the frequency of osteolytic lesions on conventional radiographs.

There was striking correlation between MRI growth patterns and those in the biopsy, as well as with the clinical and histologic staging systems (Figure 16.9).[8] The degree of infiltration in the spine as shown by MRI also correlated significantly with survival.

HAEMATOPOIESIS, STROMA, AND BONE IN MYELOMA

Myeloma cells produce a variety of cytokines that influence haematopoiesis, bone marrow stroma, and bone.

Alteration in haematopoiesis

Failure of haematopoiesis in myeloma patients is due to replacement of normal haematopoietic tissue by plasma cell infiltration, marrow atrophy possibly due to haematopoiesis-inhibiting factors produced by the myeloma cells (HIF, IL-6),[47] and, especially in previously treated patients, myelodysplasia. Reduction of the plasma cell mass with chemotherapy is usually followed by a decrease in the fatty tissue and regeneration of haematopoiesis.

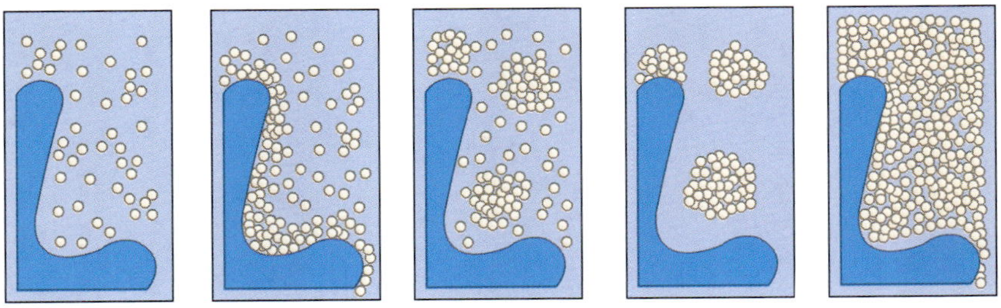

Growth pattern	Interstitial	Interstitial/ sheets	Interstitial/ nodular	Nodular	Packed
Frequency (%)	58	13	9	4	15
Osteolyses (%)	12	22	74	79	52
Survival (months)	46	31	22	20	16

Figure 16.7 Sketch of myeloma growth patterns in bone marrow biopsies, their frequencies, X-ray manifestations, and associated median survivals from time of biopsy.

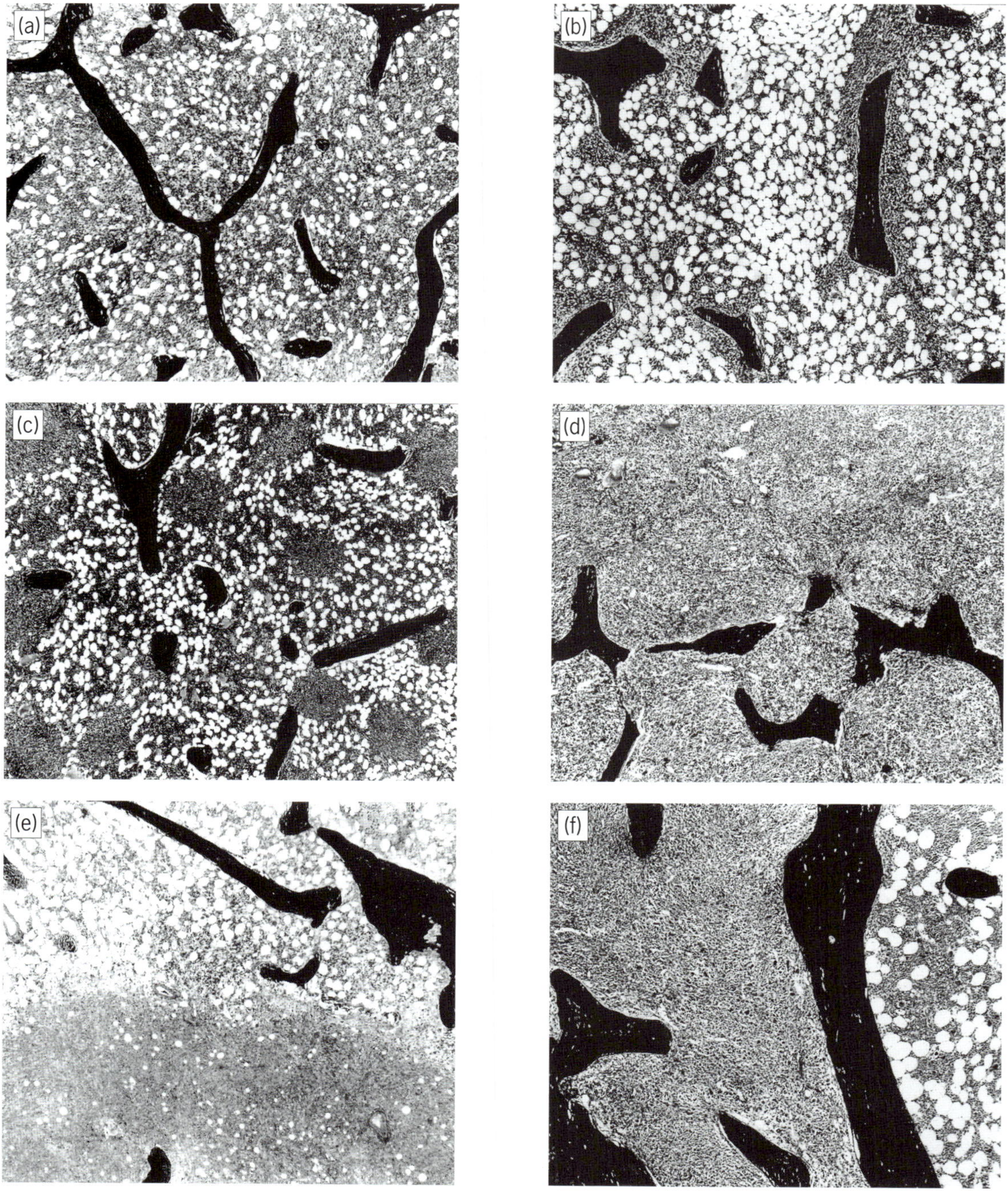

Figure 16.8 Growth patterns of myeloma in bone marrow biopsies (Gomori, ×20). (a) Interstitial, with normocellular marrow. (b) Interstitial with endosteal sheets of myeloma cells and atrophy in the central regions of the marrow cavities. (c) Multiple small nodules with interstitial infiltration. (d) Packed marrow, with absence of haematopoiesis and fat cells. Note the marked osteoclastic bone resorption, with an osteolytic lesion in the upper half. (e) Blastic-type myeloma with sarcomatous growth and osteolytic destruction of the trabeculae. (f) Strictly nodular growth of myeloma (left) and normal haematopoiesis (right), with a broad trabecula between.

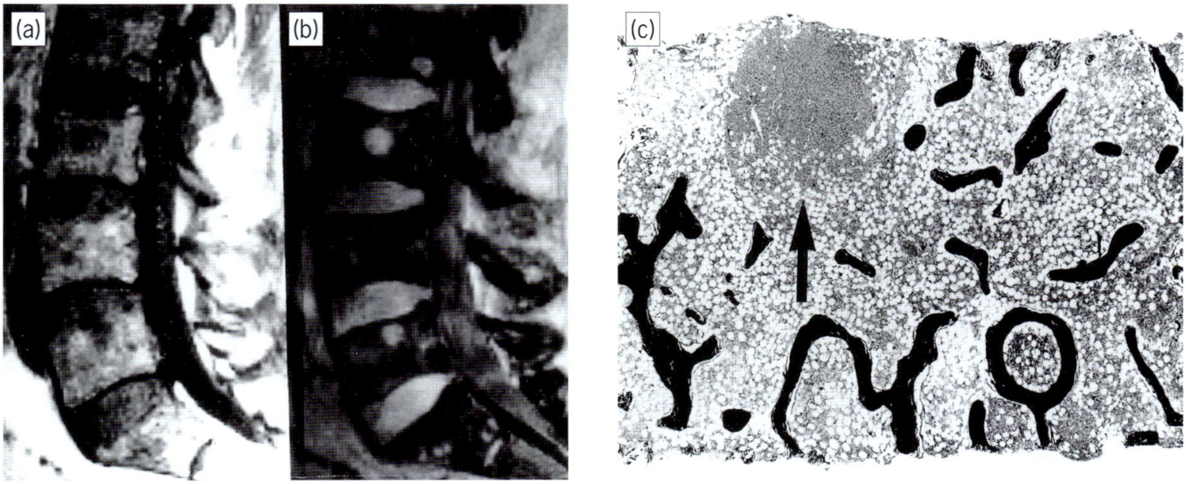

Figure 16.9 (a) *T1*-weighted spin-echo image and (b) opposed-phase gradient-echo image: combined diffuse and nodular involvement in the lumbar spine. Small myeloma nodules are distinctly shown as areas of high signal intensity on GRE images. (c) Iliac crest biopsy from the patient, with a small myeloma nodule at the arrow and a microscopic osteolytic lesion in this area, together with low interstitial infiltration in the marrow spaces (Gomori, ×20).

Alteration in the bone marrow stroma

A complex system of cellular (cytokines) and extracellular (matrix) elements normally regulate the growth and differentiation of haematopoietic cell lines in the bone marrow.[4] Under the influence of myeloma cells, the stromal cells produce large quantities of adhesion and extracellular matrix molecules, which, together with the cytokines, influence the rate and type of tumour growth in myeloma.[48] The presence of coarse fibrosis (collagen type III) accompanied by an inflammatory reaction is an unfavourable prognostic sign.[47,49–52]

Alteration in bone (Figure 16.10)

Skeletal destruction is characteristic of myeloma, and causes many of its complications, such as bone pain, pathologic fractures, hypercalcaemia and renal damage that may lead to secondary hyperparathyroidism.[3,53]

Generalized osteoporosis with or without lytic lesions is seen in 60% of patients at diagnosis. Patients with interstitial and packed marrow patterns usually have predominantly generalized osteoporosis. In smouldering myeloma, osteoporosis without any lytic lesions is seen in 40% of patients, and bone biopsy usually shows increased osteoclastic activity, indicating a 'high-turnover' status.

The presence of myeloma nodules usually correlates with osteolytic lesions. The type of skeletal lesion (osteolysis versus osteoporosis) depends mainly on the type of tumour growth: patients with interstitial and packed marrow patterns usually have diffuse rarefaction of trabecular bone (generalized osteoporosis), while patients with nodules have local osteoclastic resorption (osteolytic lesions). Therefore osteolytic lesions are a reflection of the tumour growth pattern rather than the tumour load.[38]

Osteoclast-activating factors (OAFs) produced by the myeloma cells appear to act locally, mainly in close proximity to aggregates of myeloma cells (Figure 16.11) – hence the clinical efficacy of primarily anti-osteoclastic agents such as bisphosphonates. There is a direct relationship between skeletal destruction, plasma cell burden, and the amount of OAF produced (Figure 16.12a). The type of monoclonal protein

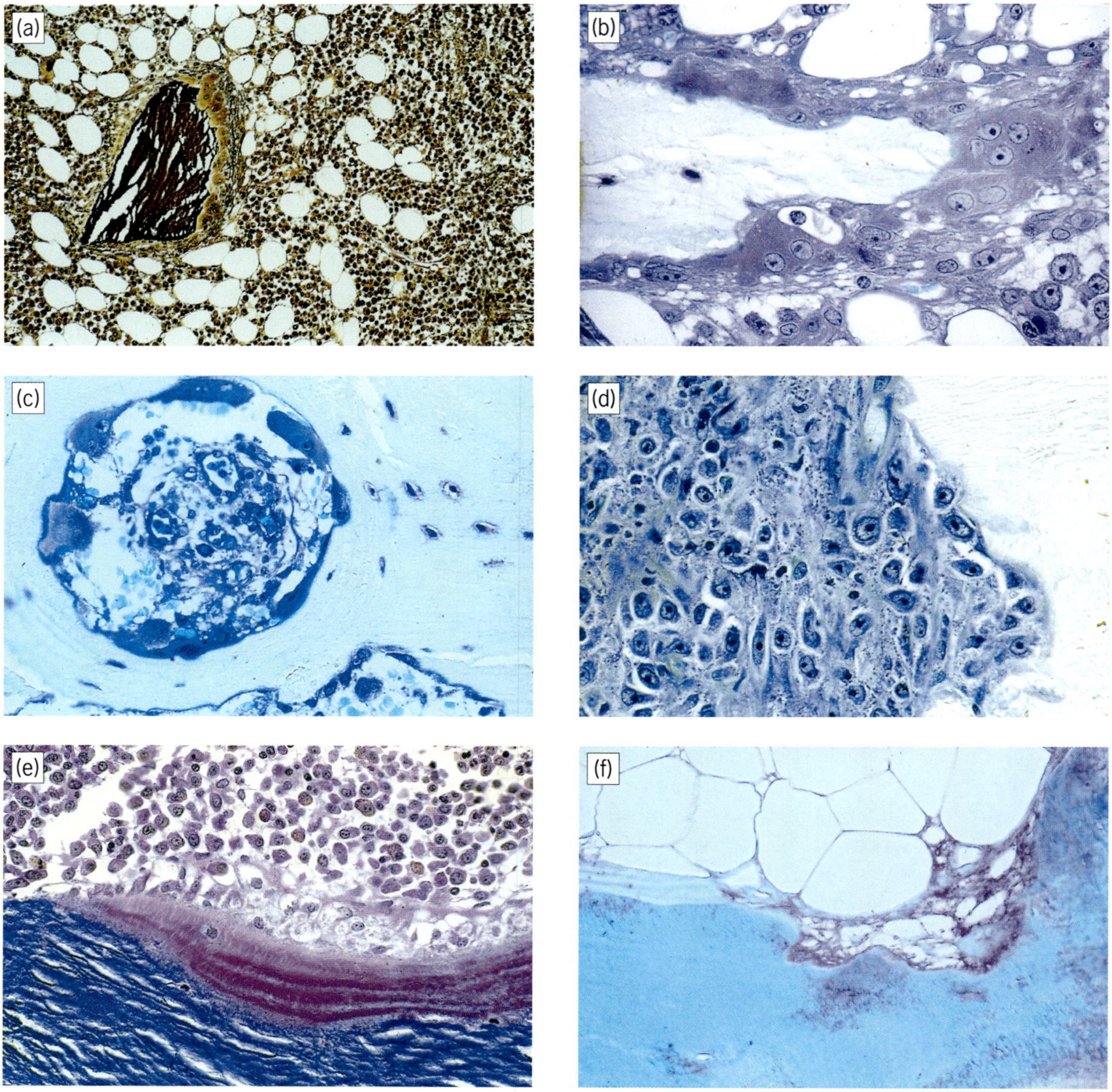

Figure 16.10 (a) Marked osteopenia with osteoclastic bone resorption of an ossicle (Gomori, ×100). (b) At higher magnification, a scalloped trabecular surface filled with active osteoclasts and separated from myeloma cells by a zone of connective tissue (Giemsa, ×400). (c) Marked osteoclastic bone resorption after radiation therapy, with oedema and necrotic material, but no residual myelomatous infiltration in the bone marrow cavity: indication for bisphosphonate therapy (Giemsa, ×250). (d) Pleomorphic myeloma cells eroding the surface of an ossicle. Note the absence of osteoclasts, indicating direct bone resorption by tumour cells (Giemsa, ×400). (e) Myeloma patient under long-term bisphosphonate therapy: ossicle covered by a broad seam of osteoid (red) and active osteoblasts. There is no osteoclastic bone resorption. Note marked myelomatous infiltration above (Ladewig, ×250).
(f) Presence of a bisphosphonate compound within a resorption cavity and an osteoclast. Biopsy taken from a myeloma patient 14 days after intravenous ibandronate (anti-ibandronate, plastic embedding, ×250).

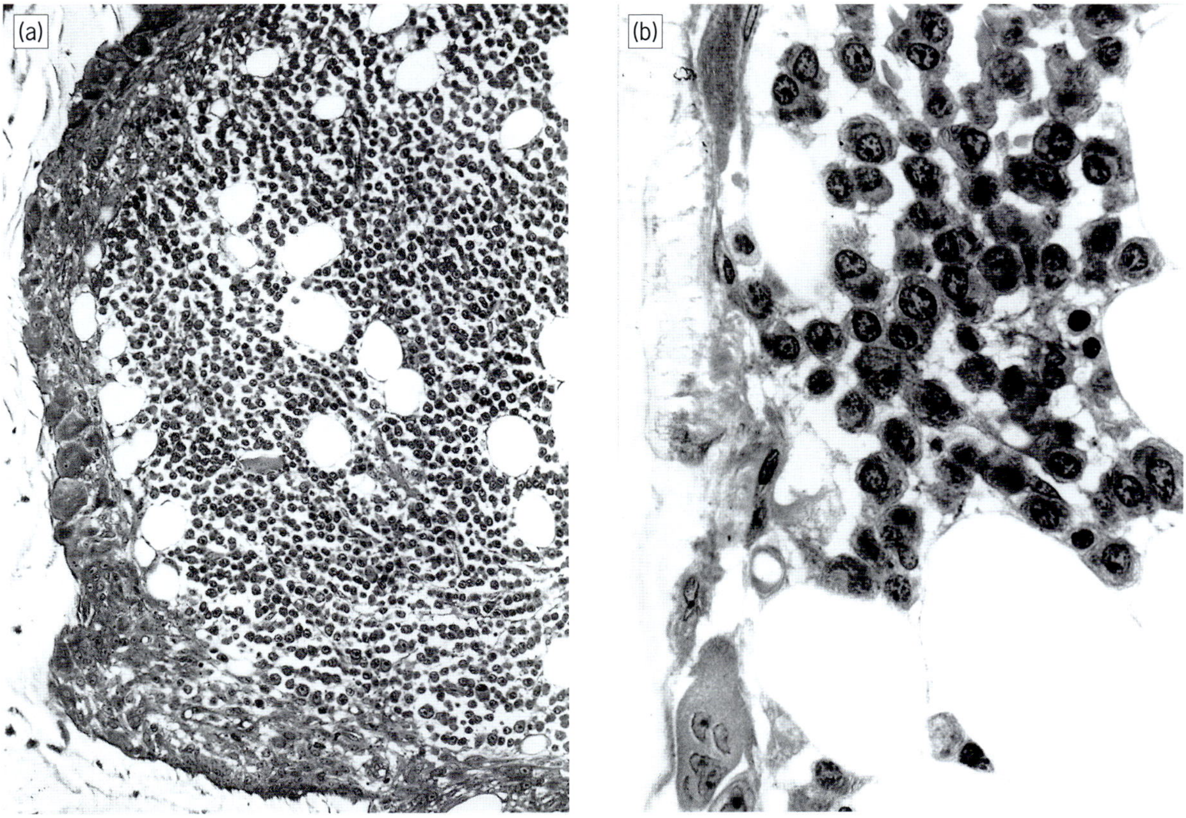

Figure 16.11 (a) Ossicle with scalloped edges lined by layers of active osteoclasts and separated from the myeloma cells by a band of fibrosis and connective tissue (Giemsa, ×100). (b) Resorption cavities filled by large multinucleated osteoclasts and surrounded by myeloma cells, Marschalko type (Giemsa, ×400).

does not influence osteoclastic activity. Direct bone resorption by myeloma cells is rare.

We have found that myeloma patients without involvement in the biopsy still have increased numbers of osteoclasts suggesting the existence of a systemic parathyroid hormone (PTH)-like factor in myeloma. Moreover, osteoblasts were inhibited, further upsetting the balance between bone resorption and bone formation (Figures 16.12(b) and 16.13).[54,55] Therapy of myeloma with corticosteroids also decreases bone formation and stimulates resorption, and so augments the osteoporosis already present.

Histomorphometric evaluation of sequential biopsies is useful to assess changes in bone remodelling with anti-osteoclastic therapy. Treatment with bisphosphonates alone also proved to have an antiproliferative effect on myeloma cells, as shown by a decline in M-protein level, especially in cases with endosteal seams of plasma cells and high osteoclastic activity (Figure 16.14).

MORPHOLOGIC CLASSIFICATION OF MYELOMA

Many studies have stressed the relationship between plasma cell morphology and prognosis in myeloma. Several morphologic classifications have recently been proposed; and prognostic cytologic features sought.[16,46,56–67]

The following features have been found to be associated with an unfavourable outcome:

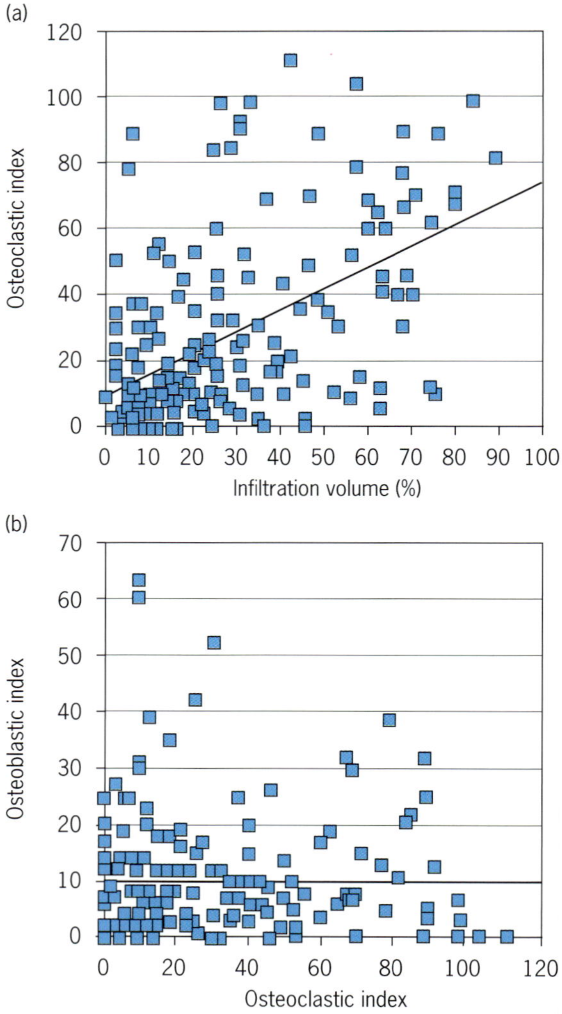

Figure 16.12 Histomorphometry of iliac crest biopsies of patients with myeloma: (a) correlation between infiltration volume and osteoclastic index; (b) correlation between osteoclastic and osteoblastic indices.

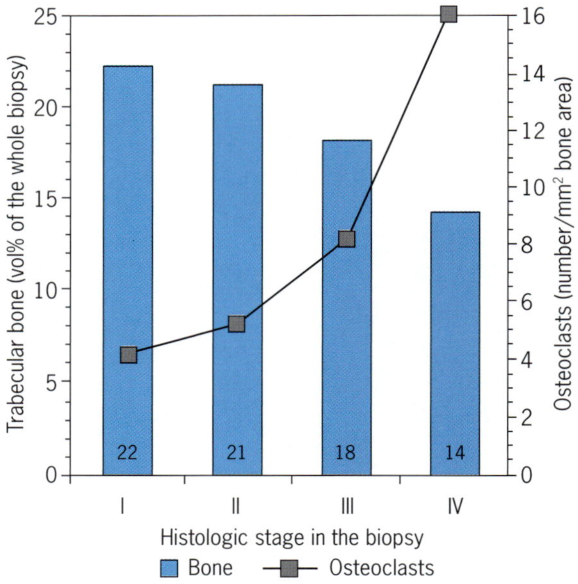

Figure 16.13 Correlation of the four histologic stages of myeloma with trabecular bone volume and osteoclastic resorption in the iliac crest biopsy.

- *plasma cell type*: nucleolated (Figure 16.15a), cleaved and large nuclei, mitotic figures in plasma cells, high PCLI, and diffuse bone marrow lymphocytosis;
- *plasma cell growth*: nodularity, packed marrow pattern (Figure 16.15b);
- *plasma cell mass*: percentages of plasma cells in smears and in sections;
- *alterations of bone and marrow*: high osteoclastic index, coarse fibrosis, marrow atrophy, myelodysplasia, amyloidosis, and secondary neoplasia.

According to the predominant plasma cell type in the aspirate and the section, the morphologic spectrum of myeloma cells can be divided into six types. These six types can be combined into three prognostic categories: low-, intermediate-, and high-grade disease[47] (Figures 16.16 and 16.17) (the values in parentheses represent overall frequency and median survival):

- *Low-grade malignancy:*
  Marschalko (59%, 38 months);
  small cell (11%, 44 months).
- *Intermediate-grade malignancy:*
  cleaved (8%, 18 months);
  polymorphous (9%, 20 months);
  asynchronous (11%, 19 months).
- *High-grade malignancy:*
  blastic (2%, 8 months).

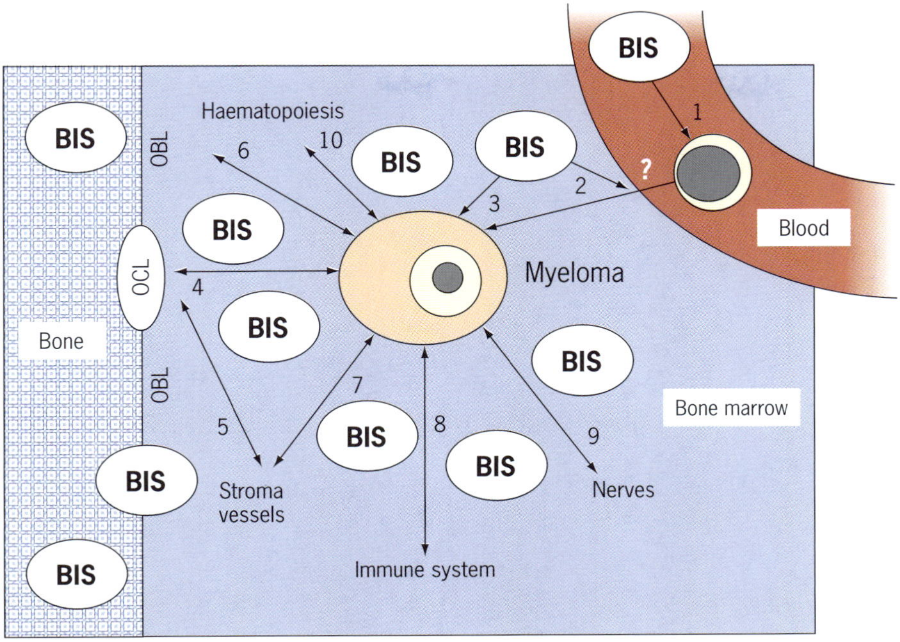

Figure 16.14 Ten actions of bisphosphonates (BIS) on myeloma cells and elements of bone and bone marrow. All the cellular and structural parameters shown in this sketch can be evaluated, quantified, and controlled in one single biopsy: myeloma cells, trabecular bone, bone cells, haematopoiesis, blood vessels, nerves, immunocytes, and stromal cells. OBL, osteoblast; OCL, osteoclast.

This morphologic classification can be applied both to smears and the sections, and has the advantage of simplicity and reproducibility. Divergent results were initially observed only in some borderline cases, in which additional counts using smears or sections, or both, subsequently established a convergent diagnosis.

Tables 16.1 and 16.2 show correlation between our classification system and immunophenotyping and other important serologic parameters. In a prospective study (German Myeloma Treatment Group, MM01), grading of the plasma cells was the most significant prognostic factor amongst all the diagnostic variables tested, and was followed by serum β_2-microglobulin, Bence Jones protein, and platelet count. The prognostic relevance of morphologic grading was confirmed in a subsequent German study (MM02; Figure 16.18).

There is no correlation between the number of nucleolated plasma cells and PCLI, indicating that nucleoli in plasma cells correlate with ribosomal activity rather than proliferative capacity or immaturity of plasma cells.

The mode of spread provides additional independent information in chronic lymphoproliferative disorders.[9,68] In contrast to CLL, in which a nodular infiltration pattern indicates an indolent course and long survival, nodularity in myeloma signals a progressive course, osteolytic lesions, and an unfavourable prognosis, thus reflecting intrinsic aggressiveness rather than the 'stage'[37,69,70] (Figure 16.19). Analogous to the Rappaport classification of the malignant lymphomas,[71] we combine plasma cell grading with the pattern of tumour growth (diffuse or nodular) in myeloma.

MORPHOLOGY IN STAGING OF MYELOMA

A relationship between the quantity of plasma cells (volume percentage, vol%) in smears and

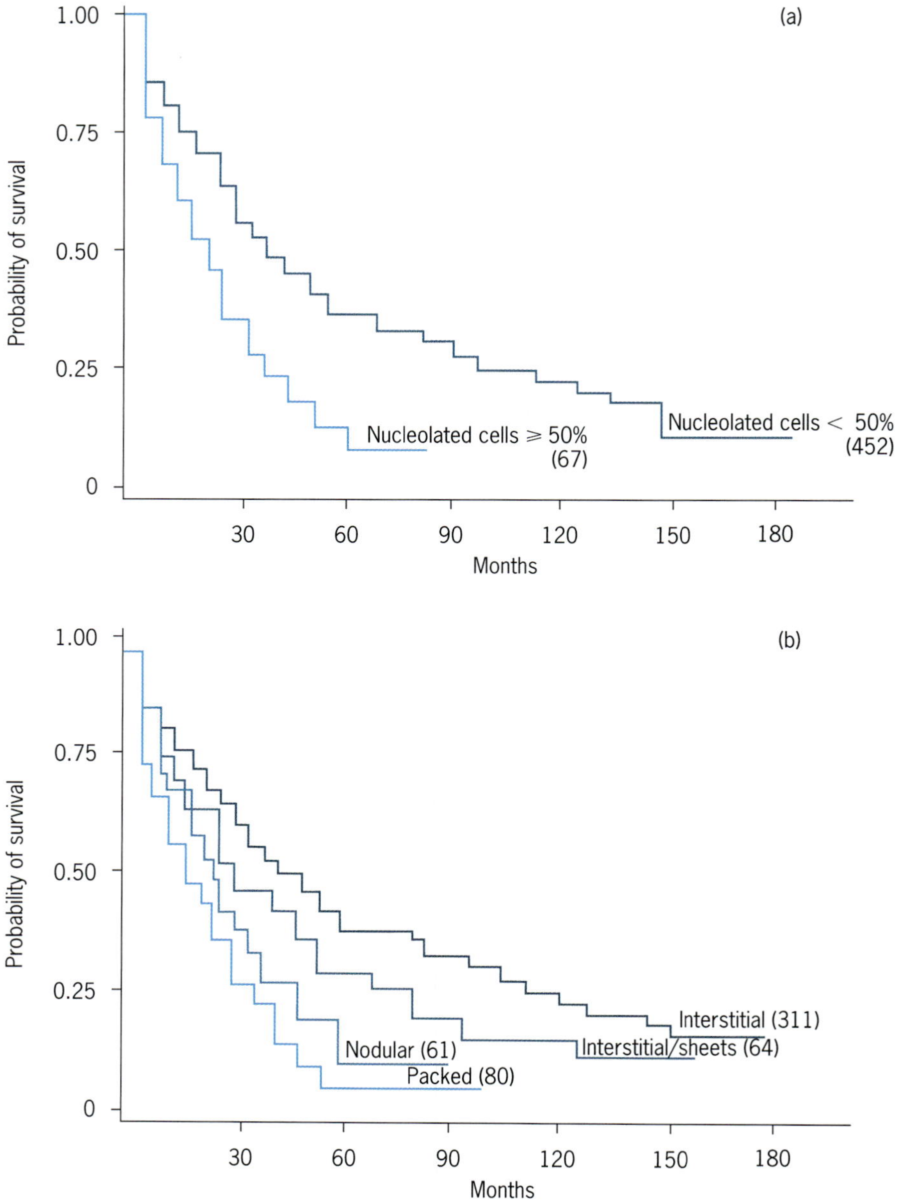

Figure 16.15 Predictive value of (a) the percentage of nucleolated myeloma cells and of (b) the growth pattern in bone marrow biopsy. The numbers of cases are shown in parentheses.

survival has been proposed,[72] but its validity has been questioned because of the possibility of over- and underestimation of the numbers of plasma cells in smears, as discussed earlier.[73–75]

In contrast, the amount of plasma cell infiltration in biopsy sections may be reliably and reproducibly estimated if the biopsy is adequate,[21] and utilized for histologic staging:

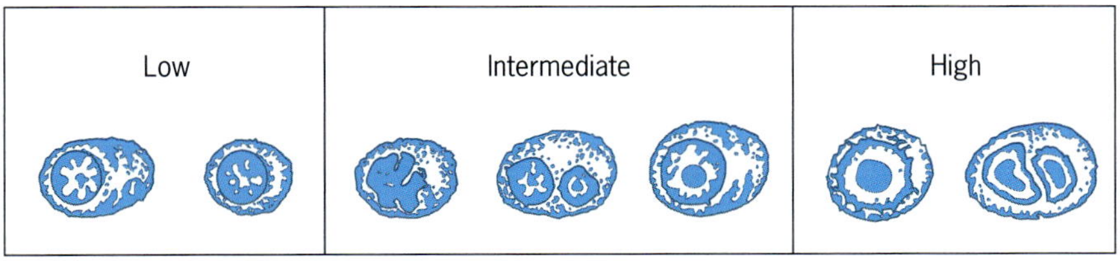

Figure 16.16 Morphologic classification of myeloma according to the predominant plasma cell type. Grouping into three grades of malignancy: *low-grade*: Marschalko and small cell type; *intermediate-grade*: cleaved, polymorphous and asynchronous type; *high-grade*: blastic and pleomorphous type.

Table 16.1 Correlation of cell grading with immunophenotyping of myeloma cells

Cell grading	No. of patients	Immunophenotype of myeloma cells				
		$CD10^{+}$	$CD19^{+}$	$CD40^{-/+}$	$CD56^{-}$	$Bcl\text{-}2^{-/+}$
Low	24	1	0	2	7	4
Intermediate	26	0	2	8	11	9
Total	50	1	2	10	18	13

Table 16.2 Correlation of morphologic cell types with plasma cell labelling index (PCLI), serum β_2-microglobulin (β_2M), and C-reactive protein (CRP)

Myeloma cell type	No. of patients	Mean PCLI (%)	Mean serum β_2M (mg/l)	Mean CRP (mg/dl)
Marschalko	72	0.6	2.5	1.8
Small cell	17	0.5	3.3	2.2
Anynchronous	25	2.5	4.0	4.8
Cleaved	6	3.1	4.4	1.6
Polymorphous	8	4.4	7.6	11.5
Total	129	1.5	3.4	3.0

- *histologic stage I*: <5 vol % plasma cells in the biopsy (14% of patients; median survival 88 months from the date of the first biopsy);
- *histologic stage II*: 5–19 vol% (28% of patients; median survival 49 months);
- *histologic stage III*: 20–50 vol% (40% of patients; median survival 27 months);
- *histologic stage IV*: >50 vol% (18% of patients; median survival 15 months).

These histologic stages also correlate well with reduction in bone mass, increase in osteoclastic activity, increase in karyotype abnormalities, and the visual rating of the tumour mass on MRI (Figure 16.20). Therefore histologic estimation of the plasma cell burden, which is easily performed by an integration disc in the microscope, supplements whatever clinical staging system is used.[76]

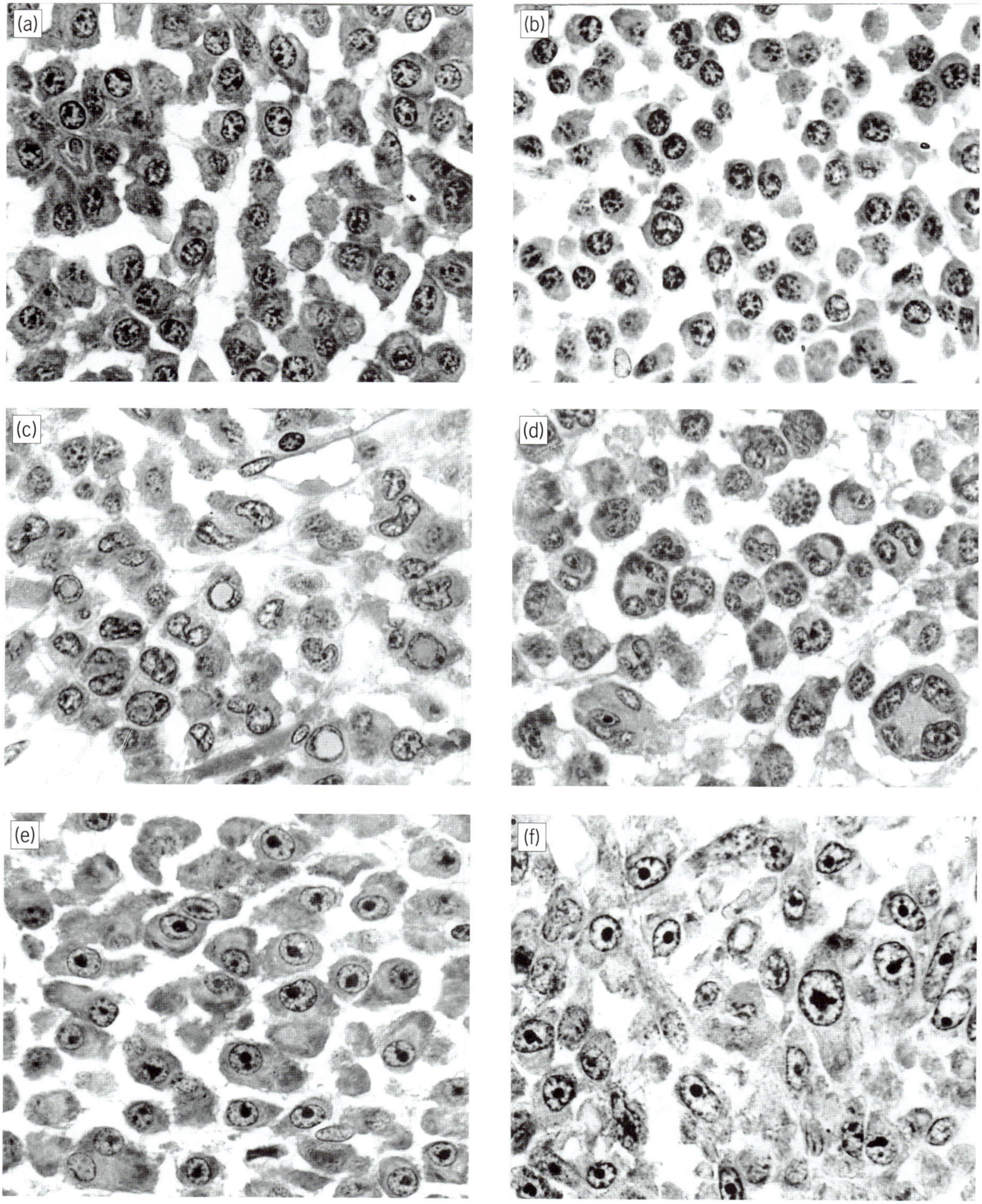

Figure 16.17 Histologic classification of myeloma according to the predominant plasma cell type: (a) Marschalko type; (b) small cell type; (c) cleaved type; (d) polymorphous type; (e) asynchronous type; (f) blastic type (Giemsa, ×300).

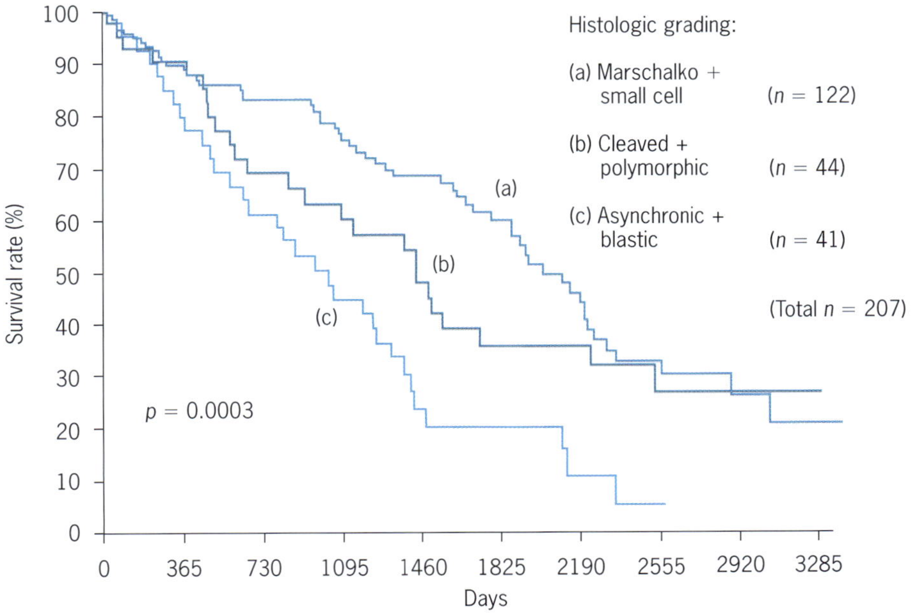

Figure 16.18 Prognostic relevance of morphologic classification, tested prospectively by the German Myeloma Treatment Group (MM-02) organized by Dr Deicher and Dr Peest, Medizinische Hochschule Hannover.

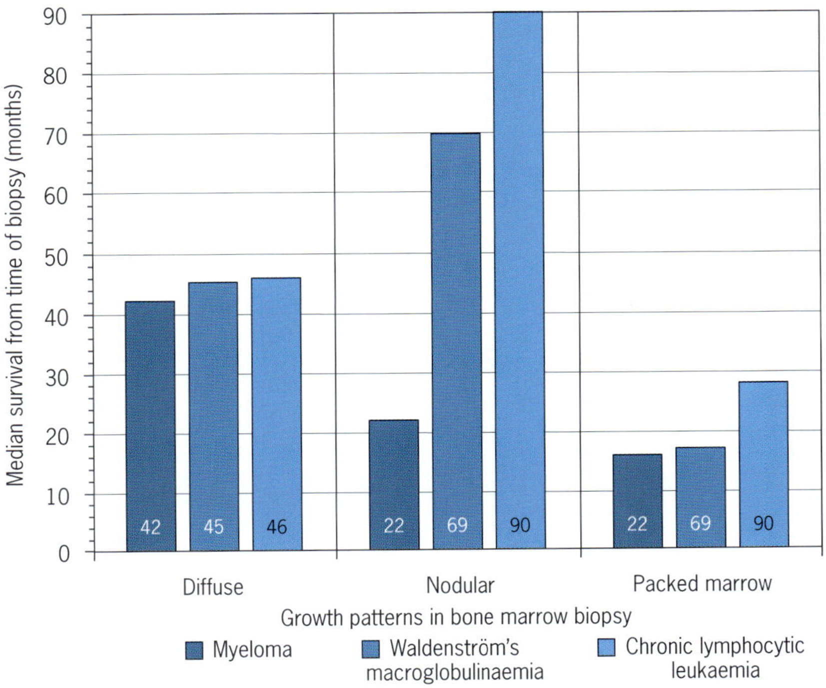

Figure 16.19 Different predictive value of growth patterns in systemic lymphoproliferative disorders.

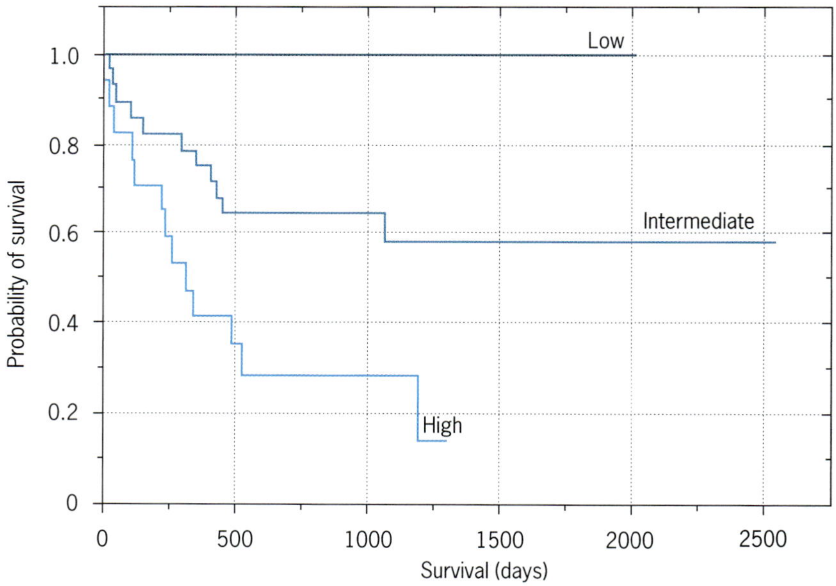

Figure 16.20 Survival curves of 53 myeloma patients correlated with visual rating of tumour mass seen on MRI.

MORPHOLOGIC FEATURES OF MYELOMA VARIANTS

Smouldering myeloma

The morphologic characteristics of smouldering myeloma are as follows (Figure 16.21):[37,47]

- minimal plasma cell infiltration (<5 vol% in biopsy and <10% plasma cells in smear);
- interstitial growth pattern;
- predominantly mature plasma cells (Marschalko);
- low PCLI (<0.8%);
- hypocellularity, with increase of fatty tissue;
- diffuse rarefaction of trabecular bone, with increased osteoclastic activity (osteoporosis).

Plasma cell leukaemia

This diagnosis requires that atypical plasma cells comprise 20% of the differential count of the peripheral blood. Bone marrow shows a packed marrow pattern and a marked infiltration of small and/or cleaved plasma cells within the sinusoids, and the PCLI is high. Sometimes these cells are lymphoplasmacytoid or even lymphoblastoid in appearance.[77]

Non-secretory myeloma

These patients have no M protein in the serum or the urine. The plasma cells either do not produce (non-producer) or do not secrete (non-secretory) monoclonal immunoglobulins or light chains.[78] There is extensive bone marrow involvement at presentation but no characteristic cytologic features or growth patterns are discernible.

Osteosclerotic myeloma

Between 1% and 2% of patients with myeloma have osteosclerotic bone lesions, possibly associated with the POEMS syndrome (polyneuropathy, organomegaly, endocrinopathy, monoclonal gammopathy, and skin changes).[79,80] In this variant, there is unbalanced activation of

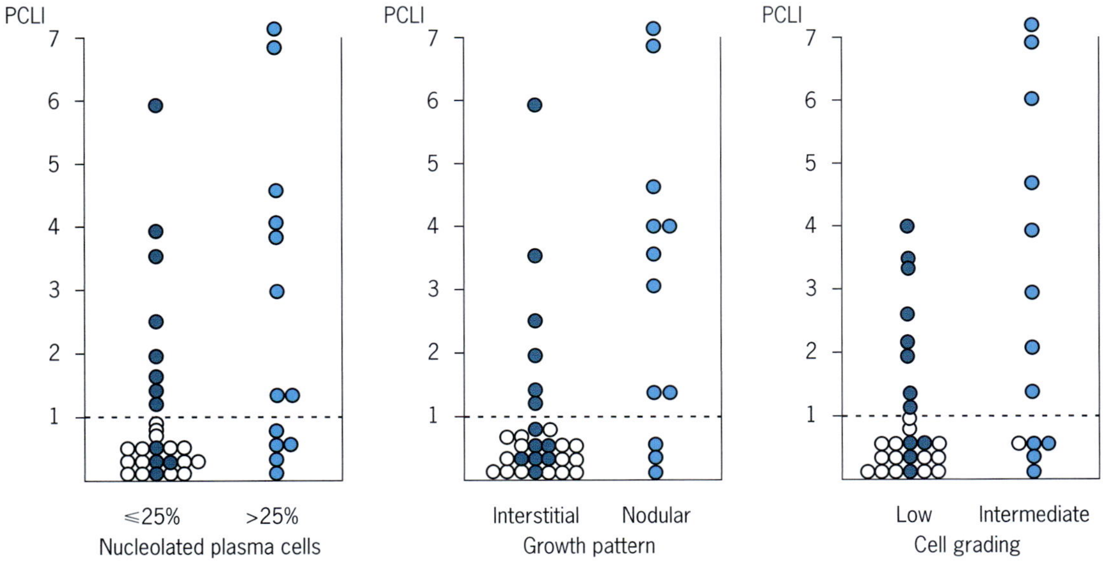

Figure 16.21 Correlation of the plasma cell labelling index (PCLI) with the amount of nucleolated myeloma cells, the growth pattern, and the cell grading of pretreatment patients with smouldering (open circles) and active (filled circles) myeloma.

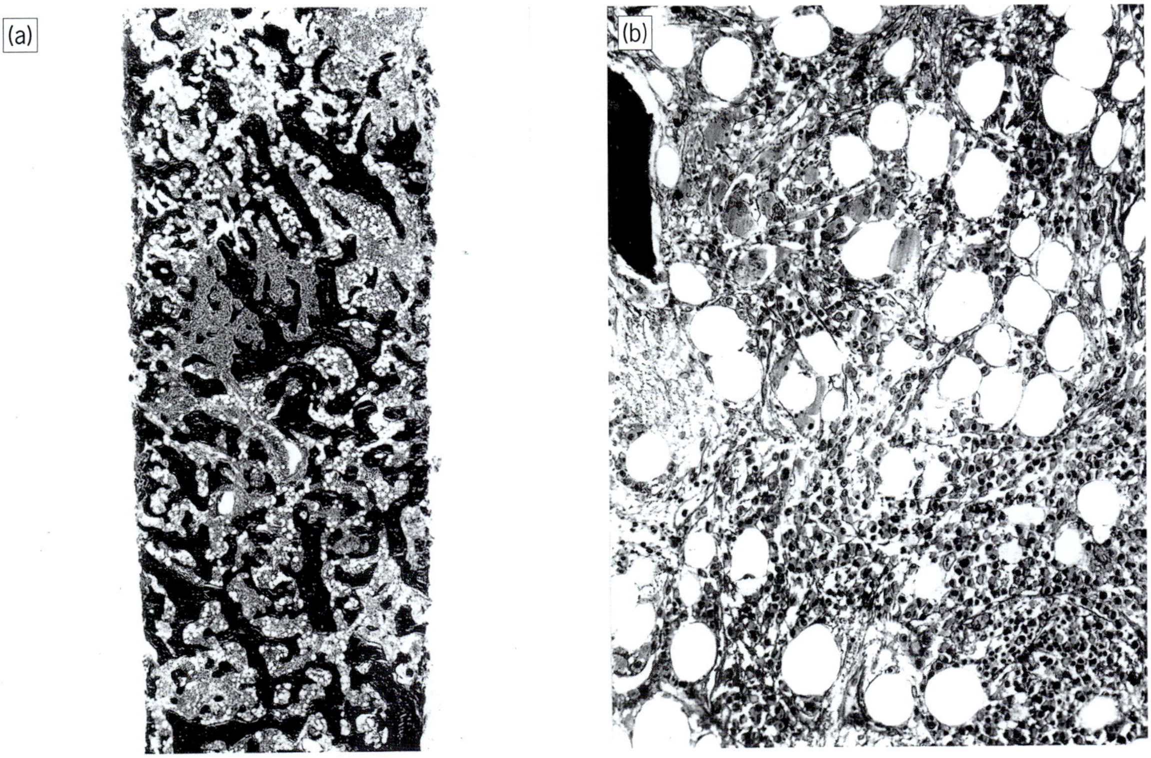

Figure 16.22 (a) Marked osteosclerotic reaction of trabecular bone in a patient with myeloma. Note the nodular myelomatous infiltration in the centre of the biopsy (Gomori, ×20). (b) Higher magnification of (a), showing concomitant plasmacellular (below) and megakaryocytic (above) infiltration, establishing the diagnosis of osteomyelosclerosis (OMS) on the basis of a concomitant myeloproliferative disorder (Gomori, ×250).

osteoblasts, but no special morphologic features of the myeloma cells have been reported. In rare cases, such as myeloma with thrombocytosis, bone marrow biopsies have revealed the coexistence of osteomyelosclerosis[81] (Figure 16.22). Osteosclerosis may also occur after chemo- and radiotherapy or administration of bisphosphonates.

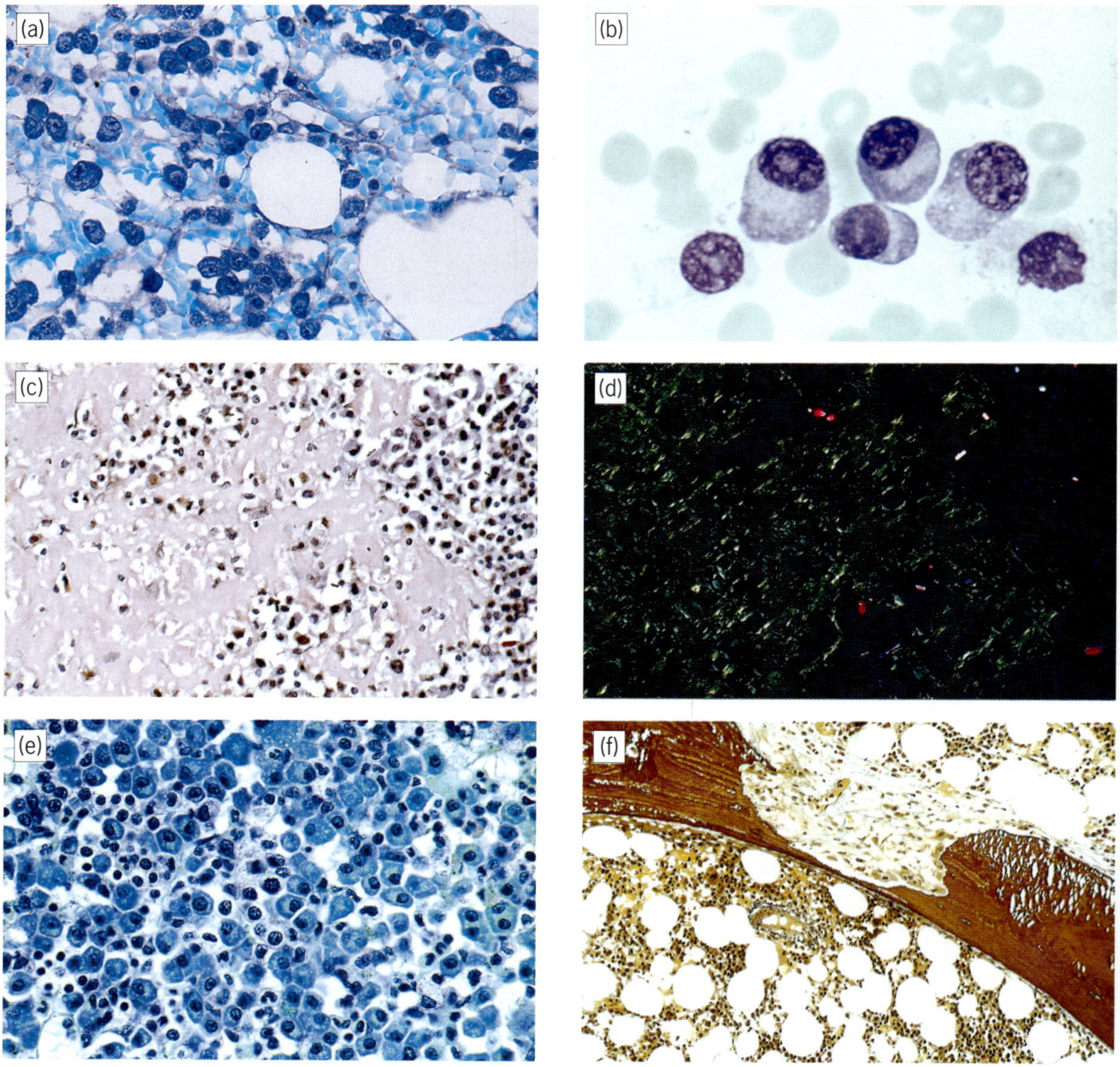

Figure 16.23 (a) Myeloma in the early treatment phase with pronounced erythrocytic extravasates and some residual mature myeloma cells (Giemsa, ×400). (b) Patient with development of plasma cell leukaemia after long-term chemotherapy. Predominance of small, lymphoplasmacytoid plasma cells in the peripheral blood film (May–Gruenwald–Giemsa, ×1000). (c) Homogenous red interstitial deposits of amyloid between myelomatous infiltrates (Congo red, ×100). (d) Same section as in (c), Congo red staining, with green amyloid deposits under polarized light. (e) Marschalko-type cells and lymphocytic infiltration predicting an unfavourable prognosis (Giemsa, ×250). (f) Ossicle showing dissecting osteoclasia without involvement in the biopsy, suggesting the existence of a systemic parathyroid hormone-related peptide (PTHrP) in myeloma (Gomori, ×250).

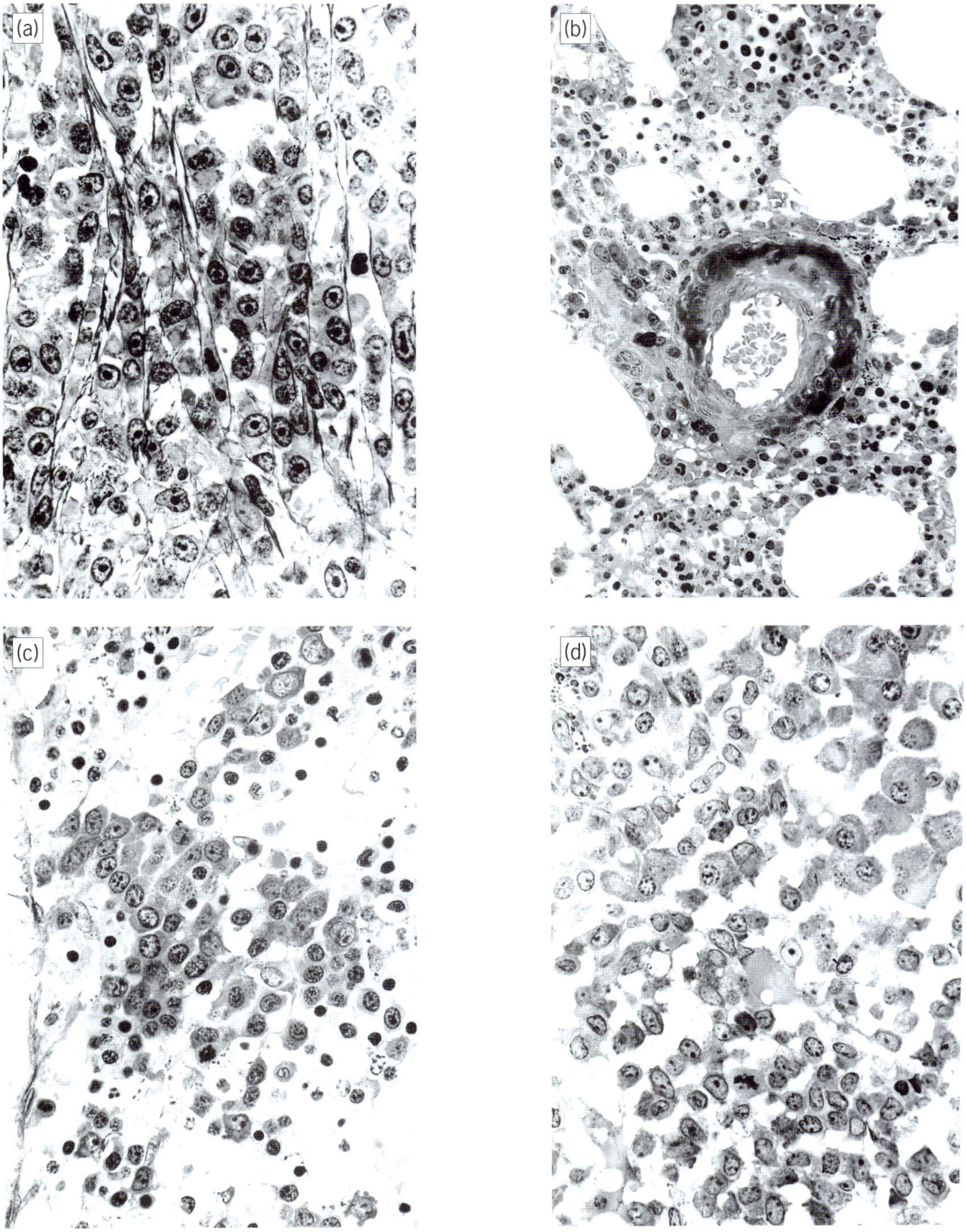

Figure 16.24 Alterations of the bone marrow in myeloma during the treatment phase. (a) Coarse fibrosis in blastic-type myeloma (Gomori, ×400). (b) Deposits of amyloidosis around a small artery (Giemsa, ×200). (c) Myelodysplasia, with marked maturation inhibition and topographic distortion especially of erythropoiesis, after long-term chemotherapy (Giemsa, ×350). (d) Acute myeloid leukaemia (AML-M2) as a second neoplasm in a patient with myeloma. Note the mixture of plasma cells and atypical myeloblasts (Giemsa, ×350).

MONITORING THE COURSE OF THE DISEASE WITH MORPHOLOGY

Initially with therapy, there is reduction of the plasma cell mass and marked oedema in sections of bone marrow biopsies (Figure 16.23). With attainment and maintenance of a stable plateau phase only a minimal residual interstitial infiltration remains. With successful chemotherapy and bisphosphonates, osteoclastic resorption is reduced, while osteoblasts, osteoid seams and trabecular bone volume are increased.

Continued or maintenance chemotherapy may have cumulative toxic effects on haematopoiesis, with a potential for the development of myelodysplasia, marrow hypoplasia or aplasia, and fibrosis. Changes in plasma cell grade and the development of nodularity signal imminent relapse. Refractory cytopenia or suspected amyloidosis are indications for taking biopsies and aspirates for clarification and appropriate therapy (Figures 16.23 and 16.24).[8,47,82] Concomitant or subsequent second neoplasias are not uncommon, and the frequency of myelodysplastic syndrome and acute leukaemia is noteworthy.

REFERENCES

1. Kyle RA, Bayrd ED. *The Monoclonal Gammopathies: Multiple Myeloma and Related Plasma-Cell Disorders* Springfield: Charles C Thomas, 1976.
2. Barlogie B, Epstein J, Selvanayagam P, Alexanian R. Plasma cell myeloma – new biological insights and advances in therapy. *Blood* 1989; **73:** 865–79.
3. Bartl R, Frisch B. *Biopsy of Bone in Internal Medicine*. Dordrecht: Kluwer Academic, 1993.
4. Frisch B, Bartl R. *Atlas of Bone Marrow Pathology*. Dordrecht: Kluwer Academic, 1990.
5. Frisch B, Lewis M, Burkhardt R, Bartl R. *Biopsy Pathology of Bone and Bone Marrow*. London: Chapman & Hall, 1985.
6. Schambeck CM, Wick M, Bartl R et al. Plasma cell proliferation in monoclonal gammopathies: measurement using BU-1 antibody in flow cytometry and microscopy: comparison with serum thymidine kinase. *J Clin Pathol* 1995; **48:** 477–81.
7. Buss DH, Prichard RW, Cooper MR. Plasma cell dyscrasias. *Hematol Oncol Clin North Am* 1988; **2:** 603–15.
8. Bartl R, Frisch B, Wilmanns W. Bone and marrow findings in multiple myeloma and related disorders. *Neoplastic Diseases of the Blood*.In: Wiernik PH, Canellos GH, Dutcher JP, Kyle RA, eds). New York: Churchill Livingstone, 1996: 477–514.
9. Bartl R, Frisch B, Burkhardt R et al. Lymphoproliferations in the bone marrow: identification and evolution, classification and staging. *J Clin Pathol* 1984; **37**: 233–54.
10. Clark P, Normansell DE, Innes DJ, Hess CE. Lymphocyte subsets in normal bone marrow. *Blood* 1986; **67:** 1600–6.
11. Turesson I. Distribution of immunoglobulin-containing cells in human bone marrow and lymphoid tissues. *Acta Med Scand* 1976; **199:** 293–304.
12. Marschalko TV. Über die sogenannten Plasmazellen, ein Beitrag zur Kenntnis der Herkunft der entzündlichen Infiltrationszellen. *Arch Dermatol Syphilol* 1895; **30:** 1–52.
13. Bartl R. Histologic classification and staging of multiple myeloma. *Hematol Oncol* 1988; **6:** 107–13.
14. Oken MM. Multiple myeloma. *Med Clin North Am* 1984; **68:** 757–87.
15. Ludwig H. *Multiples Myelom*. Berlin: Springer-Verlag, 1982.
16. Bartl R, Frisch B, Burkhardt R et al. Bone marrow histology in myeloma: its importance in diagnosis, prognosis, classification and staging. *Br J Haematol* 1982; **51**: 361–75.
17. Gavarotti P, Boccadoro M, Redoglia V et al. Reactive plasmacytosis: case report and review of the literature. *Acta Haematol* 1985; **73**: 108–10.
18. Hyun BH, Kwa D, Gabaldon H, Ashton JK. Reactive plasmacytic lesions of the bone marrow. *Am J Clin Pathol* 1976; **65:** 921–8.
19. Liu CT, Dahlke MB. Bone marrow findings of reactive plasmacytosis. *Am J Clin Pathol* 1967; **48:** 546–51.
20. Thiele J, Arenz B, Klein H et al. Differentiation of plasma cell infiltrates in the bone marrow: a clinicopathological study on 80 patients including immunohistochemistry and morphometry. *Virchows Arch A* 1988; **412:** 553–62.
21. Terpstra WE, Lokhorst HM, Blomjous F et al. Comparison of plasma cell infiltration in bone marrow biopsies and aspirates in patients with multiple myeloma. *Br J Haematol* 1992; **82:** 46–9.

22. Beltran G, Stuckey WJ. Nuclear lobulation and cytoplasmic fibrils in leukemic plasma cells. *Am J Clin Pathol* 1972; **58:** 159–64.
23. Buss DH, Reynolds GD, Cooper MR. Multiple myeloma associated with multilobated plasma cell nuclei. *Virchows Arch B* 1988b; **55:** 287–92.
24. Djaldetti M, Lewinski UH. Nuclear hypersegmentation in the myeloma cells of a patient with multiple myeloma. *Scand J Haematol* 1983; **31:** 144–8.
25. Hoffmann JJM, Breed WPM, Swaak-Lammers N. Plasma cell acid phosphatase score in multiple myeloma and related disorders. *Br J Haematol* 1985; **59:** 67–72.
26. Kurabayashi H, Miyawaki S, Murakami H et al. Ultrastructure of multi-nucleated giant myeloma cells; report of one case. *Am J Hematol* 1989; **31:** 284–5.
27. Levine SB, Bernstein LD. Crystalline inclusions in multiple myeloma. *JAMA* 1985; **254:** 1985.
28. Sivakumaran M, Parker A, Murphy et al. Multilobulated, multinucleated multiple myeloma. *Br J Haematol* 1992; **81:** 622–4.
29. Turesson I. Nucleolar size in benign and malignant plasma cell proliferation. *Acta Med Scand* 1975; **197:** 7–14.
30. Wong KF, Chan JK, Chu YC. Multiple myeloma with tadpolelike cells and rosette formation. *Am J Clin Pathol* 1992; **98:** 630–2.
31. Zukerberg LR, Ferry JA, Conlon M, Harris NL. Plasma cell myeloma with cleaved, multilobated, and monocytoid nuclei. *Am J Clin Path* 1990; **93:** 657–61.
32. Azar HA. The myeloma cell. I. In: *Multiple Myeloma and Related Disorders* (Azar HA, Potter M, eds). Hagerstown: Harper & Row, 1973: 86–152.
33. Bernier GM, Graham RC. Plasma cell asynchrony in myeloma: correlation of light and electron microscopy. *Semin Hematol* 1976; **13:** 239–45.
34. Portero JA, Martin S, Gonzales M, Miguel JF. Cytochemistry in the differential diagnosis of monoclonal gammopathies. *Br J Haematol* 1985; **60:** 768–9.
35. Saeed SM, Stock-Novack D, Pohlod R et al. Prognostic correlation of plasma cell acid phosphatase and beta-glucuronidase in multiple myeloma: a Southwest Oncology Group study. *Blood* 1991; **78:** 3281–7.
36. Bartl R, Frisch B, Burkhardt R. *Bone Marrow Biopsies Revisited: A New Dimension for Haematologic Malignancies*. Basel: Karger, 1985.
37. Bartl R, Frisch B. Bone marrow histology in multiple myeloma: prognostic relevance of histologic characteristics. *Hematol Rev* 1989; **3:** 87–108.
38. Greipp PR, Kyle RA. Clinical, morphological, and cell kinetic differencies among multiple myeloma, monoclonal gammopathy of undetermined significance, and smoldering multiple myeloma. *Blood* 1983; **62:** 166–71.
39. Bartl R, Frisch B, Diem H et al. Bone marrow histology and serum beta 2 microglobulin in multiple myeloma- a new prognostic strategy. *Eur J Haematol* 1989; **43**(Suppl 51): 88–98.
40. Greipp PR, Witzig TE, Gonchoroff NJ et al. Immunofluorescence labeling indices in myeloma and related monoclonal gammopathies. *Mayo Clin Proc* 1987; **62:** 969–77.
41. Girino M, Riccardi A, Luoni R et al. Monoclonal antibody Ki-67 as a marker of proliferative activity in monoclonal gammopathies. *Acta Haematol* 1991; **85:** 26–30.
42. Drach J, Gattringer C, Glassl H et al. The biological and clinical significance of the Ki-67 growth fraction in multiple myeloma. *Hematol Oncol* 1992; **10:** 125–34.
43. Aherne WA. The differentiation of myelomatosis from other causes of bone marrow plasmacytosis. *J Clin Pathol* 1958; **11:** 326–9.
44. Bartl R, Burkhardt R, Gierster P et al. Significance of bone marrow biopsy in the multiple myeloma. *Bibliotheca Haematol* 1978; **45:** 81–6.
45. Buss DH, Prichard RW, Hartz JW et al. Initial bone marrow findings in multiple myeloma: significance of plasma cell nodules. *Arch Pathol Lab Med* 1986; **110:** 30–3.
46. Canale DD, Collins RD. Use of bone marrow particle sections in the diagnosis of multiple myeloma. *Am J Clin Pathol* 1974; **61:** 383–92.
47. Bartl R, Frisch B, Fateh-Moghadam A et al. Histologic classification and staging of multiple myeloma. *Am J Clin Pathol* 1987; **87:** 342–55.
48. Bartl R, Frisch B, Diem H et al. Histologic, biochemical and clinical parameters for monitoring multiple myeloma. *Cancer* 1991; **68:** 2241–50.
49. Caligaris-Cappio F, Gregoretti MG, Ghia P, Bergiu L. In vitro growth of human multiple myeloma: implications for biology and therapy. *Hematol Oncol Clin North Am* 1992; **6:** 257–72.
50. Kawauchi K, Mori H, Sugiyama H et al. Multiple myeloma with coexistent myelofibrosis: improvement of myelofibrosis following recovery from multiple myeloma after treatment with melphalan and prednisolone. *Jpn J Med* 1991; **30:** 483–6.

51. Krzyzaniak RL, Buss DH, Cooper MR, Wells HB. Marrow fibrosis and multiple myeloma. *Am J Clin Pathol* 1988; **89:** 63–8.
52. Patterson KG, Treleaven JG, Zuiable A. Marrow fibrosis in myeloma: improvement by alkylating agent therapy. *Clin Lab Haematol* 1988; **10:** 221–4.
53. Riccardi A, Ucci G, Luoni R et al. Bone marrow biopsy in monoclonal gammopathies: correlations between pathologic findings and clinical data. The Cooperative Group for Study and Treatment of Multiple Myeloma. *J Clin Pathol* 1990; **43:** 469–75.
54. Witzig TE, Kyle RA, Greipp PR. Circulating peripheral blood plasma cells in multiple myeloma. *Curr Top Microbiol Immunol* 1992; **182:** 195–9.
55. Bataille R, Chappard D, Marcelli C et al. Recruitment of new osteoblasts and osteoclasts is the earliest critical event in the pathogenesis of human multiple myeloma. *J Clin Invest* 1991; **88:** 62–6.
56. Evans CE, Ward C, Rathour L, Galasko CB. Myeloma affects both the growth and function of human osteoblast-like cells. *Clin Exp Metastasis* 1992; **10:** 33–8.
57. Brink S, Bradshaw D, Rosenstrauch WJ, Van-der-Merve AM. Prognostic factors in multiple myeloma. *South African Med J* 1986; **69:** 35–8.
58. Carter A, Hocherman I, Linn S et al. Prognostic significance of plasma cell morphology in multipe myeloma. *Cancer* 1987; **60:** 1060–5.
59. Cherng NC, Asal NR, Kuebler JP et al. Prognostic factors in multiple myeloma. *Cancer* 1991; **67:** 3150–6.
60. Dehou M-F, Schots R, Lacor P et al. Diagnostic and prognostic value of the MB2 monoclonal antibody in paraffin-embedded bone marrow sections of patients with multiple myeloma and monoclonal gammopathy of undetermined significance. *Am J Clin Pathol* 1990; **94:** 287–91.
61. Fritz E, Ludwig H, Kundi M. Prognostic relevance of cellular morphology in multiple myeloma. *Blood* 1984; **63:** 1072–9.
62. Michiels JJ. Multiple myeloma: prognostic factors and treatment modalities, a review. *Neth J Med* 1992; **40:** 254–70.
63. Pasqualetti P, Casale R, Collacciani A et al. Multiple myeloma: relationship between survival and cellular morphology. *Am J Hematol* 1990; **33:** 145–7.
64. Paule B, Quillard J, Bisson M et al. Prognostic significance of plasma cell morphology in multiple myeloma. *Nouv Rev Fr Hematol* 1988; **30:** 209–12.
65. Pileri S, Poggi S, Baglioni P et al. Histology and immunohistology of bone marrow biopsy in multiple myeloma. *Eur J Haematol* 1989; **43(**Suppl 51): 52–9.
66. Riccardi A, Ucci G, Coci A, Ascari E. Bone marrow fibrosis in multiple myeloma. *Am J Clin Pathol* 1988; **90:** 753–4.
67. Schmid C, Isaacson PG. Bone marrow trephine biopsy in lymphoproliferative disease. *J Clin Pathol* 1992; **45:** 745–50.
68. Wutke K, Varbiro M, Rüdiger K-D, Kelenyi G. Cytological and histological classification of multiple myeloma. *Haematologia* 1981; **14:** 315–29.
69. Bartl R, Frisch B, Burkhardt R et al. Assessment of marrow trephine in relation to staging in chronic lymphocytic leukaemia. *Br J Haematol* 1982; **51:** 1–15.
70. Hashimoto N, Kurihara K. A histological study on the developmental process of myeloma nodules. *J Kyushu Hematol Soc* 1982; **30:** 1–8.
71. Hashimoto N, Kurihara K. The pathological significance of diffuse myeloma: two different types of compactly and sparsely diffuse myelomas. *J Kyushu Hematol Soc* 1982b; **30**: 9–20.
72. Rappaport H. *Tumours of the Hematopoietic System. Atlas of Tumor Pathology*. Washington: AFIP, 1966.
73. Vercelli D, DiGuglielmo R, Guidi G et al. Bone marrow percentage of plasma cells in the staging of monoclonal gammopathies. *Nouv Rev Fr Haematol* 1980; **22:** 139–45.
74. Cavo M, Baccarani M, Lipizer A, Tura S. Prognostic value of bone marrow plasma cell infiltration in stage I multiple myeloma. *Br J Haematol* 1983; **55:** 683–90.
75. Cavo M, Baccarani M, Gobbi M et al. Bone marrow plasma cell infiltration in multiple myeloma. Br *J Haematol* 1984; **57:** 352–3.
76. Pasqualetti P, Casale R, Collacciani A, Colantonio D. Prognostic factors in multiple myeloma: a new staging system based on clinical and morphological features. *Eur J Cancer* 1991; **27:** 1123–6.
77. Carbone A, Volpe R, Manconi R. Bone marrow pattern and clinical staging in multiple myeloma. *Br J Haematol* 1987; **65:** 502.
78. Isobe T, Ikeda Y, Ohta H. Comparison of sizes and shapes of tumor cells in plasma cell leukemia and plasma cell myeloma. *Blood* 1979; **53:** 1028–30.
79. Feng CS. Intranuclear inclusions in myeloma cells in a case of nonsecretory multiple myeloma. *Am J Hematol* 1990; **33:** 72–4.

80. Driedger H, Pruzanski W. Plasma cell neoplasms with osteosclerotic lesions: a study of 5 cases and a review of the literature. *Arch Intern Med* 1979; **139:** 144–8.
81. Miralles GD, O´Fallon JR, Talley NJ. Plasma cell dyscrasia with polyneuropathy: the spectrum of POEMS syndrome. *N Engl J Med* 1992; **327:** 1919–23.
82. Bartl R, Frisch B. Diagnostic morphology in multiple myeloma. *Curr Diagn Pathol* 1995; **2:** 222–35.

17

Imaging studies

Edgardo JC Angtuaco, Angela Moulopoulos, Theo Hronas, Ramesh Avva

CONTENTS • **Introduction** • **Radiographic skeletal survey** • **Nuclear medicine (radionuclide) scans** • **Positron emission tomography** • **Computed tomography** • **Magnetic resonance imaging** • **MRI in other plasma cell dyscrasias** • **Prognostic significance of MRI in myeloma** • **Compression fractures in myeloma** • **MRI-directed CT-guided biopsies**

INTRODUCTION

Magnetic resonance imaging (MRI) has improved the radiologic evaluation of patients with myeloma significantly. Prior to the advent of MRI, radiologic studies primarily involved conventional X-ray evaluation of the skeleton for destructive bone changes characteristic of myeloma.

Traditionally, the initial radiographic skeletal survey has been used to determine the presence of lytic bony lesions and their number to estimate the tumour burden as defined by the Durie–Salmon staging system.[1,2] Subsequent follow-up studies during and after treatment help determine disease progression by increase in the size or number of these focal lesions. Conventional radiographic studies suffer from lack of sensitivity, particularly in determining disease response. Nuclear medicine studies such as bone scans have been used but have proven to be of limited value.

The advent of MRI has made the direct evaluation of bone marrow infiltration with malignant cells possible. MRI survey of the axial skeleton in combination with bone marrow aspiration and biopsy helps define the extent of marrow involvement, and determine the presence of diffuse disease as well as the size and number of focal lesions (see Chapter 16). MRI studies can also accurately depict associated findings, such as spinal cord compression, pathologic fractures, and the effects of various therapeutic interventions on the vertebral bone marrow. Current investigations focus on its role in assessing tumour burden and prognosis, providing accurate targets for computed tomography (CT)-directed biopsies of focal lesions, and determining the effect of therapy.

Helical CT survey studies of the skeleton are currently being used in selected myeloma patients to assess lytic bony lesions, and in Waldenström's macroglobulinaemia, in the analysis of lymphadenopathy.

We have used positron emission tomography (PET) with FDG as the imaging agent to detect other sites of involvement not seen in an MRI skeletal survey. Table 17.1 shows the various imaging studies utilized in myeloma.

RADIOGRAPHIC SKELETAL SURVEY

Radiographic studies continue to be used almost universally in the initial evaluation and widely

Table 17.1 Diagnostic radiologic techniques in plasma cell dyscrasias

- Radiographic skeletal survey
- Nuclear medicine (radionuclide) scans
- Computed tomography (CT)
- Magnetic resonance imaging (MRI)
- Positron emission tomography (PET)

in the follow-up of patients with plasma cell dyscrasias.

A global skeletal survey ('metastatic bone survey') is performed in the work-up of newly diagnosed patients. This consists of radiographs of the skull, spine, pelvis, femora, humeri, and chest. Additional views of the ribs, distal extremities, hands, and feet can be performed to make the examination extensive if needed.

The findings of three or more skeletal lesions indicates high tumour burden and stage III disease.[1,2] While approximately 50% destruction of bone must occur before a lytic lesion can be visualized radiographically, diffuse osteopenia is more easily visualized. Myeloma lesions are typically osteolytic, primarily affecting the spine, pelvis, skull, ribs, sternum, and the proximal appendages[3] (Figure 17.1). Lytic lesions are usually found in 80% of patients with symptomatic myeloma at the time of diagnosis, are usually multiple, and are associated with generalized osteopenia.

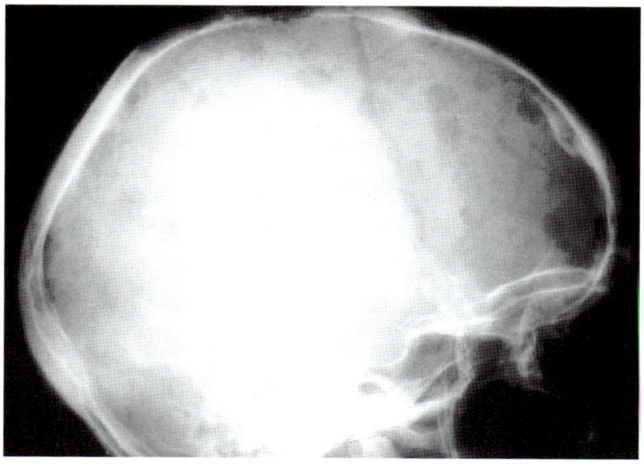

Figure 17.1 Lateral view of the skull. Multiple punched-out lytic lesions are present in the calvarium.

The multiple lytic lesions seen in patients with myeloma are radiographically difficult to differentiate from lytic lesions caused by other metastatic bone tumours. Bony sclerosis is occasionally seen (<1%); usually this is in younger patients[4] or in association with the POEMS syndrome (polyneuropathy, organomegaly, endocrinopathy, monoclonal gammopathy, and skin changes).[5]

The diagnosis of early stages of myeloma (smouldering disease) depends, in part, on the absence of lytic lesions on X rays (see Chapter 10), and these diagnoses are often difficult to make on the basis of conventional radiography. A conventional bone survey is inadequate to diagnose either monoclonal gammopathy of undetermined significance (MGUS) or solitary plasmacytoma with accuracy (see Chapters 24 and 25).

NUCLEAR MEDICINE (RADIONUCLIDE) SCANS

Bone scintigraphy is generally highly sensitive in the detection of bone metastases from malignancies such as breast and prostate cancer. However, this does not hold true in the case of myeloma. Comparative studies have repeatedly showed that conventional radiographic surveys detected more lytic lesions (sensitivity 74–82%) than bone scanning (sensitivity 37–60%).[6–8]

Most often, lesions are seen on radiographs and not on bone scans. However, in certain cases, scintigraphy identifies lesions not seen on radiography, such as those in the ribs.[9] The poor sensitivity of bone scans in myeloma can be traced to the mechanism of uptake of radioisotopes. These isotopes typically accumulate in sites of reparative bone reaction. In myeloma, bone lesions are often purely lytic with no osteoblastic response and do not attract radionuclide. It has been suggested that bone scans are useful in identifying patients with bone pain that is likely to respond to strontium therapy.[10]

Other radioisotopes have also been used to assess patients with myeloma: gallium-67 (^{67}Ga) scans may be useful in patients with fulminant disease or with extra-osseous involvement.[8,11] However, ^{67}Ga scans were found to be less sensitive than plain radiographs in screening evaluation of patients with myeloma.[8] Studies employing technetium-99m 2-methoxyisobutylisonitrile (^{99m}Tc-MIBI, ^{99m}Tc-sestamibi) have been used in the evaluation of myeloma.[12] The sensitivity of this agent is similar to that reported for radiography, but its added benefit is the ability to differentiate active lesions from healed lesions.

POSITRON EMISSION TOMOGRAPHY

The most commonly used agent in oncologic PET imaging is FDG ([^{18}F]-2-fluoro-2-deoxyglucose. This is a glucose analogue that accumulates in sites of increased glycolysis. While no prospective studies have been performed in myeloma, successful PET identification of a large lytic lesion that was negative on routine bone scan[13] and abnormalities at sites of bone pain[14] have been reported. At the Arkansas Cancer Research Center, PET scanning has been performed selectively, and has identified both osseous and extra-osseous sites of myelomatous involvement (Figure 17.2). PET imaging has also been used to determine the activity of focal lesions, primarily

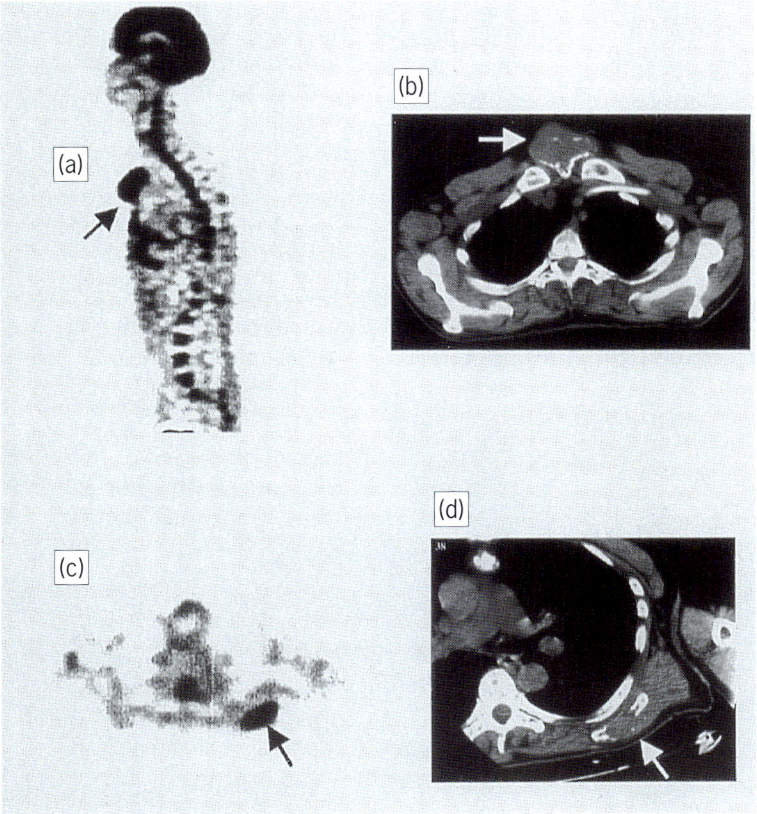

Figure 17.2 PET-identified sites of osseous myeloma with CT correlation. (a) Sagittal FDG-PET image with intense sternal uptake and (b) axial CT scan of the chest showing an expansile sternal plasmacytoma. (c) Axial FDG-PET image depicting activity in left scapula and (d) CT of the chest with lytic lesion of the left scapula.

in patients where focal lesions found on MRI persist despite successful therapy. Studies are ongoing to determine the ability of whole-body PET to qualitatively determine the extent of myelomatous spread.

COMPUTED TOMOGRAPHY

CT is highly sensitive in identifying lytic lesions in the skeleton, even before they are radiographically visible. However, it is not used routinely in the evaluation of myeloma patients because of the superiority of MRI, and the fact that it often does not alter disease stage or treatment decisions when used instead of plain radiographs.[15] It has been used in atypical presentations of the disease or as a problem-solving tool. Since MRI is confined to the axial skeleton, CT is very helpful in the evaluation of the soft tissue component of lytic lesions and extramedullary plasmacytomas arising in sites such as the chest, abdomen, and pelvis.[16–17]

Another important use of CT in myeloma is in directing imaging-guided needle biopsies. Cytology on these biopsy specimens helps in the diagnosis of solitary plasmacytoma or myeloma when the patients present with soft tissue masses.[16] In treated patients, cytology helps identify patients with persistent disease. In treated or untreated patients, cytogenetic studies on the aspiration specimen may be useful in identifying karyotype abnormalities not seen in the standard bone marrow aspirates.[18]

MAGNETIC RESONANCE IMAGING

MRI of the skeleton in myeloma offers multiple advantages (Table 17.2).

Direct visualization of the bone marrow, the ability to survey the axial skeleton for the number and size of focal lesions, and the ability to accurately assess the effects of therapy makes MRI very useful in myeloma.

Normal marrow on MRI scans

There must, however, be a clear understanding of the various MRI factors that distinguish a normal and abnormal MRI appearance of the bone marrow. In addition to the actual technique used for imaging (Table 17.3), the MRI picture is dependent upon the relative distribution of the bony trabecula, fat, and water. The predominance of these various elements contribute to the overall marrow appearance. The composition of the bone marrow changes throughout life. These changes are predictable, and it is important to distinguish age-related marrow changes from an abnormal marrow.

In the young, the bone marrow is largely haematopoietic, and starts to change in adolescence with conversion to yellow (fatty)

Table 17.2 Advantages of MRI in myeloma

- Defines the extent of disease in the axial skeleton
- Defines diffuse versus focal disease
- Assesses associated findings, such as existing or impending fractures and cord compression
- Finds areas for possible CT-guided biopsy
- Assesses response to therapy

Table 17.3 MRI parameters (techniques)

- *T1*-weighted sequence (short-*TR*–short-*TE* spin-echo)
- *T2*-weighted sequence (long-*TR*–long-*TE* spin-echo)
- STIR sequence ('short tau-inversion recovery')
- Gradient-echo sequence (short flip angle *T2* gradient-echo sequence)
- Post-contrast *T1*-weighted sequence (with intravenous administration of gadolinium-chelate compounds and fat-suppression)

marrow, which first appears in the diaphyses and epiphyses of the appendicular skeleton and eventually involves the metaphyses. By the age of 20 years, the appendicular skeleton has become mostly fatty, whereas the axial skeleton, including the spine, ribs, pelvis, and skull, and the proximal metaphyses of the femur and humerus, stays haematopoietic. The axial skeleton eventually becomes fatty, starting in the fourth decade of life, and by the sixth decade is mainly composed of fatty marrow. In both cases, predominantly haematopoietic or predominantly fatty, the appearance of the marrow is homogeneous. During the transition, when the marrow contains a mixture of both elements, it may appear inhomogeneous on MRI.

The normal bone marrow signal on *T1*-weighted MRI of the spine usually conforms to one of four distinct patterns, depending upon the age group[19] (Table 17.4). The patterns may show diffuse hypointensity or band-like hyperintensity at the endplates; the hyperintensity may be heterogeneous or uniform.

Types of MRI sequences

The imaging parameters in MRI of the bone marrow greatly affect the image (Table 17.3). The commonly used MRI sequences are *T1*-weighted, *T2*-weighted, STIR, gradient-echo, and post-contrast *T1*-weighted with fat suppression.

At our institution, the MRI survey of the axial skeleton usually consists of sagittal projections of the spine with *T1*-weighted and STIR sequences, and coronal projections of the pelvis with *T1*-weighted and STIR sequences.

Table 17.4 Patterns of normal bone marrow signal on *T1*-weighted MRI of the spine in different age groups[19]

Pattern	Marrow appearance on *T1* signal	Site	Age distribution (% of all patients with a certain pattern at a given site)
1	Hypointense except for linear areas of high intensity superior and inferior to the basivertebral vein	Cervical Thoracic Lumbar	92% <40 years 76% <30 years 99% <30 years
2	Hypointense with band-like and triangular hyperintensity at the endplates	Cervical Thoracic Lumbar	87% >40 years 88% >50 years 86% >40 years
3*	Hyperintensity	Cervical Thoracic Lumbar	75% >50 years Uniform age distribution 76% >40 years

*3a, homogeneous; 3b, heterogeneous.

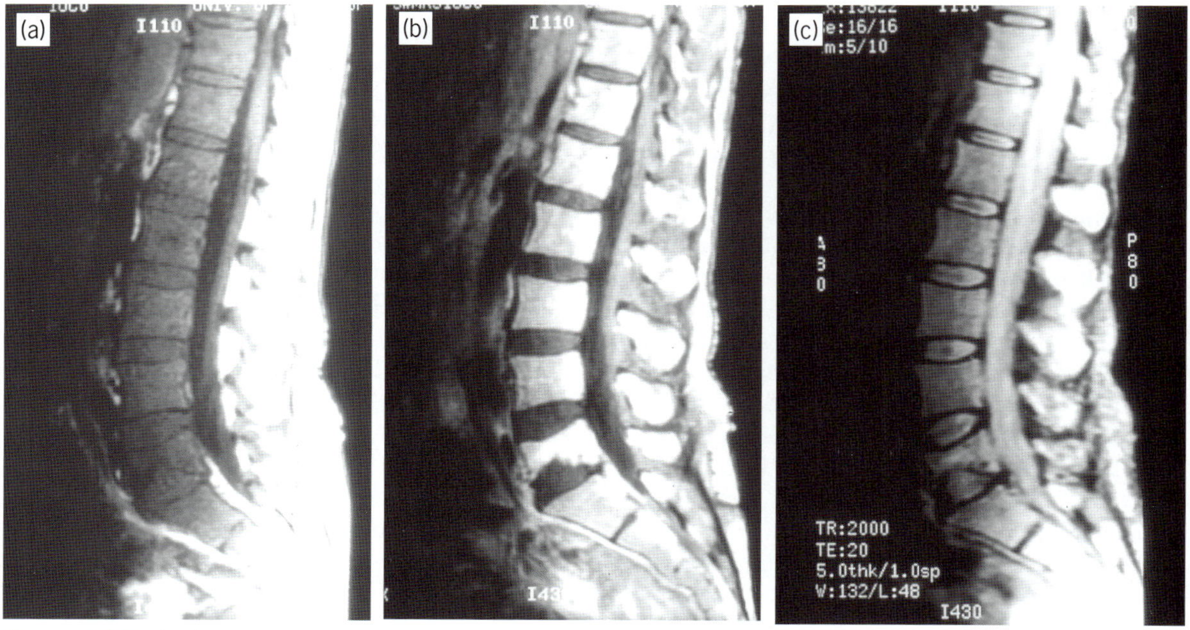

Figure 17.3 Diffuse marrow involvement. Sagittal *T1*-weighted pre-contrast, (a) post-contrast, fat-suppressed *T1*-weighted (b), and STIR (c) images of the lumbar spine.

In the initial MRI survey, we have also found the post-contrast fat-suppressed *T1* images to be helpful in locating small focal lesions in the spine. Post-contrast fat-suppressed *T1*-weighted sequences are useful for imaging the skull, coronal views for calvarial lesions, and sagittal and axial views for clival and skull base lesions.

The STIR sequence is a fat-suppression technique that allows better visualization of cellular lesions. Hence, focal and diffuse lesions stand out against the background of a suppressed marrow, and provide better contrast-to-noise ratio. This is a highly reproducible technique, permitting good accuracy when a large field of view such as the pelvis is to be imaged.

Bone marrow MRI changes in myeloma

The bone marrow may be involved in a diffuse or focal fashion in myeloma. Diffuse involvement with myeloma appears homogeneous or inhomogeneous on MRI. Diffusely abnormal marrow appears uniformly isointense with the disc interspace (intensity similar to the disc interspace) on *T1*-weighted sequence, and diffusely hyperintense in relation to the adjacent skeletal muscle (greater intensity than skeletal muscle) on STIR images. Following gadolinium contrast administration, the marrow enhances brightly when compared with the original pre-contrast *T1*-weighted image (Figure 17.3). Table 17.5 shows the differences between normal and abnormal MRI marrow appearances.

Figure 17.4 shows the various patterns of involvement of the spine on MRI. The diffusely involved marrow may also appear inhomogeneous, with scattered zones of hypointensity on the *T1*-weighted sequence within an isointense or hyperintense background, while the STIR sequence is primarily hyperintense and non-uniform. A speckled appearance of the vertebral bone marrow, with small focal areas of enhancement on the post-contrast study, suggests multiple scattered focal deposits of tumour within the marrow. Focal involvement

Table 17.5 Overall background marrow signal: comparison of normal and abnormal

	T1-weighted sequence	STIR sequence	*T1*-weighted post-contrast with fat suppression
Normal	Hyperintense	Hypointense	No enhancement seen
Abnormal	Hypointense	Hyperintense	Enhancement seen

in myeloma is variable, with single or multiple, and expansile or non-expansile, lesions. Focal lesions are hypointense on *T1*-weighted sequences, hyperintense on STIR sequences, and enhance on post-gadolinium *T1*-weighted sequences.

Other changes occurring in the bones and marrow affect the MRI in patients with myeloma. The early osteopenic fractures commonly found in patients with myeloma cause parallel zones of hypointensity along the vertebral body margins on *T1*-weighted images. Radiation to the bone marrow kills the cellular elements of the marrow and transforms it to a primarily fatty marrow. Irradiated marrow areas, particularly in the spine, are seen as distinct zones of hyperintensity on *T1*-weighted sequences. On STIR images, the converted fatty marrow is seen as a zone of hypointense signal (Figure 17.5). Severe anaemia (which stimulates haematopoietic activity in the bone marrow), diffuse marrow fibrosis, and diffuse blastic metastases to the bone marrow cause the marrow signal to be hypointense on both *T1* and STIR images.

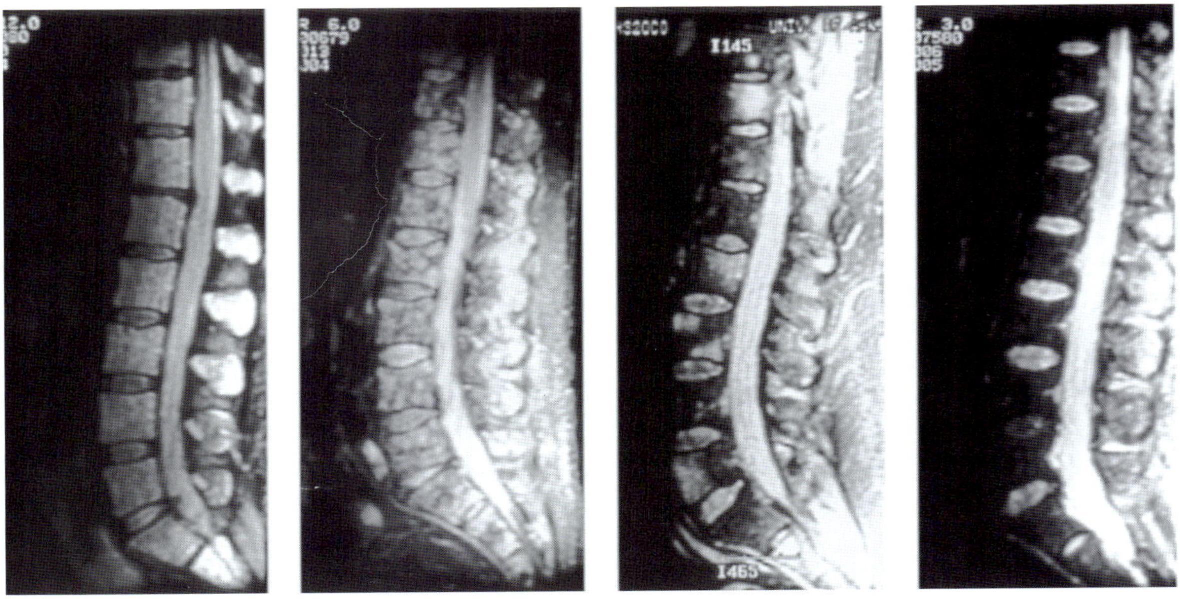

Diffuse | Heterogeneous | Focal | Normal

Figure 17.4 Patterns of spinal involvement in myeloma.

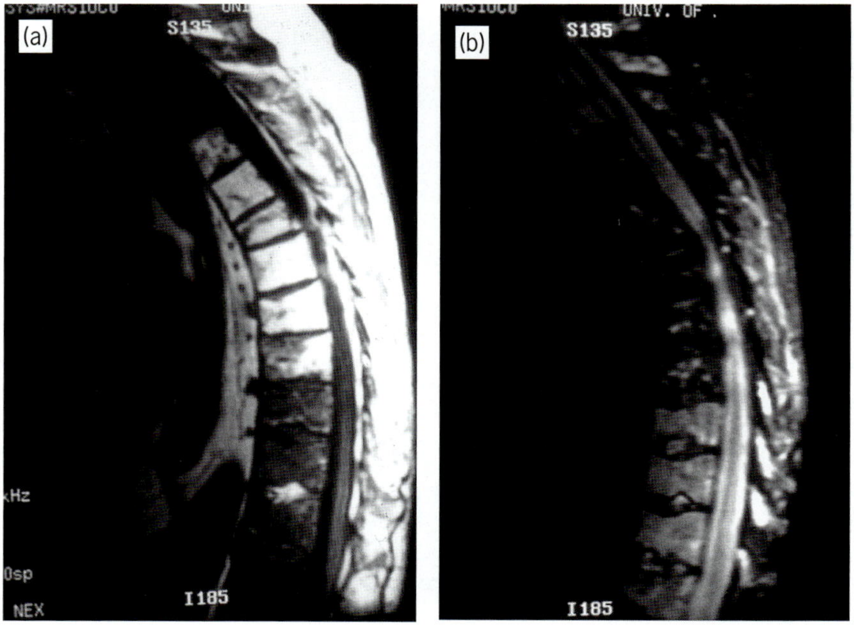

Figure 17.5 Effects of radiation on bone marrow. (a) Sagittal *T1*-weighted image of the thoracic spine shows increased signal consistent with fatty replacement. (b) Sagittal STIR image shows this same area to be hypointense.

MRI IN OTHER PLASMA CELL DYSCRASIAS

Solitary bone plasmacytoma

Solitary bone plasmacytoma is diagnosed in about 2% of patients with plasma cell dyscrasias. The diagnosis requires evidence of a tumour consisting of monoclonal plasma cells and absence of plasma cells at other sites. Tumoricidal radiotherapy usually eradicates local disease. Occult disease is probably the cause of the eventual development of myeloma in a number of patients with an initial diagnosis of a solitary bone plasmacytoma (see Chapter 25).

Indeed, 4 of 12 patients with solitary bone plasmacytoma who were examined with spinal MRI were found to have unsuspected additional lesions in the spine.[20] Three of these four patients, but none of the remainder, developed systemic disease within 18 months from diagnosis.[20] Mathieu et al,[21] reported similar findings in a group of six patients. If MRI were to include other sites such as the pelvis, skull, and proximal long bones, the number of patients with additional lesions might increase. In a recent study, seven of eight patients with solitary bone plasmacytoma staged with conventional radiographs developed myeloma, compared with only one of seven patients who were studied with both conventional radiographs and MRI.[22]

MRI should be a part of the staging of patients with suspected solitary bone plasmacytoma to limit the incidence of undetected occult disease.

MGUS

Absence of skeletal lesions is an important factor in the diagnosis of MGUS (see Chapter 10). The presence of skeletal lesions on MRI excludes MGUS and results in the diagnosis of myeloma (or solitary plasmacytoma). In patients without skeletal lesions, MRI may be useful in identifying those at greater risk of progression to myeloma.[23] Vande Berg et al[24] found bone marrow involvement on MRI in 19% of 35 patients with MGUS. None of the 30 patients with a normal MRI study of the central skeleton required treatment after a median follow-up of 30 months, whereas four of seven patients with an abnormal MRI study required treatment within five years from diagnosis. Other investigators did not detect any abnormalities on spinal MRI studies of 24 patients with MGUS.[25] Because the risk of developing myeloma increases with time after the diagnosis of MGUS, longer follow-up periods in large groups of patients with baseline MRI studies may provide more definitive information on the prognostic significance of a positive MRI study.

Indolent myeloma

About 15% of patients with myeloma are asymptomatic and the disease is discovered incidentally during a routine laboratory work-up. These patients who have asymptomatic, low-tumour-burden disease do not receive any treatment until the disease progresses. MRI of the spinal bone marrow in patients with asymptomatic myeloma shows bone marrow involvement in 30–50%.[26–28] Patients with MRI-defined marrow abnormalities have a greater probability of requiring therapy earlier.[28] MRI also permits identification of patients with otherwise indolent disease who have a large vertebral lesion compromising the integrity of the bone – such patients may require intervention for localized disease.

Waldenström's macroglobulinaemia

Waldenström's macroglobulinaemia is a lymphoproliferative disorder that always involves the bone marrow. MRI shows bone marrow abnormalities in all[29] or nearly all[30] patients. MRI patterns of marrow involvement are variegated and diffuse. Absence of focal patterns of marrow involvement correlates with the very low incidence of lytic lesions on conventional skeletal radiographs. On enhanced bone marrow MRI, grades of contrast uptake have been found to correlate with tumour burden. MRI of the bone marrow may be of use as a non-invasive tool for establishing the status of the bone marrow before and after treatment for Waldenström's macroglobulinaemia.

MRI is at least as accurate as CT in detecting enlarged lymph nodes, which may be present in about 40% of patients with Waldenström's macroglobulinaemia. However, because of the cost limitations and availability of MRI, CT remains the imaging modality of choice for the assessment of nodal disease.

PROGNOSTIC SIGNIFICANCE OF MRI IN MYELOMA

Disease progression

A number of studies have tried to define the prognostic significance of abnormal bone marrow MRI appearance study in patients with asymptomatic myeloma. The aim was to identify a group of patients with indolent disease who were at high risk for disease progression and who could perhaps benefit from early institution of chemotherapy. Patients with asymptomatic myeloma were found to develop progressive disease earlier if they had an abnormal MRI study than if they had a normal MRI study.[26,27]

Mariette et al[28] reported that MRI but not bone densitometry findings differed significantly in patients with early disease progression. MRI emerged as an independent prognostic factor, since it identified patients who were at risk for early disease progression irrespective of the presence or absence of other known adverse prognostic factors for myeloma.[27,31] MRI patterns of bone marrow involvement did not differ significantly in the group of patients with indolent disease and early progression. However, there was a trend for patients with diffuse MRI patterns to fare worse than patients with other MRI patterns of bone marrow involvement. In a longitudinal study of 101 patients with asymptomatic myeloma, MRI appearance was not one of the three independent adverse variables (serum myeloma globulin >30 g/l, IgA isotype, and Bence Jones proteinuria >50 mg/day) found to be associated with early progression. However, the presence of an abnormal MRI study in patients with one of the three adverse features helped identify patients who were at risk for imminent complications such as fractures and hypercalcaemia.[32]

Survival

In patients with symptomatic myeloma, MRI patterns of bone marrow involvement were found to correlate with several clinical indices of disease severity. Patients with diffuse patterns were found to have significantly higher bone marrow plasmacytosis and significantly lower haemoglobin values than patients with focal, variegated or normal MRI patterns.[33] Lecouvet et al[34] found significant differences in serum calcium, and β_2-microglobulin values as well, between patients with diffuse and normal or focal MRI patterns. While they reported significantly longer survival for patients with normal MRI patterns than for patients with stage III disease and abnormal MRI patterns, interestingly enough, no difference in survival was seen between patients with diffuse and focal MRI patterns.[34] Kusumoto et al[3] also reported poorer survival among patients with abnormal MRI patterns.

In a review of 90 newly diagnosed patients treated on the Total Therapy program at the University of Arkansas (see Chapter 19), serial MRI surveys of the axial skeleton were obtained at the time of diagnosis and after the second bone marrow transplant. Normalization of previously abnormal marrow appearance, 'complete remission by MR' (MR-CR), was achieved in 40 patients. The post-therapy appearance of the marrow was hyperintense homogeneous on *T1*-weighted images, and hypointense homogeneous on STIR images without focal lesions (Figure 17.6). MR-CR was associated with a superior median survival (65 months or more versus 46 months) in those without MR-CR.[35]

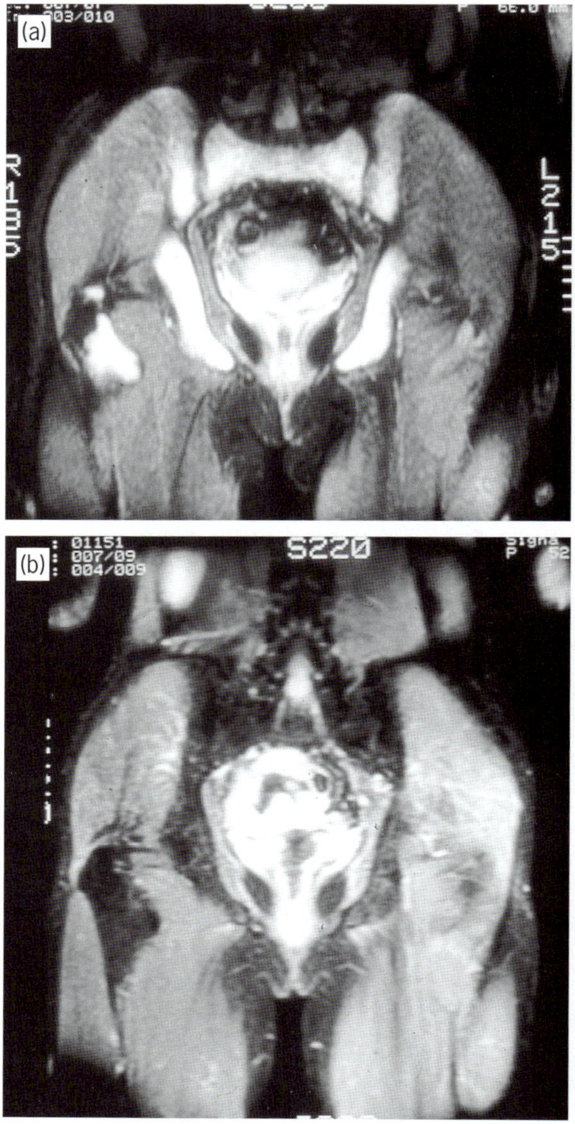

Figure 17.6 Bone marrow changes post treatment. Coronal STIR images pre-treatment (a) and post treatment (b) show the change from a diffusely involved marrow to normal bone marrow signal.

COMPRESSION FRACTURES IN MYELOMA

Development of vertebral compression fractures in myeloma is caused by replacement of the normal bone by a growing tumour mass or by osteoclastic bone resorption. Although several criteria have been proposed to differentiate benign and malignant vertebral compression, these should be applied with caution to patients with myeloma.

Normal signal intensity within a compressed vertebral body on spinal MRI does not preclude the diagnosis of myeloma. In a study of 224 vertebral fractures in patients with known myeloma, Lecouvet et al[36] found that 67% of the fractures appeared benign on MRI, and

38% of the patients had only benign-appearing fractures at diagnosis.[34] In patients with osteoporotic or post-traumatic vertebral compression fractures of recent onset, MRI will usually show inhomogeneous signal alteration that parallels one of the endplates, involves less than half of the vertebral body, does not extend to the pedicles, and enhances homogeneously after the administration of paramagnetic contrast intravenously. Diffusion-weighted MRI has been applied to the differential diagnosis of compression fractures, with promising results.[37]

It is not unusual for myeloma patients to suffer acute back pain during or at the end of chemotherapy. In responding patients, resolution of tumour mass replacing part of the vertebral body and supporting the bony cortex can cause collapse of the vertebra, as can osteopenia. Thirty-five new vertebral compression fractures were discovered on post-treatment MRI of 29 patients with myeloma in remission.[36] On the other hand, progression of the disease may also be responsible for the development of new fractures. In such a setting, MRI may be useful in obtaining information with obvious clinical and therapeutic implications.

In another study, 131 vertebral compression fractures were found to have appeared in 37 myeloma patients after the onset of therapy.[37] Patients with normal marrow appearance or less than 10 focal lesions on pretreatment MRI had a significantly longer median fracture-free interval than did those with 10 or more focal lesions or those with diffuse patterns on pretreatment MRI.[38,39]

MRI-DIRECTED CT-GUIDED BIOPSIES

MRI survey of the axial skeleton enables detection of focal lesions that are not identifiable on plain films, including those not found at the usual sites of iliac crest bone marrow biopsies. At the University of Arkansas, we have performed 87 CT-guided biopsies in 79 patients in whom MRI detected lesions in the spine and pelvis. These biopsies were performed at sites other than the iliac crest biopsies. A 20% increase in the yield of positive cytogenetic information (abnormal karyotypes) was the result.[18]

Lesions persisting on MRI after successful therapy in patients who fulfil other criteria for complete remission (CR) can also be biopsied to see if there is any evidence of active disease present. The prognostic and therapeutic implication of finding active disease in patients who are otherwise in CR are potentially interesting, and need to be studied prospectively.

REFERENCES

1. Salmon SE, Cassady JR. Plasma cell neoplasms. In: *Cancer: Principles and Practice of Oncology*, 5th edn (DeVita VT Jr, Hellman S, Rosenberg SA, eds). Philadelphia: Lippincott-Raven, 1997: 2344–87.
2. Durie BG, Salmon SE. A clinical staging system for multiple myeloma: correlation of measured myeloma cell mass with presenting clinical features, response to treatment and survival. *Cancer* 1975; **36:** 842–54.
3. Kusumoto S, Jinnai I, Itoh K et al. Magnetic resonance imaging patterns in patients with multiple myeloma. *Br J Haematol* 1997; **99:** 649–55.
4. Davies ML, Elson DL, Hertz D, McMillin JM. Syndrome of plasma cell dyscrasia, polyneuropathy, and diabetes mellitus. *West J Med* 1990; **152:** 257–60.
5. Miralles GD, O'Fallon JR, Talley NJ. Plasma cell dyscrasia with polyneuropathy: the spectrum of POEMS syndrome. *N Engl J Med* 1992; **327:** 1919–23.
6. Woolfenden JM, Pitt MJ, Durie BGM, Moon TE. Comparison of bone scintigraphy and radiography in multiple myeloma. *Radiology* 1980; **134:** 723–8.
7. Wahner HW, Kyle RA, Beabout JW. Scintigraphic evaluation of the skeleton in multiple myeloma. *Mayo Clin Proc* 1980; **55:** 739–46.
8. Waxman AD, Siemsen JK, Levine AM et al. Radiographic and radionuclide imaging in multiple myeloma: the role of gallium scintigraphy. *J Nucl Med* 1981; **22:** 232–6.
9. Leonard RCF, Owen JP, Proctor SJ, Hamilton PJ. Multiple myeloma: radiology or bone scanning? *Clin Radiol* 1981; **32:** 291–5.

10. Edwards GK, Santoro J, Taylor A. Use of bone scintigraphy to select patients with multiple myeloma for treatment with strontium-89. *J Nucl Med* 1994; **35:** 1992–3.
11. Nishiyama H, Morand TM, Seiwert VJ. Extensive skeletal involvement detected by gallium-67 citrate in a patient with multiple myeloma. *Clin Nucl Med* 1988; **13:** 179–81.
12. Tirovola EB, Biassoni L, Britton KE et al. The use of ^{99m}Tc-MIBI scanning in multiple myeloma. *Br J Cancer* 1996; **74:** 1815–20.
13. Sasaki M, Ichiya Y, Kuwabara Y et al. Fluorine-18-fluorodeoxyglucose positron emission tomography in technetium-99m-hydroxymethylene-diphosphonate negative bone tumors. *J Nucl Med* 1993; **34:** 288–90.
14. El-Shirbiny AM, Yeung H, Imbriaco M et al. Technetium-99m-MIBI versus fluorine-18-FDG in diffuse multiple myeloma. *J Nucl Med* 1997; **38:** 1208–10.
15. Schreiman JS, McLeod RA, Kyle RA, Beabout JW. Multiple myeloma: evaluation by CT. *Radiology* 1995; **154:** 483–6.
16. Leder DS, Nazarian LN, Burke M. CT of disseminated plasmacytoma in an AIDS patient. *J Comput Assist Tomogr* 1996; **20:** 468–70.
17. Moulopoulos LA, Granfield CA, Dimopoulos MA et al. Extraosseous multiple myeloma: imaging features. *AJR* 1993; **161:** 1083–7.
18. Avva R, Vanhemert RL, Barlogie B, et al. CT-guided biopsy of focal lesions in multiple myeloma patients may reveal new and more aggressive cytogenetic abnormalities. *Am J Neuroradiol* 2001; **22:** 781–8.
19. Ricci C, Cova M, Kang YS et al. Normal age-related patterns of cellular and fatty bone marrow distribution in the axial skeleton: MR imaging study. *Radiology* 1990; **177:** 83–8.
20. Moulopoulos LA, Dimopoulos MA, Weber D et al. Magnetic resonance imaging in the staging of solitary plasmacytoma of bone. *J Clin Oncol* 1993; **11:** 1311–5.
21. Mathieu D, Rahmouni A, Divine M et al. MR imaging of the spine in presumed solitary plasmacytoma. *Radiology* 1993; **189**(Suppl):119 (abst).
22. Liebross RH, Ha CS, Cox JD et al. Solitary bone plasmacytoma: outcome and prognostic factors following radiotherapy. *Int J Radiat Oncol Biol Phys* 1998; **41:** 1063–7.
23. Kyle RA. Monoclonal gammopathies of undetermined significance and solitary plasmacytoma. Implications for progression to overt multiple myeloma. *Hematol Oncol Clin North Am* 1997; **11:** 71–87.
24. Vande Berg BC, Michaux L, Lecouvet FE et al. Nonmyelomatous monoclonal gammopathy: correlation of bone marrow MR images with laboratory findings and spontaneous clinical outcome. *Radiology* 1997; **202:** 247–51.
25. Bellaiche L, Laredo JD, Liote F et al. Magnetic resonance appearance of monoclonal gammopathies of unknown significance and multiple myeloma. *Spine* 1997; **22:** 2551–7.
26. Dimopoulos MA, Moulopoulos LA, Smith T et al. Risk for disease progression in asymptomatic multiple myeloma. *Am J Med* 1993; **94:** 57–61.
27. Vande Berg BC, Lecouvet FE, Michaux L et al. Stage I multiple myeloma: value of MR imaging of the bone marrow in the determination of prognosis. *Radiology* 1996; **201:** 243.
28. Mariette X, Zagdanski AM, Guermazi A et al. Prognostic value of vertebral lesions detected by magnetic resonance imaging in patients with stage I multiple myeloma. *Br J Haematol* 1999; **104:** 723–9.
29. Duhem C, Ries F, Dicato M. Accuracy of magnetic resonance imaging (MRI) of bone marrow in Waldenström's macroglobulinemia (WM) at diagnosis and follow-up. *Blood* 1994; **84**(Suppl 1): 653a (Abst 2598).
30. Moulopoulos LA, Dimopoulos MA, Varma DGK et al. Waldenström macroglobulinemia: MR imaging of the spine and CT of the abdomen and pelvis. *Radiology* 1993; **188:** 669–73.
31. Moulopoulos LA, Dimopoulos MA, Smith TL et al. Prognostic significance of magnetic resonance imaging in patients with asymptomatic myeloma. *J Clin Oncol* 1995; **13:** 251–6.
32. Weber DM, Dimopoulos MA, Moulopoulos LA et al. Prognostic features of asymptomatic multiple myeloma. *Br J Haematol* 1997; **97:** 810–4.
33. Moulopoulos LA, Varma DGK, Dimopoulos MA et al. Multiple myeloma: spinal MR imaging in patients with untreated newly diagnosed disease. *Radiology* 1992; **185:** 833–40.
34. Lecouvet FE, Vande Berg BC, Michaux L et al. Stage III multiple myeloma: clinical and prognostic value of spinal bone marrow MR imaging. *Radiology* 1998; **209:** 653–60.

35. Angtuaco EJ, Avva R, Munshi CN et al. MR skeletal survey of the axial skeleton: a predictor of patient survival in multiple myeloma? *Radiology* 1999; **213**(Suppl): 294 (Abst 845).
36. Lecouvet FE, Vande Berg BC, Maldague BE et al. Vertebral compression fractures in multiple myeloma. Part I. Distribution and appearance at MR imaging. *Radiology* 1997; **204:** 195–9.
37. Baur A, Stabler A, Bruning R et al. Diffusion-weighted MR imaging of bone marrow: differentiation of benign versus pathologic compression fractures. *Radiology* 1998; **207:** 349–56.
38. Moulopoulos LA, Dimopoulos MA, Alexanian R et al. Multiple myeloma: MR patterns of response to treatment. *Radiology* 1994; **193:** 441–6.
39. Lecouvet FE, Malghem J, Michaux L, Michaux JL et al. Vertebral compression fractures in multiple myeloma. Part II. Assessment of fracture risk with MR imaging of the spinal bone marrow. *Radiology* 1997; **204:** 201–5.

Part 4

Therapy

18

Conventional treatment of myeloma

Athanasios Zomas, Meletios A Dimopoulos

INTRODUCTION

Myeloma is a relatively common haematologic malignancy, with an annual incidence in the United States of approximately 13 000 patients. An increasing number of patients are now diagnosed by chance (routine evaluation), and should not be treated unless there is evidence of an imminent complication or demonstration of progressive disease. However, most patients do present with symptoms and signs related to myeloma, and require prompt treatment.

Despite the significant progress achieved over the last 15 years or so, the disease remains incurable with conventional treatment, and the realistic goals of any therapeutic modality are palliation of symptoms and prolongation of life for as long as possible. The treatment of myeloma is directed at management of the complications, in addition to reduction of the malignant plasma cell mass.

High-dose therapy with haematopoietic stem cell transplantation is applicable to a substantial number of myeloma patients. The choice of first-line chemotherapy for individual patients should take into account the possibility of future high-dose therapy so that the treatment chosen does not compromise potential interventions later in the course of the disease.

SUPPORTIVE THERAPY

A number of patients present with painful bone lesions. In cases of mild or moderate pain, analgesics, a corset with plastic stays, and a rolling walker, along with systemic antimyeloma therapy, are usually adequate. Physical activity must be encouraged. Regular administration of bisphosphonates, in addition to preventing progression of skeletal events, may also improve pain control. For severe pain due to a well-defined lytic lesion, a radiotherapy dose of 30 Gy administered over 10 days is very effective. However, in patients who may be candidates for high-dose therapy in the future, the potential detrimental effects of irradiation on subsequent stem cell collection must be considered; especially if the radiation portal is wide. Fractures of the femora or humeri require prompt fixation with an intramedullary rod.

PRIMARY TREATMENT IN PATIENTS WITHOUT THE OPTION OF HIGH-DOSE THERAPY

Chemotherapy with alkylating agents is established initial treatment for symptomatic multiple myeloma in the elderly, in those who have significant medical problems unrelated to the underlying myeloma, or in those who decline or are ineligible for high-dose therapy.

Melphalan–prednisone

Intermittent courses of melphalan and prednisone (MP) have been the standard therapy for patients with myeloma for the last 30 years.[1] Melphalan (phenylalanine mustard) is usually administered at a dose of 8 mg/m^2 daily and prednisone at a dose of 60 mg/m^2 daily by mouth for 4 consecutive days. Melphalan can also be administered orally at a dose of 0.15 g/kg daily for 7 days, and prednisone at a dose of 20 mg three times a day orally for the same 7 days. Melphalan should be given before breakfast because food reduces its absorption by about 50%.[2] A fluid intake of at least 3 l per day along with allopurinol is essential, at least for the first few courses, in order to preserve renal function. If renal failure is present, the initial dose of oral melphalan should be reduced by 25% if significant myelosuppression is to be avoided.

Because gastrointestinal absorption of melphalan is unpredictable, mild cytopenia (neutrophils (1–1.5) $\times 10^9$/l or platelets 100×10^9/l) should be confirmed three weeks after administration of the drug in order to adjust the subsequent dose of melphalan. Stepwise escalation of the melphalan dose by 2–3 mg/m^2 until some haematologic toxicity is observed has been suggested to accomplish optimal drug delivery. Treatment should be repeated at intervals of four to six weeks, and (unless the disease progresses rapidly despite an adequate dose of melphalan) at least three courses of melphalan and prednisone should be given before resistance is confirmed. Melphalan appears to be equally effective when given continuously, but causes more myelosuppression and requires closer patient monitoring as well as frequent dose modification compared with the intermittent schedule.[3,4]

With MP, an objective response may not be obtained for 6–12 months in some patients. On the other hand, significant reduction of monoclonal protein early after commencing therapy (after the first or second course) may be a poor prognostic indicator because high chemosensitivity may reflect a high proliferative activity of myeloma cells with a subsequent early relapse and reduced survival.[5] However, for the minority of cases with a plasma cell labelling index (LI) of 1 or less, such a prompt response probably reflects the inherent chemosensitivity of the neoplastic clone.[5]

The MP regimen produces objective response, defined by at least 50% reduction of serum or urine myeloma protein and of bone marrow plasmatocytosis without evidence of new bone lesions, in 50–60% of patients. Lack of response was once attributed predominantly to lower melphalan levels as a result of poor drug absorption. However, a study showing equal response rates for the intravenous and oral melphalan formulations suggested that resistance of the malignant cells to chemotherapy is primarily responsible for the lack of clinical improvement.[6] Complete remission (CR), which requires disappearance of serum and urine monoclonal protein on immunofixation and a normal bone marrow biopsy, occurs in less than 5% of patients with MP. The median duration of response is about two years, and the median survival on this therapy approximately three years. Five percent of patients are alive after 10 years of treatment. It is possible that current survival rates may be better as a result of enhanced supportive care and the availability of more effective salvage regimens. It is worthwhile mentioning that before the introduction of melphalan in the 1950s, a mean survival of 7.1 months from diagnosis was reported.[7]

The relative importance of the two active agents in the MP regimen has been frequently debated. In Alexanian's original study,[1] the oral combination produced an objective response rate of 70% and a median survival of 24 months, while intermittent melphalan alone achieved a response rate of only 35% and a median survival of 18 months. The UK Medical Research Council (MRC) Myelomatosis Trial II could show no significant survival differences between oral melphalan alone versus MP.[8] In contrast, a more recent US National Cancer Institute (NCI) analysis has clearly shown the usefulness of steroids by correlating survival with prednisone dose intensity and not with the total melphalan dose.[9] In general, corticosteroids are widely accepted as an important part of primary treatment of myeloma, since a large body of both in vitro and in vivo evidence demonstrates high activity of steroids in plasma cells, with concomitant sparing of normal haematopoietic elements. They may increase the speed of response without added myelosuppression while improving the well-being of patients. Caution must be exercised in older individuals, who are at risk for infectious or gastrointestinal complications.

Other combination chemotherapy

Combination chemotherapy in myeloma was introduced in the early 1970s, a time when multidrug regimens became increasingly popular in haematologic and solid tumours on the basis of the Goldie–Coldman hypothesis.[10] Experimental observations on mouse and human plasmacytoma models as well as data from limited phase I/II clinical trials suggested that melphalan, cyclophosphamide, nitrosoureas, corticosteroids, anthracyclines, epipodophyllotoxins, interferon-α (IFN-α), and vincristine had activity in myeloma individually. Therefore, their combined use was a logical step towards the accomplishment of higher remission rates, lower resistance, and ultimately, prolongation of survival. In addition, perhaps uniquely amongst B-cell neoplasms, it was shown that resistance to one alkylating agent in myeloma did not preclude response to another with a similar mechanism of action.[11,12] This allowed for the design of regimens containing non-cross-resistant alkylating compound combinations administered concurrently, sequentially or alternatively. Table 18.1 shows some widely utilized multidrug regimens.

The combination of vincristine, carmustine (BCNU), melphalan, cyclophosphamide, and prednisone (VBMCP) has induced objective responses in approximately 70% of patients, but the median duration of survival is not significantly different from that obtained with MP.[13] The VMCP/VBAP alternating chemotherapy has been prospectively compared with melphalan and prednisone. Although the Southwest Oncology Group (SWOG) reported a response and a survival advantage for the alternating combination,[14] other randomized studies failed to confirm these data.[15,16] The MRC compared the combination of doxorubicin (Adriamycin), carmustine, cyclophosphamide, and melphalan (ABCM) with melphalan alone, and concluded that the combination was associated with a longer survival.[17] However, most investigators feel that melphalan alone was a suboptimal standard arm, even though the British group had observed no survival disadvantage with omission of steroids from the MP regimen in an earlier study.[8] A cross-trial comparison of VMCP/VBAP and ABCM suggested that these treatment schedules produce equivalent results.[18]

Melphalan–prednisone or combination chemotherapy?

Three decades later, the anticipated benefits of combination chemotherapy have not materialized, putting in doubt not only the theoretical considerations discussed above but also the value of the whole therapeutic approach in an era of tightly managed healthcare with finite resources. A recent overview by the Myeloma Trialist's Collaborative Group, which included data on 6623 patients entered in a total of 27 trials worldwide, declared MP and combination therapy to be of comparable effectiveness.[19] This report corroborated the results of an earlier meta-analysis of 18 clinical trials, which suggested that there was no survival difference between the two approaches, either overall or within any patient subgroup.[20] More importantly, both of the publications failed to confirm the long-held impression that multiagent chemotherapy conferred a survival advantage

Table 18.1 Combination chemotherapy schedules in myeloma

Regimen	Drugs	Schedule
VBMCP (M2)	Vincristine 0.03 mg/kg i.v., day 1 Carmustine (BCNU) 1 mg/kg i.v., day 1 Melphalan 0.1 mg/kg p.o., days 1–7 Cyclophosphamide 1 mg/kg i.v., day 1 Prednisone 1 mg/kg p.o., days 1–7	q 28 days
VMCP/ VBAP	Vincristine 1 mg/m^2 i.v., day 1 Melphalan 6 mg/m^2 p.o., days 1–4 Cyclophosphamide 100 mg/m^2 p.o., days 1–4 Prednisone 60 mg/m^2 p.o., days 1–4 *Alternating with* Vincristine 1 mg/m^2 i.v., day 1 Carmustine 30 mg/m^2 i.v., day 1 Doxorubicin (Adriamycin) 30 mg/m^2 i.v., day 1 Prednisone 60 mg/m^2 p.o., days 1–4	q 28 days
ABCM	Doxorubicin 30 mg/m^2 i.v., day 1 Carmustine 30 mg/m^2 i.v., day 1 Cyclophosphamide 100 mg/m^2 p.o., days 22–25 Melphalan 6 mg/m^2 p.o., days 22–25	q 5–6 weeks
MOCCA	Vincristine (Oncovin) 0.03 mg/kg i.v., day 1 Methylprednisolone 0.8 mg/kg p.o., days 1–7 Lomustine (CCNU) 40 mg p.o., day 1 Cyclophosphamide 10 mg/kg i.v., day 1 Melphalan 0.25 mg/kg p.o., days 1–4	q 35 days
EDAP	Etoposide 100 mg/m^2/day 24 h infusion, days 1–4 Dexamethasone 40 mg/day i.v./p.o., days 1–4 Cytarabine (cytosine arabinoside) 1 g/m^2 i.v., day 5 Cisplatin 25 mg/m^2/day 24 h infusion, days 1–4	q 28 days

in poor-risk patients, even though this may hold true for anthracycline-containing regimens. Gregory et al[20] also noted the variance in survival in the MP control groups (48–87%), and pointed out that an improved outcome for combination therapy was observed in studies characterized by a worse-than-expected survival in the MP arm. The reason for the inability of combination chemotherapy to translate better remissions to a survival benefit could be either that this benefit is small and becomes apparent only after long follow-up, or that the effect of continuation therapy, in the form of salvage treatment or maintenance, on the endpoint of overall survival is more important than expected and difficult to calculate.

Infusional chemotherapy

The last significant development in the evolution of myeloma chemotherapy schedules was infusional chemotherapy, aimed at targeting the slowly proliferating plasma cells. The MD Anderson group in Houston devised the VAD regimen in the early 1980s. This incorporates vincristine at 0.4 mg/day and doxorubicin at 9 mg/m^2/day, administered by continuous intravenous infusion for 4 days with oral or intravenous dexamethasone at 20 mg/m^2/day for 12 days (days 1–4, 9–12, and 17–20), every 35 days.

This regimen is often active not only in patients resistant to alkylating agents but also in a proportion of those previously failing non-infusional anthracycline–vincristine combinations. The reported response rate in chemotherapy-naive myeloma patients is approximately 60–80%, but with no obvious survival benefit when compared with standard alkylating agent-based therapies.[21–23] Still, it is important to note that 10–15% of untreated patients achieve CR.[21,22] Because the halving-time of the monoclonal protein is faster with VAD than with other regimens lacking high-dose steroids, the VAD regimen may be preferable for patients in whom rapid tumour control is desirable such as those with hypercalcaemia, renal failure, or widespread painful bone lesions. VAD produces much less myelosuppression than alkylating agent combinations, and may be conveniently applied in cases presenting with neutropenia or thrombocytopenia secondary to bone marrow infiltration. VAD is especially useful in patients with renal failure, because none of its components is excreted renally, and thus dose adjustments are not necessary. The occasional patient who presents with plasma cell leukaemia should also be treated with VAD, because standard alkylating agents are ineffective.[24]

No more than three courses of VAD are usually needed in order to confirm response or resistance to this regimen.[22] The major drawbacks of this regimen are the side-effects associated with the administration of high-dose steroids and the need for a central intravenous access. Hospitalization is unnecessary with the use of ambulatory continuous-infusion pumps attached to a central venous catheter. Nevertheless, special training of patients and nursing staff is required to safely care for catheters and pumps. In order to avoid the inconvenience of the continuous four-day infusion, VAD has also been used as a four-day outpatient schedule using intravenous bolus infusions, with responses in 67% of patients.[25] Several other modified versions of VAD have been explored in an attempt to simplify its administration or reduce toxicity (Table 18.2).

High-dose intermittent oral dexamethasone ('pulse dexamethasone') is also active as primary therapy in myeloma, with response and survival rates that are similar to those achieved with other standard regimens.[26] Because dexamethasone is not associated with myelosuppression, this agent is indicated when radiotherapy is needed for the treatment of painful bone lesions. Dexamethasone may be the primary treatment of choice in the occasional patient who presents with pancytopenia.

The role of IFN-α

The addition of IFN-α to standard chemotherapy has been considered because this agent has some activity (15%) in previously untreated patients and because it may have a different mechanism of action from classical chemotherapeutic agents.[27] The combination of VBMCP and IFN-α was associated with a modest increase in CR rates.[28] However, in three large prospective studies, the addition of IFN-α to MP[29,30] or to VBMCP[31] did not show any survival advantage when compared with MP or VBMCP alone. The comparison of an IFN-α–dexamethasone combination with dexamethasone alone in previously untreated patients indicated similar response rate and survival.[32] Moreover, the addition of interferon to VAD did not improve the response and survival rates.[33]

While a variety of opposing arguments are put forward to explain the conflicting results,

Table 18.2 The VAD regimen and its modifications

Regimen	Drugs
VAD	Vincristine 0.4 mg/day 24 h infusion, days 1–4 Doxorubicin (Adriamycin) 9 mg/m^2/day 24 h infusion, days 1–4 Dexamethasone 40 mg/day i.v./p.o., days 1–4, 9–12, 17–20 (35–day cycle)
VAMP	Vincristine 0.4 mg/day 24 h infusion, days 1–4 Doxorubicin 9 mg/m^2/day 24 h infusion, days 1–4 Methylprednisolone 1 g i.v./p.o., days 1–5
C-VAMP	Cyclophosphamide 500 mg i.v., days 1,8,15 Vincristine 0.4 mg/day 24 h infusion, days 1–4 Doxorubicin 9 mg/m^2/day 24 h infusion, days 1–4 Methylprednisolone 1 g i.v./p.o., days 1–5
DVD	Liposomal doxorubicin (Doxil) 40 mg/m^2 i.v., day 1 Vincristine 2 mg i.v., day 1 Dexamethasone 40 mg/day i.v./p.o., days 1–4
Z-Dex	Idarubicin (Zavedos) 10 mg/m^2/day p.o., days 1–4 Dexamethasone 40 mg/day i.v./p.o., days 1–4
MOD	Mitoxantrone 9 mg/m^2/day 24–h infusion, days 1–4 Vincristine (Oncovin) 0.4 mg/day 24 h infusion, days 1–4 Dexamethasone 40 mg/day i.v./p.o., days 1–4, 9–12, 17–20 (35–day cycle)

recently a Swedish group offered an interesting explanation based on a pharmacokinetic study of cyclophosphamide in patients receiving concomitant IFN-α. These investigators showed that the timing of IFN-α administration within the multidrug schedule influences the clearance rate, half-life, and peak level of the alkylating agent, affecting the drug's activity on myeloma cells and its toxicity profile on haematopoiesis.[34] An overview of data on 2469 patients included in 12 trials evaluating the addition of IFN-α to chemotherapy against a control chemotherapy arm revealed a 6% higher response rate and a six–month prolongation of the recurrence-free interval for the IFN-α-containing induction regimens.[35] Thus, compelling data supporting the addition of IFN-α to standard alkylating agent regimens are lacking. The minor, if any, benefits should be weighed against possible bone marrow or systemic toxicities and the cost. The role of interferons in treatment of myeloma is discussed further in Chapter 22.

How long should the chemotherapy be continued?

Chemotherapy should generally be continued until the patient achieves a plateau phase which is defined by stable serum and urine monoclonal protein levels for at least four to six months and no evidence of progressive disease or symptoms. In such patients chemotherapy should be discontinued because there is no evidence that maintenance chemotherapy prolongs patient survival.[36] In contrast, continued chemotherapy with alkylating agents and/or nitrosoureas may be associated with a higher frequency of myelodysplastic syndrome or acute leukaemia.[37,38] Likewise, the administration of systemic radiotherapy using double hemibody irradiation as a consolidation treatment does not prolong survival.[39]

During the plateau phase, the patient should be followed every three to four months with a physical examination, blood counts, renal function tests, and calcium, along with serum and urine electrophoretic studies. Evaluation of bone marrow and bones should also be performed wherever indicated. It should be remembered that relapse can occur with increased size and/or number of bone lesions without a corresponding increase in monoclonal protein.

PRIMARY THERAPY IN PATIENTS WITH THE OPTION OF HAEMATOPOIETIC STEM CELL TRANSPLANTATION

High-dose therapy and autologous haematopoietic stem cell transplantation (HSCT) is beneficial for many patients with myeloma. This procedure is suitable for patients younger than 70 years without significant comorbid conditions, and selected older patients. Patients who are potential candidates for high-dose therapy during some phase of their disease should not be exposed to standard melphalan-containing combinations, in order to avoid damage to haematopoietic stem cells.[40] Patients who have received standard treatment for less than one year and/or a total melphalan dose of less than 200 mg/m^2 retain a good chance of mobilizing sufficient numbers of stem cells.[41] Radiotherapy also reduces the stem cell yield, and it should be restricted to patients with an absolute indication, such as spinal cord compression.

Since a rapid response is desirable, primary therapy with VAD is a reasonable option, because it causes less damage to bone marrow progenitor cells. The UK Royal Marsden Hospital group has reported that adding weekly cyclophosphamide to the VAMP (vincristine, doxorubicin, methylprednisolone) regimen enhances responses in previously untreated patients without affecting cumulative toxicity or compromising subsequent stem cell collection.[42]

In general, collection and cryopreservation of blood stem cells should be initiated as soon as the best possible response is confirmed. In some studies, the sequential administration of VAD followed by high-dose cyclophosphamide and consolidated by the combination of etoposide, dexamethasone, cytarabine (cytosine arabinoside), and cisplatin, has increased the CR rate and has allowed the collection of adequate number of blood stem cells to support two autologous transplants.[43] Other data suggest that age more than 65 years and renal compromise are not important adverse parameters affecting the outcome of high-dose therapy and autotransplantation.[44,45] Consequently, the number of patients in whom initial therapy will have to be selected carefully because of the future possibility of high-dose therapy continues to increase. High-dose therapy with antilogons HSCT is discussed in detail in Chapter 19.

TREATMENT OF REFRACTORY MYELOMA

In order to select a second-line treatment for a patient with myeloma, the phase of the disease should be clearly defined. Primary refractory myeloma is disease not responding to adequate primary treatment. A proportion of patients with primary refractory disease exhibit 'stable' disease features without significant symptoms (non-progressors). When such patients are over 70 years of age, they are best left untreated until clear progression is confirmed. In younger patients without comorbid conditions, high-dose therapy can result in meaningful responses in 70% of cases, with a significant survival benefit.[46] Some patients have rapidly evolving myeloma whilst on induction therapy. Refractory relapse is disease that had initially responded to primary therapy, but is progressing after relapse despite administration of previously effective treatment. Finally, some patients relapse from an unmaintained response or from IFN-α maintenance.

Disease relapsing off treatment has a 50% chance of responding again to the original treatment. MP is effective in approximately 30% of patients who relapse while maintained on IFN-α.[32] For patients with disease that is primary refractory to standard alkylating agents, VAD or high-dose steroids (pulsed oral dexamethasone or intravenous methylprednisolone) can induce responses in about one-third.[47–49] A simple treatment consisting of weekly cyclophosphamide at a dose of 200–300 mg/m^2 together with alternate-day prednisone 50–100 mg can produce sustained remissions in a subgroup of patients relapsing after or resistant to melphalan.[50] This regimen combines excellent tolerability with convenience, and is particularly appealing in frail and elderly individuals unwilling or unable to receive more complex schedules.

Patients in refractory relapse are more likely to benefit from VAD, which induces responses in 40–50% with a median response duration of about one year.[47,51] The addition of IFN-α to VAD is not associated with an improved outcome.[52] The greater efficacy of VAD than dexamethasone among relapsing patients has been attributed to the greater sensitivity of proliferating tumour cells to the cell-cycle-active drugs vincristine and doxorubicin. The International Oncology Study Group tested the CEVAD combination comprising a 96-hour infusion of etoposide at a dose of 50 mg/m^2/day and bolus cyclophosphamide 1000 mg/m^2 in addition to conventional VAD plus growth factor support.[53] Despite producing responses in 40% of primary refractory cases and nearly 30% in those previously failing VAD, CEVAD was comparable to VAD in terms of overall response and survival.

The combination of bolus intravenous administration of vincristine, carmustine, and doxorubicin with oral prednisone (VBAP, Table 18.1) has been effective in 30% of patients.[54] The Finnish Leukaemia Group explored the M2 variant MOCCA (Table 18.1), which resulted in a response rate of 90% in patients relapsing off therapy and 34% in those relapsing on maintenance chemotherapy.[55] In general, patients with primary refractory myeloma tend to have lower response rates than refractory relapsed patients with all types of conventional salvage treatments, but responses may be more durable in the former group.

For patients who fail to respond to or relapse after VAD or high-dose corticosteroid therapy, non-myeloablative options are rather limited. Attempts to reverse the expression of the multidrug-resistance (MDR) gene initially focused on the addition of high-dose verapamil to VAD. This impractical regimen, which necessitates close cardiac monitoring, appeared effective for a short period in about 20% of patients with VAD-resistant myeloma.[56] A randomized trial of VAD versus VAD plus oral verapamil in alkylating agent-resistant multiple myeloma, reported similar response and survival rates.[57] Initial reports of the role of cyclosporine as an agent with clinically evident inhibition of MDR indicated that the VAD–cyclosporine combination induced responses in 40% of VAD-resistant patients.[58] A lower response rate and higher toxicity were subsequently reported.[59] Cyclosporine combined with VAD was prospectively compared with VAD in patients who were refractory or relapsing after treatment with alkylating agents. The objective response rate, median time to progression, and median survival were similar in both arms.[60] A non-immunosuppressive and non-nephrotoxic analogue of cyclosporine, PSC 833, is being investigated in an attempt to develop a less toxic and more active inhibitor of MDR. An early report of a phase II study of PSC 833 combined with VAD showed some responses in cases resistant to VAD alone.[61]

Etoposide-based regimens combining standard or escalated doses of etoposide with alkylating agents and other antineoplastics such as cytarabine or cisplatin are also frequently employed in VAD-resistant or relapsed patients. The infusional regimen EDAP, comprising etoposide, dexamethasone, cisplatin, and cytarabine, can effect responses in some VAD-resistant cases[62]. The combination of dexamethasone, cyclophosphamide, etoposide, and cisplatin (DCEP) resulted in 10% complete and 41% partial remissions among patients relapsing after autologous transplantation, but has not been properly evaluated in cohorts of patients unresponsive to conventional chemotherapy.[63] An intensified five-day schedule with etoposide, cyclophosphamide, and granulocyte–macrophage colony-stimulating factor (GM-CSF) support salvaged 42% of VAD-resistant cases, with a median remission time of eight months.[64] Patients with elevated lactate dehydrogenase (LDH) and β_2-microglobulin levels are less likely to benefit from this salvage modality. Additional high-dose alkylating programmes without stem cell support have shown respectable activity in patients with VAD-refractory myeloma. High-dose melphalan at a dose of up to 100 mg/m^2 appeared active in about one-third of patients at the expense of a 15% treatment-related mortality ratio.[65] The addition of growth factor support was able to reduce the toxic death rate.[66] Other combinations, such as high-dose cyclophosphamide–prednisone[67] or hyperfractionated cyclophosphamide plus VAD,[68] have been administered in the context of phase II studies. No more than one-third of patients seem to benefit for periods of approximately six months. The results shown by these phase II studies are likely to be difficult to reproduce, because of differences in assessing resistance to previous treatments and because of patient selection bias.

Over the last 10 years or so, several new agents have been administered to patients with myeloma. Among the most promising of these, thalidomide exerts its antimyeloma action by inhibiting angiogenesis (Chapter 8) and by modulating the synthesis of plasma cell-stimulating molecules from the bone marrow microenvironment.[69] A non-randomized single-centre study reported recently that oral thalidomide achieved 35% responses in an unfavourable group of pretreated patients, many of whom had been previously transplanted.[70] The negligible haematologic toxicity and ease of administration of this compound make it an attractive solution for multiresistant cases or those with compromised bone marrow function. Preliminary results suggest that thalidomide and steroids have a synergistic effect.[71] A pilot trial combining thalidomide with dexamethasone and four-day infusions of cisplatin, doxopubicin, cyclophosphamide, and etoposide (DT-PACE) displayed a greater than 50% resolution of myeloma activity in 68% of previously treated patients.[72] A small single-centre randomized study showing a dampening of stem cell mobilization in newly diagnosed patients suggests that this aspect of thalidomide therapy should be investigated further.[73]

All-*trans*-retinoic acid (ATRA) inhibits the growth of some human myeloma cell lines through downregulation of the interleukin-6 (IL-6) receptor. However, phase II trials both in refractory and in previously untreated patients showed no clinical activity of this agent.[74,75] The role of ATRA as a chemosensitizer along with standard chemotherapy is currently being assessed.[76]

Both organic and inorganic arsenic compounds have been found to induce apoptosis in human myeloma cell lines and freshly isolated plasma cells from resistant cases, providing the rationale for clinical use.[77,78]

The purine analogues fludarabine, pentostatin (deoxycoformycin), and cladribine (2-chlorodeoxyadenosine) have been administered to patients with previously treated myeloma, with disappointing results.[79,80,81] Paclitaxel has been evaluated both in previously treated and in newly diagnosed patients with myeloma. Despite significant haematologic toxicity, the activity of this agent was limited.[82] Of 17 patients with refractory myeloma, 2 had an objective tumour reduction after treatment with IL-2.[83]

Vinorelbine, a novel vinca alkaloid, has been administered to pretreated myeloma patients, with a 15% response rate.[84] In a phase II European study of patients with at least one line of prior treatment, vinorelbine and dexamethasone pulses produced a 77% response rate.[85]

Topotecan, a camptothecin analogue inhibiting topoisomerase I, was administered at a daily dose of 1.25 mg/m^2 over five consecutive days, with growth factor support, to relapsed or resistant myeloma patients. While myelosuppression emerged as the major toxicity, the response rate was just 16%.[86]

Idarubicin is a new anthracycline, which can be administered orally and has a long-acting metabolite, idarubicinol. Its use in patients with advanced myeloma was associated with activity in about 20% of them and in 2 of 14 cases with previous exposure to doxorubicin.[87,88] Oral idarubicin and dexamethasone with or without lomustine (CCNU) have been evaluated as oral replacements for VAD with encouraging results.[89,90]

Gruber et al studied the effect of the pyrimidine antagonist gemcitabine against myeloma cell lines that were resistant to dexamethasone.[91] Gemcitabine was found to induce a significant degree of apoptosis in all the cell lines studied at clinically attainable and tolerable concentrations, suggesting that it may have a role in salvage strategies.

The success of the anti-CD20 monoclonal antibody rituximab in lymphomas and the expression of CD20 antigen by a subpopulation of myeloma cells has prompted several investigators to use rituximab in myeloma.[92] Minor responses have been seen in a limited number of patients.[92] Interestingly, interferons were found to upregulate the expression of the CD20 molecule on malignant cells.[93]

Bisphosphonates are potent inhibitors of bone resorption and have been successfully applied in the treatment of hypercalcaemia and the prevention of skeletal complications of myeloma (Chapter 7). Second- and third-generation biphosphonates have also been shown to affect myeloma growth both directly and indirectly. A randomized study of long-term pamidronate infusions suggested a modest survival benefit for those on salvage therapy and pamidronate.[94] In addition to inducing apoptosis of myeloma cells, these agents appear to stimulate $\gamma\delta$ T cells with recognizable activity against plasma cells.[95] Occasional responses in the form of reduction of marrow plasmacytocis and/or immunoglobulin levels have been recorded with single-agent pamidronate.[96] Novel and more potent bisphosphonates are entering clinical trials, and are expected to produce more powerful inhibition of myeloma, alone or in conjunction with other biological agents or chemotherapy.

The role of radiotherapy

This is dealt with in detail in Chapter 21. Systemic radiotherapy in the form of hemibody or double-hemibody irradiation was frequently used in the past for relapsed or refractory myeloma patients, especially to those with severe bone disease. Bergsagel[97] originally suggested that the relatively prolonged doubling time of myeloma cells might permit a high logarithmic tumour cell kill with a clinically attainable radiation dose. With the advent of chemotherapy intensification and more effective means of controlling or preventing osteolytic lesions, the role of non-local radiotherapy has now become limited. However, the use of growth factors and radioprotectant agents could alleviate many of the side-effects of hemibody irradiation, and therefore this procedure could still offer marked symptomatic relief in selected multiresistant cases with generalized bone pain, on the basis that chemoresistance is usually dissociated from radiation resistance.[98]

REFERENCES

1. Alexanian R, Haut A, Khan AU et al. Treatment for multiple myeloma: combination chemotherapy with different melphalan dose regimens. *JAMA* 1969; **208:** 1680–5.
2. Alberts DS, Chang SY, Chen HS et al. Oral melphalan kinetics. *Clin Pharmacol Ther* 1979; **26:** 737–45.
3. Alexanian R, Bergsagel DE, Migliore PJ et al. Melphalan therapy for plasma cell myeloma. *Blood* 1968; **31:** 1–10.
4. McArthur JR, Athens JW, Wintrobe MM, Cartwright GE. Melphalan and myeloma. Experience with a low-dose continuous regimen. *Ann Intern Med* 1970; **72:** 665–70.
5. Boccadoro M, Marmont F, Tribalto M et al. Early responder myeloma: kinetic studies identify a patient subgroup characterized by a very poor prognosis. *J Clin Oncol* 1989; **7:** 119–25.
6. Osterborg A, Ahre A, Bjorkholm M et al. Oral versus intravenous melphalan and prednisone treatment in multiple myeoma stage II. A randomised study from the Myeloma Group of Central Sweden. *Acta Oncologica* 1990; **29:** 272.

7. Osgood EE. The survival time of patients with plasmacytic myeloma. *Cancer Chemother Rep* 1960; **9:** 1–10.
8. MRC Working Party on Leukemia in Adults. Report on the second myelomatosis trial after 5 years of follow-up. *Br J Cancer* 1980; **42:** 813–22.
9. Palmer M, Belch A, Hanson J. Dose intensity analysis of melphalan and prednisone in multiple myeloma. *J Natl Cancer Inst* 1988; **80:** 414.
10. Goldie JH, Coldman AJ, Gudauskas GA. Rationale for the use of alternating non-cross-resistant chemotherapy. *Cancer Treat Rep* 1982; **66:** 439.
11. Bergsagel DE, Ogawa M, Librach SL. Mouse myeloma: a model for studies of cell kinetics. *Arch Intern Med* 1975; **135:** 109–17.
12. Bergsagel DE, Cowan DH, Hasselback R. Plasma cell myeloma: response of melphalan resistant patients to high dose intermittent cyclophosphamide. *Can Med Assoc J* 1972; **107:** 851–5.
13. Oken MM, Harrington DP, Abramson N et al. Comparison of melphalan and prednisone with vincristine, carmustine, melphalan, cyclophosphamide, and prednisone in the treatment of multiple myeloma. Results of Eastern Cooperative Oncology Group study E 2479. *Cancer* 1997; **79:** 1561–7.
14. Salmon SE, Haut A, Bonnet JD et al. Alternating combination chemotherapy and levamisole improves survival in multiple myeloma: a Southwest Oncology Group study. *J Clin Oncol* 1983; **1:** 453–61.
15. Cooper MR, McIntyre OR, Propert KJ et al. Single, sequential and multiple alkylating agent therapy for multiple myeloma: a CALGB study. *J Clin Oncol* 1986; **4:** 1331–9.
16. Boccadoro M, Marmont F, Tribalto M et al. Multiple myeloma: VMPC/VBAP alternating combination chemotherapy is not superior to melphalan and prednisone even in high-risk patients. *J Clin Oncol* 1991; **9:** 444–8.
17. MacLennan IC, Chapman C, Dunn J et al. Combined chemotherapy with ABCM versus melphalan for treatment of myelomatosis. *Lancet* 1992; **339:** 200–5.
18. Kelly K, Durie B, MacLennan ICM. Prognostic factors and staging system for multiple myeloma: comparisons between the MRC studies in the United Kingdom and the Southwest Oncology Group studies in the United States. *Hematol Oncol* 1988; **6:** 131–40.
19. Myeloma Trialists' Collaborative Group. Combination chemotherapy versus melphalan plus prednisone as treatment for multiple myeloma: an overview of 6,633 patients from 27 randomized trials. *J Clin Oncol* 1998; **16:** 3832–42.
20. Gregory WM, Richards MA, Malpas JS. Combination chemotherapy versus melphalan and prednisolone in the treatment of multiple myeloma: an overview of published trials. *J Clin Oncol* 1992; **10:** 334–42.
21. Samson D, Gaminara E, Newland A et al. Infusion of vincristine and doxorubicin with oral dexamethasone as first-line therapy for multiple myeloma. *Lancet* 1989; **ii:** 882–5.
22. Alexanian R, Barlogie B, Tucker S. VAD-based regimens as primary treatment for multiple myeloma. *Am J Hematol* 1990; **33:** 86–9.
23. Monconduit M, Menard JF, Michaux JL et al. VAD or VMBCP in severe multiple myeloma: the Groupe d' Etudes et de Recherche sur le Myelome (GERM). *Br J Haematol* 1992; **80:** 199–204.
24. Dimopoulos MA, Palumbo A, Delasalle KB, Alexanian R. Primary plasma cell leukemia. *Br J Haematol* 1994; **88:** 754–59.
25. Segeren CM, Sonneveld P, van der Holt B et al. Vincristine, doxorubicin and dexamethasone (VAD) administered as rapid intravenous infusion for first-line treatment in untreated multiple myeloma. *Br J Haematol* 1999; **105:** 127–30.
26. Alexanian R, Dimopoulos MA, Dellasalle K, Barlogie B. Primary dexamethasone treatment of multiple myeloma. *Blood* 1992; **80:** 887–90.
27. Quesada JR, Alexanian R, Hawkins M et al. Treatment of multiple myeloma with recombinant alpha-interferon. *Blood* 1986; **67:** 275–8.
28. Oken MM, Kyle RA, Greipp PR et al. Complete remission induction with combined VBMCP chemotherapy and interferon in patients with multiple myeloma. *Leuk Lymphoma* 1996; **20:** 447–51.
29. Cooper MR, Dear K, McIntyre OR et al. A randomized clinical trial comparing melphalan/prednisone with or without interferon alfa-2b in newly diagnosed patients with multiple myeloma: a Cancer and Leukemia Group B study. *J Clin Oncol* 1993; **11:** 155–60.
30. Osterborg A, Bjorkholm M, Bjoreman M et al. Natural interferon-α in combination with melphalan/prednisone versus melphalan/prednisone in the treatment of multiple myeloma stages II and III trial. *Blood* 1995; **86**(Suppl 1): 441a.

31. Oken MM, Leong T, Kay NE et al. The effect of adding interferon or high-dose cyclophosphamide to VBMCP to treat multiple myeloma: results from an ECOG phase III trial. *Blood* 1995; **86**(Suppl 1): 441a.
32. Dimopoulos MA, Weber D, Delasalle KB, Alexanian R. Combination therapy with Interferon–dexamethasone for newly diagnosed patients with multiple myeloma. *Cancer* 1993; **72:** 2589–92.
33. Abrahamson GM, Bird JM, Newland AC et al. A randomized study of VAD therapy with either concurrent or maintenance interferon in patients with newly diagnosed multiple myeloma. *Br J Haematol* 1996; **94:** 659–64.
34. Hassan M, Nilsson C, Olsson H et al. The influence of interferon-alpha on the pharmacokinetics of cyclophosphamide and its 4–hydroxy metabolite in patients with multiple myeloma. *Eur J Haematol* 1999; **63:** 163–70.
35. Wheatley K. A meta-analysis of trials of interferon as therapy for myeloma. In: *Abstract Book of the VIIth International Multiple Myeloma Workshop,* 1999: 973.
36. Alexanian R, Gehan E, Haut A et al. Unmaintained remissions in multiple myeloma. *Blood* 1978; **51:** 1005–11.
37. Bersagel DE, Bailey AJ, Langley GR et al. The chemotherapy of plasma-cell myeloma and the incidence of acute leukemia. *N Engl J Med* 1979; **301:** 743–8.
38. Rowley JD, Golomb HM, Vardiman JW. Nonrandom chromosome abnormalities in acute leukemia and dysmyelopoietic syndromes in patients with previously treated malignant disease. *Blood* 1981; **58:** 759–67.
39. Mackenzie MR, Wold H, George C et al. Consolidation hemibody radiotherapy following induction combination chemotherapy in high-tumor burden multiple myeloma. *J Clin Oncol* 1992; **10:** 1769–74.
40. Tricot G, Jagannath S, Vesole D et al. Peripheral blood stem cell transplants for multiple myeloma: identification of favorable variables for rapid engraftment in 225 patients. *Blood* 1995; **85:** 588–96.
41. Vesole DH, Tricot G, Jagannah S et al. Auto-transplants in multiple myeloma: What have we learned? *Blood* 1996; **88:** 838–47.
42. Raje N, Powles R, Kulkarni S et al. A comparison of vincristine and doxorubicin infusional chemotherapy with methylprednisolone (VAMP) with the addition of weekly cyclophosphamide (C-VAMP) as induction treatment followed by autografting in previously untreated myeloma. *Br J Haematol* 1997; **97:** 153–60.
43. Barlogie B Jagannath S, Vesole DH et al. Superiority of tandem autologous transplantation over standard therapy for previously untreated multiple myeloma. *Blood* 1997; **89:** 789–93.
44. Tricot G, Alberts DS, Johnson C et al. Safety of autotransplants with high dose melphalan in renal failure: a pharmacokinetic and toxicity study. *Clin Cancer Res* 1996; **2:** 947–52.
45. Siegel DS, Desikan KR, Mehta J et al. Age is not a prognostic variable with autotransplants for multiple myeloma. *Blood* 1999; **93:** 51–4.
46. Alexanian R, Dimopoulos MA, Hester J et al. Early myeloablative therapy for multiple myeloma. *Blood* 1994; **84:** 4278–82.
47. Barlogie B, Smith L, Alexanian R. Effective treatment of advanced multiple myeloma refractory to alkylating agents. *N Engl J Med* 1984; **310:** 1353–6.
48. Alexanian R, Barlogie B, Dixon D. High-dose glucocorticoid treatment of resistant myeloma. *Ann Intern Med* 1986; **105:** 8–11.
49. Gertz MA, Garton JP, Greip PR et al. A phase II study of high-dose methylprednisolone in refractory or relapsed multiple myeloma. *Leukemia* 1995; **9:** 2115–8.
50. Wilson K, Shelley W, Belch A et al. Weekly cyclophosphamide and alternate-day prednisone: an effective secondary therapy in multiple myeloma. *Cancer Treat Rep* 1987; **71:** 981–2.
51. Lokhorst HM, Menwissen OJ, Bast EJ, Dekker AW. VAD chemotherapy for refractory multiple myeloma. *Br J Haematol* 1989; **71:** 25–30.
52. Alexanian R, Barlogie B, Gutterman J. Alpha-interferon combination therapy of resistant myeloma. *Am J Clin Oncol* 1991; **14:** 188–92.
53. Giles FJ, Wickham NR, Rapoport BL et al. Cyclophosphamide, etoposide, vincristine, Adriamycin, and dexamethasone (CEVAD) regimen in refractory multiple myeloma: an International Oncology Study Group (IOSG) phase II protocol. *Am J Hematol* 2000; **63:** 125–30.
54. Blade J, San Miguel, Sanz MA et al. Treatment of melphalan-resistant multiple myeloma with vincristine, BCNU, doxorubicin and high dose dexamethasone (VBAD). *Eur J Cancer* 1992; **29A:** 57–62.

55. Finnish Leukemia Group. Combination chemotherapy MOCCA in resistant and relapsing multiple myeloma. *Eur J Haematol* 1992; **48:** 37–40.
56. Salmon SE, Dalton WS, Grogan TM et al. Multidrug resistant myeloma: laboratory and clinical effects of verapamil as a chemosensitizer. *Blood* 1991; **78:** 44–50.
57. Dalton WS, Crowley J, Salmon S et al. A phase III randomized study of oral verapamil as a chemosensitizer to reverse drug resistance in patients with refractory myeloma. A Southwest Oncology Group study. *Cancer* 1995; **75:** 815–20.
58. Sonneveld P, Durie BG, Lokhorst HM et al. Modulation of multidrug-resistant multiple myeloma by cyclosporin: the Leukaemia Group of the EORTC and the HOVON. *Lancet* 1992; **340:** 255–9.
59. Weber D, Dimopoulos M, Sinicrope F, Alexanian R. VAD-cyclososporine for VAD–resistant myeloma. *Leuk Lymphoma* 1995; **19:** 159–63.
60. Sonneveld P, Suciu S, Weijermans P et al. Cyclosporin A combined with VAD vs. VAD in patients with refractory multiple myeloma. *Blood* 1997; **90**(Suppl 1): 356a.
61. Case DC, Jain V, Stiff P et al. Phase II studies of PSC 833 (PSC) and VAD chemotherapy in patients with VAD-refractory multiple myeloma (MM). *Blood* 1998; **92**(Suppl 1): 105a.
62. Barlogie B, Velasquez WS, Alexanian R, Cabanillas F. Etoposide, dexamethasone, cytarabine, and cisplatin in vincristine, doxorubicin and dexamethasone-refractory myeloma. *J Clin Oncol* 1989; **7:** 1514–7.
63. Munshi NC, Desikan KR, Jagannath S et al. Dexamethasone, cyclophosphamide, etoposide and *cis*-platinum (DCEP), an effective regimen for relapse after high-dose chemotherapy and autologous transplantation (AT). *Blood* 1996, **88**(Suppl 1): 586a.
64. Dimopoulos MA, Delassalle KB, Champlin R, Alexanian R. Cyclophosphamide and etoposide therapy with GM-CSF for VAD-resistant multiple myeloma. *Br J Haematol* 1993; **83:** 240–4.
65. Barlogie B, Alexanian R, Smallwood L et al. Prognostic factors with high-dose melphalan for refractory multiple myeloma. *Blood* 1988; **72:** 2015–9.
66. Barlogie B, Jagannath S, Dixon DO et al. High-dose melphalan and granulocyte–macrophage colony-stimulating factor for refractory multiple myeloma. *Blood* 1990; **76:** 677–80.
67. Lenhard RE, Daniels MJ, Oken MM et al. An aggressive high dose cyclophosphamide and prednisone regimen for advanced multiple myeloma. *Leuk Lymphoma* 1944; **16:** 589–92.
68. Dimopoulos MA, Weber D, Kantarjian H et al. HyperCVAD for VAD-resistant multiple myeloma. *Am J Hematol* 1996; **52:** 77–81.
69. D'Amato RJ, Loughman MS, Flynn E, Folkman J. Thalidomide is an inhibitor of angiogenesis. *Proc Natl Acad Sci USA* 1994; **91:** 4082–5.
70. Singhal S, Mehta J, Desikan R et al. Antitumor activity of thalidomide in refractory multiple myeloma. *N Engl J Med* 1999; **341:** 1565–71.
71. Weber DM, Gavino M, Delasalle K et al. Thalidomide alone or with dexamethasone for multiple myeloma. *Blood* 1999; **94**(Suppl 1): 604a.
72. Munshi N, Desikan R, Zangari M et al. Chemoangiotherapy with DT-PACE for previously treated multiple Myeloma (MM). *Blood* 1999; **94**(Suppl 1): 123a.
73. Munshi N, Desikan R, Anaissie E et al. Peripheral blood stem cell collection (PBSC) after CAD + G-CSF as part of Total Therapy II in newly diagnosed multiple myeloma (MM): influence of thalidomide (THAL) administration. *Blood* 1999; **94**(Suppl 1): 578a.
74. Siegel D, Niesvizky R, Miller WH et al. All-*trans* retinoic acid (ATRA) and interferon α (IFNα) synergistically inhibit myeloma cell growth and induce retinoic acid receptor α (RARα) expression. *Blood* 1992; **80**(Suppl 1): 12a.
75. Weber DM, Bseiso A, Wood A et al. All-*trans* retinoic acid for multiple myeloma. *Blood* 1997; **90**(Suppl 1): 357a.
76. Koskela K, Pelliniemi TT, Pulkki K et al. Treatment of multiple myeloma with all-*trans* retinoic acid alone and in combination with chemotherapy: a phase I/II trial. In: *Abstract Book of the VIIth International Multiple Myeloma Workshop*, 1999: 140.
77. Munshi N, Desikan R, Zangari M et al. Marked antitumor effect of arsenic trioxide (AS2O3) in high risk refractory multiple myeloma. *Blood* 1999; **94**(Suppl 1): 123a.
78. Pearse R, Bajenova O, Feinman R et al. Arsenic compounds induce apoptosis in multiple myeloma (MM): role of NFκB–RIP pathway. *Blood* 1999; **94**(Suppl 1): 309a.
79. Belch AF, Henderson JF, Brox LW. Treatment of multiple myeloma with deoxycoformycin. *Cancer Chemother Pharmacol* 1985; **14:** 49–52.

80. Lichtman SM, Mittelman A, Budman DR et al. Phase II trial of fludarabine phosphate in multiple myeloma using a loading dose and continuous infusion schedule. *Leuk Lymphoma* 1991; **6:** 61–3.
81. Dimopoulos MA, KantarjianH, Estey EH, Alexanian R. 2-Chlorodeoxyadenosine in the treatment of multiple myeloma. *Blood* 1992; **80:** 1626.
82. Dimopoulos MA, Arbuck S, Huber M et al. Primary therapy of multiple myeloma with paclitaxel. *Ann Oncol* 1994; **5:** 757–9.
83. Peest D, Leo R, Bloche S et al. Low dose recombinant interleukin-2 therapy in advanced multiple myeloma. *Br J Haematol* 1995; **89:** 328–37.
84. Harousseau JL, Maloisel F, Sotto JJ et al. Vinorelbine in patients with recurrent multiple myeloma: a phase II study. *Proc Am Soc Clin Oncol* 1997; **16:** 11a.
85. Dammacco F, San Miguel JF, Attal M et al. Vinorelbine (VRL) plus high dose dexamethasone (DEX) for treatment of relapsing multiple myeloma (MM): a phase II study. *Blood* 1998; **92**(Suppl 1): 319a.
86. Kraut EH, Crowley JJ, Wade JL et al. Evaluation of topotecan in resistant and ralapsing multiple myeloma: a Southewest Oncology Group Study. *J Clin Oncol* 1998; **16:** 589–92.
87. Chisesi T, Capnist G, De Dominicis E, Dini E. A phase II study of idarubicin (4-demethoxydaunorubicin) in advanced myeloma. *Eur J Cancer Clin Oncol* 1988; **24:** 681–4.
88. Sumpter K, Powles R. Raje N et al. Oral idarubicin as single agent therapy for patients with relapased multiple myeloma. *Blood* 1997; **90** (Suppl 1): 310b.
89. Cook G, Sharp RA, Tansey P, Franklin IM. A phase I/II trial of Z-Dex (oral idarubicin and dexamethasone) an oral equivalent of VAD, as initial therapy at diagnosis or progression in multiple myeloma. *Br J Haematol* 1996; **93:** 931–4.
90. Gupta d, Kelsey SM, Littlewood TJ, et al. Oral idarubicin with CCNU and dexamethasone for relapsed myeloma – an effective oral regimen with minimal toxicity. *Br J Haematol* 1996; **93:** 313.
91. Gruber J, Geisen F, Sgonc R et al. 2′,2′-Difluorodeoxycytidine (gemcitabine) induces apoptosis in myeloma cell lines resistant to steroids and 2-chlorodeoxyadenosine (2-CdA). *Stem Cells* 1996; **14:** 351–62.
92. Treon SP, Grossbard ML, Doss DS et al. Phase II study of rituximab in previously treated patients with multiple myeloma (MM): progress report. *Blood* 1999; **94**(Suppl 1): 312a–13a.
93. Treon SP, Shima Y, Raje N et al. Interferon-γ induces CD20 expression on multiple myeloma cells via induction of Pu.1 and augments rituximab binding to myeloma cells. *Blood* 1999; **94**(Suppl 1): 119a.
94. Berenson JR, Lightenstein A, Porter L et al. Long-term pamidronate treatment of advanced multiple myeloma patients reduces skeletal events. *J Clin Oncol* 1998; **16:** 593–602.
95. Kunzmann V, Bauer E, Feurle J et al. Stimulation of T-cells by aminobisphosphonates and induction of antiplasma cell activity in multiple myeloma. *Blood* 2000; **96:** 384–92.
96. Dhodapkar MV, Singh J, Mehta J et al. Anti-myeloma activity of pamidronate in vivo. *Br J Haematol* 1998; **103:** 530–2.
97. Bergsagel DE. Total body irradiation for myelomatosis. *BMJ* 1971; **2:** 325.
98. McSweeney EN, Tobias JS, Blackman G et al. Double hemibody irradiation (DHBI) in the management of relapsed and primary chemoresistant multiple myeloma. *J Clin Oncol* 1993; **5:** 378–83.

19

High-dose therapy and autologous transplantation

Seema Singhal

INTRODUCTION

Response rates with conventional chemotherapy are low in myeloma.[1,2] The attainment of sustained remission with high-dose therapy and syngeneic bone marrow transplantation (BMT) showed that there was a dose–response relationship in myeloma.[3] Later, McElwain and Powles [4] demonstrated the profound activity of high-dose melphalan in myeloma and plasma cell leukemia, obtaining excellent responses, including near-complete remission (CR), with 100–140 mg/m^2 melphalan as a single agent.

Although most patients treated with high-dose melphalan as primary therapy by the UK Royal Marsden Hospital group had excellent responses, the majority eventually relapsed.[5,6] However, a small number of the responses were durable: of 61 patients receiving 140 mg/m^2 melphalan as initial therapy, 9 patients were alive at a median of over 11 years with 3 in continuous CR at 10–12 years (Figure 19.1). The major problem with this therapy, pioneered in the pre-growth-factor era, was prolonged pancytopenia.

The advent of myeloid growth factor support, initially with granulocyte–macrophage colony-stimulating factor (GM-CSF) and then with granulocyte colony-stimulating factor (G-CSF), made high-dose chemotherapy safer by ensuring prompt hematologic recovery.[7] The addition of autologous marrow support[8] permitted escalation of the melphalan dose to 200 mg/m^2.

Despite high CR rates and prolongation of survival[9] with high-dose therapy, this approach is not widely accepted as part of the routine therapy of myeloma. However, it has been an integral part of the front-line treatment of the disease at some centers for years[10,11] and is increasing in acceptance. With the recognition that biologic factors pertaining to the disease affect the prognosis more than other factors, high-dose therapy is also being used in patients over the age of 65 years[12,13] and in those with abnormal renal function[14] – groups that have usually been excluded from high-dose therapy-based treatment plans in the past.

It is also important to recognize that while autotransplantation is probably not curative in myeloma in the conventional sense, because of

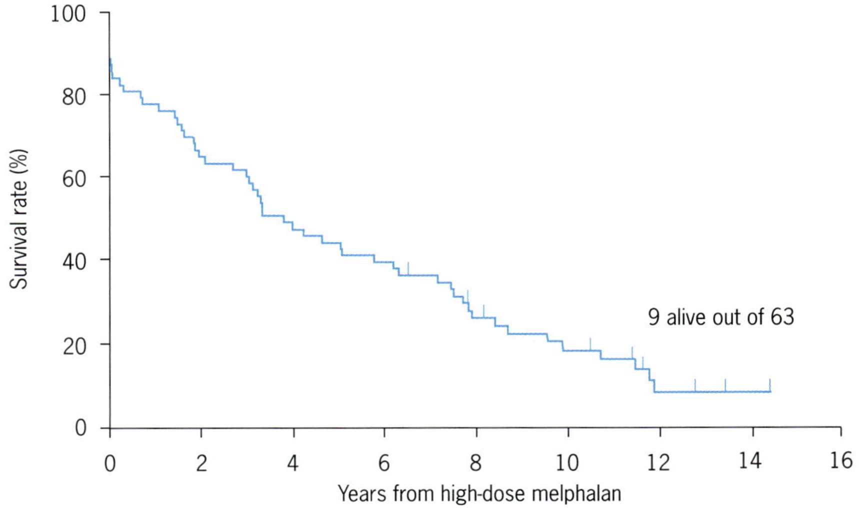

Figure 19.1 Long-term follow-up of 63 patients receiving 140 mg/m^2 melphalan without hematopoietic stem cell rescue or growth factor support. Therapy at relapse was variable. Data from the Royal Marsden Hospital, UK. (Courtesy of Professor Ray Powles.)

benefits in terms of extension of survival with good quality of life, some patients may be 'operationally cured'.[15] 'Operational cure' is a term that we have developed to denote a continuous first remission lasting 10 years or more.

COMPARISON OF HIGH-DOSE THERAPY AND CONVENTIONAL CHEMOTHERAPY

High-dose chemoradiotherapy and conventional chemotherapy have been compared prospectively by the Intergroupe Français du Myelome (IFM).[9] In the IFM study, 200 previously untreated patients received four to six cycles of conventional induction chemotherapy (alternating VMCP–BVAP; see Chapter 18). After this, they were randomized to continued conventional therapy or autologous BMT (ABMT) following a cytoreductive regimen comprising high-dose melphalan and total-body irradiation (TBI). Although only 74 of the 100 patients assigned to the ABMT arm were actually transplanted, high-dose therapy was associated with a significantly higher response rate (81% versus 57%, $p < 0.001$) on an intent-to-treat basis. While the actuarial 5-year event-free survival (EFS) rate (28% for high-dose therapy versus 10% for conventional chemotherapy) was not significantly different between the groups, the 5-year overall survival (OS) rate (52% versus 12%; $p = 0.03$) was superior for patients in the ABMT group (Figure 19.2).

A retrospective comparison[16] of 116 newly diagnosed patients who received conventional chemotherapy on various Southwest Oncology Group (SWOG) protocols with pair-matched control patients who underwent tandem high-dose chemotherapy cycles with autotransplantation showed that OS (62 months or more versus 48 months; $p = 0.01$) and EFS (49 months versus 22 months; $p = 0.0001$) were higher in the transplanted patients.

Dose intensification of melphalan to non-myeloablative levels is also beneficial. A recent retrospective study from Italy showed that patients receiving two or three courses of 100 mg/m^2 melphalan had superior CR rates, OS, and EFS compared with pair-matched control patients receiving standard-dose melphalan and prednisone.[13] While these courses of melphalan were supported with stem cells, 100 mg/m^2 melphalan is unlikely to require stem cell support if growth factors are administered – and may offer a non-transplant avenue to intensify the dose.

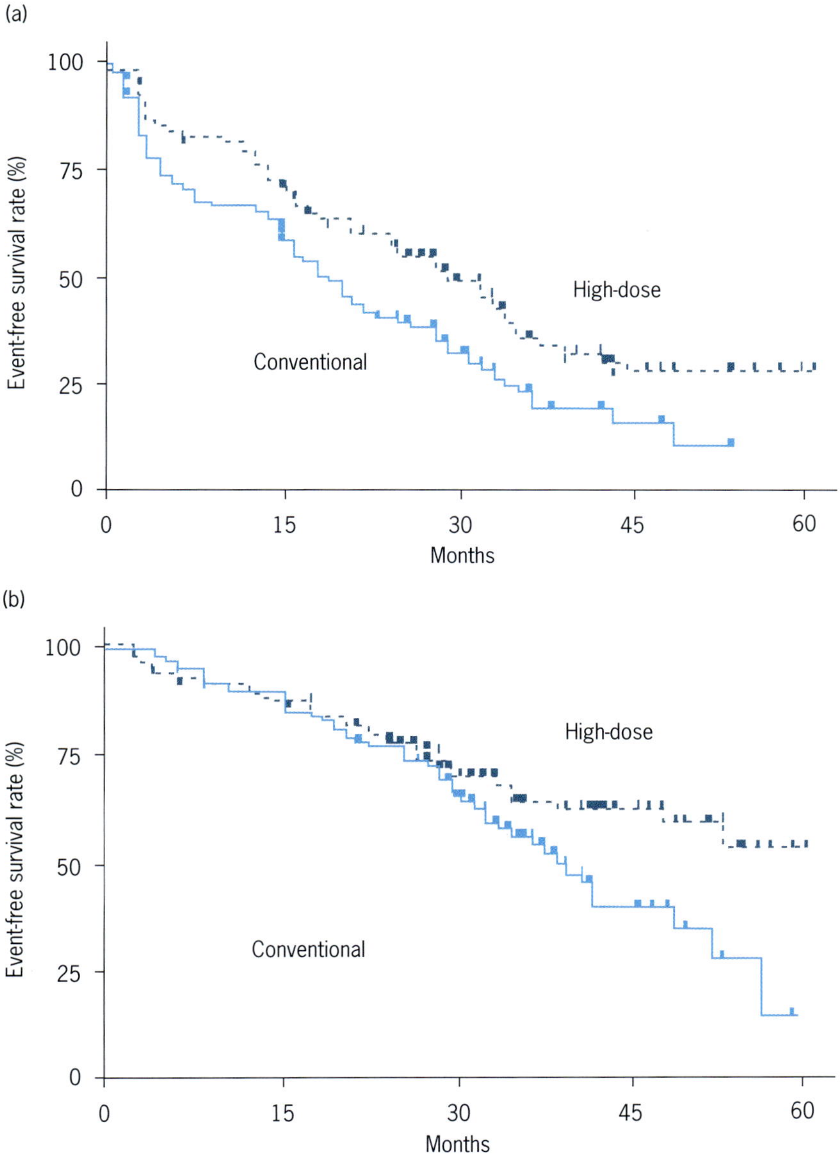

Figure 19.2 Comparison of conventional and high-dose chemotherapy: (a) event-free and (b) overall survival. (Used with permission from Attal M, Harousseau JL, Stoppa AM et al. A prospective, randomized trial of autologous bone marrow transplantation and chemotherapy in multiple myeloma. Intergroupe Français du Myelome. *N Engl J Med* 1996; **335:** 91–7.)

OTHER STUDIES OF HIGH-DOSE THERAPY

A number of other phase II studies have also shown encouraging results with high-dose therapy and autotransplantation in newly diagnosed as well as previously treated patients with myeloma.[10,17–29] Table 19.1 summarizes the results from some of the reports.

There are two noteworthy features common to all these reports: variable response rates, and a steady decline in OS and EFS with time. There are a number of reasons for the variable response rates: heterogeneous patient populations, especially with reference to disease chemosensitivity, different conditioning regimens, and varying definitions of response.[30] The lack of a plateau on the survival curves suggests that autotransplantation, including tandem autotransplantation,[11] is unlikely to be curative in myeloma.

Table 19.1 Results of phase II studies of high-dose therapy with autotransplantation (Tx) in myeloma

Authors	No. of patients	Chemosensitive disease	Median age (years)[a]	Conditioning regimen[b]	Purging[c]	Overall CR[d]	Tx-related mortality	Post-Tx IFN[e]	Overall survival	Event-free survival
Allegre et al[27]	259	81%	52 (23–67)	Various (87% Mel-based)	—	51%	4%	44%	50% at 3 yrs	35% at 3 yrs
Barlogie et al[29]	133 (63 transplanted; 70 other high-dose therapy)	26%	59% >50 yrs	Various (86% Mel-based)	—	12%	17%	No	5–23% at 7 yrs depending on conditioning	3–13% at 7 yrs depending on conditioning
Bensinger et al[26]	63	35%	51 (31–66)	Bu-Cy (29%), Bu-Cy-TBI (57%), Bu-Mel-thiotepa (14%)	—	30%	25%	Yes	43% at 3 yrs	21% at 3 yrs
Björkstrand et al[20]	15 (Tx1) 11 (Tx2)	100%	49 (40–57)	Mel (Tx1) Mel-TBI (Tx2)	— —	50% 73%	7% —	No Yes (PR)	NS	78% at 2 yrs (from Tx1)
Cunningham et al[22]	53	89%	52 (30–69)	Mel-methylprednisolone	—	77%	2%	No	63% at 3 yrs	30% at 3 yrs
Dimopoulos et al[19]	40	43%	49 (34–64)	Bu-Cy-thiotepa	CD19-coated magnabeads in 28%	29%	13%	Yes	NS	88% at 1 yr (PR), 55% at 1 yr (prim. refr.), 0% at 1 yr (refr. rel.)
Fermand et al[17]	63	30%	44 (29–58)	Carmustome-toposide-Mel-TBI (+ Cy in 41%)	—	20%	11%	Yes	69% at 3 yrs	53% at 3 yrs
Harousseau et al[21]	133	77%	52 (26–66)	Various (75% TBI)	—	37%	4%	Yes	43% at 5 yrs	NS
Marit et al[25]	73 (72 transplanted)	67%	54 (32–65)	Mel-TBI	—	45%	1%	NS	66% at 3 yrs	35% at 3 yrs
Powles et al[10]	195 (141 high-dose therapy)	71%	52 (31–70)	Mel (112: 200 mg/m^2, 23: 140 mg/m^2), Bu (6)	—	53%	5%	29%	45% at 5 yrs	20% at 5 yrs
Reece et al[18]	14	100%	48 (24–60)	Mel-Bu-Cy	4-HC	57%	21%	10%	10% at 3 yrs	10% at 3 yrs
Schiller et al[28]	55	100%	52 (34–69)	Bu-Cy	CD34$^+$ selection	8%	11%	NS	47% at 3 yrs	29% at 3 yrs
Seiden et al[23]	36	100%	48 (32–65)	Mel-TBI, Cy-TBI	MoAb	50%	6%	NS	70% at 3 yrs	42% at 3 yrs
Vesole et al[24]	496 (470 Tx1) (363 Tx2)	62%	54% >50 yrs	Mel (Tx1) Mel, Mel-Cy, Mel-TBI (Tx2)	— — —	36% (24% after Tx1) (43% after Tx2)	7%	±	60% at 3 yrs (from Tx1)	35% at 3 yrs (from Tx1)

[a] Range in parentheses. [b] Mel, melphalan; Bu, busulfan; Cy, cyclophosphamide; TBI, total-body irradiation. [c] 4-HC, 4-hydroperoxycyclophosphamide; MoAb, monoclonal antibody.
[d] Complete remission. [e] Interferon. *Other abbreviations:* NS, not specified; PR, partial remission; prim. refr., primary refractory; refr. rel., refractory relapse.

Fermand et al[17] autografted 63 patients after high-dose chemotherapy and TBI. The transplant-related mortality rate was relatively high at 11%, but all the surviving patients (including those with refractory disease) responded, and were in remission 6 months post transplant. The median OS and EFS after transplantation were 59 and 43 months respectively, with an actuarial 3-year OS rate of 69%.

The MD Anderson Cancer Center group in Houston,[19] evaluated the combination of thiotepa, busulfan, and cyclophosphamide with autologous blood or marrow support in 40 patients. Sixty-five percent of the patients responded, including 85% of patients in partial remission (PR) and 48% of patients with refractory disease, with an overall CR rate of 53%. While the patients treated in refractory relapse had short-lived responses (median 4 months), none of the patients transplanted in remission had experienced disease progression by 4–20 months post transplant (at the time of the report).

Björkstrand et al[20] treated 15 patients with 200 g/m^2 melphalan and ABMT. Eleven of these had a second autograft after conditioning with 140 mg/m^2 melphalan and 1000 cGy TBI. Amongst the latter, molecular CR was seen in 4 of 5 patients tested for the immunoglobulin heavy-chain (IgH) rearrangement using PCR. While the molecular remission was sustained at a relatively limited follow-up of 17–33 months, longer follow-up will be needed to see if what the eventual CR durations are and if any of these patients remain in long-term CR.

A cooperative group study from 18 French centers[21] on 133 patients autografted after initial induction chemotherapy reported an overall response rate of 83% and a CR rate of 37%. The median OS was 46 months: 54 months for patients with chemosensitive disease and 30 months for non-responders.

The Royal Marsden Hospital group[22] autografted 53 previously untreated patients using 200 mg/m^2 melphalan and 7.5 g (1.5 g/day x 5 days) methylprednisolone as conditioning. Patients had previously received infusional induction chemotherapy. CR was seen in 75% of the patients. Patients in CR had significantly longer survival than those not attaining CR, suggesting that achievement of CR (i.e. maximal cytoreduction) may be of benefit.

Marit et al[25] autografted 72 patients after melphalan-based conditioning regimens, resulting in CR in 32 patients and PR in 36 patients. The transplant-related mortality rate was low (1%), and the 3–year probability of OS was 66%.

The use of busulfan-based conditioning regimens in Seattle resulted in considerable treatment-related mortality (25%) amongst 63 patients, with CR and PR being seen in 30% and 37% of patients, respectively.[26]

Amongst 195 consecutive newly diagnosed patients under the age of 70 years seen at the Royal Marsden Hospital between 1986 and 1995 (including those reported by Cunningham et al,[22] see above), 112 (57%) were autografted after 200 mg/m^2 melphalan, 29 (15%) received 140 mg/m^2 melphalan or 16 mg/kg busulfan, and 28% did not proceed to high-dose therapy.[10] All patients received infusional induction chemotherapy comprising vincristine, doxorubicin, and methylprednisolone with (C-VAMP) or without (VAMP) cyclophosphamide. The CR rate was 53% for the whole group and 74% for patients receiving 200 mg/m^2 melphalan. The median OS (Figure 19.3) and EFS for the whole group from the time of the initial infusional chemotherapy were 4 years and 25 months respectively. The outcome of patients receiving 200 mg/m^2 melphalan was significantly better, with median OS and EFS of 6 years and 27 months, respectively, from the time of transplantation (see below).

The University of Arkansas *Total Therapy* program comprised remission induction with non-cross-resistant combination chemotherapy (two or three cycles of vincristine–doxorubicin–dexamethasone (VAD), high-dose cyclophosphamide with GM-CSF for leukapheresis, and etoposide–dexamethasone–cytarabine–cisplatin (EDAP)), followed by tandem autotransplantation (200 mg/m^2 melphalan $\times$ 2 or second transplant with added TBI or cyclophosphamide in patients not achieving a PR after the first transplant) and maintenance therapy with interferon-α2b (IFN-α2β).[11] Two hundred

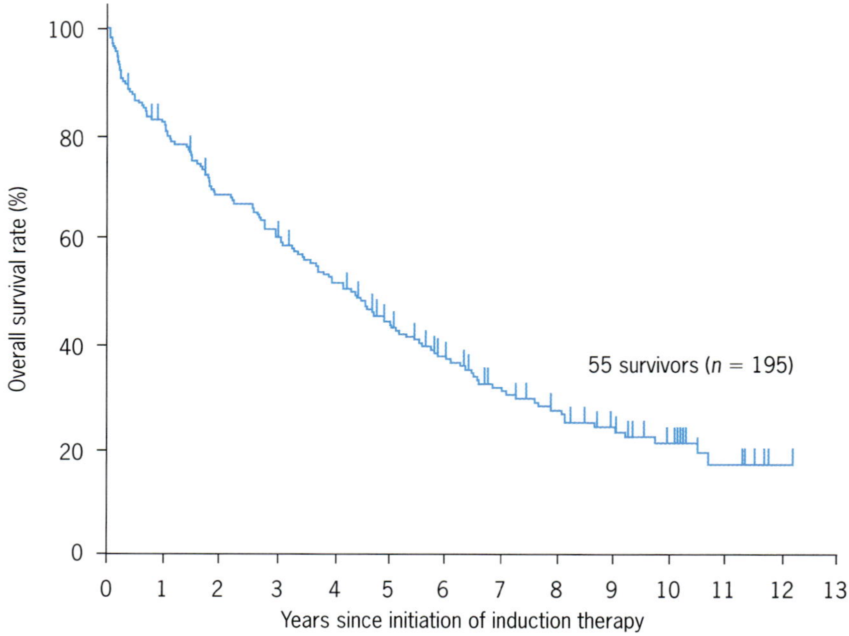

Figure 19.3 Overall survival of 195 consecutive newly diagnosed patients seen at the Royal Marsden Hospital, UK between 1986 and 1995. (Courtesy of Professor Ray Powles.)

and thirty-one patients were enrolled, two-thirds of whom had previously been untreated. The number of patients completing the first and the second transplants and eventually receiving IFN-α2b were 195 (84%), 165 (71%), and 128 (55%), respectively. An incremental response (CR as well as PR) was seen with each stage of therapy, with final CR and PR rates of 41% and 42% for the entire group of 231 patients, and 51% and 44% for the 165 patients completing two transplants. The median OS and EFS were 5.7 and 3.6 years, respectively, and the median CR duration was close to 4 years (Figure 19.4).[12] However, the noteworthy feature seen in the figures is the lack of a plateau on the survival or the relapse curves, despite the intensity of the treatment. Also, the median survival of this tandem transplant group is identical with that of patients undergoing a single autograft after 200 mg/m^2 melphalan at the Royal Marsden Hospital, suggesting that tandem transplantation has no demonstrable benefit in myeloma at present.

Of 496 consecutive patients treated at the University of Arkansas on clinical studies of tandem transplantation (including *Total Therapy*[12]),[24] 470 (95%) received 200 mg/m^2 prior to the first autotransplant, and 363 (73%) received high-dose melphalan with or without additional cytoreductive agents (usually cyclophosphamide or TBI) and a second transplant. The median interval between the two transplants was 5 months. The treatment-related mortality rate during the first year after transplantation was 7%, and CR was seen in 36%. The median durations of EFS and OS from the first transplant were 26 and 41 months, respectively.

A report[29] on 133 patients with advanced myeloma who received various types of high-dose therapy regimens between 1985 and 1990 at the MD Anderson Cancer Center provided long-term follow-up on outcome of dose-

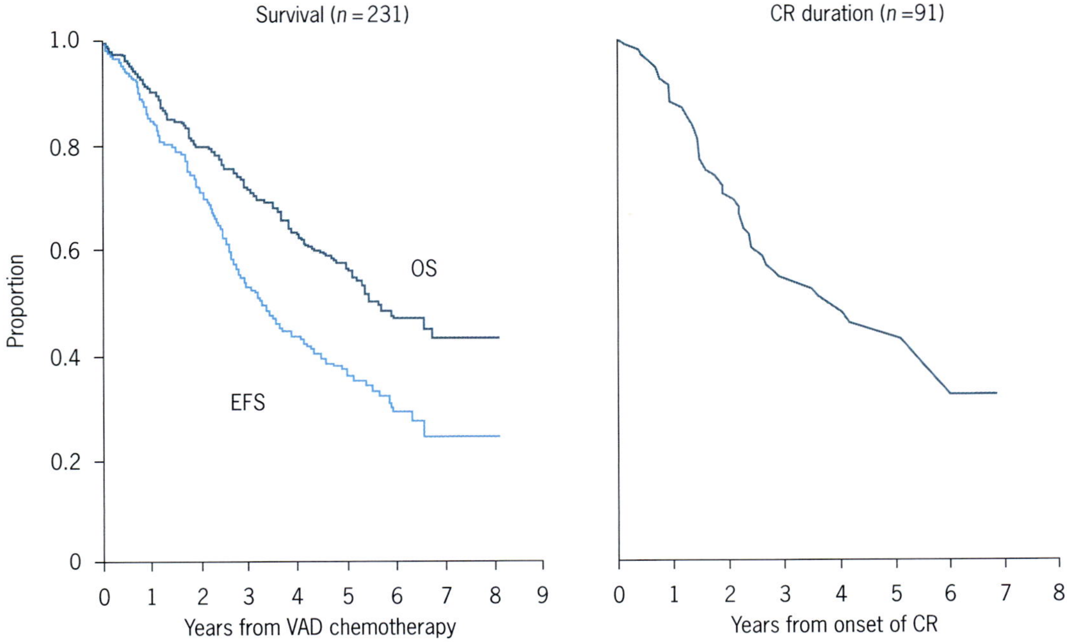

Figure 19.4 Outcome of the University of Arkansas *Total Therapy* program: there is no evidence of a plateau on the survival or relapse curves despite intensive combination chemotherapy including tandem transplantation. (Used with permission from Mehta J, Singhal S, Desikan K et al. High-dose therapy and stem cell support in myeloma. In: *PPO Updates*, Vol 13 (De Vita VT Jr, Hellman S, Rosenberg SA, eds). Philadelphia: Lippincott Williams & Wilkins, 1999: 1–12.)

intensified therapy: up to 100 mg/m^2 melphalan (46 patients), 100 mg/m^2 melphalan with GM-CSF (24 patients), 140 mg/m^2 melphalan with ABMT (8 patients), 140 mg/m^2 melphalan and 850 cGy TBI with ABMT (37 patients), and 750 mg/m^2 thiotepa and 850 cGy TBI with ABMT (18 patients). Four of 16 patients attaining CR remained in CR at 10 years. The median EFS and OS were 6 and 15 months, respectively. EFS and OS were favorably influenced by β_2-microglobulin 2.5 mg/l or less, age 50 years or less, absence of refractory relapse, and ABMT/GM-CSF support.

The bulk of the published literature suggests that all patients can potentially benefit from high-dose therapy. This counters previous observations made on small numbers of patients that those with more than a year's prior history of conventional chemotherapy[31] or those with responsive disease transplanted within a year[32] derive limited benefit from high-dose therapy.

SOURCE OF STEM CELLS

Blood-derived stem cells result in faster hematologic recovery than marrow.[33,34] In patients receiving adequate quantities of blood stem cells[35], additional marrow infusion makes no difference to hematologic recovery. Blood cell transplantation is also less expensive owing to the lower cost of supportive therapy.[36]

The tumor cell content of marrow harvests is higher than that of blood cell harvests from the same patients.[37] However, the clinical significance of this observation is unclear. It is possible to obtain adequate stem cells by leukapheresis after mobilization with chemotherapy plus growth factor or growth factor alone in patients with significant marrow infiltration with plasma cells. This is unlikely to be practical with marrow harvests.

EFS and OS appear to be identical with blood- and marrow-derived stem cells in myeloma.[33,34]

Therefore, because of more rapid engraftment, peripheral blood is the preferred source of stem cells.

COLLECTION OF STEM CELLS

There is a significant correlation between the number of $CD34^+$ peripheral blood stem cells infused and the speed of hematologic recovery.[35,38] Exposure to as little as six months of conventional chemotherapy with alkylating agents prior to stem cell collection affects the harvest and post-transplant recovery adversely.[35,39–41] Stem cell-damaging agents such as melphalan and the nitrosoureas should not be used in patients who may be candidates for autotransplantation; alternatively, stem cells should be collected prior to commencement of such therapy. Prior IFN-α therapy has been found to affect stem cell yields adversely in patients harvested after having undergone an autotransplant.[42] It is possible that interferon-induced marrow damage may be seen even in patients who have not been transplanted. Extensive local radiation also compromises stem cell collection.

For patients collected after high-dose cyclophosphamide and GM-CSF, the minimum number of $CD34^+$ cells necessary for prompt engraftment was 2×10^6/kg for patients with up to 24 months of prior chemotherapy, and 5×10^6/kg for those with more extensive prior chemotherapy.[35] The number of $CD34^+$ cells required for prompt engraftment in patients mobilized with G-CSF as a single agent may be lower. In a comparative study, although the number of $CD34^+$ cells collected was higher after high-dose cyclophosphamide and GM-CSF compared with that collected after G-CSF alone, engraftment kinetics were similar and G-CSF was better tolerated.[43] Similarly, while the number of $CD34^+$ cells collected after cyclophosphamide and G-CSF was higher than that collected after G-CSF alone,[44] engraftment kinetics were similar, and the morbidity of G-CSF alone was considerably less.

In extensively pretreated patients, the use of stem cell factor (SCF; also known as c-Kit ligand and Steel factor) in combination with G-CSF with or without chemotherapy may be more successful at mobilizing stem cells than G-CSF alone with or without chemotherapy.[45] Unfortunately, studies showing superiority of combined SCF and G-CSF over G-CSF alone have not employed very high doses of G-CSF, and therefore the possibility remains that single-agent G-CSF at doses of 16–20 μg/kg or even higher may be sufficient to collect stem cells in some patients with compromised marrow function. Figure 19.5 shows the potential approach to a patient with compromised marrow function in whom stem cells need to be collected.

The usual practice is to harvest sufficient stem cells for one transplant (or two if on a tandem transplant protocol) and use them all up for the planned procedures. While this is appropriate in diseases such as leukemia, it may not be appropriate in myeloma, where repeat high-dose therapy procedures are feasible for relapsed disease. Therefore, it is worthwhile collecting extra cells and cryopreserving them for potential future use. While it is possible to harvest stem cells in previously autografted patients, the cell yields are quantitatively and qualitatively poor.[42]

Some investigators have reported differential mobilization of normal and malignant cells during recovery from chemotherapy-induced myelosuppression,[46] but others have not found this to be the case.[47] Since there is little evidence supporting the role of reinfused malignant cells in myeloma relapse following autotransplantation, differential mobilization is likely to be of limited value.

CONDITIONING REGIMENS

In patients with advanced disease, 100 mg/m^2 melphalan without transplantation and melphalan–TBI with transplantation were associated with a 20–25% treatment-related mortality rate.[48] The four series using busulfan-based regimens[18,19,26,28] reported treatment-related mortality rates of 11–25% (Table 19.1), which are far in excess of those seen with high-dose melphalan.

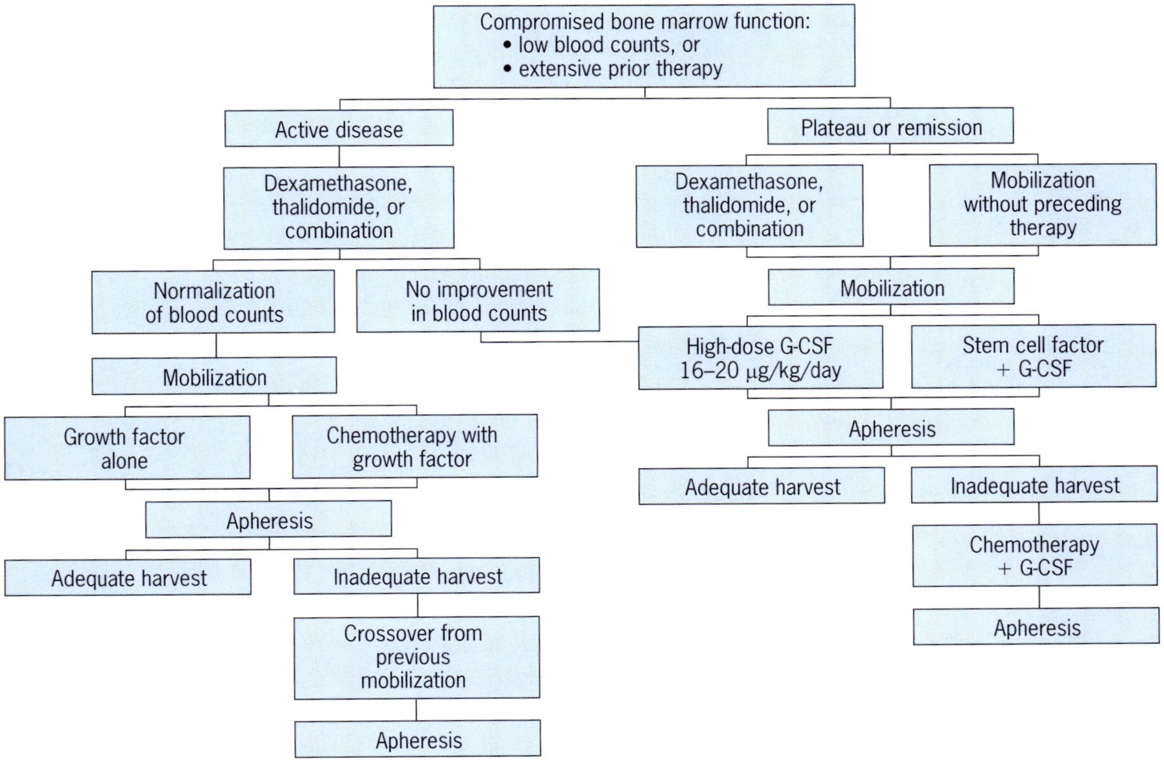

Figure 19.5 Approach to stem cell collection in a myeloma patient with compromised marrow function.

The availability of growth factors, the use of blood-derived stem cells, and improved supportive care has made single-agent melphalan very safe, with treatment-related mortality rates of 1–5%, even in patients with advanced disease.[48]

Relatively poor response rates and survival after regimens such as high-dose busulfan,[11,49] busulfan–cyclophosphamide,[18,26] and high-dose etoposide combinations[50] suggest a limited role for these regimens in myeloma. A European Blood and Marrow Transplant group (EBMT) study of 130 autografted patients[20] found that high-dose melphalan singly or in combination appeared to be superior to other regimens. Similarly, amongst patients undergoing tandem autotransplantation, after a first autograft with 200 mg/m^2 melphalan, patients receiving alternative regimens such as melphalan–TBI or melphalan–cyclophosphamide for the second transplant were reported to have a shorter response duration than those who received 200 mg/m^2 melphalan for the second transplant.[51] This is somewhat difficult to explain, since the melphalan dose in patients receiving melphalan–cyclophosphamide was also 200 mg/m^2. Figure 19.6 shows data from the Royal Marsden Hospital demonstrating superior OS after 200 mg/m^2 melphalan compared with high-dose busulfan or 140 mg/m^2 melphalan.

The combination of cyclophosphamide, carboplatin, and etoposide has been used for patients with advanced, refractory myeloma who had relapsed following a preceding transplant. The antitumor efficacy was poor in most patients, and the toxicity was significant in the setting of compromised renal function.[52] Carmustine, etoposide, cytarabine, and melphalan (BEAM) is being investigated as a conditioning regimen for patients with more aggressive disease with features resembling non-Hodgkin's lymphoma (unpublished data).

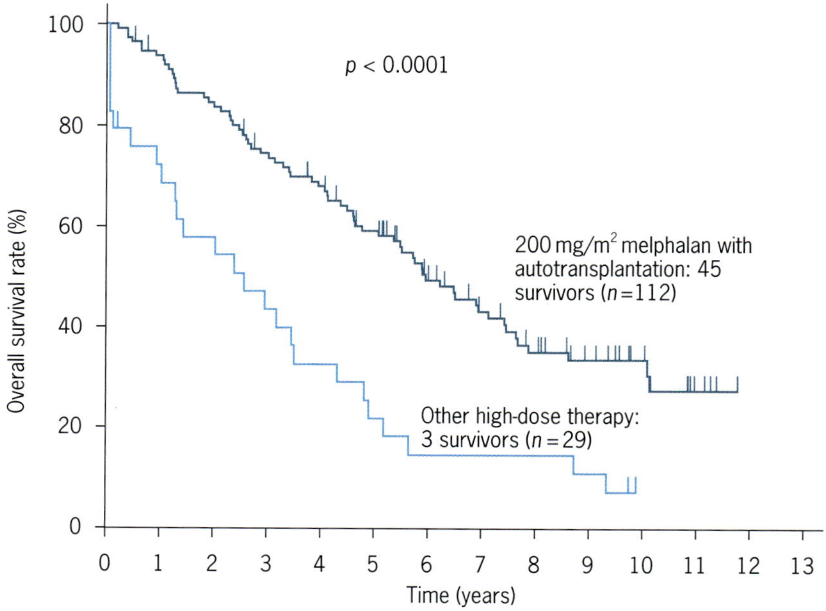

Figure 19.6 Superior overall survival amongst patients treated with high-dose melphalan compared with other high-dose therapy regimens. Data from the Royal Marsden Hospital, UK. (Courtesy of Professor Ray Powles.)

An interesting approach under evaluation currently is to administer bone-seeking compounds conjugated with radioisotopes to deliver radiation to bone and bone marrow preferentially.[53] This could allow dose escalation without excessive extramedullary toxicity.

For the moment, high-dose melphalan appears to be the most active regimen, with no obvious additional benefit coming from more complex combination regimens. Pharmacokinetic studies suggest that the terminal half-life of melphalan ranges from 50 to 170 minutes,[54,55] and the drug is not detectable in the plasma 24 hours after intravenous administration. It is thus safe to reinfuse hematopoietic stem cells 24 hours after the administration of melphalan[10] rather than waiting an additional day.[11] From the published studies as well as unpublished observations, there appears to be no difference between a single dose of melphalan and two divided doses 24 hours apart in terms of regimen-related toxicity, haematopoietic recovery or antitumor efficacy. While 200 mg/m^2 is the commonly used dose of melphalan, 220 mg/m^2 has also been administered; albeit with a high incidence of severe mucositis.[54] A dose of 240 mg/m^2 has been used as a conditioning regimen for allogeneic transplantation for haematologic malignancies, and should, in theory, be feasible for autotransplantation in myeloma.[56] The availability of potential chemoprotectants such as amifostine and newer growth factors such as keratinocyte growth factor may help reduce mucositis and other toxicity.

PURGING AND POSITIVE SELECTION

Increased quantities of monoclonal plasma cells amongst the harvested stem cells have been associated with an increased probability of disease progression.[57] However, this observation may be an indication of aggressive disease behavior rather than evidence that reinfused malignant cells contribute to relapse. In fact, the high relapse rates observed after syngeneic[58,59] and allogeneic[60] transplantation suggest that failure to eradicate residual disease within the patient is usually the problem.

Nevertheless, attempts have been made to obtain tumor-free stem cells by purging with monoclonal antibodies[23] or 4-hydroperoxycyclophosphamide (4-HC),[18] and by selection of CD34$^+$ progenitor cells.[28,61–65] The latter approach is based upon the observation that myeloma cells do not express the CD34 antigen.[66]

The Dana-Farber group[23] autografted 36 patients using marrow purged with a combination of three anti-B cell monoclonal antibodies. Engraftment was slow, with a median of 24 days to 0.5×10^9/l neutrophils and 40 days to 20×10^9/l platelets. One patient died of toxicity. Chemosensitive disease contributed to excellent response rates, with 50% CR and 44% PR. The 3-year probabilities of OS and EFS were 70% and 40%, respectively.

Reece et al[18] autografted 14 patients with responsive disease using marrow purged with 4-HC following a conditioning regimen containing busulfan, cyclophosphamide, and melphalan. Three patients died of toxicity, and 11 responded to the transplant. Seven patients progressed subsequently, and 4 were reported to be progression-free at a median of 20 months (range 6–42 months).

CD34$^+$ selection procedures reduce the malignant cell content of the graft by 2–5 logs,[28,61–65] usually without affecting engraftment.[61] Whether these procedures reduce relapse rates is not known. Schiller et al[28] treated 51 patients with high-dose chemotherapy and CD34$^+$ selected peripheral blood progenitor cell transplants. With a median follow-up of 33 months for the 31 surviving patients, the actuarial 3-year EFS and OS rates were 29% and 47%, respectively. These outcomes are similar to those seen with unmanipulated transplants (Table 19.1). In a small retrospective study, Gupta et al[62] found that EFS was not significantly different between CD34$^+$ selected and unselected groups (median 21 and 26 months respectively). Long-term follow-up of a randomized study[61] shows no survival benefit from CD34$^+$ selection.[66] Therefore, the utility of purging and positive selection remains questionable.

Indeed, there are potential problems with transplantation of selected CD34$^+$ progenitor cells: it has been found to be associated with slow reconstitution of cellular and humoral immunity in some reports,[67,68] but not in others.[69] Not only can the compromised immune status put patients at risk of opportunistic infections (reference 68 and unpublished observations) but it can also potentially increase relapse by eliminating tumor immune surveillance. These patients are also poor candidates for experimental post-transplant immune approaches to eliminate residual disease, because they are incapable of mounting an immune response. A better approach would be to engineer the graft to retain or even enhance the immune effector cells while depleting tumor cells.[70]

PROGNOSIS

A number of studies have shown that the attainment of CR is an independent favorable prognostic factor for OS and EFS after high-dose therapy.[11,22,24] Logically, achievement of CR is a *sine qua non* for long-term disease-free survival or cure. However, it is possible that achievement of CR is a surrogate marker for the biological nature of the disease activity and simply identifies patients with less aggressive disease who are likely to enjoy longer disease-free survival. For the moment, a sequence of treatment steps aimed at increasing CR rates is probably an appropriate approach for most patients.

A number of variables have been found to be predictive of prognosis in patients undergoing high-dose therapy. These include the chromosomal karyotype (cytogenetic abnormalities), β_2-microglobulin at the time of initial presentation or the autograft, C-reactive protein at the time of initial presentation, and the duration of standard therapy prior to high-dose therapy.[11,12,24,71–73]

While the immunologic subtype of myeloma has not been found to influence prognosis in some series, others have found IgA to be an adverse prognostic feature. Lactate dehydrogenase (LDH) levels have rarely been shown to have an independent adverse influence when a comparison is made between patients with normal and abnormal LDH at presentation. In our experience (unpublished observations), presentation LDH that is more than 2.5–3-fold higher than the upper limit of normal is associated with extremely poor prognosis after autotransplantation, with relapse and death within two years of diagnosis being the norm.

Figure 19.7 shows the influence of chromosome 13 abnormalities, and β_2-microglobulin and C-reactive protein levels at presentation in patients undergoing sequential induction and high-dose chemotherapy. Patients in whom all the variables are favorable have low-risk disease, those with one adverse feature have medium-risk disease, and those with two or three adverse features have high-risk disease.[74] In patients with previously treated disease (in whom biochemical values at the time of presentation may not be available), a similar model can be constructed based on cytogenetics, β_2-microglobulin level at the time of the transplant, and the duration of standard chemotherapy prior to the transplant.[2,75]

The Mayo Clinic group found that the presence of any cytogenetic abnormalities was associated with a poorer prognosis compared with abnormal karyotype.[73] Others have found that partial or complete deletion of chromosome 13, abnormalities of chromosome 11q and all translocations are associated with poor prognosis.[71,72] Further work is required to identify the specific karyotype abnormalities associated with poor outcome.

The idea of identifying high-risk disease is to suitably intensify the treatment: patients with higher-risk disease could be subjected to allogeneic transplantation rather than autologous, or could receive intensive post-transplant maintenance therapy to prolong response duration.[74,75]

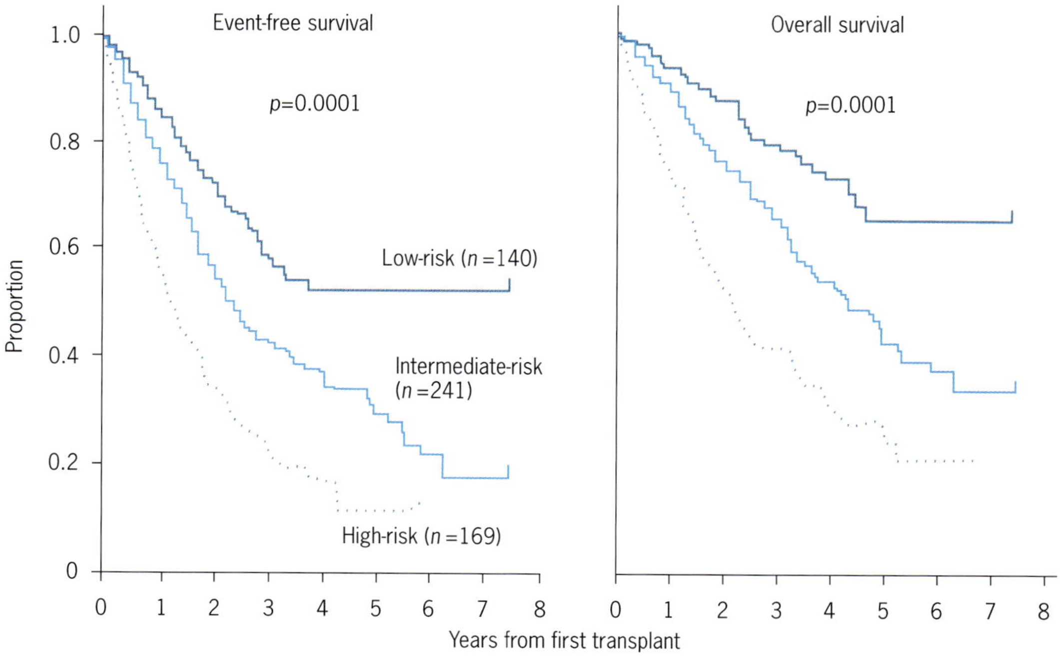

Figure 19.7 Influence of chromosome 13 abnormalities, and β_2-microglobulin and C-reactive protein levels at presentation in patients undergoing sequential induction and high-dose chemotherapy. See the text for the relationship between prognostic factors and risk status. (Used with permission from Mehta J, Singhal S, Desikan K et al. High-dose therapy and stem cell support in myeloma. In: *PPO Updates*, Vol 13 (De Vita VT Jr, Hellman S, Rosenberg SA, eds). Philadelphia: Lippincott Williams & Wilkins, 1999:1–12.)

PATIENTS WITH RENAL IMPAIRMENT

Melphalan was originally thought to be excreted by the kidneys, and therefore was avoided in patients with renal impairment. Patients with compromised renal function were treated with high-dose busulfan, with acceptable toxicity[49] but poor eventual outcome because of suboptimal antitumor effects.[11] More recent data suggest that renal dysfunction does not alter melphalan pharmacokinetics.[76]

High-dose melphalan is therefore routinely offered at some institutions to patients with renal failure, including those on dialysis.[15] A comparison of 42 renal failure patients and 84 matched controls with normal renal function receiving 200 mg/m^2 melphalan showed comparable transplant-related mortality rate (7% versus 6%) and response rates (64% versus 65%). Overall, 50% of patients experienced improved renal function, including one-third of the dialysis-dependent patients, who stopped requiring dialysis. The OS and EFS of the two groups were comparable. However, these data are preliminary and are yet to be confirmed; especially with regard to safety issues. Patients with renal failure have substantially higher morbidity with high-dose therapy, including central nervous system changes, cardiac dysrhythmias, and, occasionally, unexpected mortality (unpublished observations).

Melphalan at a dose of 200 mg/m^2 cannot be considered routine therapy for patients with renal failure at the moment. Until safety concerns have been addressed, dose-intensive therapy should probably be avoided in patients who have responded well to initial chemotherapy – or employed at a reduced dose of 100 mg/m^2. Patients who have not responded sufficiently could receive 100–140 mg/m^2 melphalan with stem cell support.

Busulfan and cyclophosphamide have also been administered to a small number of patients with renal failure without problems [77]. However, amongst relapsed patients undergoing repeat autotransplantation after conditioning comprising cyclophosphamide, carboplatin, and etoposide, those with impaired renal function had a higher incidence of complications and mortality.[52] Thus, the role of regimens other than high-dose melphalan is even less clear in myeloma patients with renal dysfunction.

OLDER PATIENTS

Age does not affect the outcome of myeloma, provided that appropriate therapy is delivered.[13] The difficulty is in delivering intensive treatment to older patients. The upper age limit for the administration of high-dose melphalan has generally been increased to 65 years, although some centers have routinely used this in patients over the age of 70 years.[13]

Morbidity is usually considerably higher for individuals aged over 70 years. While mortality also appears to be higher (unpublished observations), the differences have not reached statistical significance, because of relatively small patient numbers.[13] Rather than administering 200 mg/m^2 melphalan to all patients over the age of 70 years, a more judicious approach would be to use a lower dose of 100–140 mg/m^2 to improve tolerance. It is possible that cytoprotective agents such as amifostine and cytokines such as epidermal growth factor or keratinocyte growth factor would reduce the extramedullary toxicity of high-dose therapy in older patients.

At the moment, routine use of high-dose therapy in all older individuals cannot be justified. Prospective evaluation of high-dose chemotherapy in patients over the age of 70 years must address morbidity and quality-of-life issues rather than just disease-related endpoints.[12,13]

LONG-TERM CONSEQUENCES

Myelodysplastic syndrome (MDS) and secondary acute myeloid leukemia (AML) have been described in autografted myeloma patients.[78–80] Although an early study based on limited data concluded that these complications were seen exclusively in patients previously treated with conventional-dose alkylating agent chemotherapy,[78] a review of serial karyotype data from 868 autografted patients (including those reported in the previous study[78]) revealed cytogenetic changes typical of MDS in 133 patients.[79] Forty-four patients had only myelodysplastic karyotype abnormalities and 89 patients had myelodysplastic as well as typical myeloma-type karyotype abnormalities within the same metaphases. The actuarial 5-year probabilities of the development of cytogenetic MDS and combined cytogenetic MDS-myeloma were 5% and 10%, respectively, and appeared to increase with longer follow-up. Prolonged duration of pre-transplant chemotherapy was the most important risk factor for the development of MDS, followed by greater age and a low number of infused $CD34^+$ cells.[79] It is possible that this extraordinarily high rate of myelodysplastic charges is the result of two autotransplants in comparison with the more commonly employed single autograft.

Although most patients tolerate two autografts well, there is evidence of development of late renal dysfunction signified by decreased creatinine clearance and increasing non-specific proteinuria that cannot be attributed to the disease in a few patients (unpublished observations). This is especially likely in patients who have received periodic post-transplant maintenance/intensification chemotherapy (see below) with the combination of cyclophosphamide, dexamethasone, etoposide, and cisplatin (unpublished observations). Administration of this combination chemotherapy repeatedly post transplant may also increase the incidence of myelodysplasia.

Bone density improves in patients who have responded to high-dose chemotherapy even if they do not receive bisphosphonates, and administration of drugs such as pamidronate provides additive benefit.

Patients autografted for other diseases such as acute leukemia using more intensive conditioning regimens lose their immunity from childhood immunizations.[81] Whether this happens in myeloma patients or not and what the optimum re-immunization schedule after high-dose chemotherapy is in these patients unknown.[81]

UNANSWERED QUESTIONS

Time of transplantation

A French study has compared early with late autotransplantation. Patients autografted early received high-dose therapy as consolidation of response to conventional therapy, and those autografted late received it as salvage therapy after disease progression following initial conventional chemotherapy.[82] While OS was not influenced by the time of transplantation, the early-transplant group had superior EFS. The potential disadvantages of waiting until disease progression include longer time on chemotherapy (maintenance chemotherapy after initial induction therapy), continued loss of bone density with potential development of fractures, development of renal failure, and a higher risk of eventual MDS. The potential advantage of waiting is avoidance of (or rather delay in) transplantation in a small number of patients who may survive for several years without disease progression. In the French study,[82] 78% of patients in the late-transplant group were eventually transplanted, and only 12% were alive without disease progression. Clearly, early transplantation would appear to be the approach of choice.

One transplant or two?

The proportion of patients attaining CR has been reported to increase progressively through the various courses of therapy, including from the first transplant to the second in a program of tandem transplantation.[12,24] Since attainment of CR has been identified as an independent indicator of favorable outcome (with limitations that have been discussed earlier),[11,21,24] one would expect tandem autotransplantation with a higher CR rate to be superior to a single transplant. The timely completion of two autotransplants within six months is reportedly associated with better OS and EFS.[24] However, there are no data showing that patients who did undergo timely double transplants had disease that was biologically similar to those who did not, and the possibility remains that the difference is at least partly attributable to differences in disease characteristics. There are no controlled data comparing one and two autografts. A cooperative French study is evaluating this question prospectively.

To complicate the issue, it is not known whether tandem transplantation (two elective autografts a few months apart) is superior to one transplant followed by a salvage second transplant as therapy of progressive disease.[83–85] Since a second high-dose therapy procedure is an effective salvage treatment for relapse after one autograft, it may be acceptable to do just one autograft in the beginning. In fact, in theory, if adequate numbers of stem cells were available, one could serially administer high-dose chemotherapy with stem cell support every time the disease relapsed in an attempt to prolong the natural course of the disease.[86] Eventually, there would be problems with cumulative toxicity and resistance.[86] Anecdotally, this has been done four times over a period of 15 years in a young patient who eventually died of recurrent disease (Professor Ray Powles, personal communication).

In view of the lack of published data showing a benefit of tandem autografts over single, and the comparable outcomes with single and double crossplants in large series of patients,[10,11] tandem autografts should not be performed routinely in all myeloma patients. We confine the use of tandem autografts to the 20–25% of patients who have responded to the first autograft but are not in CR or near-CR.

DECREASING RELAPSE AFTER HIGH-DOSE THERAPY

Almost all autografted patients eventually experience disease progression, and it is not known if this procedure cures anyone with myeloma. However, it is possible to extend the duration of remission after transplantation. Various approaches have been tried to reduce or delay relapse after transplantation.

IFN-α2b has been used as maintenance therapy after autografting in myeloma.[11,12] The Royal Marsden Hospital group performed a randomized study of maintenance IFN-α2b (3 MU/m^2 three times a week) or no therapy after high-dose melphalan (140–200 mg/m^2) or busulfan (16 mg/kg) in 85 patients.[87] The median EFS of interferon-treated patients was 46 months, compared with 27 months for the controls. Because of the decreased early disease progression, the OS was significantly superior for the interferon arm at a median follow-up of 52 months. However, almost all patients in both arms eventually experienced disease progression, and eventually the OS and EFS differences between the two groups ceased to be significant. One of the reasons for this may have been that patients in the control arm went on to interferon at the time of disease progression, resulting in a narrowing of the survival difference between the two groups. Another interesting observation in this study was that the benefit of interferon was confined to patients attaining CR, although interferon administration did not influence the probability of attaining CR.[88] When all autografted patients from the Royal Marsden Hospital, including those not on the randomized trial,[87] were studied, there was a beneficial effect of interferon administration on OS as well as EFS (Professor Ray Powles, personal communication; see Chapter 22). The role of interferon in the management of myeloma is discussed comprehensively in Chapter 22.

Dexamethasone at a dose of 20–40 mg daily for four days every three or four weeks is an alternative maintenance approach, especially in patients with significantly compromised renal function or poor hematopoietic recovery following the transplant. Dexamethasone may not be useful as maintenance therapy in patients whose disease is unresponsive to corticosteroids pretransplant. The combination of dexamethasone and interferon may be superior for maintenance of remission following high-dose therapy, as it is following conventional therapy.[89]

Thalidomide is a remarkably active drug in advanced myeloma,[90] possibly through inhibition of angiogenesis. Limited data suggest that patients attaining CR after an autograft continue to exhibit increased microvessel density.[91] Based upon these observations, thalidomide is administered as standard post-autograft maintenance therapy in selected patient populations at the Northwestern University Medical School: (a) disease known to be sensitive to thalidomide pre transplant, (b) disease poorly responsive to dexamethasone pre transplant, and (c) inability to tolerate dexamethasone or interferon. The role of thalidomide in myeloma is discussed in Chapter 8.

Intensive chemotherapy is being explored after autotransplantation to prolong remission duration.[92,93] Preliminary data suggest that four courses of DCEP chemotherapy (dexamethasone, cyclophosphamide, etoposide, and cisplatin) decrease relapse rates and improve survival over the short term,[92] whereas one course of acute lymphoblastic leukemia-type chemotherapy has no effect.[93] Both types of therapy are tolerated reasonably well. However, long-term follow-up is needed to see if the benefits seen with DCEP are sustained. There is already some indication that repeated cycles of DCEP chemotherapy increase long-term toxicity such as renal dysfunction (unpublished observations) and possibly MDS. Since DCEP chemotherapy only delays relapse rather than preventing it, its exact place in the post-transplant treatment of myeloma needs to be looked at closely.

Cyclosporine administration after autotransplantation can induce a clinical syndrome resembling graft-versus-host disease (GVHD) in a minority of patients and histologic changes (usually cutaneous) of GVHD in about half.[94] However, no data exist showing the efficacy of this reaction in controlling residual disease or preventing/delaying relapse. The apparent decline of paraprotein in one reported case[95] may have been related to corticosteroid therapy administered for cutaneous GVHD rather than any immunologic effect.[60]

The other potential approaches in the setting of minimal residual disease applicable after autologous transplantation include idiotype vaccination and infusion of idiotype-pulsed dendritic cells.[96–98] These are aimed at generating specific cell-mediated as well as humoral immunity, and are discussed in depth in Chapter 6.

Table 19.2 summarizes maintenance-therapy approaches following autotransplantation in patients with myeloma. Long-term administration of bisphosphonates such as pamidronate or zoledronate should be considered standard in patients even after high-dose therapy because of ongoing benefits on reversing bone loss as well as potential antimyeloma action.

OUTCOME OF RELAPSE AFTER TRANSPLANTATION

Relapse is almost inevitable after autotransplantation – single or double/tandem. However, disease relapsing after autotransplantation can be treated with further autologous[52,83–86] or allogeneic[84,99] transplantation, conventional chemotherapy,[83] or investigational agents such as thalidomide.[90] Subgroups of patients with relapsing disease may still have relatively long survival with appropriate therapy. What treatment is appropriate for a particular patient is determined by patient-related (age, performance status, extent of prior therapy, availability of autologous cells, availability of HLA-matched donors) and disease-related (biologic nature, sensitivity to prior therapy) factors.

Table 19.2 Potential maintenance therapy after high-dose therapy and autotransplantation in myeloma

Maintenance therapy	Supportive evidence
Dexamethasone	Good
Interferon	Good
Thalidomide	Limited
Combination	Limited
Bisphosphonates	Limited
Periodic intensive chemotherapy	Limited
Idiotype vaccination	Limited
Dendritic cell infusions	Limited

Since myeloma patients can attain a second (or even subsequent) CR with appropriate salvage therapy following relapse, the usual measure of disease control, namely continuous CR, is inadequate to assess outcome. We use 'discontinuous CR' (DCR) to quantify this (unpublished). DCR is the total duration from the first day of the first CR or the last day of the last CR.

CONCLUSIONS

High-dose therapy and autologous transplantation is almost universally applicable in myeloma, and is generally very safe. Disease recurrence remains a problem, and strategies to increase CR rates are required along with post-transplant immunologic or chemotherapeutic maneuvers to eliminate residual disease. Thalidomide and other inhibitors of angiogenesis may have a very significant role to play in the future management of myeloma in conjunction with high-dose therapy.

REFERENCES

1. Mehta J, Powles RL. Autologous blood and marrow transplantation. In: *Leukaemia and Associated Diseases* (Whittaker JA, Holmes JA, eds). Oxford: Blackwell Science, 1998: 455–81.
2. Singhal S, Mehta J, Barlogie B. Advances in the treatment of multiple myeloma. *Curr Opin Hematol* 1997; **4:** 291–7.
3. Fefer A, Cheever MA, Greenberg PD. Identical-twin (syngeneic) marrow transplantation for hematologic cancers. *J Natl Cancer Inst* 1986; **76:** 1269–73.
4. McElwain TJ, Powles RL. High-dose intravenous melphalan for plasma-cell leukaemia and myeloma. *Lancet* 1983; **2:** 822–4.
5. Cunningham D, Paz-Ares L, Gore ME et al. High-dose melphalan for multiple myeloma: long-term follow-up data. *J Clin Oncol* 1994; **12:** 764–8.
6. Powles R, Cunningham D, Gore M et al. Long-term follow-up of myeloma patients treated with 140 mg/m^2 melphalan without autologous transplantation. *Blood* 1997; **90**(Suppl 1): 356a.
7. Barlogie B, Jagannath S, Dixon DO et al. High-dose melphalan and granulocyte-macrophage colony-stimulating factor for refractory multiple myeloma. *Blood* 1990; **76:** 677–80.
8. Barlogie B, Hall R, Zander A et al. High-dose melphalan with autologous bone marrow transplantation for multiple myeloma. *Blood* 1986; **67:** 1298–301.
9. Attal M, Harousseau JL, Stoppa AM et al. A prospective, randomized trial of autologous bone marrow transplantation and chemotherapy in multiple myeloma. Intergroupe Français du Myelome. *N Engl J Med* 1996; **335:** 91–7.
10. Powles R, Raje N, Milan S et al. Outcome assessment of a population-based group of 195 unselected myeloma patients under 70 years of age offered intensive treatment. *Bone Marrow Transplant* 1997; **20:** 435–43.
11. Barlogie B, Jagannath S, Desikan KR et al. Total therapy with tandem transplants for newly diagnosed multiple myeloma. *Blood* 1999; **93:** 55–65.
12. Siegel DS, Desikan KR, Mehta J et al. Age is not a prognostic variable with autotransplants multiple myeloma. *Blood* 1999; **93:** 51–4.
13. Palumbo A, Triolo S, Argentino C et al. Dose-intensive melphalan with stem cell support (Mel100) is superior to standard treatment in elderly myeloma patients. *Blood* 1999; **94:** 1248–53.
14. Mehta J, Ayers D, Mattox S et al. High-dose melphalan and autotransplantation in myeloma with renal impairment: a matched-pair comparison with patients without renal failure. *Blood* 1997; **90**(Suppl 1): 419a.
15. Powles R, Sirohi B, Treleaven J et al. Continued first complete remission in multiple myeloma for over 10 years: a series of 'operationally cured' patients. *Blood* 2000; **96**(Suppl 1): abst 2215.
16. Barlogie B, Jagannath S, Vesole DH et al. Superiority of tandem autologous transplantation over standard therapy for previously untreated multiple myeloma. *Blood* 1997; **89:** 789–93.
17. Fermand JP, Chevret S, Ravaud P et al. High-dose chemoradiotherapy and autologous blood stem cell transplantation in multiple myeloma: results of a phase II trial involving 63 patients. *Blood* 1993; **82:** 2005–9.
18. Reece DE, Barnett MJ, Connors JM et al. Treatment of multiple myeloma with intensive chemotherapy followed by autologous BMT using marrow purged with 4-hydroperoxycyclophosphamide. *Bone Marrow Transplant* 1993; **11:** 139–46.

19. Dimopoulos MA, Alexanian R, Przepiorka D et al. Thiotepa, busulfan, and cyclophosphamide: a new preparative regimen for autologous marrow or blood stem cell transplantation in high-risk multiple myeloma. *Blood* 1993; **82:** 2324–8.
20. Björkstrand B, Goldstone AH, Ljungman P et al. Prognostic factors in autologous stem cell transplantation for multiple myeloma: an EBMT Registry Study. European Group for Bone Marrow Transplantation. *Leuk Lymphoma* 1994; **15:** 265–72.
21. Harousseau JL, Attal M, Divine M et al. Autologous stem cell transplantation after first remission induction treatment in multiple myeloma: a report of the French Registry on autologous transplantation in multiple myeloma. *Blood* 1995; **85:** 3077–85.
22. Cunningham D, Paz-Ares L, Milan S et al. High-dose melphalan and autologous bone marrow transplantation as consolidation in previously untreated myeloma. *J Clin Oncol* 1994; **12:** 759–63.
23. Seiden MV, Schlossman R, Andersen J et al. Monoclonal antibody-purged bone marrow transplantation therapy for multiple myeloma. *Leuk Lymphoma* 1995; **17:** 87–93.
24. Vesole DH, Tricot G, Jagannath S et al. Autotransplants in multiple myeloma: what have we learned? *Blood* 1996; **88:** 838–47.
25. Marit G, Faberes C, Pico JL et al. Autologous peripheral-blood progenitor-cell support following high-dose chemotherapy or chemoradiotherapy in patients with high-risk multiple myeloma. *J Clin Oncol* 1996; **14:** 1306–13.
26. Bensinger WI, Rowley SD, Demirer T et al. High-dose therapy followed by autologous hematopoietic stem-cell infusion for patients with multiple myeloma. *J Clin Oncol* 1996; **14:** 1447–56.
27. Alegre A, Diaz-Mediavilla J, San Miguel J et al. Autologous peripheral blood stem cell transplantation for multiple myeloma: a report of 259 cases from the Spanish Registry. Spanish Registry for Transplant in MM (Grupo Espanol de Trasplante Hematopoyetico–GETH) and PETHEMA. *Bone Marrow Transplant* 1998; **21:** 133–40.
28. Schiller G, Vescio R, Freytes C et al. Autologous CD34-selected blood progenitor cell transplants for patients with advanced multiple myeloma. *Bone Marrow Transplant* 1998; **21:** 141–5.
29. Barlogie B, Jagannath S, Naucke S et al. Long-term follow-up after high-dose therapy for high-risk multiple myeloma. *Bone Marrow Transplant* 1998; **21:** 1101–7.
30. Blade J, Samson D, Reece D et al. Criteria for evaluating disease response and progression in patients with multiple myeloma treated by high-dose therapy and haemopoietic stem cell transplantation. *Br J Haematol* 1998; **102:** 1115–23.
31. Alexanian R, Dimopoulos M, Smith T et al. Limited value of myeloablative therapy for late multiple myeloma. *Blood* 1994; 83:512–516.
32. Alexanian R, Dimopoulos MA, Hester J et al. Early myeloablative therapy for multiple myeloma. *Blood* 1994; **84:** 4278–82.
33. Harousseau JL, Attal M, Divine M et al. Comparison of autologous bone marrow transplantation and peripheral blood stem cell transplantation after first remission induction treatment in multiple myeloma. *Bone Marrow Transplant* 1995; **15:** 963–9.
34. Raje N, Powles R, Horton C et al. Comparison of marrow vs blood-derived stem cells for autografting in previously untreated multiple myeloma. *Br J Cancer* 1997; **75:** 1684–9.
35. Tricot G, Jagannath S, Vesole D et al. Peripheral blood stem cell transplants for multiple myeloma: identification of favorable variables for rapid engraftment in 225 patients. *Blood* 1995; **85:** 588–96.
36. Duncan N, Hewetson M, Powles R et al. An economic evaluation of peripheral blood stem cell transplantation as an alternative to autologous bone marrow transplantation in multiple myeloma. *Bone Marrow Transplant* 1996; **18:** 1175–8.
37. Henry JM, Sykes PJ, Brisco MJ et al. Comparison of myeloma cell contamination of bone marrow and peripheral blood stem cell harvests. *Br J Haematol* 1996; **92:** 614–9.
38. Millar BC, Millar JL, Bell JB et al. Role of CD34+ cells in engraftment after high-dose melphalan in multiple myeloma patients given peripheral blood stem cell rescue. *Bone Marrow Transplant* 1996; **18:** 871–8.
39. Goldschmidt H, Hegenbart U, Wallmeier M et al. Factors influencing collection of peripheral blood progenitor cells following high-dose cyclophosphamide and granulocyte colony-stimulating factor in patients with multiple myeloma. *Br J Haematol* 1997; **98:** 736–44.
40. Gertz MA, Lacy MQ, Inwards DJ et al. Factors influencing platelet recovery after blood cell transplantation in multiple myeloma. *Bone Marrow Transplant* 1997; **20:** 375–80.

41. Bensinger WI, Longin K, Appelbaum F et al. Peripheral blood stem cells (PBSCs) collected after recombinant granulocyte colony stimulating factor (rhG-CSF): an analysis of factors correlating with the tempo of engraftment after transplantation. *Br J Haematol* 1994; **87:** 825–31.
42. Singhal S, Mehta J, Desikan K et al. Collection of peripheral blood stem cells after a preceding autograft: unfavorable effect of prior interferon-α therapy. *Bone Marrow Transplant* 1999; **24:** 13–7.
43. Alegre A, Tomas JF, Martinez-Chamorro C et al. Comparison of peripheral blood progenitor cell mobilization in patients with multiple myeloma: high-dose cyclophosphamide plus GM-CSF vs G-CSF alone. *Bone Marrow Transplant* 1997; **20:** 211–7.
44. Desikan KR, Barlogie B, Jagannath S et al. Comparable engraftment kinetics following peripheral-blood stem-cell infusion mobilized with granulocyte colony-stimulating factor with or without cyclophosphamide in multiple myeloma. *J Clin Oncol* 1998; **16:** 1547–53.
45. Facon T, Harousseau JL, Maloisel F et al. Stem cell factor in combination with filgrastim after chemotherapy improves peripheral blood progenitor cell yield and reduces apheresis requirements in multiple myeloma patients: a randomized, controlled study. *Blood* 1999; **94:** 1218–25.
46. Gazitt Y, Tian E, Barlogie B et al. Differential mobilization of myeloma cells and normal hematopoietic stem cells in multiple myeloma after treatment with cyclophosphamide and granulocyte-macrophage colony-stimulating factor. *Blood* 1996; **87:** 805–11.
47. Lemoli RM, Fortuna A, Motta MR et al. Concomitant mobilization of plasma cells and hematopoietic progenitors into peripheral blood of multiple myeloma patients: positive selection and transplantation of enriched CD34+ cells to remove circulating tumor cells. *Blood* 1996; **87:** 1625–34.
48. Vesole DH, Barlogie B, Jagannath S et al. High-dose therapy for refractory multiple myeloma: improved prognosis with better supportive care and double transplants. *Blood* 1994; **84:** 950–6.
49. Mansi J, Da Costa F, Viner C et al. High-dose busulfan in patients with myeloma. *J Clin Oncol* 1992; **10:** 1569–73.
50. Long GD, Chao NJ, Hu WW et al. High dose etoposide-based myeloablative therapy followed by autologous blood progenitor cell rescue in the treatment of multiple myeloma. *Cancer* 1996; **78:** 2502–9.
51. Desikan KR, Fassas A, Siegel D et al. Superior outcome with melphalan 200 mg/m^2 (Mel 200) for scheduled second autotransplant compared with Mel + TBI or CTX for myeloma (MM) in pre-Tx2 PR. *Blood* 1997; **90**(Suppl 1): 231a.
52. Mehta J, Jagannath S, Tricot G et al. High-dose chemotherapy with carboplatin, cyclophosphamide and etoposide and autologous transplantation for multiple myeloma relapsing after a previous transplant. *Bone Marrow Transplant* 1997; **20:** 113–6.
53. Bayouth JE, Macey DJ, Boyer AL, Champlin RE. Radiation dose distribution within the bone marrow of patients receiving holmium-166-labeled-phosphonate for marrow ablation. *Med Phys* 1995; **22:** 743–53.
54. Moreau P, Kergueris MF, Milpied N et al. A pilot study of 220 mg/m^2 melphalan followed by autologous stem cell transplantation in patients with advanced haematological malignancies: pharmacokinetics and toxicity. *Br J Haematol* 1996; **95:** 527–30.
55. Pinguet F, Martel P, Fabbro M et al. Pharmacokinetics of high-dose intravenous melphalan in patients undergoing peripheral blood hematopoietic progenitor-cell transplantation. *Anticancer Res* 1997; **17:** 605–11.
56. Singhal S, Powles R, Treleaven J et al. Melphalan alone prior to allogeneic bone marrow transplantation from HLA-identical sibling donors for hematologic malignancies: alloengraftment with potential preservation of fertility. *Bone Marrow Transplant* 1996; **18:** 1049–55.
57. Gertz MA, Witzig TE, Pineda AA et al. Monoclonal plasma cells in the blood stem cell harvest from patients with multiple myeloma are associated with shortened relapse-free survival after transplantation. *Bone Marrow Transplant* 1997; **19:** 337–42.
58. Bensinger WI, Demirer T, Buckner CD et al. Syngeneic marrow transplantation in patients with multiple myeloma. *Bone Marrow Transplant* 1996; **18:** 527–31.
59. Gahrton G, Svensson H, Björkstrand B et al. Syngeneic bone marrow transplantation in multiple myeloma. *Bone Marrow Transplant* 1997; **19**(Suppl 1): S88.
60. Mehta J, Singhal S. Graft-versus-myeloma. *Bone Marrow Transplant* 1998; **22:** 835–43.

61. Vescio R, Schiller G, Stewart AK et al. Multicenter phase III trial to evaluate CD34(+) selected versus unselected autologous peripheral blood progenitor cell transplantation in multiple myeloma. *Blood* 1999; **93:** 1858–68.
62. Gupta D, Bybee A, Cooke F et al. CD34+-selected peripheral blood progenitor cell transplantation in patients with multiple myeloma: tumour cell contamination and outcome. *Br J Haematol* 1999; **104:** 166–77.
63. Voso MT, Hohaus S, Moos M et al. Autografting with CD34+ peripheral blood stem cells: retained engraftment capability and reduced tumour cell content. *Br J Haematol* 1999; **104:** 382–91.
64. Thunberg U, Banghagen M, Bengtsson M et al. Linear reduction of clonal cells in stem cell enriched grafts in transplanted multiple myeloma. *Br J Haematol* 1999; **104:** 546–52.
65. Tricot G, Gazitt Y, Leemhuis T et al. Collection, tumor contamination, and engraftment kinetics of highly purified hematopoietic progenitor cells to support high dose therapy in multiple myeloma. *Blood* 1998; **91:** 4489–95.
66. Stewart AK, Vescio R, Schiller G et al. Purging of autologous peripheral-blood stem cells using CD34 selection does not improve overall or progression-free survival after high-dose chemotherapy for multiple myeloma: Results of a multicenter randomized controlled trial. *J Clin Oncol* 2001; **19**: 3771–9.
67. Siegel D, Mehta J, Anaissie E et al. Prolonged immunosuppression after CD34+ or CD34+/Thy-1+/Lin- selected autologous peripheral blood stem cell (PBSC) transplants (Tx) for multiple myeloma. *Blood* 1997; **90**(Suppl 1): 112a.
68. Rossi JF, Legouffe E, Fegueux N et al. Autologous transplantation (AT) of CD34+ peripheral blood progenitor cells (PBPC) after double (D) high dose chemotherapy (HDC) in multiple myeloma (MM) is followed by severe immunodeficiency (ID) and high production of interleukin-6 (IL-6)-related C-reactive protein (CRP) requiring additive immunotherapy (IT). *Blood* 1996; **88**(Suppl 1): 132a.
69. Freytes CO, Stewart AK, Vescio R et al. CD34 selection did not delay immune recovery nor increase frequency of infections in multiple myeloma patients transplanted on a phase III trial. *Blood* 1998; **92**(Suppl 1): 660a.
70. Mehta J, Powles R. The future of bone marrow transplantation. In: *Clinical Bone Marrow and Stem Cell Transplantation: A Reference Textbook*, 2nd edn (Atkinson K, ed). Cambridge: Cambridge University Press, 2000: 1457–65.
71. Tricot G, Barlogie B, Jagannath S et al. Poor prognosis in multiple myeloma is associated only with partial or complete deletions of chromosome 13 or abnormalities involving 11q and not with other karyotype abnormalities. *Blood* 1995; **86:** 4250–6.
72. Tricot G, Sawyer JR, Jagannath S et al. Unique role of cytogenetics in the prognosis of patients with myeloma receiving high-dose therapy and autotransplants. *J Clin Oncol* 1997; **15:** 2659–66.
73. Rajkumar SV, Fonseca R, Lacy MQ et al. Abnormal cytogenetics predict poor survival after high-dose therapy and autologous blood cell transplantation in multiple myeloma. *Bone Marrow Transplant* 1999; **24:** 497–503.
74. Mehta J, Singhal S, Desikan K et al. High-dose therapy and stem cell support in myeloma. In: *PPO Updates*, Vol 13 (De Vita VT Jr, Hellman S, Rosenberg SA, eds). Philadelphia: Lippincott Williams & Wilkins, 1999; 1–12.
75. Singhal S, Mehta J, Jagannath S, Barlogie B. Hematopoietic stem cell transplantation for myeloma. In: *Current Therapy in Cancer*, 2nd edn (Foley JF, Vose JM, Armitage JO, eds). Philadelphia: WB Saunders, 1999: 475–84.
76. Kergueris MF, Milpied N, Moreau P et al. Pharmacokinetics of high-dose melphalan in adults: influence of renal function. *Anticancer Res* 1994; **14:** 2379–82.
77. Ballester OF, Tummala R, Janssen WE et al. High-dose chemotherapy and autologous peripheral blood stem cell transplantation in patients with multiple myeloma and renal insufficiency. *Bone Marrow Transplant* 1997; **20:** 653–6.
78. Govindarajan R, Jagannath S, Flick JT et al. Preceding standard therapy is the likely cause of MDS after autotransplants for multiple myeloma. *Br J Haematol* 1996; **95:** 349–53.
79. Drach J, Ayers D, Govindarajan R et al. MDS-associated cytogenetic abnormalities (CGA) in both hematopoietic and neoplastic cells after autotransplants (AT) in 868 patients with multiple myeloma (MM). *Blood* 1998; **92** (Suppl 1): 97a.
80. Saso R, Kulkarni S, Powles R et al. Secondary MDS/AML in patients treated for myeloma. *Blood* 1998; **92**(Suppl 1): 455a.
81. Singhal S, Mehta J. Reimmunization after blood or marrow stem cell transplantation. *Bone Marrow Transplant* 1999; **23:** 637–46.

82. Fermand JP, Ravaud P, Chevret S et al. High-dose therapy and autologous peripheral blood stem cell transplantation in multiple myeloma: up-front or rescue treatment? Results of a multicenter sequential randomized clinical trial. *Blood* 1998; **92:** 3131–6.
83. Tricot G, Jagannath S, Vesole DH et al. Relapse of multiple myeloma after autologous transplantation: survival after salvage therapy. *Bone Marrow Transplant* 1995; **16:** 7–11.
84. Mehta J, Tricot G, Jagannath S et al. Salvage autologous or allogeneic transplantation for multiple myeloma refractory to or relapsing after a first-line autograft? *Bone Marrow Transplant* 1998; **21:** 887–92.
85. Kulkarni S, Powles R, Singhal S et al. Second autografts for relapsed multiple myeloma: Is tandem autotransplantation better? *Blood* 1998; **92**(Suppl 1): 344b.
86. Singhal S, Mehta J, Hood S et al. Third transplants for myeloma relapsing after two prior autografts. *Blood* 1997; **90**(Suppl 1): 547a.
87. Cunningham D, Powles R, Malpas J et al. A randomized trial of maintenance interferon following high-dose chemotherapy in multiple myeloma: long-term follow-up results. *Br J Haematol* 1998; **102:** 495–502.
88. Singhal S, Powles R, Milan S et al. Kinetics of paraprotein clearance after autografting for multiple myeloma. *Bone Marrow Transplant* 1995; **16:** 537–40.
89. Salmon SE, Crowley JJ, Balcerzak SP et al. Interferon versus interferon plus prednisone remission maintenance therapy for multiple myeloma: a Southwest Oncology Group Study. *J Clin Oncol* 1998; **16:** 890–6.
90. Singhal S, Mehta J, Desikan R et al. Anti-tumor activity of thalidomide in refractory multiple myeloma. *N Engl J Med* 1999; **341**: 1565–71.
91. Rajkumar SV, Fonseca R, Witzig TE et al. Bone marrow angiogenesis in patients achieving complete response after stem cell transplantation for multiple myeloma. *Leukemia* 1999; **13:** 469–72.
92. Desikan R, Siegel D, Fassas A et al. DCEP consolidation after tandem autotransplants in (AT) in high risk multiple myeloma (MM) – improved prognosis compared to matched historical controls. *Blood* 1998; **92**(Suppl 1): 660a.
93. Powles R, Sirohi B, Kulkarni S et al. Acute lymphoblastic leukemia-type intensive chemotherapy to eliminate minimal residual disease after high-dose melphalan and autologous transplantation in multiple myeloma – a phase I/II feasibility and tolerance study of 17 patients. *Bone Marrow Transplant* 2000; **25**: 949–56.
94. Giralt S, Weber D, Colome M et al. Phase I trial of cyclosporine-induced autologous graft-versus-host disease in patients with multiple myeloma undergoing high-dose chemotherapy with autologous stem-cell rescue. *J Clin Oncol* 1997; **15:** 667–73.
95. Byrne JL, Carter GI, Ellis I et al. Autologous GVHD following PBSCT, with evidence for a graft-versus-myeloma effect. *Bone Marrow Transplant* 1997; **20:** 517–20.
96. Osterborg A, Yi Q, Bergenbrant S et al. Idiotype-specific T cells in multiple myeloma stage I: an evaluation by four different functional tests. *Br J Haematol* 1995; **89:** 110–6.
97. MacKenzie M, Strang G, Peshwa M et al. Phase I/II trial of immunotherapy with idiotype-loaded autologous dendritic cells (APC8020) for refractory multiple myeloma. *Blood* 1998; **92**(Suppl 1): 108a.
98. Reichardt VL, Okada CY, Liso A et al. Idiotype vaccination using dendritic cells after autologous peripheral blood stem cell transplantation for multiple myeloma – a feasibility study. *Blood* 1999; **93:** 2411–19.
99. Kulkarni S, Powles RL, Treleaven JG et al. Impact of previous high-dose therapy on outcome after allografting for multiple myeloma. *Bone Marrow Transplant* 1999; **23:** 675–80.

20

Allogeneic hematopoietic stem cell transplantation in myeloma

Jayesh Mehta

INTRODUCTION

High-dose chemotherapy without[1] or with[2] autologous hematopoietic stem cell support improves complete remission (CR) rates and survival in myeloma. A small minority do survive long term ('operational cure'),[3] but there is no evidence that there is a true cure, because relapses have been described even in the minority of patients who have been in remission for a decade following high-dose therapy[3–6] (see Chapter 19).

However, allogeneic transplantation in myeloma results in molecular remission of the disease as well as long-term survival in a minority of patients. This points to the existence of immunologic graft-versus-tumor effects ('graft-versus-myeloma', GVM), which can eradicate residual disease and potentially result in a cure.[7,8]

Allogeneic transplantation has been used in myeloma for over 15 years now.[9–13] However, despite its curative potential, allogeneic transplantation has been utilized sparingly in myeloma until recently because of very poor results.

While it has been argued that myeloma patients are unusually susceptible to toxicity of an allograft, it is far likelier that poor patient selection has been responsible for unacceptable results. Allogeneic transplantation has been reserved for patients with terminal disease, who typically have organ dysfunction and a poor performance status – factors that increase treatment-related mortality dramatically.

Of course, prolonged exposure to steroids and compromised pulmonary function due to collapsed vertebrae, which is unique to myeloma, also probably contribute to some extent to increased toxicity.[14]

The recent improvement in results is attributable to better patient selection, improved supportive care, and modified conditioning regimens, which we have advocated repeatedly.[4–8,14–17]

GRAFT-VERSUS-MYELOMA

An attempt was made to harness GVM over a decade ago at the Hadassah University Hospital in Jerusalem, when a patient with recurrent multiple extramedullary plasmacytomas and IgA paraprotein, who had relapsed after conventional chemotherapy, underwent a T-cell-depleted allograft from her HLA-identical brother. The transplant was followed by donor leukocyte infusions (DLI) in graded increments at weekly intervals to elicit GVM. Although no graft-versus-host disease (GVHD) was seen, CR was attained 6 weeks after transplantation.[18] The patient remains alive in continuous CR 12 years post transplant (Shimon Slavin, personal communication).

Multiple lines of clinical and laboratory evidence support the existence of GVM:

- Allogeneic transplantation results in relapse rates that are significantly lower than those seen after autotransplantation (Figure 20.1) in patients with biologically comparable disease.[15,19,20]
- A plateau has been observed in relapse rates (Figure 20.1)[15] and survival[20] after allografts but not after autografts.
- Achievement of molecular CR is significantly more frequent after allogeneic than autologous transplantation, despite comparable conditioning regimens.[21,22]
- Myeloma relapsing after allogeneic transplantation has been brought under control once again through the use of cell- or cytokine-mediated immunotherapy to stimulate graft-versus-tumor effects.[7,8,23–26]

CLINICAL RESULTS OF CONVENTIONAL TRANSPLANTATION

Until recently, myeloma patients were always allografted using regimens and techniques that were similar to those employed for leukemia. These intensive regimens aimed to cause myeloablation and severe immunosuppression to permit engraftment of allogeneic cells. The intensity of the regimens was, in large part, responsible for the poor results of conventional allogeneic transplantation in myeloma (Table 20.1).

As Table 20.1 shows, the results of conventional allografts in myeloma are variable, with

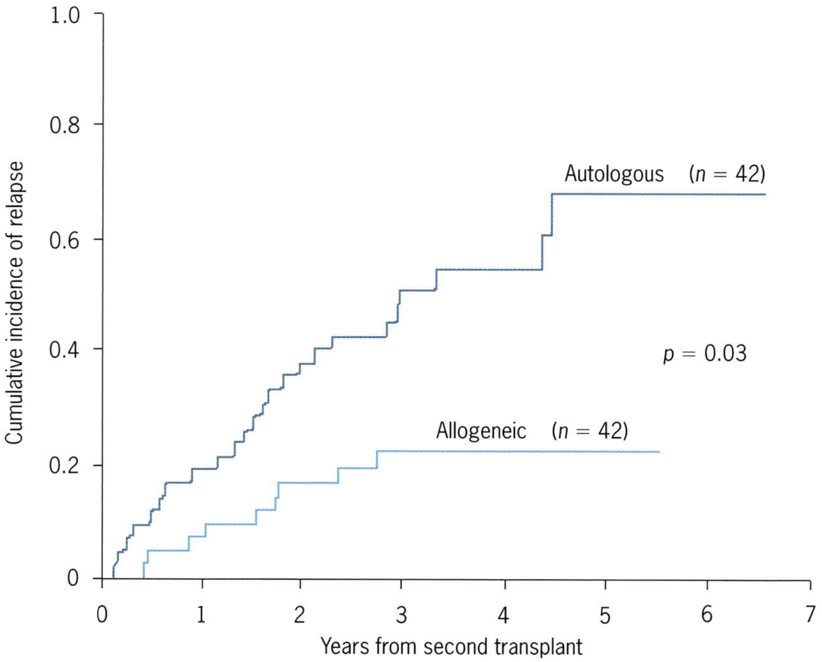

Figure 20.1 Evidence of graft-versus-myeloma: comparison of relapse rates after autologous blood stem cell and allogeneic bone marrow transplantation in patients with disease progression after a preceding autograft. (Used with permission from Mehta J, Tricot G, Jagannath S et al. Salvage autologous or allogeneic transplantation for multiple myeloma refractory to or relapsing after a first-line autograft? *Bone Marrow Transplant* 1998; **21:** 887–92.)

Table 20.1 Results of conventional allogeneic transplantation in myeloma

Authors	No. of patients	Median age (years)	Previous autograft	Source of cells	T-cell depletion	Conditioning regimen (variable doses)[a]	Transplant-related deaths	Progressive disease	Event-free survival	Overall survival	Comments
Bensinger et al[27]	80	44	None	Marrow	1%	71% Bu-Cy 29% Bu-Cy-TBI	58%	40% at 4 yrs	20% at 4 yrs	24% at 4 yrs	6% mismatched and 11% unrelated donors
Cavo et al[28]	19	43	None	Marrow	16%	Bu-Cy	37%	42%	21% at 4 yrs	26% at 4 yrs	
Couban et al[29]	22	43	None	Marrow (91%) Blood (9%)	No	59% Cy-TBI 36% Bu-Cy 5% Mel-TBI	59%	23% at 3 yrs	22% at 3 yrs	32% at 3 yrs	Age at diagnosis
Gahrton et al[30]	162	43	Not specified	Marrow	55%	Variable 72% with TBI 28% without TBI	25%	Not specified	34% at 6 yrs for the 72 patients in CR post BMT	32% at 4 yrs	Retrospective multicenter analysis from EBMT
Huff et al[31]	51	49	None	Marrow	100%	Bu-Cy	24%	51%	20% at 4 yrs	59%	
Kulkarni et al[16]	33	38	36%	Marrow (88%) Blood (12%)	3%	67% Mel-TBI 15% other with Mel 18% other without Mel	55%	6%	36% at 3 yrs	36% at 3 yrs	3% haploidentical and 12% unrelated donors
Majolino et al[32]	10	45	40%	Blood	No	90% Bu-Mel 10% Bu-Cy	20%	10%	70%	80%	Prior autografts done after intermediate-dose therapy
Mehta et al[15]	97	45	68%	Marrow	29%	36% with TBI 64% without TBI	54% at 3 yrs	60% at 3yrs	12% at 3 yrs	18% at 3yrs	18% unrelated donors
Reece et al[33]	26	48	4%	Marrow	No	54% Bu-Mel-Cy 31% Bu-Cy 15% Cy-TBI	31%	19%	40% at 3 yrs	47% at 3 yrs	12% mismatched and 15% unrelated donors
Russell et al[34]	13	49	None	Marrow (92%) Blood (8%)	No	92% Mel-TBI 8% Cy-TBI	23%	8%	67% at 3 yrs	67% at 3 yrs	
Seiden et al[35]	21	43	None	Marrow	100%	90% Cy-TBI	10%	57%	33% at 2 yrs	60% at 2 yrs	

[a] Bu, busulfan; Cy, cyclophosphamide; Mel, melphalan; TBI, total-body irradiation.

the treatment-related mortality rate varying from 10% to almost 60%. The likelihood of disease progression as well as disease-free and overall survival are highly variable too. Prognostic factors that have been found to affect the outcome of allogeneic transplantation are shown in Table 20.2. The patient populations reported in the studies summarized in Table 20.1 were quite heterogeneous with respect to the prognostic factors outlined in Table 20.2, and also employed differing sources of stem cells, conditioning regimens, modes of GVHD prophylaxis, and supportive therapy. These factors explain the variable results reported.[15,16,27–36]

Some of the reports summarized in Table 20.1 are discussed further here.

The Seattle group[27] reported on 80 myeloma patients who were conditioned with busulfan–cyclophosphamide with or without total-body irradiation (TBI) and received marrow from allogeneic donors. Seventy-one percent of the patients had refractory disease. Forty-six patients (58%) died of treatment-related causes, 35 within the first 100 days. The actuarial probabilities of survival and event-free survival at 4 years were 24% and 20%, respectively. Achievement of CR after the transplant, seen in 36% of the patients, resulted in better overall (50%) and event-free (43%) survival. Longer diagnosis–transplant intervals were associated with higher treatment-related mortality and lower survival, higher β_2-microglobulin levels with lower survival, stage III disease with lower event-free survival, and increasing extent of prior therapy and donor–recipient sex mismatch (female patients with male donors) with higher relapse rates in multivariate analysis. The extent of prior therapy was crucial, because patients transplanted within a year of diagnosis had a treatment-related mortality rate of under 20%.

Table 20.2 Factors adversely affecting the outcome of allogeneic transplantation in myeloma

Advanced Durie–Salmon stage
Extensive prior therapy
High β_2-microglobulin
High lactate dehydrogenase (LDH)
Long diagnosis–transplant interval
Low albumin
Prior autograft
Refractory disease
Renal dysfunction

Cavo et al[28] treated 19 patients with 16 mg/kg busulfan and 200 mg/kg cyclophosphamide, followed by allogeneic bone marrow transplantation (BMT). Two-thirds of the patients had resistant disease. The transplant-related mortality rate was 37%, and 42% achieved CR. The actuarial probabilities of survival and event-free survival at 4 years were 26% and 21%, respectively. The outcome of patients with chemosensitive disease was superior, with a treatment-related mortality rate of 14%, an overall CR rate of 86%, and an actuarial 4-year event-free survival rate of 57%.

In a report from the European Blood and Marrow Transplant Group (EBMT) spanning procedures performed between 1983 and 1993,[30] allogeneic BMT from HLA-matched siblings in 162 patients was associated with a remission rate of 44%. One-fourth of the patients died of toxicity. The overall survival rate of 32% at 4 years declined to 28% at 7 years. However, patients in CR at the time of BMT had a 3-year survival rate of 64%, and those in CR after BMT had an event-free survival rate of 34% at 6 years. Female sex, stage I disease at diagnosis, limited prior treatment, CR at the time of BMT, IgA disease, and low β_2-microglobulin level were associated with a favorable outcome. Attainment of CR after BMT was also associated with good outcome, whereas the development of grade III–IV acute GVHD influenced the survival adversely.

The Johns Hopkins group[31] employed elutriation to deplete T cells prior to allogeneic BMT in 51 patients from June 1991 to April 2000. The conditioning regimen was busulfan (16 mg/kg) and cyclophosphamide (200 mg/kg). Thirteen patients developed GVHD, and two died of GVHD. Overall, 12 patients died of treatment-related causes. Of the 39 surviving patients, 26 relapsed at a median of one year. There was a trend for patients who developed GVHD to do better: patients with GVHD had an event-free survival rate of 40% at 40 months, versus 18% at 40 months for patients without GVHD.

The UK Royal Marsden Hospital group[16] reported that previous high-dose chemotherapy and autotransplantation affected the outcome of allogeneic transplantation adversely because of significantly higher treatment-related mortality (Figure 20.2) and lower survival (Figure 20.3). Renal function as measured by EDTA clearance also affected outcome, with significantly poorer survival amongst patients with EDTA clearance under 100 ml/min/1.73 m^2. This group updated their experience recently,[36] confining the analysis to 18 patients receiving peripheral blood stem cells (PBSC) after melphalan–TBI (16 patients) or busulfan–cyclophosphamide (2 patients). Ten of these patients had been autografted previously. Treatment-related mortality occurred in 7 (39%), and was significantly higher with prior autograft and low albumin.

The Arkansas group[15] allografted 97 patients between 1988 and 1996, two-thirds after one or two preceding autografts. Thirty-one percent of the patients died of toxicity within 2 months, and the overall treatment-related mortality rate was about 50%. Most deaths occurred as a result of infections or GVHD. The overall response rate was 57%. Thirty-one percent experienced disease progression at a median of 5 months post transplant, most dying of progressive disease or toxicity of further therapy. At the time of the report, 25 patients (26%) were alive, including 19 patients in continuous CR or partial remission (PR). The use of TBI-containing conditioning regimens and elevated lactate dehydrogenase (LDH) were associated with higher treatment-related mortality and poorer overall survival. Patients with refractory disease and those with elevated β_2-microglobulin levels also had higher treatment-related mortality. Those with low albumin levels and refractory disease had a higher probability of disease progression.

Reece et al[33] evaluated 65 myeloma patients aged 55 years or less over a 6-year period for allogeneic transplantation, and 26 of these were actually allografted. Only 3 of those not allografted

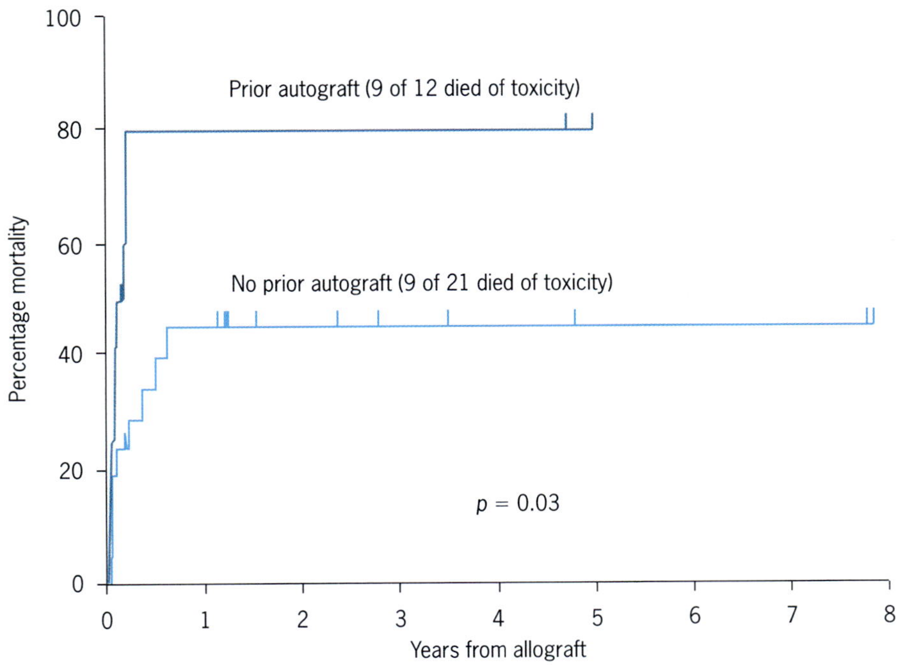

Figure 20.2 Effect of prior high-dose therapy (autograft or non-myeloablative high-dose melphalan) on treatment-related mortality after allogeneic bone marrow transplantation. (Data from the Royal Marsden Hospital, UK; courtesy of Professor Ray Powles.)

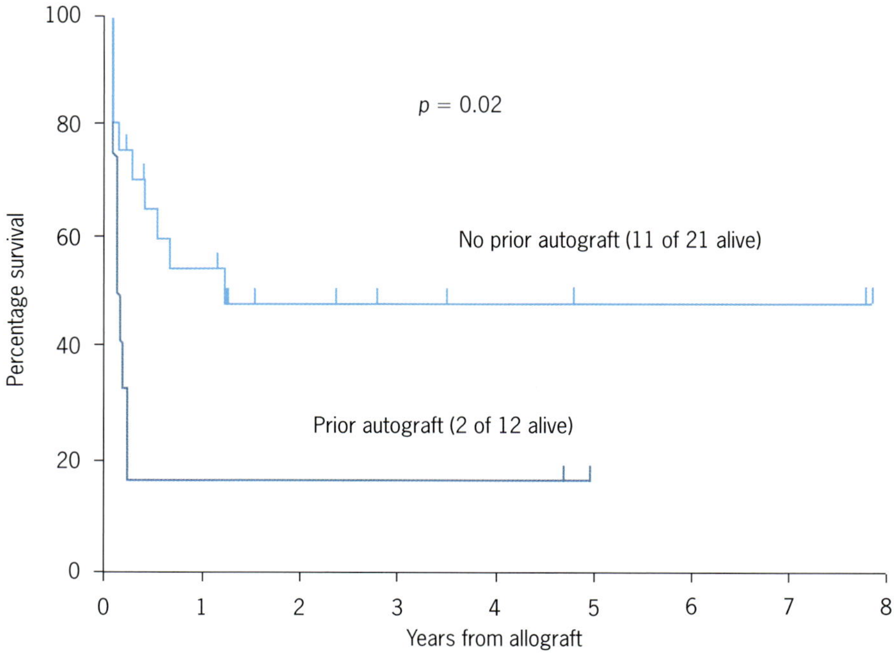

Figure 20.3 Effect of prior high-dose therapy (autograft or non-myeloablative high-dose melphalan) on overall survival after allogeneic bone marrow transplantation (Data from the Royal Marsden Hospital, UK; courtesy of Professor Ray Powles.)

were excluded because of medical reasons (renal dysfunction and amyloidosis[37]). Over 80% of patients had chemosensitive disease. Grade II–IV acute GVHD was seen in 20 patients. Six patients died of acute or chronic GVHD. The event-free survival rate was 52% at 3 years in patients with sensitive disease, compared with 0% in those with resistant disease ($p = 0.007$).

The Dana-Farber group[35] reported 21 patients with chemosensitive disease who underwent BMT from HLA-identical siblings. The marrow was depleted of T cells with an anti-CD6 monoclonal antibody. Two patients died of toxicity, 81% responded (33% CR), and 62% were alive at a median of 20 months. Selective T-cell depletion resulted in the elimination of GVHD as a significant cause of problems; only two patients developed severe GVHD, and no deaths were attributable to GVHD.

An International Bone Marrow Transplant Registry (IBMTR) analysis[38] of 247 patients allografted between 1988 and 1993 showed a 5-year survival rate of 24%. Better performance status and sensitive disease were associated with higher survival, whereas TBI and diagnosis-transplant interval had no impact on survival. No data were available on toxic deaths or disease progression.

CLINICAL RESULTS OF NON-MYELOABLATIVE TRANSPLANTATION

Slavin et al[39] showed that reduction in the intensity of the conditioning regimen could ameliorate treatment-related toxicity and mortality without compromising engraftment of allogeneic cells. These non-myeloablative transplants, because of the ease with which they can be performed, have become increasingly popular. Their attraction in a disease such as myeloma, where results of conventional allografts have been poor, is obvious.

However, apart from demonstrating successful engraftment and short-term disease control, available data support no other conclusions. The exact place of non-myeloablative transplants in clinical practice remains to be determined.

Table 20.3 shows reported results of non-myeloablative transplants in myeloma reported at the 42nd Annual Meeting of the American Society of Hematology.

Table 20.3 Primary results of non-myeloablative ('mini') allografts in myeloma presented in abstract form[a]

Authors	No. of patients	Median age	Previous autograft	Conditioning regimen[b]	GVHD prophylaxis[c]	Response rate[d]	Transplant-related deaths	Progressive disease	Overall survival	Comments
Badros et al[40]	16	57	100%	Mel	CsA	44% CR/NRC 13% PR	19%	38%		Multiple stem cell infusions described elsewhere[7,41] (Figure 20.3)
Lalancette et al[43]	50	48		Variable	Variable	33% CR 35% PR	32%	13% at 1 yr	40% at 2 yrs	12% unrelated donors. CR/PR rates exclude patients in CR/PR at the time of transplantation, respectively
Molina et al[43]	12	49	100% (planned)	TBI	CsA-MMF	50% CR 33% PR	17%	8%	75%	The contribution of the preceding autograft to response was not specified
Peggs et al[44]	23	47	43%	Mel-Flu-Campath-1H		18% CR	17% at 1 yr	42% at 1 yr	62% at 1 yr	26% unrelated donors. CR rate excludes 2 patients in CR at the time of transplantation
Schaefer et al[45]	22	54	86%	TBI-Cy-Flu	CsA-ATG	38% PR	32%			73% unrelated donors

[a] These studies were presented at the 42nd Annual Meeting of the American Society of Hematology. Information on vital factors such as conditioning regimens, GVHD prophylaxis, and stem cell source was limited and variable.

[b] Mel, melphalan; TBI, total-body irradiation; Flu, fludarabine; Cy, cyclophosphamide.

[c] CsA, cyclosporine; MMF, mycophenolate mofetil; ATG, anti-thymocyte globulin.

[d] CR, complete remission;

[e] The status of patients with persistent (but not progressive) disease is not clarified in most reports. The disease progression figure probably excludes such patients.

We have developed a novel non-myeloablative transplant protocol ('microallograft'),[7,41] which has been utilized successfully in a number of myeloma patients. Figure 20.4 shows the protocol scheme. The unique aspect of this protocol is the repeated infusion of stem cells, which may compensate for the minimal cytoreduction by exerting a powerful GVM effect. We have recently added mycophenolate mofetil to this. Additional cyclophosphamide (50 mg/kg) is administered to patients who have not previously been autografted.

COMPARISON OF AUTOLOGOUS AND ALLOGENEIC TRANSPLANTATION

A number of retrospective analyses comparing autografts and allografts in myeloma have shown higher treatment-related mortality, lower relapse, and poorer survival with allogeneic transplantation.[14,19,20,46]

On behalf of the EBMT, Björkstrand et al[19] compared 189 allografted myeloma patients with 189 autograft recipients who were matched on the basis of sex and the number of lines of therapy pre transplant, although allografted patients were younger. The treatment-related mortality rate was significantly higher in the allograft group (41% versus 13% at 3 years; $p = 0.0001$), and the rate of disease progression lower (50% versus 70% at 4 years; $p = 0.04$). The overall survival rate was significantly better after autografting (50% versus 40% at 3 years; $p = 0.001$); but the survival advantage was confined to males. Interestingly, because of fewer events in the allograft group beyond a year, amongst patients alive at 1 year, allograft recipients had better event-free and overall survival.

In a three-center study, Varterasian et al[20] compared 24 autografted patients with 24 allografted patients. The treatment-related mortality rate was 12.5% in the autograft group and 25% in the allograft group. With a limited median follow-up of just over a year, there was no difference in overall or event-free survival between the groups. However, there appeared to be a plateau in survival in the allografted patients, whereas none was seen in the autograft group.

A rigorous comparison of autologous and allogeneic transplantation in myeloma was reported by Mehta et al.[14] In this single-center comparison, 42 patients who had received 200 mg/m^2 melphalan followed by an autograft and had not attained a partial remission or had experienced disease progression after the autograft were studied. These patients underwent allogeneic transplantation as salvage therapy, and were compared with 42 pair-matched controls who underwent salvage autotransplantation under identical conditions after having failed an initial autograft. The groups were well matched for critical prognostic factors such as albumin, C-reactive protein, creatinine, disease sensitivity, duration of standard therapy prior to the first transplant, Ig isotype, karyotype, LDH, and response to the first transplant. The allografted patients were younger, had lower β_2-microglobulin, and had a longer interval between the two

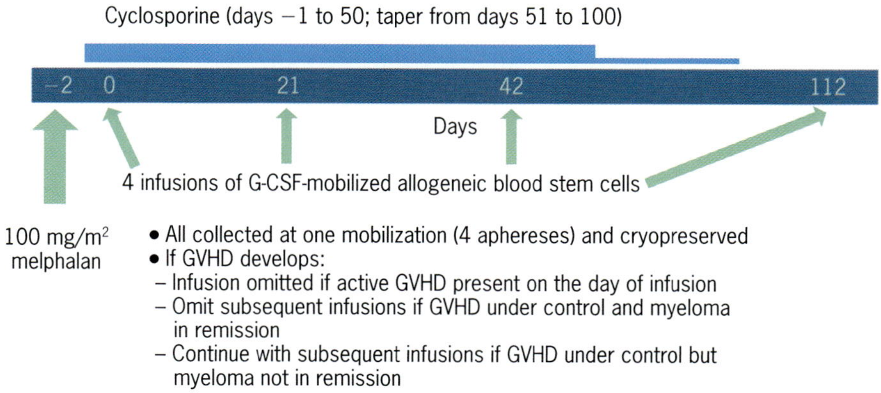

Figure 20.4
Microallograft for myeloma.[7,41] See also text. (G-CSF, granulocyte colony-stimulating factor.)

transplants. Amongst evaluable patients (alive at least 2 months after transplantation), the CR rate was 53% after allogeneic and 36% after autologous transplantation ($p = 0.15$). The 3-year probability of disease progression was significantly lower after allogeneic transplantation (31% versus 72%; $p = 0.03$; Figure 20.1), but the 1-year probability of treatment-related mortality was significantly higher amongst allograft recipients (43% versus 10%; $p = 0.0001$; Figure 20.5). Because both groups had a high incidence of one of the two forms of treatment failure, the event-free survival rates were comparable (25% after autografting and 20% after allografting; Figure 20.6a). However, since relapsed myeloma patients can still live for a period of time after disease progression, the 3-year probability of survival was significantly higher after autotransplantation (54% versus 29%; $p = 0.01$; Figure 20.6b). It was noteworthy that no progression was seen in the allograft group beyond 20 months, whereas progressive disease continued to be seen amongst autografted patients more than 4 years following the transplant (Figure 20.1).

A retrospective comparison of syngeneic transplantation with autologous and allogeneic transplantation in myeloma from the EBMT[46] found that response rates were comparable for all three. However, relapse rates after syngeneic and allogeneic transplantation were lower than those seen after autotransplantation. The overall and event-free survival rates with syngeneic transplantation were better than those with autologous and allogeneic transplantation.

Corradini et al[21] showed that amongst patients in CR by conventional criteria after high-dose therapy and transplantation, only 7% of the autografted patients attained molecular remission. In comparison, 50% of the allografted patients achieved molecular remission. These findings were confirmed by Martinelli et al.[22] These observations are important, because eradication of all detectable disease using sensitive techniques would appear to be a natural prerequisite for cure.

The development of myelodysplasia and secondary acute myeloid leukemia (AML) is a long-term complication of myeloma therapy, especially autotransplantation, which has been seen by the Arkansas group at an extraordinarily

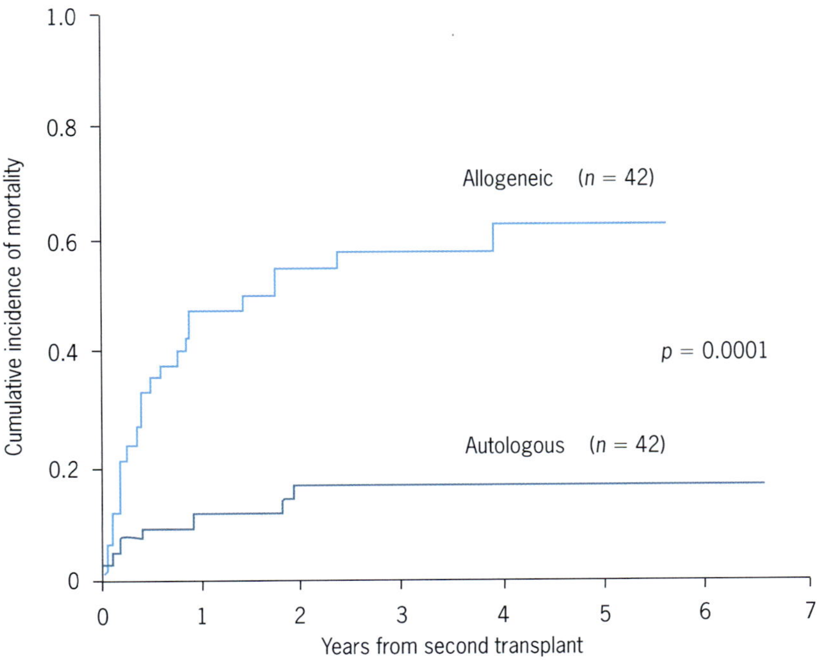

Figure 20.5
Comparison of treatment-related mortality after autologous blood stem cell and allogeneic bone marrow transplantation with disease progression after a preceding autograft. (Used with permission from Mehta J, Tricot G, Jagannath S et al. Salvage autologous or allogeneic transplantation for multiple myeloma refractory to or relapsing after a first-line autograft? *Bone Marrow Transplant* 1998; **21:** 887–92.)

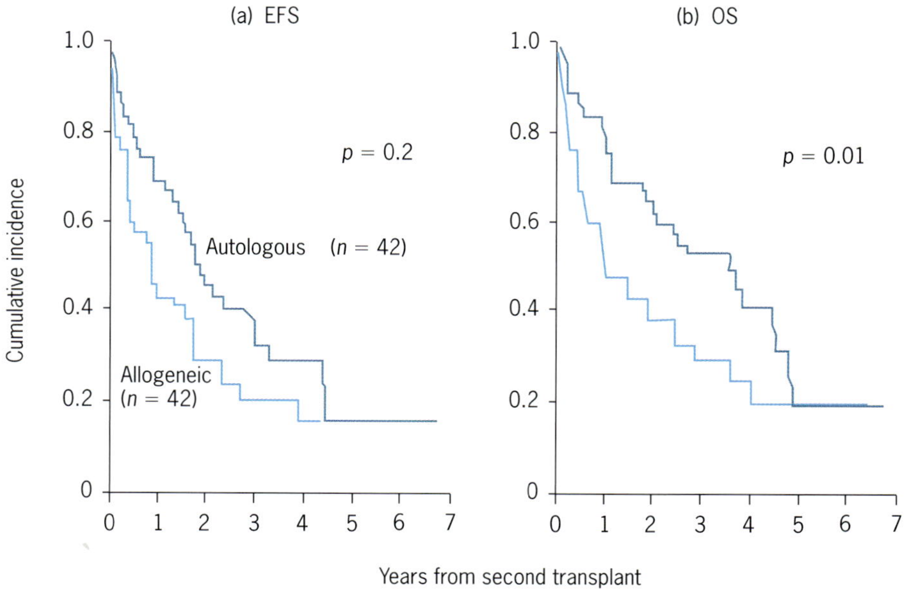

Figure 20.6 Comparison of event-free survival (a) and overall survival (b) after autologous blood stem cell and allogeneic bone marrow transplantation with disease progression after a preceding autograft. (Used with permission from Mehta J, Tricot G, Jagannath S et al. Salvage autologous or allogeneic transplantation for multiple myeloma refactory to or relapsing after a first line autograft? *Bone Marrow Transplant* 1998; **21:** 887–92.)

high frequency.[47,48] Another potential advantage of allogeneic transplantation is that the replacement of the chemotherapy-treated host hematopoietic system by an untreated normal-donor hematopoietic system will almost certainly eliminate this complication.

ENHANCING GRAFT-VERSUS-MYELOMA

Source of allogeneic cells

The use of PBSC has been found to reduce relapse rates compared with marrow[49] in patients with hematologic malignancies, including myeloma. Substitution of marrow with blood as the source of allogeneic cells therefore may be a relatively simple way of improving results by reducing relapse rates.

Vaccination strategies

The idiotype of the myeloma paraprotein can be used as a unique tumor-specific antigen. Immunization of the donor with the recipient's idiotype protein prior to the harvest can augment T-cell-mediated specific immunity against the idiotype.[50] There is evidence in a murine B-cell lymphoma model that reconstitution with marrow from idiotype-immune donors can confer protection against subsequent lethal tumor challenge.[51] If the anti-idiotype response is similarly protective in myeloma, immunization of the donor before harvest and/or before collecting cells for DLI could selectively boost GVM. Infusion of dendritic cells loaded with the myeloma protein post transplant is another potential way of enhancing GVM effects of allogeneic transplantation by stimulating T-cell-mediated specific immunity.

Adjuvant post-allograft therapy

While a substantial proportion of patients attains CR after allogeneic transplantation, a number of patients do not do so. Additionally, relapse rates may also be high. Interferon-α2b (IFN-α2b) has been used after autografts to increase response duration successfully (although it does not *prevent* relapse). Interferon therefore has been explored as a post-allograft adjuvant agent in myeloma to improve CR rates as well as long-term disease-free survival.[52,53]

Seventeen patients received IFN-α2b three months after allogeneic transplantation in a pilot EBMT study.[52] No problems were seen in five at the dose of 1 MU three times a week. One of seven patients receiving 2 MU three times a week developed fatal acute GVHD, whereas at the dose of 3 MU three times a week, four of five patients developed GVHD. This was primarily a feasibility study, and no efficacy data were available.

Byrne et al[53] administered IFN-α at a dose of 3 MU three times a week to five patients, starting a median of 4 months (range 4–7.5) post transplant. One had clearly progressive disease and four had persistent disease. No acute GVHD was seen, but one patient developed chronic GVHD. CR was seen in two patients within 2 months and in two more within 9 months, whereas the patient with progressive disease did not respond. Myeloma, like other low-grade lymphoid malignancies, often takes time to respond following transplantation. Because of this, it is a little difficult to ascertain the exact contribution of interferon to the achievement of CR in these patients.

In our experience, chronic GVHD is almost universal in myeloma (unpublished observations) and leukemia[54] patients receiving IFN-α after allogeneic transplantation as immunotherapy for relapse. Based on the limited data that are available, it is difficult to recommend the use of interferon after allogeneic transplantation in myeloma on a routine basis. A case could be made for using it in patients who do not have GVHD, are off GVHD prophylaxis, and whose disease is in a clear plateau phase (i.e. the paraprotein is not declining) following an allograft.

Enhancing immune reconstitution

We have shown that lower lymphocyte counts 4 weeks after allogeneic transplantation for AML is associated with a significantly higher risk of relapse and poorer survival.[55] Recently, the Mayo Clinic group has made a similar observation in patients autografted for non-Hodgkin's lymphoma and myeloma.[56] It is possible that achieving faster immune reconstitution after allogeneic transplantation may help enhance GVM and reduce relapse rates. This can be achieved by the use of PBSC rather than marrow, which results in faster immune recovery.[49] DLI or the use of cytokines may be another way to enhance immune reconstitution.

GRAFT-VERSUS-MYELOMA INDEPENDENT OF ALLOGENEIC TRANSPLANTATION

As Table 20.3 shows, even non-myeloablative transplantation is associated with some risk of treatment-related mortality. Attempts have therefore been made to exploit allogeneic GVM outside the setting of allogeneic transplantation to avoid morbidity and mortality.

Attempts have been made to exploit what we have termed 'hit-and-run' graft-versus-tumor effects[7,8,57,58] by infusing haploidentical donor cells in conjunction with a conventional autograft. This was initially tried by the Hadassah University Hospital Group in a small number of patients with leukemia, with no success.[59]

It was subsequently attempted at the University of Arkansas in a small number of patients who were being transplanted for the second or third[60] time. Fatal toxicity, including GVHD, was a serious problem in patients receiving this therapy with their third autografts. Although survival of donor cells for several weeks was seen in the few patients receiving this therapy with their second autografts, all patients eventually relapsed, and the efficacy of this treatment could not be judged.

A similar strategy was employed recently[61] with the use of DLI and interleukin-2 (IL-2) in conjunction with conventional autologous transplantation. Self-limited so-called hyperacute GVHD was seen in some patients. However, no donor cell chimerism could be demonstrated. One patient died, one was inevaluable, two attained partial response, and three attained CR. The authors attributed this to the immunotherapeutic intervention. However, such a clinical GVHD-like syndrome can result from IL-2 administration itself, and the response seen in this small group of patients can be attributed to the conditioning regimen. Thus, in the absence of demonstrable chimerism, it is impossible to conclude that the immunotherapeutic intervention helped.

Infusion of mononuclear cells from HLA-identical sibling donors has been tried without any preceding conditioning therapy.[62] Whilst almost all patients had donor cells detectable immediately after infusion, only one-fourth had donor cells detectable over 4 weeks following the infusion, and all of these developed GVHD. There appeared to be transient antitumor response in two patients, including one with myeloma, during GVHD. These data are too limited to evaluate the efficacy of this approach.

IMPROVING OUTCOME

The factors responsible for poor outcome are those related to the underlying disease, the patient's condition, and the treatment regimen, including supportive therapy. The factors included in the first two categories have been summarized in Table 20.2. Of course, some of the biologic factors are not modifiable and cannot be manipulated to improve the outcome of allogeneic transplantation in myeloma.

Patient selection (disease- and patient-related factors)

Patients with a higher risk of disease progression (e.g. high-risk cytogenetoic abnormalities, high LDH, plasma cell leukemia, central nervous system involvement,[63] etc.) should be considered for allogeneic transplantation early in the course of the disease rather than being autografted – a relatively ineffective procedure (under the circumstances), which may select for resistant malignant clones.

Patients eligible for allogeneic transplantation should be allografted before their condition and performance status deteriorate as a result of excessive therapy, organ dysfunction (particularly renal failure), or infections, as well as progressive disease.

Treatment-related factors

The use of blood-derived stem cells may make allogeneic transplantation safer because of the higher numbers of $CD34^+$ and nucleated cells infused.[64,65]

It is not necessary to go from the extreme intensity of conventional allogeneic transplantation to the minimal intensity of non-myeloablative transplantation to make the procedure safer.

Modest attenuation in the dose intensity of a conventional conditioning regimens can lead to dramatic decreases in treatment-related mortality and improvement in survival,[66] as shown by the Royal Marsden Hospital group in AML.

Application of the above measures in addition to rigorous GVHD prophylaxis and stringent prophylaxis against opportunistic infections[67] can result in improvement in the outcome of allogeneic transplantation in myeloma (Figures 20.7 and 20.8; unpublished observations).

MANAGEMENT OF RELAPSE AFTER ALLOGENEIC TRANSPLANTATION

The four broad alternatives in patients relapsing after an allograft for myeloma are supportive therapy only, conventional therapy, measures to incite GVM, and novel therapies.

Supportive therapy

This line of action is probably the least detrimental option for the patient's quality of life in the short term. However, it is unlikely to result in substantial prolongation of life, much less long-term disease control. Since allogeneic transplantation is performed with curative intent,

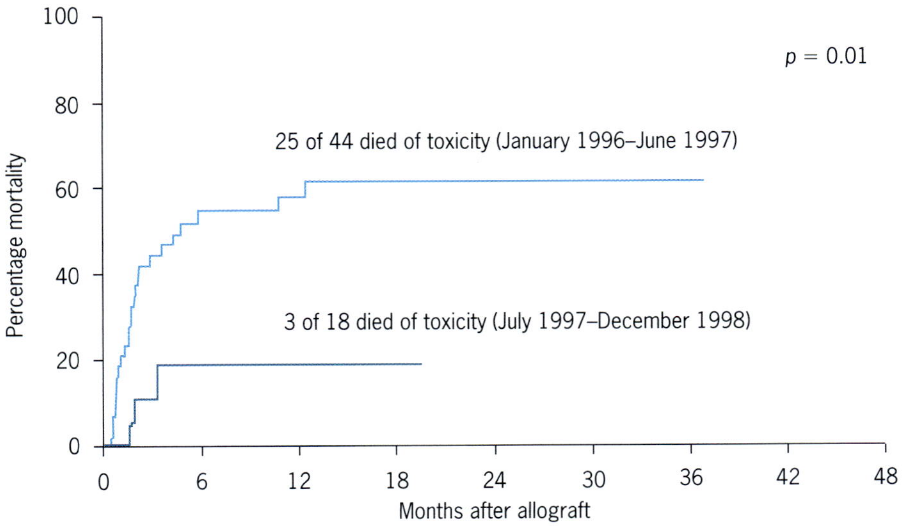

Figure 20.7 Reduction in transplant-related mortality after allogeneic transplantation in myeloma with the use of peripheral blood stem cells, attenuated (but not non-myeloablative) conditioning regimens, and improved supportive care at the University of Arkansas (modeled on the Royal Marsden Hospital experience).[66]

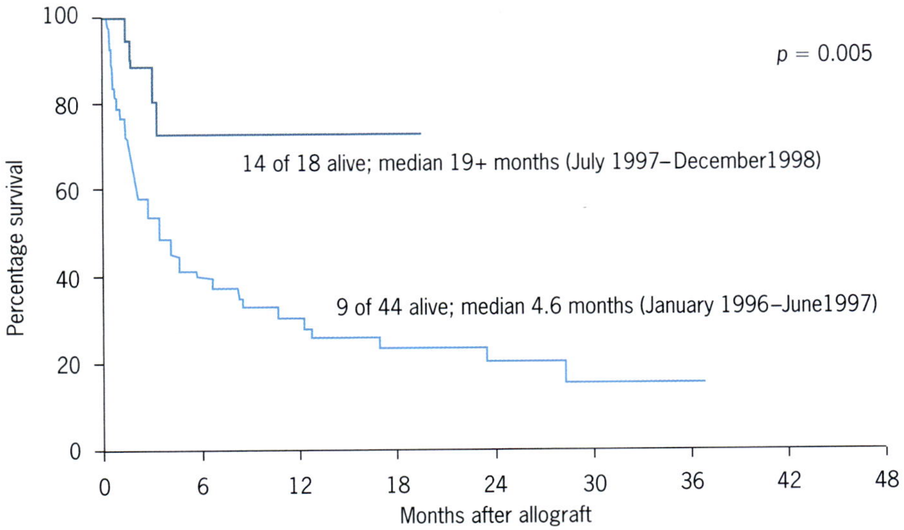

Figure 20.8 Improvement in survival after allogeneic transplantation in myeloma with the use of peripheral blood stem cells, attenuated (but not non-myeloablative) conditioning regimens, and improved supportive care at the University of Arkansas (modeled on the Royal Marsden Hospital experience).[66]

choosing this alternative is usually not appropriate as a first choice. In patients failing other courses of action, it may be a reasonable choice.

Conventional therapy

This comprises standard therapy such as pulse dexamethasone, melphalan–prednisone, and vincristine–doxorubicin–dexamethasone (VAD) (see Chapter 18). Depending upon the tempo of the disease, this option may result in disease control for a reasonable period of time. However, it is unlikely to help with aggressive relapse or result in long-term disease control. The major problem is that all conventional treatment approaches are likely to terminate any GVM reactions, and consequently antagonize the very foundation on which allogeneic transplantation is based.

Graft-versus-myeloma

Exploitation of GVM is the most obvious choice, since it aims to harness the same biologic reactions that the original allograft was intended to. The intervention depends upon the tumor load, ongoing immunosuppression, ongoing GVHD, and the type of transplant.

Measures to evoke GVM include cessation of immunosuppression, use of DLI (with or without preceding chemotherapy), and administration of cytokines such as IFN-α and IL-2 singly or in combination. Published results of GVM have been reviewed.[7] The best approach has not been determined, but an algorithm has been suggested[7] based upon the published results of GVM as well as success of the approach in patients with acute leukemia.[68]

Unfortunately, the relationship between GVM and GVHD appears to be close.[7] In a review of GVM reports published until 1998,[7] 18 of 22 patients developing GVHD were found to respond, compared with 2 of 7 not developing GVHD ($p = 0.02$; Fisher's exact test). In fact, we have observed an undesirable separation of GVM and GVHD in a number of patients with advanced, aggressive disease – who developed significant GVHD without any evidence of GVM.

Novel therapies

Thalidomide has recently been shown to be dramatically active in myeloma.[69] Interestingly, the first patient to have responded to thalidomide (and the second to have been treated with the drug) had relapsed after an allograft and had failed to respond to measures to elicit GVM. The mechanism of action of thalidomide is still not well defined (see Chapter 8), but it is possible that its immunomodulating actions do not compromise GVM reactions while acting directly against myeloma. We have seen no relapses in leukemia patients receiving thalidomide successfully for chronic GVHD,[70] a preliminary observation that has led us to speculate that the anti-angiogenesis activity of thalidomide may make up for loss of graft-versus-tumor effects as GVHD comes under control.

REFERENCES

1. McElwain TJ, Powles RL. High-dose intravenous melphalan for plasma-cell leukaemia and myeloma. *Lancet* 1983; **ii**: 822–4.
2. Attal M, Harousseau JL, Stoppa AM et al. A prospective, randomized trial of autologous bone marrow transplantation and chemotherapy in multiple myeloma. Intergroupe Français du Myelome. *N Engl J Med* 1996; **335**: 91–7.
3. Powles R, Sirohi B, Treleaven J et al. Continued first complete remission in multiple myeloma for over 10 years: a series of 'operationally cured' patients. Blood 2000; **96**(Suppl 1): Abst 2215.
4. Mehta J, Singhal S, Desikan K et al. High-dose therapy and stem cell support in myeloma. In: *PPO Updates*, Vol. 13 (De Vita VT Jr, Hellman S, Rosenberg SA, eds). Philadelphia: Lippincott Williams & Wilkins, 1999: 1–12.
5. Singhal S, Mehta J, Jagannath S, Barlogie B. Hematopoietic stem cell transplantation for myeloma. In: *Current Therapy in Cancer*, 2nd edn

(Foley JF, Vose JM, Armitage JO, eds). Philadelphia: WB Saunders, 1999: 475–84.
6. Singhal S, Mehta J, Barlogie B. Advances in the treatment of multiple myeloma. *Curr Opin Hematol* 1997; **4**: 291–7.
7. Mehta J, Singhal S. Graft-versus-myeloma. *Bone Marrow Transplant* 1998; **22**: 835–43.
8. Mehta J. The graft-versus-myeloma effect. In: *Allogeneic Immunotherapy for Malignant Diseases* (Barrett AJ, Jiang YZ, eds). New York: Marcel Dekker, 2000: 223–38.
9. Yee GC, McGuire TR. Allogeneic bone marrow transplantation in the treatment of hematologic diseases. *Clin Pharm* 1985; **4**: 149–60.
10. Gahrton G, Ringden O, Lonnqvist B et al. Bone marrow transplantation in three patients with multiple myeloma. *Acta Med Scand* 1986; **219**: 523–7.
11. Gallamini A, Buffa F, Bacigalupo A et al. Allogeneic bone marrow transplantation in multiple myeloma. *Acta Haematol* 1987; **77**: 111–14.
12. Gahrton G, Tura S, Flesch M et al. Allogeneic bone marrow transplantation in 24 patients with multiple myeloma reported to the EBMT registry. *Hematol Oncol* 1988; **6**: 181–6.
13. Nikoskelainen J, Koskela K, Katka K et al. Allogeneic bone marrow transplantation in multiple myeloma: a report of four cases. *Bone Marrow Transplant* 1988; **3**: 495–500.
14. Mehta J, Tricot G, Jagannath S et al. Salvage autologous or allogeneic transplantation for multiple myeloma refractory to or relapsing after a first-line autograft? *Bone Marrow Transplant* 1998; **21**: 887–92.
15. Mehta J, Ayers D, Mattox S et al. Allogeneic bone marrow transplantation in multiple myeloma: single-center experience of 97 patients. *Blood* 1997; **90**(Suppl 1): 225a.
16. Kulkarni S, Powles RL, Treleaven JG et al. Impact of previous high-dose therapy on outcome after allografting for multiple myeloma. *Bone Marrow Transplant* 1999; **23**: 675–80.
17. Mehta J, Powles R. The future of bone marrow transplantation. In: *Clinical Bone Marrow and Blood Stem Cell Transplantation*, 2nd edn (Atkinson K, ed). Cambridge: Cambridge University Press, 2000: 1457–65.
18. Or R, Mehta J, Naparstek E et al. Successful T cell-depleted allogeneic bone marrow transplantation in a child with recurrent multiple extramedullary plasmacytomas. *Bone Marrow Transplant* 1992; **10**: 381–2.
19. Björkstrand BB, Ljungman P, Svensson H et al. Allogeneic bone marrow transplantation versus autologous stem cell transplantation in multiple myeloma: a retrospective case-matched study from the European Group for Blood and Marrow Transplantation. *Blood* 1996; **88**: 4711–18.
20. Varterasian M, Janakiraman N, Karanes C et al. Transplantation in patients with multiple myeloma: a multicenter comparative analysis of peripheral blood stem cell and allogeneic transplant. *Am J Clin Oncol* 1997; **20**: 462–6.
21. Corradini P, Voena C, Tarella C et al. Molecular and clinical remissions in multiple myeloma: role of autologous and allogeneic transplantation of hematopoietic cells. *J Clin Oncol* 1999; **17**: 208–15.
22. Martinelli G, Terragna C, Zamagni E et al. Molecular remission after allogeneic or autologous transplantation of hematopoietic stem cells for multiple myeloma. *J Clin Oncol* 2000; **18**: 2273–81.
23. Pavord S, Sivakumaran M, Durrant S, Chapman C. The role of alpha interferon in the pathogenesis of GVHD. *Bone Marrow Transplant* 1992; **10**: 477.
24. Kolb HJ, Mittermüller J, Hertenstein H et al. Adoptive immunotherapy in human and canine chimeras – the role of interferon alfa. EBMT Chronic Leukemia Working Party. *Semin Hematol* 1993; **30**(Suppl 3): 37–9.
25. Collins RH Jr, Pineiro LA, Nemunaitis JJ et al. Transfusion of donor buffy coat cells in the treatment of persistent or recurrent malignancy after allogeneic bone marrow transplantation. *Transfusion* 1995; **35**: 891–8.
26. Verdonck LF, Lokhorst HM, Dekker AW et al. Graft-versus-myeloma effect in two cases. *Lancet* 1996; **347**: 800–1.
27. Bensinger WI, Buckner CD, Anasetti C et al. Allogeneic marrow transplantation for multiple myeloma: an analysis of risk factors on outcome. *Blood* 1996; **88**: 2787–93.
28. Cavo M, Bandini G, Benni M et al. High-dose busulfan and cyclophosphamide are an effective conditioning regimen for allogeneic bone marrow transplantation in chemosensitive multiple myeloma. *Bone Marrow Transplant* 1998; **22**: 27–32.
29. Couban S, Stewart AK, Loach D et al. Autologous and allogeneic transplantation for multiple myeloma at a single centre. *Bone Marrow Transplant* 1997; **19**: 783–9.
30. Gahrton G, Tura S, Ljungman P et al. Prognostic factors in allogeneic bone marrow transplantation

for multiple myeloma. *J Clin Oncol* 1995; **13**: 1312–22.
31. Huff CA, Noga SJ, Jones RJ et al. Allogeneic bone marrow transplantation (allo BMT): role of T cell depletion (TCD) and graft versus host disease (GVHD). *Blood* 2000; **96**(Suppl 1): Abst 862.
32. Majolino I, Corradini P, Scime R et al. Allogeneic transplantation of unmanipulated peripheral blood stem cells in patients with multiple myeloma. *Bone Marrow Transplant* 1998; **22**: 449–55.
33. Reece DE, Shepherd JD, Klingemann HG et al. Treatment of myeloma using intensive therapy and allogeneic bone marrow transplantation. *Bone Marrow Transplant* 1995; **15**: 117–23.
34. Russell NH, Miflin G, Stainer C et al. Allogeneic bone marrow transplant for multiple myeloma. *Blood* 1997; **89**: 2610–11.
35. Seiden MV, Schlossman R, Andersen J et al. Monoclonal antibody-purged bone marrow transplantation therapy for multiple myeloma. *Leuk Lymphoma* 1995; **17**: 87–93.
36. Cheung B, Ackers C, Powles R et al. Allogeneic peripheral blood stem cell transplantation (PBSCT) for patients with multiple myeloma (MM) – single centre experience. *Blood* 2000; **96**(Suppl 1): Abst 5276.
37. Mehta J, Nagler A, Slavin S. Marrow transplantation for multiple myeloma. *N Engl J Med* 1992; **326**: 1087–8.
38. Durie BGM, Gale RP, Horowitz MM. Allogeneic and twin transplants for multiple myeloma: an IBMTR analysis. *Blood* 1994; **84**(Suppl 1): 202a.
39. Slavin S, Nagler A, Naparstek E et al. Non-myeloablative stem cell transplantation and cell therapy as an alternative to conventional allogeneic bone marrow transplantation with lethal cytoreduction for the treatment of malignant and nonmalignant hematologic diseases. *Blood* 1998; **91**: 756–63.
40. Badros A, Tricot G, Morris C et al. Significant graft-vs-myeloma (GVM) effect after non-myeloablative allogeneic transplantation in multiple myeloma (MM). *Blood* 2000; **96**(Suppl 1): Abst 5273.
41. Singhal S, Safdar A, Chiang KY et al. Non-myeloablative allogeneic transplantation (micro-allograft) for refractory myeloma after two preceding autografts: feasibility and efficacy in a patient with active aspergillosis. *Bone Marrow Transplant* 2000; **26**: 1231–3.
42. Lalancette M, Rezvani K, Szydlo R et al. Excellent outcome of non-myeloablative stem cell transplant (NMSCT) for good risk myeloma: the EBMT experience. *Blood* 2000; **96**(Suppl 1): Abst 872.
43. Molina A, Sahebi F, Maloney DG et al. Non-myeloablative peripheral blood stem cell (PBSC) allografts following cytoreductive autotransplants for treatment of multiple myeloma (MM). *Blood* 2000; **96**(Suppl 1): Abst 2063.
44. Peggs KS, Williams CD, Chopra R et al. Non-myeloablative allogeneic transplantation with adjuvant dose escalated donor lymphocyte infusions for multiple myeloma. *Blood* 2000; **96**(Suppl 1): Abst 3379.
45. Schaefer H, Bader P, Hebart H et al. Mini-allografts as salvage therapy in patients with heavily pretreated multiple myeloma. *Blood* 2000; **96**(Suppl 1): Abst 5066.
46. Gahrton G, Svensson H, Björkstrand B et al. Syngeneic transplantation in multiple myeloma – a case-matched comparison with autologous and allogeneic transplantation. European Group for Blood and Marrow Transplantation. *Bone Marrow Transplant* 1999; **24**: 741–5.
47. Govindarajan R, Jagannath S, Flick JT et al. Preceding standard therapy is the likely cause of MDS after autotransplants for multiple myeloma. *Br J Haematol* 1996; **95**: 349–53.
48. Drach J, Ayers D, Govindarajan R et al. MDS-associated cytogenetic abnormalities (CGA) in both hematopoietic and neoplastic cells after autotransplants (AT) in 868 patients with multiple myeloma (MM). *Blood* 1998; **92**(Suppl 1): 97a.
49. Powles R, Mehta J, Kulkarni S et al. Allogeneic blood and bone-marrow stem-cell transplantation in haematological malignant diseases: a randomised trial. *Lancet* 2000; **355**: 1231–7.
50. Kwak LW, Taub DD, Duffey PL et al. Transfer of myeloma idiotype-specific immunity from an actively immunised marrow donor. *Lancet* 1995; **345**: 1016–20.
51. Kwak LW, Pennington R, Longo DL. Active immunization of murine allogeneic bone marrow transplant donors with B-cell tumor-derived idiotype: a strategy for enhancing the specific antitumor effect of marrow grafts. *Blood* 1996; **87**: 3053–60.
52. Samson D, Volin L, Schanz U et al. Feasibility and toxicity of interferon maintenance therapy after allogeneic BMT for multiple myeloma: a pilot

study of the EBMT. *Bone Marrow Transplant* 1996; **17**: 759–62.

53. Byrne JL, Carter GI, Bienz N et al. Adjuvant alpha-interferon improves complete remission rates following allogeneic transplantation for multiple myeloma. *Bone Marrow Transplant* 1998; **22**: 639–43.
54. Singhal S, Powles R, Kulkarni S et al. Long-term follow-up of relapsed acute leukemia treated with immunotherapy after allogeneic transplantation: the inseparability of graft-versus-host disease and graft-versus-leukemia, and the problem of extramedullary relapse. *Leuk Lymphoma* 1999; **32**: 505–12.
55. Powles R, Singhal S, Treleaven J et al. Identification of patients who may benefit from prophylactic immunotherapy after bone marrow transplantation for acute myeloid leukemia on the basis of lymphocyte recovery after transplantation. *Blood* 1998; **91**: 3481–6.
56. Porrata LF, Gertz MA, Inwards DJ et al. Early lymphocyte recovery predicts superior survival after autologous hematopoietic stem cell transplantation in multiple myeloma or non-Hodgkin's lymphoma. *Blood* 2000; **96**(Suppl 1): Abst 2398.
57. Mehta J, Powles R, Singhal S et al. Outcome of autologous rescue after failed engraftment of allogeneic marrow. *Bone Marrow Transplant* 1996; **17**: 213–17.
58. Mehta J, Singhal S. Graft failure: diagnosis and management. In: *The Clinical Practice of Stem Cell Transplantation* (Barrett J, Treleaven JG, eds). Oxford: Isis Medical Media, 1998: 645–58.
59. Nagler A, Ackerstein A, Or R et al. Adoptive immunotherapy with mismatched allogeneic peripheral blood lymphocytes (PBL) following autologous bone marrow transplantation (ABMT). *Exp Hematol* 1992; **20**: 705.
60. Singhal S, Mehta J, Hood S et al. Third transplants for myeloma relapsing after two prior autografts. *Blood* 1997; **90**(Suppl 1): 547a.
61. Ballester O, Fang T, Bruno G et al. Adoptive immunotherapy with donor lymphocyte infusions (DLI) and IL-2 after high-dose therapy (HDT) and autologous stem cell (ASC) rescue for relapsed/refractory multiple myeloma. *Blood* 2000; **96**(Suppl 1): Abst 839.
62. Porter DL, Connors JM, Doyle B et al. Donor leukocyte infusions as primary allogeneic adoptive immunotherapy for patients with malignancies. *Blood* 1997; **90**(Suppl 1): 549a.
63. Singhal S, Siegel D, Mattox S et al. Central nervous system involvement in multiple myeloma. *Blood* 1996; **88**(Suppl 1): 218b.
64. Mehta J, Powles R, Treleaven J et al. Number of nucleated cells infused during allogeneic and autologous bone marrow transplantation: an important modifiable factor influencing outcome. *Blood* 1997; **90**: 3808–10.
65. Singhal S, Powles R, Treleaven J et al. A low CD34+ cell dose results in higher mortality and poorer survival after blood or marrow stem cell transplantation from HLA-identical siblings: Should 2×10^6 CD34+ cells/kg be considered the minimum threshold? *Bone Marrow Transplant* 2000; **26**: 489–96.
66. Wilson K, Powles R, Treleaven J et al. Allografting after melphalan-total body irradiation for first remission acute myeloid leukemia. *Blood* 1996; **88**(Suppl 1): 613a.
67. Mehta J, Powles R, Singhal S et al. Antimicrobial prophylaxis to prevent opportunistic infections in patients with chronic lymphocytic leukemia after allogeneic blood or marrow transplantation. *Leuk Lymphoma* 1997; **26**: 83–8.
68. Mehta J, Powles R, Treleaven J et al. Induction of graft-versus-host disease as immunotherapy of leukemia relapsing after allogeneic transplantation: single-center experience of 32 adult patients. *Bone Marrow Transplant* 1997; **20**: 129–35.
69. Singhal S, Mehta J, Desikan R et al. Antitumor activity of thalidomide in refractory multiple myeloma. *N Engl J Med* 1999; **341**: 1565–71.
70. Kulkarni S, Powles R, Mehta J et al. Thalidomide in GVHD – Is anti-GVHD effect separable from the antiangiogenesis? *Blood* 1998; **92**(Suppl 1): 344b.

21

The role of radiotherapy

Dennis C Shrieve

CONTENTS • **Introduction** • **Basic radiobiological principles** • **Solitary plasmacytomas** • **Myeloma** • **New directions** • **Conclusions**

INTRODUCTION

Radiotherapy plays an important role in the treatment of patients with plasma cell tumors. Radiotherapy may be delivered for the following reasons:

- definitive treatment for potential cure of patients with solitary plasmacytoma;
- in combination with chemotherapy in patients with systemic disease;
- as part of a pre-transplant conditioning regimen in the form of total-body irradiation;
- for palliation of pain, neurologic compromise, or structural instability from focal disease.

BASIC RADIOBIOLOGICAL PRINCIPLES

Cells irradiated in vitro demonstrate a characteristic radiation dose–response relationship for cell survival (Figure 21.1a). The hallmark of the curve for survival following graded doses of radiation is the curvilinear nature of the dose–response relationship. The most common interpretation of this shape is the production of two types of lesions in the cellular target (DNA): sublethal, reparable lesions; and lethal lesions produced by a single ionizing event. Cell death occurs at a rate that depends on the production of single lethal events (α-type damage) proportional to dose (D) and the interaction of sublethal events to create a lethal lesion (β-type damage) proportional to the square of the dose (D^2). This may be thought of as the production of double-strand breaks in DNA by either a single event or the combination of two sublethal single-strand breaks occurring in close proximity on complementary strands of DNA (Figure 21.2).

Cell survival (or other effects of radiation) may be expressed using the linear–quadratic formula

$$\text{surviving fraction} = \exp[-(\alpha D + \beta D^2)]$$

where α and β are characteristic of the cell type or tissue being irradiated. The ratio α/β is a measure of the relative contributions of α-type and β-type damage to the effect under study. α/β has units of dose and is equivalent to the dose at which $\alpha D = \beta D^2$.

When radiation dose is fractionated, as in clinical radiotherapy, sublethal damage is repaired between doses, with a half-time of 1–2 hours.[1] Therefore, when fractionated radiotherapy is

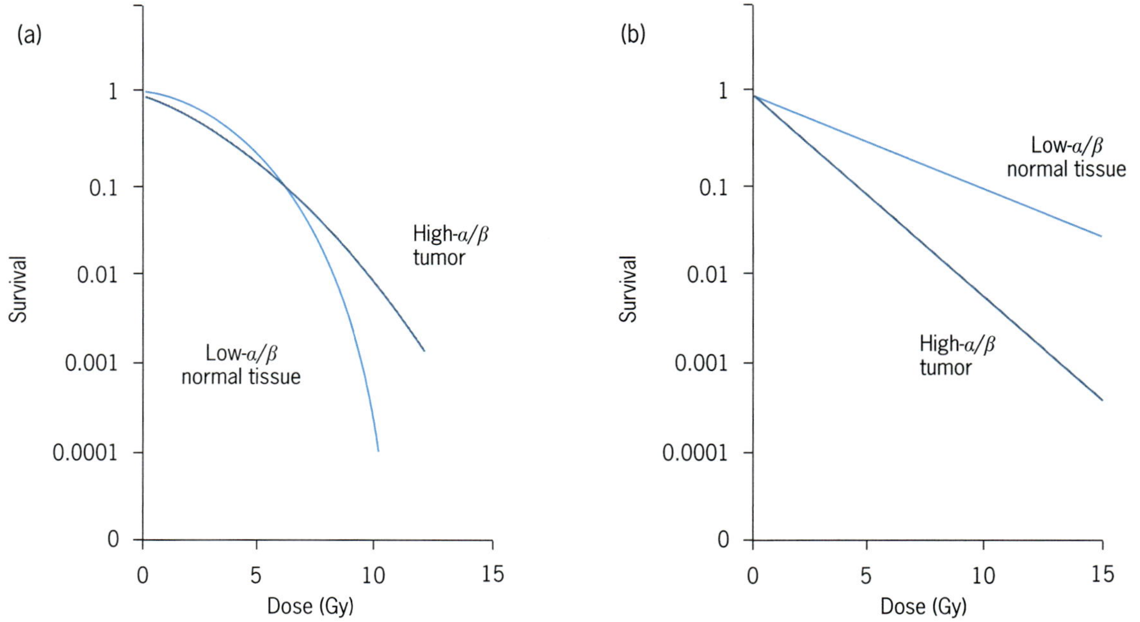

Figure 21.1 (a) Generalized survival curve for mammalian cells following exposure to graded single doses of ionizing radiation. Curves are shown for early-responding, rapidly proliferating tissues with $\alpha/\beta = 10$ Gy (high α/β) and for late-responding, slowly or non-proliferating tissues with $\alpha/\beta = 2$ (low α/β). (b) Generalized survival curves for mammalian cells irradiated with multiple 2 Gy fractions separated by sufficient time for complete repair of sublethal damage between doses. When low daily doses are used, as in standard fractionation, the small differential effect seen in the low-dose region of (a) is amplified.

employed, higher total doses must be used to achieve the same level of response relative to single doses (Figure 21.1b). Different tissues may demonstrate varying degrees of sparing by dose fractionation, depending on α/β (Figure 21.3a). In general, rapidly proliferating tissues such as bone marrow stem cells, intestinal crypt cells, mucosa, and most malignant tumor cells (high α/β) demonstrate relatively little sparing effect of fractionation compared with slowly proliferating or quiescent normal tissues, such as nerve, brain, lung, and kidney (low α/β) (Figure 21.3b).[2]

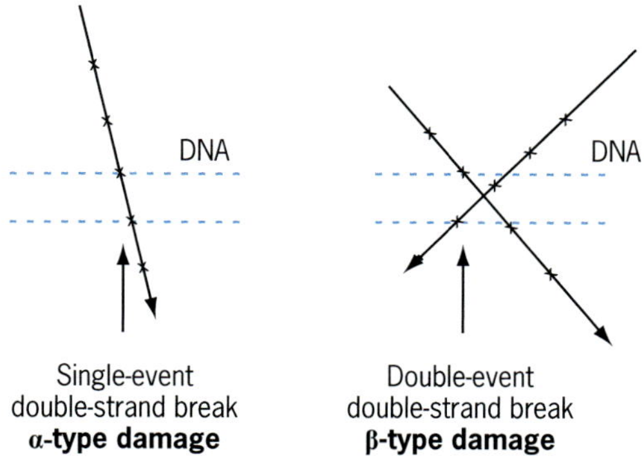

Figure 21.2 Diagrammatic representation of production of double-strand breaks in DNA by a single photon or interaction of damage produced by two photons.

Myeloma cells irradiated in vitro demonstrate the curvilinear dose–response relationship described above when clonogenic survival is the endpoint used. The narrow width of the shoulder region is indicative of a relatively small capacity to accumulate sublethal damage in myeloma cells, and therefore relatively little sparing with fractionation of dose (Figure 21.4).[3] A measure of shoulder width, the extrapolation number ($\tilde{n}$), is smaller than those found for most

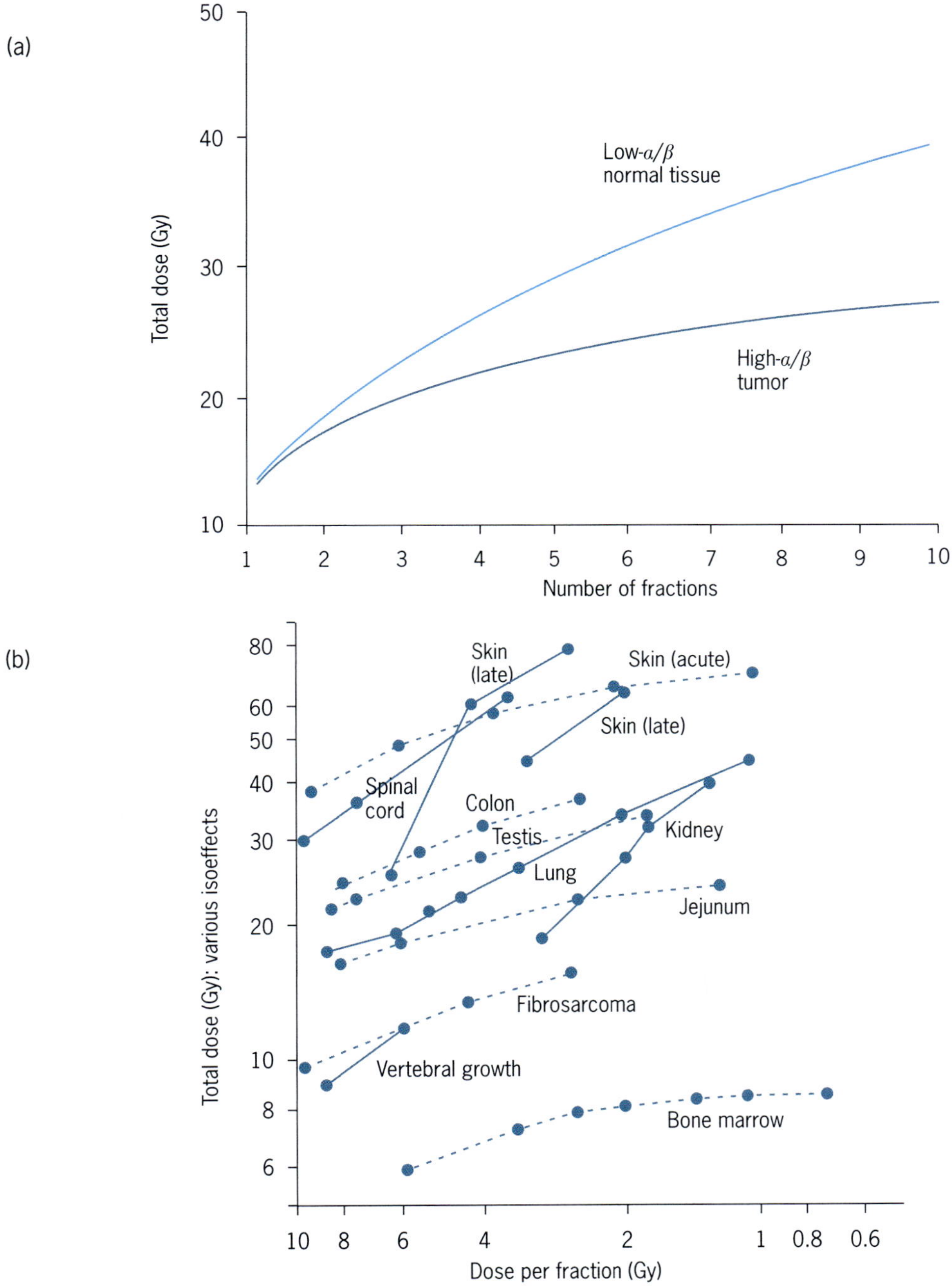

Figure 21.3 (a) Isoeffect plots for tissues with low and high α/β. The curves represent combinations of total doses and fraction size required to achieve the same biologic effect as 12 Gy in a single dose. (b) Data from various animal experiments demonstrating isoeffect curves for various normal tissues and tumor. Early-responding tissues (dashed lines) have a shallow slope, demonstrating that a modest increase in total dose required as dose per fraction is decreased. Late-responding tissues (solid lines) demonstrate a steeper slope, indicating a more rapid rise in total dose required for a given effect as dose per fraction is decreased, producing a greater sparing of late-responding tissues by dose fractionation. (From Withers.[2])

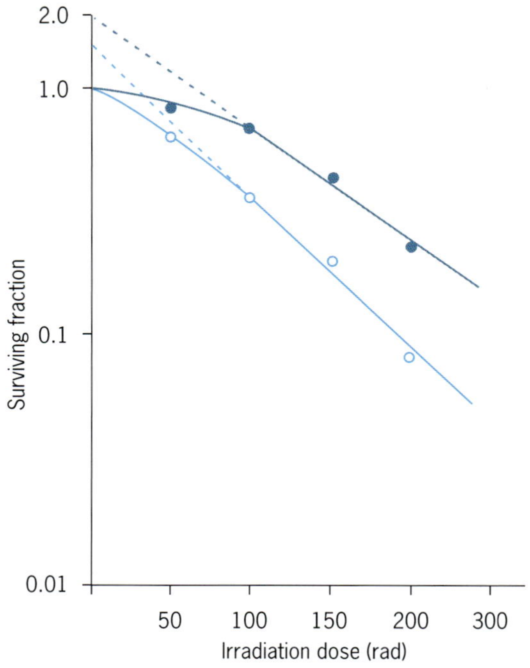

Figure 21.4 Survival curves for two myeloma cell lines irradiated in vitro. (From Shimizu et al.[3])

human tumor cell lines. Shimizu et al[3] found extrapolation numbers of 1.6 and 2.0 for two human myeloma cell lines (Figure 21.4). Freshly explanted human tumors, including cancers of the bronchus, breast, endometrium, ovary, and stomach, and melanoma, exhibited extrapolation numbers of 19–125.[4] Consequently, as expected, comparison of dose–response curves for human myeloma cell lines irradiated with single doses or multiple 2 Gy fractions separated by 12 hours revealed very little sparing by dose fractionation.[5]

Programmed cell death, or apoptosis, is a second important mode of cell death following irradiation. Apoptotic death can be induced by low doses of radiation (<1 Gy), and may require a functioning *p53* tumor suppressor gene.[6] Some cells, including myeloma cell lines, have demonstrated an adaptive response to even very low doses of radiation, leading to little or no programmed cell death from subsequent radiation. This adaptive response may be blocked by an inhibitor of poly(ADP-ribose)polymerase, such as 3-aminobenzamide, or okadaic acid, an inhibitor of protein phosphatase.[7] Further elucidation of the pathways of programmed cell death, the mechanisms of the adaptive response, and effective manipulation of these processes may lead to important means of modulating therapeutic response to radiation.

SOLITARY PLASMACYTOMAS

Approximately 5% of patients with plasma cell tumors present with apparently localized disease of bone or soft tissue (solitary plasmacytoma). Approximately 70% of solitary plasma cytomas occur in bone (SPB) and the remainder are extramedullary (EMP). Clearly, the diagnosis of 'solitary plasmacytoma' implies that an appropriate work-up has been done to rule out systemic myeloma (see Chapter 25).

Local control

Radiotherapy has been used as definitive treatment of solitary plasma cell tumors for more than 50 years. Corwin and Lindberg[8] reported on 24 highly selected patients treated with RT for solitary plasmacytoma at the MD Anderson Hospital, Houston, between 1948 and 1977. These were selected from among 288 patients. All had biopsy-proven plasma cell tumors, hemoglobin 13 g% or more, normal serum protein or serum electrophoresis (or decreasing monoclonal peak after radiotherapy), no Bence Jones protein in urine, and normal distant bone marrow. All 12 patients with SPB were controlled locally. Two of 12 patients with EMP had local failure. These two patients were treated with doses of 50 Gy or more. Subsequent reports in the era of computed tomography/magnetic resonance imaging (CT/MRI) have confirmed the excellent local control rates of 88–100% for osseous lesions and 80–100% for extramedullary lesions (Tables 21.1 and 21.2). Most local failures are reported to be in patients receiving lower radiation doses or with unusually long overall treatment times. It may be

Table 21.1 Local control of solitary plasmacytoma of bone by radiotherapy

Institution	No. of patients	Local control rate (%)
Mayo Clinic[9]	46	89
MD Anderson Cancer Center[10]	45	96
Stanford[11]	20	95
Princess Margaret Hospital[12]	25	100
University of Florida[13]	27	96
Iowa[14]	17	88
Mallinkrodt[15]	32	94
Trivandrum[16]	20	100

Table 21.2 Local control of extramedullary plasmacytoma by radiotherapy

Institution	No. of patients	Local control rate (%)
MD Anderson Cancer Center[8]	12	83
Stanford[17]	10	80
Princess Margaret Hospital[12]	25	100
University of Florida[13]	10	100
Iowa[14]	13	92
Mallinkrodt[15]	14	93
Trivandrum[16]	7	86

possible to salvage such patients with further radiation.[13]

Intracranial plasmacytomas may affect the meninges, skull, or brain. Since these lesions are usually initially approached surgically, they are more likely to be completely excised than plasmacytomas in other sites. This approach raises two issues: is complete surgical excision necessary or is biopsy followed by radiotherapy sufficient; and if a complete surgical resection is achieved, is adjuvant radiotherapy necessary?

Bindal et al[18] addressed these issues in their report on eight patients with intracranial plasmacytoma. Four of these patients were found to have myeloma in the immediate postoperative period. Of the remaining four patients, local control was obtained in three in whom a total tumor resection was achieved followed by radiotherapy. The fourth patient had radiotherapy following a subtotal resection, and required further surgery and radiation 7 years later. The authors suggest that 'the only definitive treatment for intracranial plasmacytoma is complete surgical resection followed by radiation therapy'. However, it is not clear that this combined approach results in better local control than radiotherapy alone (see Tables 21.1 and 22.2).

Treatment volume

Carefully planned treatment is essential in order to treat the entire lesion adequately while sparing as much normal tissue as possible. Osseous lesions may have a soft tissue component best evaluated by CT. Diligence in establishing the true tumor extent will avoid 'marginal misses' and underdosing. Use of CT-based three-dimensional treatment planning when appropriate will allow full coverage of the tumor volume without excessive irradiation of normal tissues (Figure 21.5).

Some authors advocate the treatment of the entire involved bone when treating osseous lesions.[19] While this may be necessary and reasonable in some sites, it is not clear that the entire bone need be treated in all cases. Catell et al[20] reviewed the results in patients treated between 1971 and 1994. The institutional policy had been not to treat the entire extremity but only the 'symptomatic area' plus a margin of 1–2 cm. Twenty-seven patients were treated to 41 sites in long bone extremity sites. The mean length of fields for femoral lesions was 18 cm, representing 42% of total femur length. For humeral lesions, the mean field length was 20 cm, representing 68% of overall length. Only four patients developed disease in the treated bone outside the irradiated field.

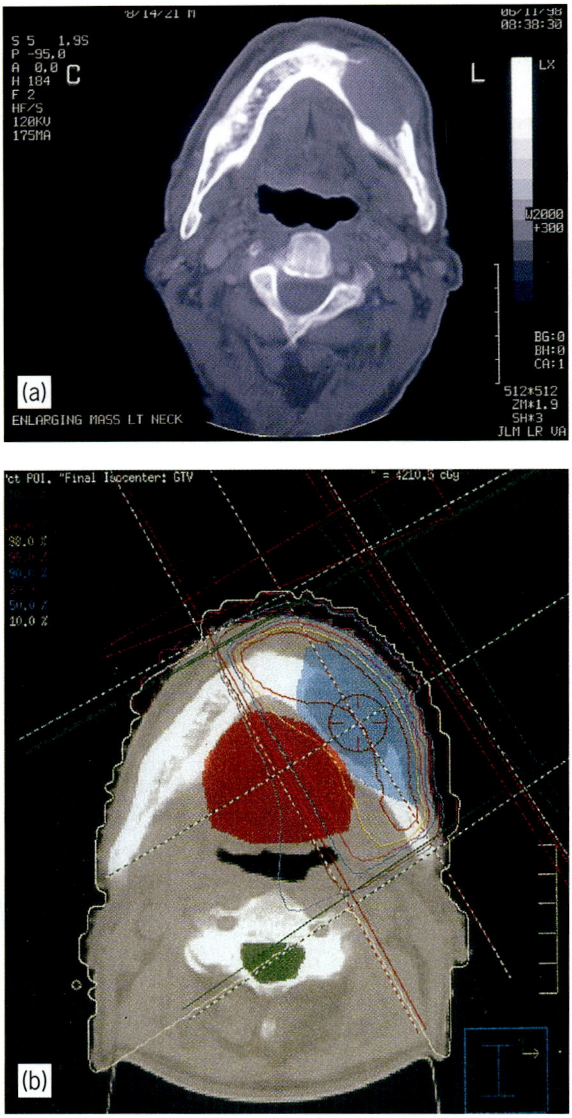

Figure 21.5 (a) CT of the mandible of a 78-year-old male with a painful mass in his left lower jaw. Biopsy demonstrated a plasma cell tumor. Work-up revealed no other masses. The patient was referred for local radiotherapy. (b) CT-based treatment plan of the same patient. An aquaplast mask was used for immobilization, and a CT was made with the patient in the treatment position. The tumor was outlined (blue), and the tongue (red) and spinal cord (green) were outlined as normal tissues. Using computer-generated blocking to shape the fields, a wedge pair field arrangement was used to treat the tumor, with a 2 cm margin. A dose of 4000 cGy was prescribed in 20 daily fractions. Most of the tongue received less than 50% of the prescribed dose, while the spinal cord received less than 10%. Two years following treatment, the patient has no local tumor, but has developed evidence of myeloma.

Liebross et al[21] have updated the MD Anderson experience in treating solitary plasmacytomas of bone. Their policy was to treat the entire tumor with generous margins, but not to routinely treat the entire bone. Local control was obtained in 55 of 57 patients (96%).

The vast majority of EMP involve upper respiratory tract sites. The incidence of nodal failure in patients initially deemed to be free of nodal involvement may be more than 20%.[14] For this reason, most authors advocate elective regional nodal irradiation.[13,14,19] Others have recommended against routine regional nodal irradiation if there is no bulky primary disease present.[17] There are few data on patients with EMP of the upper aerodigestive tract treated in the CT era. Our policy is to fully assess the extent of disease with CT and/or MRI. In patients without radiographic evidence of nodal spread, the regional nodes are not included in the treatment portal. However, in the case of bulky primary disease, regional nodes will often be included in a portal covering the primary with margin. In these cases, it is reasonable to extend the field slightly to adequately cover the draining lymph nodes.

Radiation dose

With radiotherapy in doses of 40 Gy or more, there have been reports of local control rates of 88–100% in osseous sites and 80–100% in soft tissue sites (Tables 21.1 and 21.2). A review of 114 cases by Bataille and Sany[22] suggested that radiation doses below 35 Gy may not be as efficacious as higher doses in achieving local control in SPB. Mendenhall et al[23] analyzed 81 cases from the literature, and found 96% local control in cases where doses of 40 Gy or more were used. These high rates of local control are found in previously untreated patients, and may not be applicable to lesions treated in patients who have previously received multiple courses of chemotherapy. At the University of Arkansas, we recommend a dose of 40 Gy for most cases of solitary plasmacytoma. This dose results in high rates of local control and allows for further treatment in the form of total-body irradiation should the patient progress to myeloma and require high-dose chemotherapy and bone marrow transplantation.

Outcome following radiotherapy for SPB or EMP

Nearly all patients presenting with SPB will progress to myeloma, with a median myeloma-free interval of approximately 10 years with adequate local therapy. True solitary plasmacytoma is a rare event. Knowling et al[12] reported on 822 patients with plasma cell tumors, of whom 25 (3%) had EMP and 25 (3%) SPB. All others had myeloma and a median age of 61 years, while the group of patients with EMP or SPB had a median age of 50 years. There were distinct differences in outcome between the groups of patients with SPB and EMP. Twenty percent of patients with EMP progressed following radiotherapy: two developed myeloma, while two recurred as EMP and one as SPB. Twelve patients (48%) with SPB developed myeloma, with a median time to progression of 6.5 years. Bolek et al[13] reported actuarial rates of progression to myeloma and survival for patients with EMP and SPB. The risk of conversion at 10 years was 54% for patients treated for SPB, compared with 11% for patients with EMP (Figure 21.6a).

The survival rate of patients presenting with SPB was 23% at 15 years, compared with 80% for patients presenting with EMP (Figure 21.6b). Patients presenting with SPB also had a poorer prognosis following progression to myeloma than did patients with EMP (Figure 21.7). Liebross et al[21] found that the disappearance of M protein following radio therapy of SPB was a significant positive prognostic indicator. Two of 11 patients with complete resolution of the M-protein peak progressed to myeloma at 2 and 11 years. Seventeen of 30 patients with a persistent M protein progressed to myeloma, with a median actuarial time to progression of about 4.5 years.

MYELOMA

Palliative radiotherapy

As with solitary plasmacytoma, radiotherapy is a very effective palliative modality for symptomatic osseous or extramedullary manifestations of myeloma. Since palliation rather than cure is the goal of treatment in these cases, lower radiation doses are usually used.

Mill and Griffith[24] studied 116 patients treated for palliation of painful bony lesions. Doses of a few grays up to 44 Gy were used. Ninety-one percent of patients reportedly had relief of symptoms. Analysis of minimum doses producing pain relief revealed that a majority of patients were palliated with doses of 15–20 Gy. These authors recommended doses in this range for the purpose of palliation.

Leigh et al[25] reported on palliative treatment for 101 patients with myeloma. A total of 316 sites were treated with radiotherapy. Of these, 306 sites were treated for palliation of pain and were evaluated for response. Tumors were treated with doses ranging from 6 Gy to 60 Gy. Relief of symptoms was obtained in 97% of patients: 26% with complete and 71% with partial pain relief. No significant dose response was evident with regard to relief of symptoms, probability of relapse, or time to relapse. All relapses were successfully retreated with radiation.

Palliative radiation treatment for myeloma must be individualized. The palliative regimen of 30 Gy in 10 fractions commonly used to treat metastatic disease may not be appropriate for all patients. Lower doses of 10–20 Gy will afford palliation in the vast majority of patients, while allowing for retreatment in those few in whom it is required. There are two situations in which higher total doses may be recommended: (i) neurologic compromise resulting from tumor impingement on spinal cord or cranial nerve; (ii)

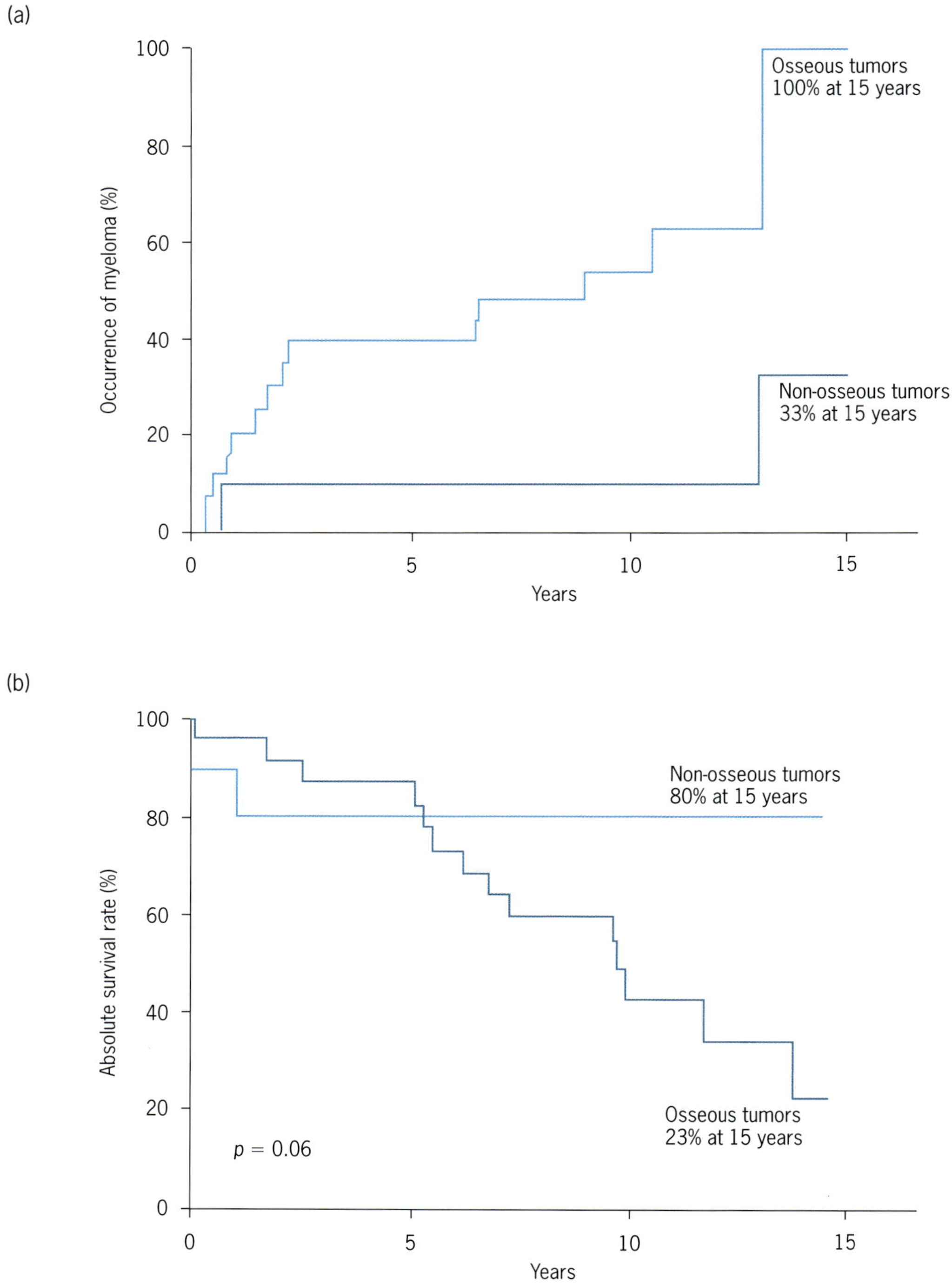

Figure 21.6 (a) Actuarial risk of occurrence of myeloma as a function of time following diagnosis and treatment of SPB and EMP. (b) Survival of patients following diagnosis and treatment of SPB and EMP. (From Bolek et al.[13])

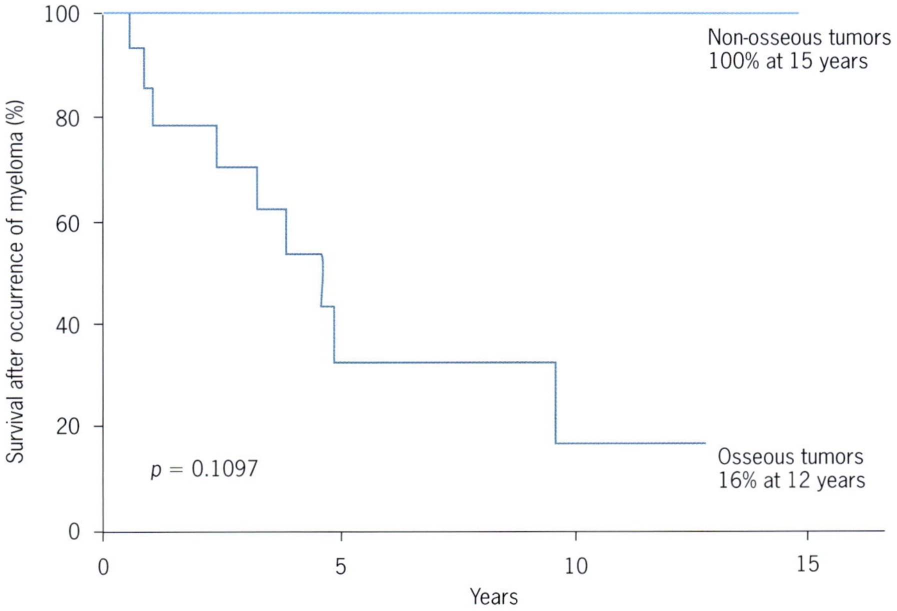

Figure 21.7 Survival of patients with SPB or EMP following occurrence of myeloma. (From Bolek et al.[13])

involvement of weight-bearing bones and impending pathologic fracture. In these cases, it is recommended that higher total doses of 30–40 Gy be used in standard fractionation (2 Gy per fraction) in order to obtain the best probability of durable reversal of symptoms in the former case and tumor eradication and bone healing in the latter.

Care must be taken not to treat unnecessarily large fields including large amounts of bone marrow. When treating for palliation of pain, it is not recommended to treat the entire involved bone. Most patients will have received multiple courses of chemotherapy or will require systemic treatment in the future. It is extremely important to preserve marrow function in these patients to avoid pancytopenia and not to compromise the ability to collect stem cells for future transplantation.

Hemibody irradiation

The disseminated nature and radiosensitivity of myeloma provide the rationale for the use of hemibody radiotherapy. The use of hemibody irradiation has been proposed as second-line therapy for chemotherapy-resistant myeloma. Singer et al[26] treated 41 patients who had progressive, melphalan-resistant disease with either single half-body (HBI) or double half-body (DHBI) radiotherapy. Failure of melphalan treatment was based on one of the following factors: (i) an increase in paraprotein despite three courses of chemotherapy; (ii) failure of paraprotein levels to fall by at least 25% after therapy; (iii) progressive pain or pathologic fractures and a reduction of less than 50% in paraprotein levels; or (iv) progressive local disease. Patients were evaluated and grouped into one of three prognostic groups using the UK Medical Research Council's classification criteria based on blood urea nitrogen (BUN), hemoglobin, and performance status.[27]

Radiotherapy was delivered in a single fraction using ^{60}Co through an anteroposterior field at a dose rate of 0.25 Gy/min. Median doses were 7.5 Gy (range 5–10 Gy) for upper HBI and 8.5 Gy (range 5–10 Gy) for lower HBI. All patients were a minimum of 6 weeks from the most recent chemotherapy, and no chemotherapy was given concomitant with HBI. When DHBI was planned, the more symptomatic hemibody was treated first, and the second HBI was delivered as soon as peripheral blood counts allowed, typically 7–10 weeks.

Two patients in Group I (better prognosis) received DHBI for increasing paraprotein following 6 and 10 courses of melphalan and prednisolone. These two patients were 'alive and well' 30 and 31 months following DHBI, with paraprotein reductions of 36% and 46%. Thirteen of 18 patients in Group II (intermediate prognosis) received DHBI, while 4 received lower HBI and 1 upper HBI alone. Six of 21 Group III (poor prognosis) patients received DHBI, while 8 were treated with lower HBI and 7 with upper HBI.

Of patients treated for palliation of pain, 88% reported prompt pain relief following DHBI and 54% following HBI. Seventy-two percent of patients reduced or discontinued use of pain medication. A significant reduction in paraprotein (>25%) was achieved in 64% of patients. This response was greater and more durable in patients receiving DHBI with less than 6 months between HBI fractions.

The median survival of all 41 patients was 4.5 months. The two patients in Group I were 'alive and well' 30 and 31 months following DHBI. Median survival of Group II patients was 17 months, with 3 (17%) alive after 18 months. Patients in Group III had a median survival of 3.5 months.

Complications were significant, with 14% of patients receiving upper HBI developing pneumonitis, 10% becoming infected, 5% with pancytopenia, and 7% with bleeding, and there was 1 (2%) treatment-related death. The authors suggest HBI as an alternative to second-line chemotherapy in these patients, citing effective palliation of pain, delay of disease progression, and durable response in a significant proportion of better-prognosis patients without maintenance chemotherapy.

A phase III protocol sponsored by the Southwest Oncology Group randomized 180 patients with chemoresponsive myeloma to either further chemotherapy (VMCP: vincristine, melphalan, cyclophosphamide, and prednisone) or sequential DHBI as consolidative therapy.[28] Both freedom from relapse and overall survival were superior following consolidative chemotherapy (medians 26 and 36 months, respectively) than for sequential DHBI (medians 20 and 28 months, respectively) ($p = 0.04$). Sixty-six partial or non-responders were also treated with HBI. Twenty-four percent of PR patients were converted to complete remission (CR) status following HBI. Only 5% of patients unresponsive to chemotherapy achieved CR following HBI. Overall, the authors concluded that the use of HBI in myeloma was not supported by their results. At our institution, HBI is reserved for palliation of diffuse disease in patients with disease refractory to chemotherapy. We prefer to use localized radiation portals to preserve marrow function and the ability to deliver chemotherapy. However, fractionated total-body irradiation as part of a bone marrow transplantation regimen plays an important role in the treatment of our patients.

Total-body irradiation

The use of total-body irradiation (TBI) as part of a preparative regimen for bone marrow transplantation (BMT) is well established.[29] The purpose of TBI is to treat the malignancy and to aid engraftment through immunosuppressive effects. The latter effect is mediated through cytotoxicity of TBI to lymphocytes. TBI is used in preparative regimens for BMT of radiosensitive diseases such as the leukemias, lymphomas, neuroblastoma, Ewing's sarcoma, and myeloma.

At our institution, TBI is most commonly employed in myeloma patients receiving an allogeneic BMT. The conditioning regimen most commonly used is melphalan 110 mg/m^2 on day −4 followed by 1000 cGy TBI in 8 fractions over days −3 to 0. Infusion of marrow of peripheral stem cells takes place immediately following the last TBI dose. In patients receiving a T-cell-depleted preparation, a dose of 1120 cGy is used. (All patients are treated with twice-daily fractionation, with a minimum of 6 hours between TBI fractions to allow for maximal repair of normal tissues and potential sparing of normal tissue from late toxicity.)

Patients are treated in the lateral decubitus position with a horizontal beam orientation. On the first treatment session, radiographs are taken of the torso with the patient in the treatment position. Partial-transmission filters are designed to cover all but the periphery of both lungs in the anteroposterior (AP) and posteroanterior (PA) projections. The thickness of these filters is designed to allow the central portion of the lungs to receive a dose of 700 cGy. The transmission through the patient with and without the lung filters in place is measured using electronic diode dosimetry. All subsequent treatments are made with the partial-transmission filters in place. The patient also undergoes a CT scan of the abdomen in the treatment position for localization of the kidneys. Posterior kidney blocks are used to limit the dose to the kidneys to 700 cGy. In some cases, the spleen may overlie the left kidney in the PA projection. In these cases, the spleen and left kidney are not shielded.

All patients are treated using 18 MV_p photons at a distance of 5 m. Dose rates are measured for individual patients, and vary from 8 to 12 cGy/min. A Lucite 'beam spoiler' is placed adjacent to the patient to increase the surface dose. Patients receive 8 fractions over 4 days. Placement of lung blocks are verified prior to delivery of each TBI dose. Each alternate fraction is delivered AP or PA, with the exception of the first and last fractions, which are delivered half through the AP and half through the PA portals.

Acute reactions to TBI

The most common acute side-effects of TBI are nausea and vomiting, mucositis, diarrhea, and parotiditis. The incidence of these acute reactions has been shown to be greatly reduced with fractionated schedules compared with single-dose TBI.[30] Nausea and vomiting are usually well controlled by premedication with antiemetics. The incidence of parotiditis is nearly zero in fractionated regimens, but may be as high as 40% with single-dose TBI.[31] The TBI regimen used at our institution is extremely well tolerated by patients over the acute period of treatment. This is likely a reflection of the twice-daily fractionation with a minimum 6-hour interfraction interval and the use of routine premedication with antiemetics and dexamethasone. All patients are likely to experience some fatigue during TBI. There is usually some degree of skin erythema, followed by hyperpigmentation. Severe skin reactions in the acute setting are unusual.

Late toxicity of TBI

Interstitial pneumonitis (IP) has been a major factor leading to transplant-related mortality. The incidence of IP has been reported to be up to 20% in patients in whom TBI was not part of the conditioning regimen,[32] and as high as 70% when conditioning included TBI delivered as a single dose.[29] Factors that increase the risk of IP are greater patient age, male gender, body surface area in excess of 1.5 m^2, and a diagnosis of chronic myeloid leukemia.[33,34]. The occurrence of graft-versus-host disease (GVHD) appears to be related to an increased incidence of IP.[33] Depletion of T cells greatly reduces the incidence of GVHD and IP.[35] However, there is a concomitant increase in graft failure and possibly a higher incidence of relapse.[29] TBI-related factors also influence the incidence of IP. The most important are the use of fractionated dose regimens and the inclusion of partial shielding for the lungs. Fractionated regimens have uniformly resulted in lower incidences of IP compared with the use of single-dose TBI regimens (Figure 21.8). In a large series of non-randomized studies, single-dose regimens resulted in an average incidence of IP that was 2.5 times higher than that following fractionated regimens.[30,32,36–42] Many of the fractionated regimens also utilized partial-transmission filters over the lungs. Labar et al[43] compared the incidence of IP in two groups of patients receiving the identical TBI regimen with or without lung blocks. IP was reduced to 8% in the group in which the lung dose was reduced with partial shielding,

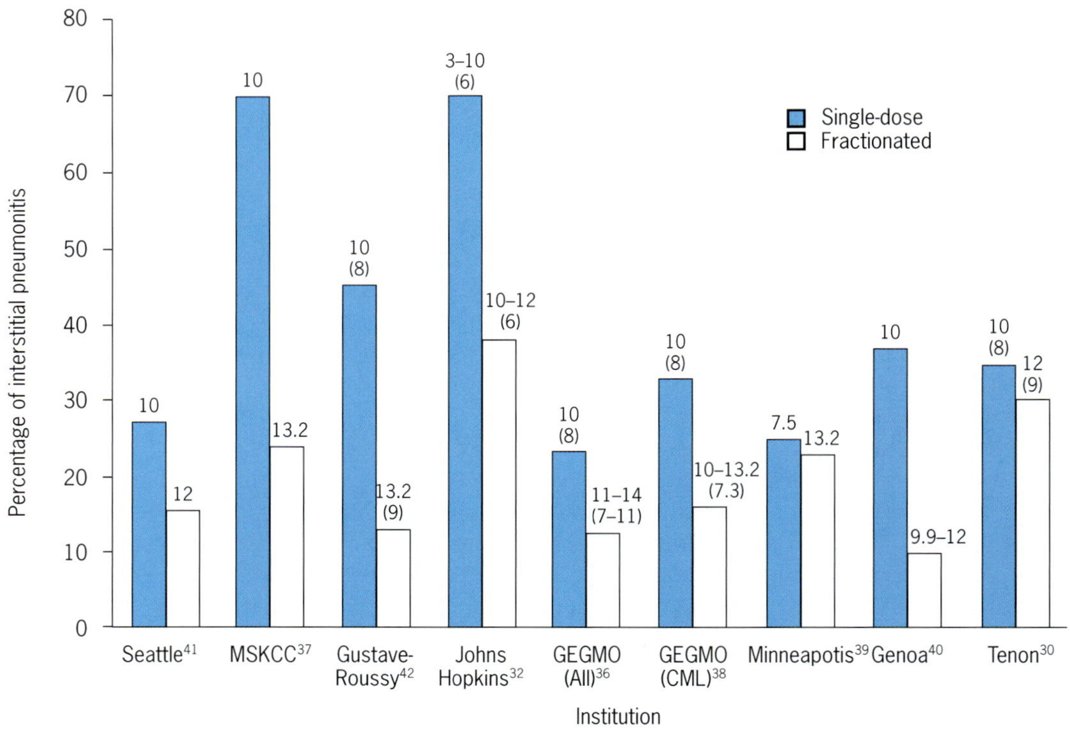

Figure 21.8 The incidence of interstitial pneumonitis in patients receiving total-body irradiation, either single-dose or fractionated, in various institutional reports. The total dose appears above each bar. The total lung dose appears in parentheses when lung blocks were used and the doses reported. (After Shank.[29])

compared with 27% without lung blocks. IP can be fatal in up to two-thirds of patients in which it occurs. Reduction of the lung dose with partial-transmission filters, delivery of fractionated TBI, and successful treatment of IP in its early stages with antivirals and immunoglobulin have reduced both the incidence and the mortality rate of IP in BMT patients.

Veno-occlusive disease of the liver (VOD) is a potentially fatal complication of BMT. The incidence of VOD has increased with increasingly intensive preparative regimens. The incidence of VOD may be increased in patients treated with single-dose regimens compared with fractionated TBI regimens, those receiving doses of more than 12 Gy, or those treated with dose rates above 0.1 Gy/min in single-dose regimens. There does not appear to be a dose-rate effect on the incidence of VOD when TBI is fractionated.[30]

BMT and TBI will exert late effects through impairment of endocrine function. Changes in thyroid function have been demonstrated following TBI and BMT.[44] Single-dose regimens (10 Gy) have been shown to result in an increased incidence of both subclinical hypothyroidism and clinical hypothyroidism compared with fractionated regimens (12–15.75 Gy) in the pediatric population.[41,45]

The incidence of gonadal dysfunction is higher in patients treated with single-dose TBI as measured by serum luteinizing hormone and follicle-stimulating hormone. In female patients, the incidence of infertility is nearly 100%, with only anecdotal reports of successful pregnancies following TBI and BMT.

Growth retardation following TBI is affected by reduction in growth hormone production and direct inhibition of bone growth. Most fractionated dose regimens using total doses of 12–15 Gy will have minimal effects on epiphyseal growth plates.

The human kidney is generally considered to be tolerant of the doses usually delivered in TBI. However, the group from Boston's Children's Hospital demonstrated renal dysfunction at a rate of 35% in pediatric patients following TBI and bone marrow transplant for acute lymphoblastic leukemia.[46] Moulder et al[47] have reported on the effect of chemotherapeutic agents in contributing to renal dysfunction at earlier times following lower doses of TBI. Late manifestation of renal injury following TBI has been reported in up to 45% of patients.[48–50] Conditioning regimens containing melphalan and TBI have been shown to pose a higher risk of nephrotoxicity compared with cyclophosphamide–TBI regimens.[51]

Radiation-induced renal injury has been demonstrated to be highly dependent on fraction size and on repair of sublethal radiation damage, which occurs in the kidney with a half-time of about 2 hours.[52] Deleterious effects of TBI on the kidney may therefore be reduced by fractionated regimens with sufficient time between fractions for complete repair. Partial blocking of kidneys during TBI may reduce the risk of late renal dysfunction.[53]

NEW DIRECTIONS

Administration of bone-seeking compounds conjugated with radionuclides can allow escalation of the dose of radiation delivered to the marrow significantly while sparing other organs.[54–56] In a preliminary study, six myeloma patients received holmium-166 (^{166}Ho)-DOTMP (1,4,7,10-tetraazacyclododecane-1,4,7,10-tetramethylenephosphonic acid) as the conditioning regimen. The radiation absorbed dose delivered to the bone marrow ranged from 15.0 to 46.3 Gy, which is considerably higher than can be delivered during TBI. Radioactivity concentration in skeletal regions predominantly composed of trabecular bone was five- to sixfold higher than that in cortical regions. The distribution of the absorbed marrow dose was heterogeneous: 15–20% of the marrow received an absorbed dose significantly larger than the average value, while 5–10% of the marrow received a substantially lower dose.[56] This approach is currently being evaluated by itself and in addition to standard high-dose chemotherapy to augment the conditioning regimen.

CONCLUSIONS

Radiotherapy plays a central and diverse role in the management and care of patients with solitary plasmacytoma and myeloma. Whether for palliation or for cure, directed at a focal site of disease or total-body, treatment should be based on modern imaging and careful planning. With an increased understanding of the biology of plasma cell tumors and the development of improved systemic treatments, local control of focal disease by radiation may further contribute to prolonged patient survival.

REFERENCES

1. Hall E. *Radiobiology for the Radiologist*, 4th edn. Philadelphia: JB Lippincott, 1994.
2. Withers H. Biologic basis for altered fractionation schemes, *Cancer* 1985; **55**: 2086–95.
3. Shimizu T, Motoji T, Oshimi K et al. Proliferative state and radiosensitivity of human myeloma stem cells. *Br J Cancer* 1982; **45**: 679–83.
4. Fertil B, Malaise E-P. Inherent cellular radiosensitivity as a basic concept for human tumor radiosensitivity. *Int J Radiat Oncol Biol Phys* 1981; **7**: 621–9.
5. Glück S, Van Dyk J, Messner HA. Radiosensitivity of human clonogenic myeloma cells and normal bone marrow precursors: effect of different dose rates and fractionation. *Int J Radiat Oncol Biol Phys* 1994; **28**: 877–82.
6. Lowe SW, Schmitt EM, Smith SW et al. p53 is required for radiation-induced apoptosis in mouse thymocytes. *Nature* 1993; **362**: 847–9.
7. Filippovich IV, Sorokina NI, Robillard N et al. Radiation-induced apoptosis in human tumor cell lines: adaptive response and split-dose effect. *Int J Cancer* 1998; **77**: 76–81.

8. Corwin J, Lindberg RD. Solitary plasmacytoma of bone vs. extramedullary plasmacytoma and their relationship to multiple myeloma. *Cancer* 1979; **43**: 1007–13.
9. Frassica DA, Frassica FJ, Schray MF et al. Solitary plasmacytoma of bone: Mayo Clinic experience. *Int J Radiat Oncol Biol Phys* 1989; **16**: 43–8.
10. Dimopoulos MA, Goldstein J, Fuller L et al. Curability of solitary bone plasmacytoma. *J Clin Oncol* 1992; **10**: 587–90.
11. Chak LY, Cox RS, Bostwick DG et al. Solitary plasmacytoma of bone: treatment, progression, and survival. *J Clin Oncol* 1987; **5**: 1811–15.
12. Knowling MA, Harwood AR, Bergsagel DE. Comparison of extramedullary plasmacytomas with solitary and multiple plasma cell tumors of bone. *J Clin Oncol* 1983; **1**: 255–262.
13. Bolek TW, Marcus RB, Mendenhall NP. Solitary plasmacytoma of bone and soft tissue. *Int J Radiat Oncol Biol Phys* 1996; **36**: 329–33.
14. Mayr NA, Wen BC, Hussey DH et al. The role of radiation therapy in the treatment of solitary plasmacytoma. *Radiother Oncol* 1990; **17**: 293–303.
15. Holland J, Trenkner DA, Wasserman TH et al. Plasmacytoma: treatment results and conversion to myeloma. *Cancer* 1992; **69**: 1513–17.
16. Jyorthirmayi R, Gangadharan VP, Nair MK. Radiotherapy in the treatment of solitary plasmacytoma. *Br J Radiol* 1997; **70**: 511–16.
17. Bush SE, Goffinet DR, Bagshaw MA. Extramedullary plasmacytoma of the head and neck. *Radiology* 1981; **140**: 801–5.
18. Bindal AK, Bindal RK, van Lovern H et al. Management of intracranial plasmacytoma. *J Neurosurg* 1995; **83**: 218–21.
19. Wasserman TH. Myeloma and plasmacytomas. In: *Principles and Practice of Radiation Oncology* (Perez CA, Brady LW, eds). Philadelphia: Lippincott-Raven, 1997: 2013–23.
20. Catell D, Kogen Z, Donahue B et al. Multiple myeloma of an extremity: Must the entire bone be treated? *Int J Radiat Oncol Biol Phys* 1998; **40**: 117–19.
21. Liebross RH, Ha CS, Cox JD et al. Solitary plasmacytoma: outcome and prognostic factors following radiotherapy. *Int J Radiat Oncol Biol Phys* 1998; **41**: 1063–7.
22. Bataille R, Sany J. Solitary myeloma: clinical and prognostic features of a review of 114 cases. *Cancer* 1981; **48**: 845–51.
23. Mendenhall CM, Thar TL, Million RR. Solitary plasmacytoma of bone and soft tissue. *Int J Radiat Oncol Biol Phys* 1980; **6**: 1497–501.
24. Mill WB, Griffith R. The role of radiation therapy in the management of plasma cell tumors. *Cancer* 1980; **45**: 647–52.
25. Leigh BR, Kurtts TA, Mack CF et al. Radiation therapy for palliation of multiple myeloma. *Int J Radiat Oncol Biol Phys* 1993; **25**: 801–4.
26. Singer CRJ, Tobias JS, Giles F et al. Hemibody irradiation. *Cancer* 1989; **63**: 2446–51.
27. Medical Research Council's Working Party on Leukaemia in Adults. Prognostic features in the third MRC myelomatosis trial. *Br J Cancer* 1980; **42**: 831–40.
28. Salmon SE, Tesh D, Crowley J et al. Chemotherapy is superior to sequential hemibody irradiation for remission consolidation in multiple myeloma: a Southwest Oncology Group study. *J Clin Oncol* 1990; **8**: 1575–84.
29. Shank B. Total body irradiation. In: *Textbook of Radiation Oncology* (Leibel S, Phillips TL, eds). Philadelphia: WB Saunders, 1998: 253–75.
30. Ozsahin M, Pene F, Touboul E et al. Total-body irradiation before bone marrow transplantation; results of two randomized instantaneous dose rates in 157 patients. *Cancer* 1992; **69**: 2853–65.
31. Valls A, Granena A, Carreras E et al. Total body irradiation in bone marrow transplantation: fractionated vs single dose. Acute toxicity and preliminary results. *Bull Cancer* 1989; **76**: 797–804.
32. Pino y Torres JL, Bross DS, Lam W-C et al. Risk factors in interstitial pneumonitis following allogeneic bone marrow transplantation. *Int J Radiat Oncol Biol Phys* 1982; **8**: 1301–7.
33. Granena A, Carreras E, Rozman C et al. Interstitial pneumonitis after BMT: 15 years experience in a single institution. *Bone Marrow Transplant* 1993; **11**: 453–8.
34. Petersen FB, Bearman SI. Preparative regimens and their toxicity. In: *Bone Marrow Transplantation* (Forman SJ, Blume KG, eds). Boston: Blackwell Scientific, 1994: 79–95.
35. Latini P, Aristei C, Aversa F et al. Interstitial pneumonitis after hyperfractionated total body irradiation in HLA-matched T-depleted bone marrow transplantation. *Int J Radiat Oncol Biol Phys* 1992; **23**: 401–5.
36. Sutton L, Kuentz M, Cordonnier C et al. Allogeneic bone marrow transplantation for adult acute lymphoblastic leukemia in first complete remission: factors predictive of transplant-related mortality and influence of total body irradiation modalities. *Bone Marrow Transplant* 1993; **12**: 583–9.

37. Shank B, Chu FCH, Dinsmore R et al. Hyperfractionated total body irradiation for bone marrow transplantation. Results in seventy leukemia patients with allogeneic transplants. *Int J Radiat Oncol Biol Phys* 1981; **9**: 1607–11.
38. Socie G, Devergie A, Girinsky T et al. Influence of the fractionation of total body irradiation on complications and relapse rate for chronic myelogenous leukemia. *Int J Radiat Oncol Biol Phys* 1991; **20**: 397–404.
39. Kim TH, McGlave PB, Ramsay N et al. Comparison of two total body irradiation regimens in allogeneic bone marrow transplantation for acute non-lymphoblastic leukemia in first remission. *Int J Radiat Oncol Biol Phys* 1990; **19**: 889–97.
40. Bacigalupo A, Van Lint MT, Frassoni F et al. Late complications of allogeneic bone marrow transplantation. *Med Oncol Tumor Pharmacother* 1991; **8**: 261–3.
41. Thomas BC, Stanhope R, Plowman PN et al. Endocrine function following single fraction and fractionated total body irradiation for bone marrow transplantation in childhood. *Acta Endocrinol* 1993; **128**: 508–12.
42. Cosset JM, Baume D, Pico JL et al. Single versus hyperfractionated total body irradiation before allogeneic bone marrow transplantation: a non-randomized comparative study of 54 patients at the Institut Gustave Roussy. *Radiother Oncol* 1989; **15**: 151–60.
43. Labar B, Bogdanic V, Nemet D et al. Total body irradiation with and without lung shielding for allogeneic bone marrow transplantation. *Bone Marrow Transplant* 1992; **9**: 343–7.
44. Carlson K, Lonnerholm G, Smedmyr B et al. Thyroid function after autologous bone marrow transplantation. *Bone Marrow Transplant* 1992; **10**: 123–7.
45. Sanders JE. The impact of marrow transplant preparative regimens on subsequent growth and development. *Semin Hematol* 1991; **8**: 244–9.
46. Tarbell NJ, Guinan EC, Niemeyer C et al. Late onset of renal dysfunction in survivors of bone marrow transplantation. *Int J Radiat Oncol Biol Phys* 1988; **41**: 63–6.
47. Moulder JE, Fish BJ, Abrams RA. Renal toxicity following total body irradiation in syngeneic bone marrow transplantation. *Transplantation* 1987; **43**: 589–92.
48. Chappell ME, Keeling DM, Prentice HG et al. Haemolytic uraemic syndrome after bone marrow transplantation: an adverse effect of total body irradiation? *Bone Marrow Transplant* 1988; **3**: 339–47.
49. Guinan EC, Tarbell NJ, Niemeyer CM et al. Intravascular hemolysis and renal insufficiency after bone marrow transplantation. *Blood* 1988; **72:** 451–5.
50. Lawton CA, Cohen EP, Barber-Derus SW et al. Late renal dysfunction in adult survivors of bone marrow transplantation. *Cancer* 1991; **67**: 2795–800.
51. Helenglass G, Powles RL, McElwain JJ et al. Melphalan and total body irradiation (TBI) versus cyclophosphamide and TBI as conditioning for allogeneic matched sibling bone marrow transplant for acute myeloblastic leukemia in first remission. *Bone Marrow Transplant* 1988; **3**: 21–9.
52. Van Rongen E, Kuijpers WC, Madhuizen HT. Fractionation effects and repair kinetics in rat kidney. *Int J Radiat Oncol Biol Phys* 1990; **18**: 1093–106.
53. Lawton CA, Barber Derus SW, Murray KJ et al. Influence of renal shielding on the incidence of late renal dysfunction associated with T-lymphocyte depleted bone marrow transplantation in adult patients. *Int J Radiat Oncol Biol Phys* 1992; **23**: 681–6.
54. Appelbaum FR, Brown PA, Sandmaier BM et al. Specific marrow ablation before marrow transplantation using an aminophosphonic acid conjugate ^{166}Ho-EDTMP. *Blood* 1992; **80**: 1608–13.
55. Parks NJ, Kawakami TG, Avila MJ et al. Bone marrow transplantation in dogs after radio-ablation with a new Ho-166 amino phosphonic acid bone-seeking agent (DOTMP). *Blood* 1993; **82**: 318–25.
56. Bayouth JE, Macey DJ, Boyer AL, Champlin RE. Radiation dose distribution within the bone marrow of patients receiving holmium-166-labeled-phosphonate for marrow ablation. *Med Phys* 1995; **22**: 743–53.

22

Role of interferons

Bhawna Sirohi, Jennifer Treleaven, Ray Powles

INTRODUCTION

Interferon-α (IFN-α) possesses antitumour activity against a number of haematologic neoplasms, including hairy cell leukaemia, chronic myeloid leukaemia, and myeloma. Although it was first introduced as a treatment for myeloma over 20 years ago,[1] its place in the treatment of patients with myeloma is still not entirely defined. The controversy concerning the in vivo use of IFN-α is further emphasized by in vitro studies showing that, under various conditions, IFN-α can either stimulate or inhibit the growth and proliferation of myeloma cells.[2–6]

Studies assessing the value of continuing chemotherapy after patients with myeloma have attained a plateau phase have not shown any benefit on survival.[7] In view of the relative lack of efficacy of chemotherapy for relapsing or refractory patients with myeloma, attempts have been made to investigate the role of biologic response modifiers in this disease.

Issacs and Lindenmann[8] in 1957 demonstrated that when chicken egg chorioallantoic membranes were exposed to a heat-inactivated influenza virus, a factor was released that could protect fresh tissues from viral infection with live influenza. The factor was termed interferon (IFN). It was not until 20 years later that sufficient supplies of partially purified human IFNs were available for evaluation in a variety of human tumours, although crude preparations had been administered to cancer patients as early as 1966.[9]

Weissman successfully isolated and cloned the gene for human IFN-α in 1979. Using recombinant DNA technology, this gene was introduced into *Escherichia coli*. Supplies of human IFN manufactured by recombinant DNA techniques and purified to homogeneity became available in 1981, permitting evaluation of the effects of single IFN species in the absence of contaminating proteins.[10]

'Inducible inducers'

IFNs have been referred to as 'inducible inducers', since their production can be induced in cells by a wide variety of agents, including viruses, polyribonucleotides, certain fungal extracts, bacteria and bacterial products, mitogens, and specific antigens, and, in turn, their application to cells induces the production of a wide range of substances, including various proteins, enzymes, prostaglandins, and histocompatibility antigens, that may mediate many of the effects seen with IFN therapy.[10]

CHARACTERIZATION AND NOMENCLATURE

The interferons are a group of proteins and glycoproteins, subdivided according to differences in antigenic, biologic, and chemical properties. The three distinct antigenic types of IFN are α, β and γ.[11]

Genes encoding IFNs are located on human chromosomes 9 (α and β), 2 (β), 5 (β), and 12 (γ). The molecular cloning of human IFNs in *E. coli* has permitted the large-scale production of highly purified single molecular species of various IFNs (α, β, and γ).

Type I

The alpha-IFNs are a family of at least 14 highly homogeneous species (with approximately 75% homology in their amino acid sequences) of about 166 amino acids and a molecular weight of 15–26 kDa that are produced by a variety of cell types, including macrophages, null cells, and B-cell lines, upon exposure to viruses or synthetic polynucleotides. IFN-α2b is a 98% pure preparation of a single species of human alpha-IFN with a specific activity of 2×10^8 IU/mg protein. The molecule consists of 165 amino acids, has a molecular weight of 20 kDa, and is the main preparation used in patients with myeloma.

IFN-β is also a protein, with 166 amino acids and a molecular weight of 15–22 kDa, which is naturally produced by fibroblasts and epithelial cells. It is induced by viruses or synthetic polynucleotides. Both of these interferons are acid-stable and relatively heat-resistant.

Type II

Also called immune IFN, IFN-γ is secreted by both sensitized and unsensitized T lymphocytes. It has different physicochemical properties (146 amino acids and a molecular weight of 17 kDa) and different inducers, and uses a different cellular receptor than do IFN-α and -β.

MECHANISM OF ACTION

The specific mechanisms of action of the IFNs are not very clearly defined, but the role of IFN receptors does explain the numerous biochemical processes brought about by IFNs.[12] Once IFN binds to the specific receptor (one receptor for α and β with the coding gene on chromosome 21, and another for γ with the coding gene on chromosome 6), the IFN–receptor complex is internalized. IFN is partially degraded, while the receptor is returned to the cell surface. Within the cell, IFN exerts its action by altering the expression of genes and up- or downregulating their expression.

Antitumour effect

IFNs have the capacity to alter the relationship between host and tumour by augmentation of host effector mechanisms or by direct effects on the tumour, involving changes in the state of differentiation or in the expression of tumour-associated antigens.

Direct antitumour effects may be through induction of apoptosis, and indirect effects, mediated through the host, may be through inhibition of angiogenesis or immunomodulation.

The relative importance of direct versus host-mediated effects in the expression of the antitumour activity of IFNs in the clinical setting remains undefined. It is likely that the exact mechanism varies from patient to patient, depending principally upon the immune status of the host and the biochemical characteristics of the tumour, including the presence or absence of IFN receptors and the ability of the tumour to inactivate IFN by release of proteases.

The inhibitory effect of IFNs is more prominent in non-cycling tumour cells (G_0–G_1), and in some cases an accumulation of cells in G_0 has been seen accompanied by a decrease in transition to G_1 and the arrest of some cell types in G_1.[13,14]

Among the various mechanisms postulated to explain the antiproliferative effect of IFNs have been inhibition of c-*myc* and c-*fos*, induction of 2′–5′ A synthetase, and a protein kinase-inhibiting translation and inhibition of the gene for ornithine decarboxylase, which explains the effect of IFN-α on the overall slowing of the cell cycle and arrest of cell division during G_0.[15,16]

PRECLINICAL BIOLOGY OF THE ALPHA INTERFERONS

Two models that have provided an insight into the preclinical biology of the IFNs have been the human tumour clonogenic assay and human tumour xenografts in immunodeficient mice.[17] These models indicated that the use of IFNs would likely be effective treatment for a broad range of malignancies and that response would be highly dependent upon the type of IFN as well as on the dose schedule and route of administration. Both models provided evidence that IFN-α may demonstrate a synergistic or additive interaction with standard chemotherapeutic agents such as cyclophosphamide and doxorubicin.

IMMUNE MODULATION

IFNs have immunomodulating effects, enhance phagocytosis by macrophages, and increase the target cell-specific cytotoxicity exerted by lymphocytes, IFN-γ being more active than IFN-α.[11] IFN-γ increases the expression of class I major histocompatibility complex (MHC) molecules on tumour cells, rendering them more susceptible to destruction by T lymphocytes. It also increases class II MHC antigen expression on monocytes, T lymphocytes, fibroblasts, and endothelial cells.[18]

IFNs also increase the expression of receptors for the Fc fragment of IgG on the surface of lymphocytes and macrophages, enhancing the tumoricidal activity of these cells.[19,20] IFNs may modify the expression of cell surface antigens on tumour cells, rendering them more susceptible to control by existing immune effector mechanisms. IFN-α also activates natural killer cells. The mechanism if action of IFN-α in hairy cell leukaemia is still unclear, but much of the evidence favours a direct antiproliferative effect rather than an upregulation of the immune response.[21]

IN VITRO EFFECTS OF INTERFERON ON MYELOMA CELL LINES

Myeloma was one of the malignancies where results of IFN treatment in small numbers of patients were initially encouraging.[1] Subsequent studies have confirmed that IFN-α is capable of producing regression in myeloma and other tumours.

In a clonogenic assay, myeloma and other tumour cells were tested with recombinant IFNα-2b, melphalan, doxorubicin, cyclophosphamide, and other cytotoxic agents. Low concentrations of IFN resulted in a reduction in myeloma cell colony numbers, and the combination of IFN and melphalan apparently had a synergistic effect on tumour cell colony reduction.

As a single agent, IFN-α2b showed maximum tumour cell colony reduction when used in higher concentrations with continuous cell exposure, whereas short-term exposure did not produce significant tumour cell colony reduction.[22]

Tanaka et al[23] studied the effects of IFN-α on in vitro proliferation and M-protein secretion in human myeloma cells, and suggested that IFN-α had a more pronounced inhibitory effect on M-protein secretion than on cell proliferation.

In vitro studies of the effect of IFN-α on five human myeloma cell lines[24] demonstrated enhancement of myeloma cell apoptosis induced by IFN-α. Cell cycle analysis revealed an accumulation of myeloma cells in the G_1 fraction and reduction of S-phase cells, with an increase in hypodiploid apoptotic cells. This implied that IFN-α not only has cytoreductive effects on myeloma cells by bringing about apoptotic cell death but also has a cytostatic function, as seen by the arrest of cells in G_1. Thus, the use of IFN-α may improve response rates as well as helping to maintain a plateau phase. [25–28]

In vitro data support the belief that the principal effect of IFNs is to increase the length of all phases of the cell cycle and not to cause a selective accumulation of cells in G_2, as shown on fibroblasts and epithelial cells from normal, hyperplastic, and neoplastic human breast tissue. At an IFN concentration of 1000 IU/ml, the inhibitory effects on monolayer growth were completely reversible, but the growth potential of cells at lower density in colony-forming cultures was not completely recovered.[29] IFNs also decrease both the labelling index of myeloma cells[30] and their clonogenic potential.[31]

INTERFERONS AND INTERLEUKIN-6

IFN-α induces autocrine production of interleukin-6 (IL-6) in myeloma cell lines, raising the question of IFN-α possibly inducing myeloma cells to produce their own tumour growth factor in vitro.[4] Recently, it has been shown that IFN-α is a survival factor for IL-6-dependent myeloma cell lines that are induced to apoptose when IL-6 is removed.[32]

However, other studies have shown that IFN-α inhibits the growth of IL-6-dependent myeloma cell lines,[33,34] and downregulates the IL-6 receptor.[35,36] In addition, IFN-β, which shares a common receptor with IFN-α, interrupts the IL-6-dependent signalling pathway.[6]

Cell lines in which growth is actually stimulated by IFN-α have also been reported.[4,5,37] The exact interaction of IFN-α and IL-6 in the cytokine network surrounding myeloma cells is not well defined.

INTERFERON AND β_2-MICROGLOBULIN

An increase in serum β_2-microglobulin (β_2M) can be induced by IFN-α in myeloma. This should be taken into consideration when using β_2M for the assessment of tumour response during IFN therapy. In general, the limited value of β_2M in following therapy and response (see Chapter 15) is lost with IFN-α therapy.[38]

CLINICAL TRIALS

IFN-α and -β both inhibit the growth of myeloma colony-forming cells and reduce the self-renewal capacity of these cells, suggesting that IFNs may be better at prolonging remission than at inducing remission.[39] Clinical trials of IFNs, however, have evolved through various stages.

Interferon alone as induction therapy

The efficacy of IFN in myeloma was initially demonstrated in four patients in 1979, who received the drug as single-agent induction therapy. Although it induced complete remission (CR) in two cases and partial remission (PR) in the other two, it has subsequently been shown to be less effective than melphalan–prednisolone[40] or combination chemotherapy (VMCP: vincristine, melphalan, cyclophosphamide, and prednisone)[41] as induction therapy. Thus, the use of IFN-α alone for remission induction is not recommended.

Interferon in combination with other agents as induction therapy

The first study[42] using IFN-α2b (2 MU/m^2 three times a week for 2 weeks of a 28-day cycle) along with melphalan–prednisone (MP) resulted in an overall response rate of 75%. This high response rate was subsequently confirmed by an Eastern Cooperative Oncology Group (ECOG) study,[28] which used IFN at a dose of 5 MU/m^2 three times a week for 3 weeks, alternating with

VBMCP (vincristine, carmustine, melphalan, cyclophosphamide, and prednisone). The overall response rate was 80%, with 30% of patients attaining CR.

These preliminary studies prompted randomized trials, which have yielded conflicting results, with some studies showing no survival benefit or improvement in response rate from the addition of IFN to induction chemotherapy.[26,43]

A Cancer and Leukemia Group B (CALGB) study,[26] which used IFN-α2b at a dose of 2 MU three times a week, randomized 278 patients to MP alone or MP with IFN-α2b. The response rates were comparable (44% for MP and 37% for MP + IFN-α2b), as were the median survival durations (3.12 years with MP and 3.05 years with MP + IFN-α2b). Thus, it appeared that there was no advantage in the concomitant administration of IFN-α2b and standard MP in the initial treatment of myeloma.

Other studies have reported better survival and increased response rates with the addition of IFN to MP[44] or other combination chemotherapy[28] as initial treatment of myeloma. A Swedish study[45] showed in a randomized trial that patients receiving IFN-α and MP had a response rate of 68%, compared with 42% in the group receiving MP alone ($p = 0.0001$), although there was no difference in overall survival between the two groups. Scheithauer et al[46] and Montuoro et al[47] also showed a better response rate as well as survival benefit with the addition of IFN-α to VMCP and MP, respectively.

Ludwig et al[48] have pooled and analysed data from 16 trials where 2286 patients were randomized to receive induction chemotherapy alone or induction chemotherapy combined with IFN. The total weekly IFN dose ranged between 4.8 and 18.7 MU. The overall response rate was 54.4% for patients treated with IFN and chemotherapy, compared with 45.9% for patients treated with chemotherapy alone. The improvements in relapse-free and overall survival were 6 and 5 months, respectively, with the addition of IFN.

Normal or malignant plasma cells do not usually express CD20. However, a minority of patients with myeloma who have $CD20^+$ cells can respond to the anti-CD20 monoclonal antibody rituximab. IFN-γ can induce CD20 expression on the surface of plasma cells, which may make them sensitive to the lytic action of rituximab.

Interferon as maintenance therapy

Cell cycle analysis carried out by Otsuki et al[24] revealed an accumulation of myeloma cells in the G_1 phase and a reduction of S-phase cells, with an increase in hypodiploid apoptotic cells. This implied that IFN-α not only had cytoreductive effects on myeloma cells through apoptotic cell death but also had a cytostatic function, as shown by the G_1 arrest of the cells. Thus, it is possible that the use of IFN-α can improve the frequency and quality of remission and help maintain the plateau phase.[25–27,49]

The role of IFNs in maintenance therapy is still open to debate because of the various conflicting data published.

Mandelli et al[50] were the first to assess the use of IFN-α2b during the plateau phase. In a randomized study of 101 patients, maintenance IFN-α2b (50 patients) was found to be of greatest benefit in patients with the lowest tumour burdens at the start of therapy. IFN-α2b was beneficial in terms of response duration in all patients ($p = 0.0002$) and superior survival in responders ($p = 0.04$). The updated results of this study 9 years after randomization[51] confirm a significant prolongation of response duration in the patients who received IFN-α2b maintenance, with the median response duration being 24 months in the IFN-α2b arm versus 13 months in the no-IFN arm ($p = 0.002$) (Figure 22.1). The median overall survival durations were not significantly different at 50 months (IFN) and 39 months (no IFN) ($p = 0.2$), but amongst patients who had experienced a greater than 50% reduction in paraprotein, the median overall survival durations were 50 and 35 months, respectively ($p = 0.07$). In this study, IFN maintenance therapy appeared to significantly prolong the duration of response in patients benefiting from earlier induction chemotherapy, while the effect on survival was less clear. The study concluded

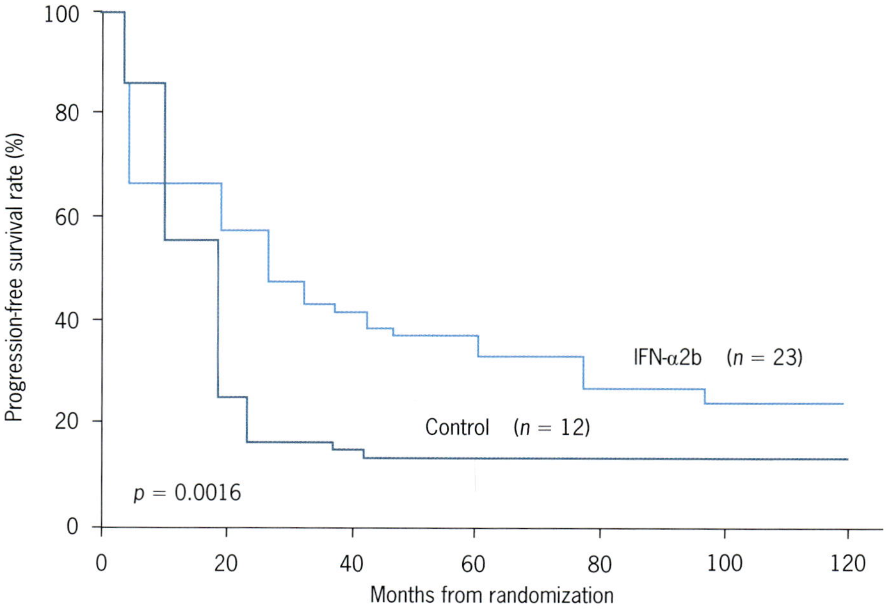

Figure 22.1 Long-term follow-up of patients randomized to maintenance IFN-α2b or no therapy after initial conventional-dose chemotherapy. (From: Pulsoni A, Avvisati G, Petrucci MT et al. The Italian experience on interferon as maintenance treatment in multiple myeloma: ten years after. *Blood* 1998; **92:** 2184–5. Copyright American Society of Hematology, used by permission.)

that IFN maintenance was appropriate in responsive myeloma patients, because delaying relapse would result in improved quality of life (QOL). Accurate QOL evaluation is required in these patients to confirm this assumption.

Other major studies conducted after the initial study are summarized in Table 22.1.

In the UK Medical Research Council (MRC) IFN trial,[52] 284 myeloma patients in plateau phase were randomized to receive IFN-α or no maintenance therapy. IFN-α did not prolong overall survival in this study, but there was a non-significant trend towards longer relapse-free survival in patients receiving IFN-α. It was noted that disease relapse in patients receiving IFN-α was more aggressive, with greater elevations in serum paraprotein and β_2M.

IFN-α maintenance therapy had no effect on progression-free or overall survival in a German study where 117 of 406 untreated myeloma patients reached the stage of randomization to IFN-α or no IFN.[53]

A randomized study conducted at the UK Royal Marsden Hospital[54] used IFN-α as maintenance treatment following high-dose chemotherapy, mostly with autotransplantation, in 84 patients. At a median follow-up of 52 months, the median progression-free survival was 46 months in the IFN-α arm versus 27 months in the control arm ($p < 0.025$). For the 65 patients who achieved CR after high-dose treatment, there was a significant prolongation of remission duration ($p < 0.03$), and 49% of the patients who received IFN-α maintenance were still in remission 4 years after high-dose therapy. This prolongation of remission duration was not seen in partial responders and non-responders. Overall survival was significantly longer in the IFN-α arm ($p = 0.006$). However, at a median follow-up of 77 months, most patients had relapsed and died, and the survival advantage noted earlier was no longer apparent. For the 65 CR patients, only a trend towards improved progression-free survival was noted ($p = 0.09$) (Figure 22.2). These data clearly indicate that IFN-α delays, but does not prevent, disease progression.

A retrospective comparison from the European Blood and Marrow Transplant group (EBMT)[55] of 473 patients who received IFN maintenance after autologous transplantation with 419 patients who did not receive IFN showed that overall survival (78 months versus 47 months; $p = 0.006$) and progression-free survival (29 months versus 20 months; $p = 0.01$) were significantly better in

Table 22.1 Summary of interferon (IFN) maintenance trials

		Overall survival (months)			Response duration (months)		
Study	**No. of patients**	**IFN**	**No IFN**	***p* value**	**IFN**	**No IFN**	***p* value**
Italian[50,51]	101	50	39	0.21	24	13	0.0016
MRC[52]	284	41.2	34.5	0.57	16.9	12.7	0.2
German[53]	117	45	45	NS	13	13	NS
RMH[54]	84	80	68	0.1	43	27	0.11
Canadian[56]	176	44	33	0.049	18	13	<0.003
Spanish[57]	92	38.8	32.7	0.12	13	7.7	0.042
SWOG[58]	193	32	38	NS	12	11	NS
Austrian[65]	100	50.6	34.4	<0.05	17.8	8.2	<0.01
Nordic[67]	319	—	—	NS	19	14	NS

NS, not significant.

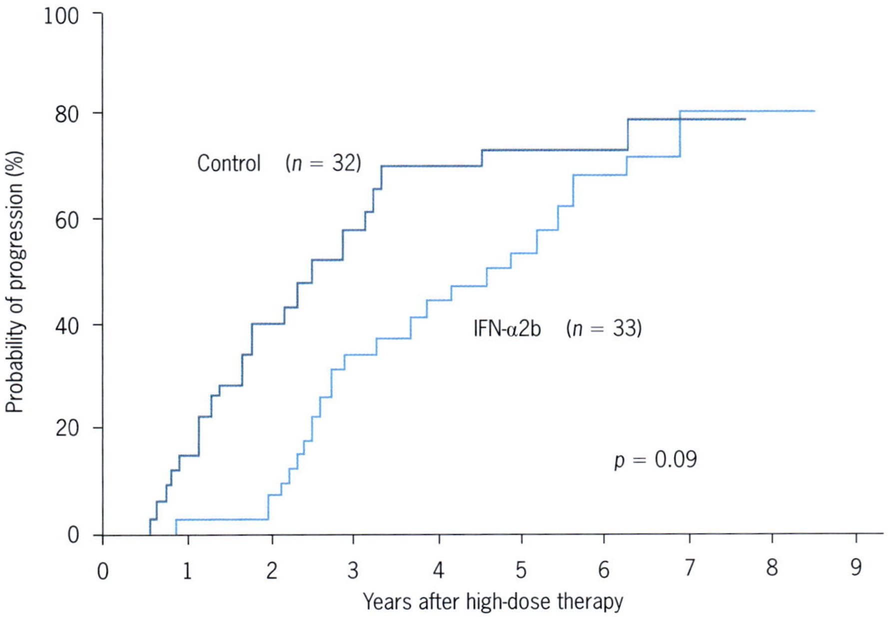

Figure 22.2 Progression-free survival after randomization to IFN-α2b or no maintenance amongst patients achieving CR after high-dose chemotherapy. (From Cunningham et al,[54] with permission from the *British Journal of Haematology*.)

the IFN group. The difference in overall survival was most pronounced in patients who were in PR after the autograft ($p < 0.0001$), while it was of borderline statistical significance in the CR patients ($p = 0.05$). Progression-free survival was significantly better in PR patients receiving IFN ($p < 0.0001$), while no difference was seen in patients who attained CR. This is in contrast to the Royal Marsden study, where benefit was confined to CR patients.

A Canadian study[56] of 176 patients responding to MP who were randomized to receive either

IFN 2 MU/m^2 three times a week (85 patients) or no maintenance treatment (91 patients) showed no apparent benefit for IFN (median overall survival 43 months compared with 35 months for patients not receiving IFN; $p = 0.16$). However, when adjusted for chance imbalances in baseline prognostic factors, particularly performance status, the median overall survival was 44 months in the IFN arm versus 33 months in the control arm ($p = 0.05$). Progression-free survival was also favourably influenced by IFN (unadjusted $p < 0.002$; adjusted $p < 0.003$). IFN toxicity caused 58% of patients to reduce the dose, although 84% of these were able to return to the original dose while 14% had to discontinue IFN treatment completely.

A Spanish study[57] of 92 patients with an objective response to 12 courses of VMCP/VBAP (vincristine, carmustine, doxorubicin, and prednisone) who were randomized to receive maintenance therapy with IFN-α2b (50 patients) or not (41 patients) showed no prolongation of survival ($p = 0.12$). However, IFN-α2b recipients experienced a significantly longer duration of response (13 months versus 7.7 months; $p = 0.04$).

A study from the Southwestern Oncology Group (SWOG)[58] included 193 patients who had attained remission and were randomized to receive IFN-α 3 MU three times a week. IFN-α did not result in any improvement in relapse-free or overall survival when compared with observation alone, and additionally, QOL was poorer.

However, the meta-analysis conducted by Ludwig et al,[48] which evaluated IFN maintenance therapy from eight randomized trials comprising 929 patients, has demonstrated benefit for IFN therapy in terms of prolongation of remission duration and survival. IFN maintenance treatment appeared to prolong the average relapse-free survival by 7 months and the average overall survival by 5 months. Younger patients, those with a good performance status, and those with a low tumor burden appear to benefit most from IFN maintenance.

Another meta-analysis evaluated 24 randomized IFN trials (12 induction and 12 maintenance), which included 4012 patients.[59] Overall survival was better with IFN; the 3-year survival rate being 53% with IFN and 49% without IFN ($p = 0.01$). An effect of similar magnitude was observed in both induction and maintenance trials, with increases in median survival of about 2 and 7 months, respectively. Progression-free survival was significantly better with IFN in both induction ($p = 0.0003$) and maintenance ($p < 0.0001$) trials. However, survival after recurrence was worse ($p = 0.02$) with IFN. The conclusion was that the benefits of IFN therapy must be weighed against its cost and its effect on patients' quality of life.

INTERFERON FOLLOWING ALLOGENEIC TRANSPLANTATION

Relapse is still a major cause of treatment failure in patients undergoing allografts for myeloma. In a pilot study, Byrne et al[60] used IFN-α as adjuvant therapy in patients failing to achieve CR following allogeneic transplantation. The rationale was that IFN-α could have a dual effect by acting directly on residual myeloma cells and by augmenting the graft-versus-myeloma effect. Five out of 13 evaluable patients who were all in PR received IFN-α at a dose of 3 MU three times a week starting at a median of 4 months post transplant. No increased toxicity occurred in terms of a worsening of graft-versus-host disease. Durable CRs were achieved in two patients within 8 weeks of therapy, while two more attained CR after 36 and 30 weeks. Thus, IFN after allogeneic transplantation may be an effective adjuvant treatment for patients who fail to attain CR. See Chapter 20 for a full discussion of interferon in the setting of allogeneic transplantation for myeloma.

REFRACTORY AND RESISTANT MYELOMAS

IFN was originally used successfully in the setting of refractory disease.[61] Since then, several other studies have been published on the use of IFN as salvage treatment, with conflicting results.

Alexanian et al[62] used IFN-α combined with either VAD (vincristine, doxorubicin, and dexamethasone) or dexamethasone, and showed that response rates and survival times did not improve with the addition of IFN. They felt that the use of IFN with salvage chemotherapy was inappropriate. However, data from a Spanish group[63] indicated that IFN-α combined with dexamethasone was beneficial in patients with refractory myeloma.

IFN may induce objective responses in a small proportion of resistant patients and a larger proportion of those who relapse, but as salvage treatment it should be combined with other forms of therapy.

OPTIMUM DOSE, PREPARATIONS, AND ADMINISTRATION

Most of the published trials have used a dose of 3 MU/m^2 three times a week, but this may require reduction if the patient is unable to tolerate the full dose.

The preferred mode of administration is subcutaneous. When given intravenously, all IFNs have a short plasma half-life, ranging from 0.2 (IFN-α) to 2 hours (IFN-β). With intramuscular administration, the half-life is prolonged to 6 hours, or even 7 hours if the IFN is administered subcutaneously.

Two recombinantly produced products are available: IFN-α2a and IFN-α2b, which differ by only one amino acid residue.

A randomized multicentre study including 52 patients[64] compared two schedules of IFN-α2b maintenance therapy (3 MU three times a week and 3 MU daily) in plateau-phase myeloma. Patients receiving daily IFN-α2b had a significantly longer progression-free survival ($p = 0.004$), but overall survival was not significantly different. The toxicity of the two dose schedules was similar.

MYELOMA ISOTYPE AND RESPONSE TO INTERFERON

The Swedish group[45] reported a low response to IFN-α induction therapy in IgG disease, whereas response rates with IgA and light-chain disease were comparable to that seen in patients receiving MP. To study this phenomenon further, they treated 50 previously untreated IgA and light-chain disease patients with 10 MU/day IFN-α2b intramuscularly for 7 days every 3 weeks. The response rate was 36% (41% with IgA disease and 23% with light-chain disease), implying that IFN might be particularly active in these isotypes and in patients with a low tumour burden (stage I/II).[65]

The same group corroborated[45] these findings in a randomized trial involving patients with IgA and light-chain myeloma using IFN-α concomitantly with induction chemotherapy: 85% of IgA and 71% of light-chain disease patients responded to MP plus IFN-α, compared with 48% and 27% response rates, respectively, to MP alone ($p = 0.001$). Overall survival was significantly prolonged in patients who received MP plus IFN-α (median 32 months), compared with those who received MP alone (median 17 months; $p < 0.05$).

It has also been noted in several studies that patients who have the greatest serological response benefit most from the addition of IFN.[50,66,67]

ADVERSE EFFECTS

Phase I and II trials have defined a wide spectrum of side-effects associated with IFN treatment.[68] Nearly all patients experience some degree of toxicity at some time during therapy, because side-effects are so common.

Flu-like symptoms are virtually universal, particularly when therapy starts. The severity of symptoms tends to increase with higher doses, although symptoms are usually controlled by paracetamol (acetaminophen) or by dose reduction, and are rapidly reversible within one to two days of treatment cessation. Also, symptoms may improve without dose reduction as patients acclimatise to the medication.

Progressive fatigue is another common dose-limiting side-effect when IFN is administered chronically. Various central nervous system disorders, of which depression is common, also appear to be dose-related. Haematologic toxicity may manifest with granulocytopenia and thrombocytopenia, both of which reflect bone marrow suppression. This is also dose-related and rapidly reversible on stopping IFN, which should be started at a lower dose after the bone marrow has recovered.

Hypothyroidism can occasionally be seen, and monitoring thyroid function once or twice a year is warranted. Avascular necrosis of the femoral head has also been described.

Table 21.2 summarizes the principal side-effects associated with IFN, although some, such as hair loss and skin problems, are relatively uncommon.

Table 22.2 Adverse effects of interferon

Constitutional	**Haematologic**
Fever[a] Chills[a] Myalgias[a] Arthralgias Anorexia[a] Fatigue, weakness Altered taste Weight loss	Neutropenia Thrombocytopenia[a] Anaemia Coagulation abnormalities **Hepatic** Elevated transaminases Altered drug metabolism (suppression of cytochrome P450 activity)
Cardiovascular	**Nervous System**
Hypertension Hypotension (orthostatic) Arrhythmias Myocardial infarction **Gastrointestinal** Nausea Vomiting Diarrhoea	Headache Lethargy[a] Confusion Decreased concentration[a] Mood alterations (especially depression) EEG abnormalities Seizures Peripheral neuropathy
Renal/metabolic	**Other**
Hypocalcaemia Hyperkalaemia Azotaemia Proteinuria Interstitial nephritis	Antibodies to interferon Hair loss Impotence Rashes Hypothyroidism Avascular necrosis of the femoral head

[a] Common side-effects.

Patient preferences

In a survey in the USA, 350 myeloma patients were interviewed by telephone[69] to obtain information that might facilitate medical decision-making. Without identifying IFN as the treatment agent, interviewers described the adverse effects, cost, self-injection, and the results of the meta-analysis by Ludwig et al.[48] Approximately half of the patients accepted the unidentified treatment if remission or survival improved by 6 months.

Effect of prior interferon therapy on stem cell collection

Singhal et al[70] attempted to collect peripheral blood stem cells with granulocyte colony-stimulating factor (G-CSF) stimulation in 88 myeloma patients who had been autografted previously. Amongst the factors that adversely affected the quantity of $CD34^+$ cells collected, IFN therapy for over 6 months was found to be significant ($p = 0.03$).

Serum neutralizing activity

In 1981, Vallbracht et al[71] reported that patients treated with human fibroblast IFN had developed detectable levels of IgG antibodies that could neutralize human IFN-β. Later, Trown et al[72] described a patient who developed IgG antibodies to human leukocyte IFN-α. However, phase I–II studies with IFN-α2b have reported no development of serum neutralizing factors.

CONCLUSIONS

Many attempts have been made to define the role of IFNs in the treatment of myeloma so that they may be exploited to maximum effect. Overall, their use appears to be beneficial, and IFN-α currently plays a role as part of standard myeloma treatment, mostly as maintenance therapy. Future studies involving large patient numbers will further clarify the areas where IFNs can be used with maximum impact on survival.

REFERENCES

1. Mellstedt H, Bjorkholm M, Johansson B et al. Interferon therapy in myelomatosis. *Lancet* 1979; i: 245–8.
2. Brenning G, Ahre A, Nilsson K. Correlation between in vitro and in vivo sensitivity to human leukocyte interferon in patients with multiple myeloma. *Scand J Haematol* 1985; **35**: 543–50.
3. Palumbo A, Battaglio P, Napoli P et al. Recombinant interferon-g inhibits the in vitro proliferation of human myeloma cells. *Br J Haematol* 1994; **86**: 726–34.
4. Jourdan M, Zhang XG, Portier M et al. IFN-α induces autocrine production of IL-6 in myeloma cell lines *J Immunol* 1991; **147**: 4402–7.
5. Jelinek DF, Aagaard-Tillery KM, Arendt BK et al. Differential human multiple myeloma cell line responsiveness to interferon-α. Analysis of transcription factor activation and interleukin 6 receptor expression. *J Clin Invest* 1997; **99:** 447–56.
6. Berger LC, Hawley RG. Interferon-β interrupts interleukin 6 dependent signaling events in myeloma cells. *Blood* 1997; **89**: 261–71.
7. Warburton P, Dunn JA, MacLennan ICM. *Cambridge Medical Reviews: Hematological Oncology*, Vol 3. Cambridge: Cambridge University Press, 1994: 95–114.
8. Isaacs A, Lindenmann J. Virus interference. *Proc R Soc Lond, Ser B* 1957; **147**: 249–67.
9. Falcoff E, Falcoff R, Fournier F et al. Production en masse, purification partielle et caractérisation d'un interferon destiné à des essais thérapeutiques humans. *Ann Inst Pasteur* 1972; **111**: 562–9.
10. Figlin RA. Biotherapy with interferon – 1988. *Semin Oncol* 1988; **15**: 3–9.
11. Stewart WE 2nd. Interferon nomenclature recommendations. *J Infect Dis* 1980; **142**: 643.
12. Aguet M, Morgensen KE. Interferon receptors. *Interferon* 1983; **5**: 1–22.
13. Creasey AA, Bartholomew JC, Merigan TC. Role of G0–G1 arrest in the inhibition of tumor cell growth by interferon. *Proc Natl Acad Sci USA* 1980; **77**: 1471–5.

14. Horoszewicz JS, Leong SS, Carter WS. Noncycling tumor cells are sensitive targets for the antiproliferative activity of human interferon. *Science* 1979; **206**: 1091–3.
15. Kimchi A. Autocrine interferon and the suppression of the c-myc nuclear oncogene. *Interferon* 1987; **8**: 85–110.
16. Holdener EE, Schnell P, Spieler P, Senn H. In vitro effect of interferon-alpha on human granulocyte/macrophage progenitor cells and human clonogenic tumor cells. *Rec Res Cancer Res* 1984; **94**: 205–19.
17. Trotta PP. Preclinical biology of alpha interferons. *Semin Oncol* 1986; **13**(Suppl 2): 3–12.
18. Rosa FM, Fellous M. Regulation of HLA-DR gene by IFN-gamma. Transcriptional and post-transcriptional control. *J Immunol* 1988; **140**: 1660–4.
19. De Maeyer-Guingard J, De Maeyer E. Immunomodulation by interferons: recent developments. *Interferon* 1985; **6**: 69–91.
20. Fertsch D, Vogel SN. Recombinant interferons increase macrophage Fc receptor capacity. *J Immunol* 1984; **132**: 2436–9.
21. Huddlestone JR, Merigan TC, Oldstone MB. Induction and kinetics of natural killer cells in humans following interferon therapy. *Nature* 1979; **282**: 417–19.
22. Welander CE. Overview of preclinical and clinical studies of interferon alfa-2b in combination with cytotoxic drugs. *Invest New Drugs* 1987; **5**(Suppl): S47–59.
23. Tanaka H, Tanabe O, Iwato K et al. Sensitive inhibitory effect of interferon-alpha on M-protein secretion of human myeloma cells. *Blood* 1989; **74**: 1718–22.
24. Otsuki T, Yamada O, Sakaguchi H et al. Human myeloma cell apoptosis induced by interferon-α. *Br J Haematol* 1998; **103**: 518–29.
25. Alexanian R, Gutterman J, Levy H. Interferon treatment for multiple myeloma. *Clin Hematol* 1982; **11**: 211–20.
26. Cooper MR, Dear K, McIntyre OR et al. A randomized clinical trial comparing melphalan/prednisolone with or without interferon alpha-2b in newly diagnosed patients with multiple myeloma: a Cancer and Leukemia Group B study. *J Clin Oncol* 1993; **11**: 155–60.
27. Niesvizky R, Siegel D, Michaeli J. Biology and treatment of multiple myeloma. *Blood Rev* 1993; **7**: 24–33.
28. Oken MM. Standard treatment of multiple myeloma. *Mayo Clin Proc* 1994; **69**: 781–6.
29. Balkwill FR, Watling D, Taylor-Papadimitriou J. Inhibition by lymphoblastoid interferon on growth of cells derived from the human breast. *Int J Cancer* 1978; **22**: 258–65.
30. Salmon SE, Durie BGM, Young L et al. Effects of cloned leukocyte interferons in the human tumor stem cell assay. *J Clin Oncol* 1983; **1**: 217–25.
31. Brenning G. The in vitro effect of leucocyte alpha-interferon on human myeloma cells in a semisolid agar culture system. *Scand J Haematol* 1985; **35**: 178–85.
32. Ferlin-Bezombes M, Jourdan M, Liautard J et al. IFN-α is a survival factor for human myeloma cells and reduces dexamethasone induced apoptosis. *J Immunol* 1998; **161**: 2692–9.
33. Kubonishi I, Seto M, Shimamura T et al. The establishment of an IL-6 dependent myeloma cell line (FLAM-76) carrying t(11;14)(q13;q32) chromosome abnormality from an aggressive nonsecretory plasma cell leukemia. *Cancer* 1992; **70**: 1528–35.
34. Goto H, Shimazaki C, Tatsumi T et al. Establishment of a novel myeloma cell line KPMM2 carrying t(3;14)(q21;q32), which proliferates specifically in response to interleukin 6 through an autocrine mechanism. *Leukemia* 1995; **9**: 711–18.
35. Schwabe M, Brini AT, Bosco MC et al. Disruption by interferon alpha of an autocrine interleukein 6 growth loop in IL-6 dependent U266 myeloma cells by homologous and heterologous down regulation of the IL-6 receptor alpha- and beta-chains. *J Clin Invest* 1994; **94**: 2317–25.
36. Anthes JC, Zhan Z, Gilchrest H et al. Interferon-alpha down-regulates the interleukin-6 receptor in a human multiple myeloma cell line, U266. *Biochem J* 1995; **309**: 175–80.
37. Westendorf JJ, Ahmann GJ, Greipp PP et al. Establishment and characterization of three myeloma cell lines that demonstrate variable cytokine responses and abilities to produce autocrine interleukin-6. *Leukemia* 1996; **10**: 866–76.
38. Tienhaara A, Remes K, Pelliniemi TT. Alpha interferon raises serum beta-2-microglobulin in patients with multiple myeloma. *Br J Haematol* 1991; **77**: 335–8.
39. Bergsagel DE, Haas RH, Messner HA. Interferon alfa-2b in the treatment of chronic granulocytic leukemia. *Semin Oncol* 1986; **13**(Suppl 2): 29–34.

40. Ahre A, Bjorkholm M, Mellstedt H et al. Human leukocyte interferon and intermittent high-dose melphalan–prednisolone administration in the treatment of multiple myeloma: a randomized clinical trial from the Myeloma Group of Central Sweden. *Cancer Treat Rep* 1984; **68**: 1331–8.
41. Ludwig H, Cortelezzi A, Scheithauer W et al. Recombinant interferon alfa-2c versus polychemotherapy (VMCP) for treatment of multiple myeloma: a prospective randomized trial. *Eur J Cancer Clin Oncol* 1986; **22**: 1111–16.
42. Cooper MR, Fefer A, Thompson J et al. Alpha-2–interferon/melphalan/prednisone in previously untreated patients with multiple myeloma: a phase I–II trial, *Cancer Treat Rep* 1986; **70**: 473–6.
43. Corrado C, Flores A, Pavlovsky S et al. Randomized trial of melphalan (L-PAM)–prednisone (PRED) with or without recombinant alpha 2 interferon (ra2 IFN) in multiple myeloma. *Proc Am Soc Clin Oncol* 1991; **10**: 304.
44. Mellstedt H, for the Myeloma Group of Central Sweden. MP versus MP/IFN as induction therapy: a randomized trial in multiple myeloma. In: *Proceedings of the 5th Hannover Interferon Workshop*, 1990: 44.
45. Osterborg A, Bjorkholm M, Bjoreman M et al. Natural interferon-α in combination with melphalan/prednisone versus melphalan/prednisone in the treatment of multiple myeloma stage II and III: a randomized study from the myeloma group of central Sweden. *Blood* 1993; **81**: 1428–34.
46. Scheithauer W, Cortelezzi A, Fritz E et al. Combined α-2c interferon/VMCP polychemotherapy versus VMCP polychemotherapy as induction therapy in multiple myeloma: a prospective randomized trial. *J Biol Response Modif* 1989; **8**: 109–15.
47. Montuoro A, De Rosa L, De Blasio A et al. Alpha-2a interferon/melphalan/prednisone versus melphalan/prednisone in previously untreated patients with multiple myeloma. *Br J Haematol* 1990: **76**: 365–8.
48. Ludwig H, Fritz E, Zulian GB, Browman GP. Should alpha-interferon be included as standard treatment in multiple myeloma? *Eur J Cancer* 1998; **34**: 12–24.
49. Oken MM. Standard treatment of multiple myeloma. *Mayo Clin Proc* 1994; **69**: 781–6.
50. Mandelli F, Avvisati G, Amadori S et al. Maintenance treatment with recombinant interferon alpha 2b in patients with multiple myeloma responding to conventional induction chemotherapy. *N Engl J Med* 1990; **322**: 1430–4.
51. Pulsoni A, Avvisati G, Petrucci MT et al. The Italian experience on interferon as maintenance treatment in multiple myeloma: ten years after. *Blood* 1998; **92**: 2184–5.
52. Drayson MT, Chapman CE, Dunn JA et al. MRC trial of α2b-interferon maintenance therapy in first plateau phase of multiple myeloma. *Br J Haematol* 1998; **101**: 195–202.
53. Peest D, Deicher H, Coldewey R et al. A comparison of polychemotherapy and melphalan/prednisolone for primary remission induction, and interferon-alpha for maintenance treatment, in multiple myeloma. A prospective trial of the German Myeloma Treatment Group. *Eur J Cancer* 1995; **31A**: 146–51.
54. Cunningham D, Powles R, Malpas J et al. A randomized trial of maintenance interferon following high-dose chemotherapy in multiple myeloma: long-term follow-up results. *Br J Haematol* 1998; **102**: 495–502.
55. Bjorkstrand B, Svensson H, Goldschmidt H et al. Interferon maintenance treatment after autologous stem cell transplantation – a retrospective case–control study from the EBMT. In: *Proceedings of the VIIth International Myeloma Workshop, Stockholm*, 1999: 99.
56. Browman GP, Bergsagel D, Sicheri D et al. Randomized trial of interferon maintenance in multiple myeloma: a study of the National Cancer Institute of Canada Clinical Trials Group. *J Clin Oncol* 1995; **13**: 2354–60.
57. Blade J, San Miguel JF, Escudero ML et al. Maintenance treatment with interferon alpha-2b in multiple myeloma: a prospective randomized study from PETHEMA (Program for the Study and Treatment of Hematological Malignancies, Spanish Society of Hematology). *Leukemia* 1998; **12**: 1144–8.
58. Salmon SE, Crowley JJ, Grogan TM et al. Combination chemotherapy, glucocorticoids and interferon alfa in the treatment of multiple myeloma: a Southwest Oncology Group study. *J Clin Oncol* 1994; **12**: 2405–14.
59. Wheatley K. A meta-analysis of trials of interferon as therapy for myeloma. In: *Proceedings of the VIIth International Myeloma Workshop, Stockholm*, 1999: 97.

60. Byrne JL, Carter GI, Bienz N et al. Adjuvant α-interferon improves complete remission rates following allogeneic transplantation for multiple myeloma. *Bone Marrow Transplant* 1998; **22**: 639–43.
61. Idestrom K, Cantell K, Killander D et al. Interferon therapy in multiple myeloma. *Acta Med Scand* 1979; **205**: 149–54.
62. Alexanian R, Barlogie B, Gutterman J. Alpha interferon combination therapy of resistant myeloma. *Am J Clin Oncol* 1991; **14**: 188–92.
63. San Miguel JF, Moro M, Blade J et al. Combination of interferon and dexamethasone in refractory multiple myeloma. *Hematol Oncol* 1990; **8**: 185–9.
64. Offidani M, Oliveri A, Montillo M et al. Two dosage interferon-α2b maintenance therapy in patients affected by low-risk multiple myeloma in plateau phase: a randomized trial. *Haematologica* 1998; **83**: 40–7.
65. Ludwig H, Cohen AM, Polliack A et al. Interferon-alpha for induction and maintenance in multiple myeloma: results of two multicentre randomized trials and summary of other studies. *Ann Oncol* 1995; **6**: 467–6.
66. Powles R, Raje N, Horton C et al. Comparison of interferon tolerance after autologous bone marrow or peripheral blood stem cell transplants for myeloma patients who have responded to induction therapy. *Leuk Lymphoma* 1995; **18**: 179–84.
67. Wislaff F, Hjorth M, Kassa S, Westin J. Effect of interferon on the health-related quality of life of multiple myeloma patients: results of a Nordic randomized trial comparing melphalan–prednisolone to melphalan–prednisolone + α-interferon. *Br J Haematol* 1996; **94**: 324–32.
68. Speigel RJ. Intron A (interferon alpha 2β): clinical overview and future directions. *Semin Oncol* 1986; **13**(3 Suppl 2): 89–101.
69. Ludwig H, Fritz E, Neuda J et al. Patient preferences for interferon alfa in multiple myeloma. *J Clin Oncol* 1997; **15**: 1672–9.
70. Singhal S, Mehta J, Desikan K et al. Collection of peripheral blood stem cells after a preceding autograft: unfavorable effect of prior interferon-α therapy. *Bone Marrow Transplant* 1999; **24**: 13–17.
71. Vallbracht A, Treuner J, Flehmig B et al. Interferon neutralizing antibodies in patients treated with human fibroblast interferon. *Nature* 1981; **299**: 496–7.
72. Trown PW, Kramer MJ, Dennin RA et al. Antibodies to human leukocyte interferon in cancer patients. *Lancet* 1983; **i**: 81–84.

23

Supportive therapy

Heinz Ludwig, Elke Fritz

INTRODUCTION

During the course of the disease, patients with myeloma experience a number of complications that are secondary to the widespread immunologic, haematologic, and hormonal/cytokine abnormalities seen in plasma cell dyscrasias. These include infections, hypercalcaemia, anaemia, pain, and fractures. Adequate prophylaxis and therapy of these complications is essential to improve patients' quality of life, ensure adequate delivery of cytoreductive therapy, and, sometimes, to prevent fatal consequences.

INFECTIONS

The susceptibility of myeloma patients to infections and its consequences as well as management are dealt with in depth in Chapter 14. We summarize some of the important issues here.

Infections, particularly bacterial, are frequent in myeloma, and are amongst the predominant causes of death in myeloma patients.[1] Susceptibility to infections in myeloma patients stems mainly from granulocytopenia and deficiencies in humoral and/or cellular immunity (Table 23.1).[2–5]

Table 23.1 Factors underlying the increased risk of infections in myeloma

Neutropenia

- Nadir neutrophil count
- Duration of neutropenia

Immunosuppression

- Impaired T-cell function
  - Suppressed natural killer (NK)-cell activity
  - Reduced proliferative response to mitogenic stimulation
- Impaired B-cell function
  - Suppressed production of polyclonal immunoglobulins
- Damage to mucosal or skin barriers
- Chemotherapy- or radiation-induced mucositis
- Catheter-related bacteraemia

The risk of infection is about four times higher during active disease than during remission.[6] During the first two months of induction chemotherapy, bacterial infections occur twice as frequently as during the rest of the disease course. A number of these early infections are fatal, and others can prevent adequate administration of chemotherapy.[7] Myeloma patients who have reached a plateau phase of their disease are at increased risk of serious infection if they show poor IgG responses to exogenous antigens, such as pneumococcal capsular polysaccharides or tetanus and diphtheria toxoids.[6]

The spectrum of microorganisms changes during the course of the disease. In early-stage myeloma, the most common infections occur in the respiratory tract, and lead to bronchitis and pneumonia. They are predominantly caused by *Haemophilus influenzae* or *Streptococcus pneumoniae*. In patients with advanced myeloma and during phases of neutropenia following intensive chemotherapy, *Staphylococcus aureus* and Gram-negative bacteria are more common. However, in recent years, Gram-positive bacteria have been increasingly observed in neutropenic myeloma patients – for instance, in the majority of episodes of sepsis observed in 20–40% of patients after high-dose therapy and autotransplantation.[8,9] Advanced myeloma may be complicated by infections of the urinary tract and by septicaemia. Mortality from infection is particularly high in immunosuppressed patients after receiving allografts from unrelated donors.[10]

Early diagnosis and treatment of infections is important in myeloma. Diagnostic procedures should include differential blood counts, urine tests, bacterial cultures from blood, urine, and other specimens, chest X-rays, serum electrophoresis, and quantitative assessment of immunoglobulins. Neutropenic patients, who are at risk of severe infections, often lack the usual symptoms of sepsis. In these patients, fever during a 12-hour period may be the only presenting symptom of infection. Intensive broad-spectrum antibiotic treatment is essential in these cases.

Infections in myeloma patients can be prevented to some degree by the administration of immunoglobulin preparations. A randomized placebo-controlled trial of monthly immunoglobulin infusions (0.4 g/kg body weight) for one year in plateau-phase patients found significant reductions in the frequency and severity of infections. Patients who responded poorly to pneumococcal immunization benefited most from immunoglobulin infusions.[11] Regular immunoglobulin substitution should be considered for all myeloma patients suffering from recurrent infections. A randomized trial yielded significant benefits of nebulizations with IgA (every 12 hours for 3 months) in preventing respiratory infections or delaying the onset of infection in patients with lymphoproliferative syndromes or myeloma.[12]

Prophylactic administration of trimethoprim–sulfamethoxazole (co-trimoxatole, 160 mg/800 mg orally twice a day) during the first 2 months of initial chemotherapy was found to decrease the frequency and severity of bacterial infections significantly in a randomized study.[7] The efficacy of antibiotic treatment of infections in severely granulocytopenic patients after high-dose chemotherapy may be improved by the addition of granulocyte colony-stimulating factor (G-CSF). One randomized trial in myeloma patients showed that the addition of G-CSF 5 μg/kg/day to broad-spectrum antibiotics improved clinical response to antibiotic treatment, decreased superinfections, mortality, and length of hospital stay, and prevented fungal infections.[13] However, similar placebo-controlled randomized trials in febrile neutropenic cancer patients[14,15] receiving antibiotic treatment in combination with G-CSF[14] or granulocyte–macrophage colony-stimulating factor (GM-CSF)[15] failed to confirm these benefits. G-CSF-treated patients showed significant reductions in the time to resolution of febrile neutropenia, but not in days of fever or hospitalization.[14] The addition of GM-CSF to antibiotics significantly improved response rates, but failed to improve survival.[15]

Table 23.2 lists microorganisms frequently responsible for infections in myeloma patients. Fungal infections are common during high-dose dexamethasone or other glucocorticoid medications. Invasive aspergillosis and infections with other filamentous fungi may occur in neutropenic patients, particularly after allogeneic transplantation, and are associated with a high mortality rate.[16,17] Cerebral abscesses and pulmonary aspergillosis lesions in the vicinity of the pulmonary artery require emergency surgical interventions in addition to antifungal medication.[18] Amphotericin B is still considered the

Table 23.2 Microorganisms frequently responsible for infections in myeloma

Class	Organism	Source
Gram-negative bacteria	*Escherichia coli, Klebsiella pneumoniae, Pseudomonas aeruginosa*	Gastrointestinal tract
Gram-positive bacteria	*Staphylococcus aureus*	Oropharynx, skin, catheters
	Streptococcus pneumoniae	Respiratory tract
	Haemophilus influenzae	Respiratory tract
Fungi	*Candida* spp.	Cutaneous and mucosal surfaces; especially after broad-spectrum antibiotics
	Aspergillus spp.	Respiratory tract
Viruses	Herpes simplex, varicella zoster, cytomegalovirus	Reactivation of latent infections
	Adenovirus	Respiratory tract

gold standard in the treatment of invasive fungal infections. The degree of in vitro susceptibility or resistance of the invading *Aspergillus* sp. to amphotericin B is a reliable predictor of clinical outcome.[16] Amphotericin B or imidazoles are also used as prophylaxis against fungal infections in neutropenic patients. In severely neutropenic patients, combination with G-CSF is recommended.[16] Acyclovir is given to prevent infections with herpes simplex virus, which may particularly threaten patients undergoing allogeneic transplantation.

The introduction of the haematopoietic growth factors GM-CSF and G-CSF has helped to control chemotherapy-induced neutropenia. GM-CSF and G-CSF may prevent infections, or at least support their treatment. Although these growth factors have been reported to stimulate the growth of myeloma cells in vitro,[19] this effect has not been observed in vivo.[20]

HYPERCALCAEMIA

Hypercalcaemia is the most frequent metabolic complication of myeloma. It is caused by tumour-induced bone resorption, and may be aggravated by reduced renal calcium excretion in patients with impaired kidney function. In myeloma patients, bone resorption is mediated by tumour necrosis factor (TNF)-α, interleukin (IL)-1, IL-6, vascular endothelial growth factor (VEGF), and prostaglandins – the so-called 'osteoclast-activating factors'.

The diagnosis of hypercalcaemia is usually readily based on serum calcium levels. However, the low serum albumin level common in myeloma may result in underestimation of biologically active calcium, because albumin binds circulating calcium. For more accurate results, the concentration of ionized calcium should be determined or the calcium level should be corrected as follows:[21]

$$\text{corrected serum calcium (mmol/l)} = \text{measured serum calcium (mmol/l)} - [0.025 \times \text{albumin (g/l)}] + 1$$

The characteristic symptoms of hypercalcaemia are shown in Table 23.3. The frequency and intensity of the symptoms depend upon the degree of hypercalcaemia. Patients with slightly

Table 23.3 Characteristic symptoms of hypercalcaemia

Gastrointestinal	Anorexia Nausea Vomiting Constipation
Renal	Polyuria Polydipsia Nocturia Thirst and dryness of mouth
Cardiac	Increased diastolic blood pressure Increased myocardial contractility Shortened ventricular systole Shortened QT interval Tachycardia
Neurologic	Fatigue Weakness Drowsiness Lethargy Confusion Depression Coma

increased calcium levels (< 3 mmol/l) are often asymptomatic. More pronounced hypercalcaemia (3–4 mmol/l) induces more severe symptoms, such as anorexia, nausea, vomiting, constipation, depression, confusion, psychological alterations, coma, general malaise, and fatigue. Dry mouth, polydipsia and polyuria are also characteristic symptoms of hypercalcaemia. Above levels of 4 mmol/l, a hypercalcaemic crisis with severe symptoms may develop, and may be rapidly fatal if not treated promptly.

Successful treatment of the underlying myeloma is the best and the only definitive therapy of hypercalcaemia. However, except in very mild cases, myeloma patients presenting with hypercalcaemia need immediate symptomatic treatment of this metabolic condition in order to avoid severe consequences.

The therapy should start with intravenous saline (3–6 litres daily) for restoration of extracellular fluid and induction of calcium diuresis. This measure alone may reduce calcium levels by 0.3–0.5 mmol during the first 48 hours.

Additional treatment, particularly in patients who are at risk of developing hypercalcaemic crisis, comprises calcitonin for rapid reduction of calcium levels. Calcitonin inhibits osteoclastic bone resorption effectively and inhibits renal tubular calcium reabsorption. It can reduce serum calcium levels within 2 hours. The effect of calcitonin on bone resorption is transient, because receptors on osteoclasts become down-regulated. Its effect on renal tubular calcium excretion is prolonged, and accounts for adequate control of hypercalcaemia during longer time periods.[22]

Alternatively, in severe cases of hypercalcaemia, forced saline diuresis in combination with high doses of loop diuretics (furosemide 80–100 mg/day) can be used to induce a sodium-linked calcium diuresis (Table 23.4). This measure requires careful central venous pressure monitoring, frequent serum electrolyte measurements, and electrolyte replacements as needed. Under such intensive care conditions, the intravenous fluid load can be increased to 500–750 ml/h. However, if patients are treated with only moderate quantities of saline under routine monitoring conditions, diuretics are not recommended, since they may aggravate volume depletion.

In recent years, the use of saline replenishment and bisphosphonates such as pamidronate or clodronate has become the standard treatment of hypercalcaemia.[23] Bisphosphonates have been shown to inhibit bone resorption by osteoclasts.[24] Clodronate is used as a single infusion of 1200 mg over 6 hours or repeatedly at daily doses of 300–600 mg. Pamidronate may be given as a single 4-hour infusion of 60–90 mg. However, the onset of the effect of bisphosphonates is delayed, and 2–3 days may elapse before calcium levels drop appreciably. The effect is more sustained than that of calcitonin; 10–14 days for clodronate and 20–30 days for pamidronate. Bisphosphonate treatment should be continued with oral clodronate (400 mg three times a day) or intermittent monthly clodronate (600–1200 mg) or pamidronate (60–90 mg).

Table 23.4 Treatment of hypercalcaemia

Treatment	Dose	Comments
Hydration		
Normal saline	3–6 litres/day	Monitor fluid balance
Bisphosphonates		
Pamidronate	60–90 mg in 1 litre saline over 4 h	Start after replacement of fluid deficit; effect will take 24–48 h
Clodronate	600–1200 mg in 500 ml saline over 4 h	
Ibandronate	4–8 mg as slow intravenous injection	
Zoledronate	4 mg as 15-minute infusion	
Calcitonin	5–10 U/kg in 500 ml saline over 6 h, followed by the same dose once or twice daily subcutaneously	Causes a rapid drop in the calcium level, but tachyphylaxis occurs rapidly
Forced saline diuresis		
Normal saline	500 ml/h	Start furosemide after replacement of fluid deficit. Monitor and replace electrolytes (especially potassium and magnesium)
Furosemide	20–40 mg/h	

Transient pyrexia may occur as an adverse effect of pamidronate.

Previously used options for the treatment of hypercalcaemia, such as intravenous phosphate infusions, mithramycin, and gallium nitrate, have become obsolete and have largely been replaced by bisphosphonate therapy. Ibandronate and zoledronate are third-generation bisphosphonates that not only are more potent than pamidronate,[25] but also have the advantage of shorter infusion times. Ibandronate may be given by slow intravenous injection. A dose of 4–8 mg results in a significant reduction of calcium levels within 3–4 days and lasting up to 30 days.[26] Zoledronate, at a dosage of 4 mg and given as a 15-minute infusion, induces a higher rate of calcium normalization and longer times to relapse than pamidronate, while maintaining an excellent safety profile.[26,27] Additional studies will clarify whether the enhanced capacity of zoledronate to decrease calcium levels is mirrored in a superior effect in malignant bone disease, as compared with clondronate, ibandronate, and pamidronate.

Corticosteroids, which are part of most chemotherapy regimens for the treatment of myeloma, inhibit bone resorption to some degree, and also exert an inhibitory effect on intestinal calcium absorption. They are often used as part of the combination therapy of hypercalcaemia.

ANAEMIA

Anaemia is a common complication of advanced myeloma, and 20% of patients have anaemia at the time of diagnosis. In myeloma patients, the anaemic state is most often caused by inadequate erythropoietin (EPO) production.[28] EPO deficiency occurs in practically all patients with impaired kidney function, and in about 25% of those with normal creatinine levels.[29] Other causes of myeloma-associated anaemia are decreased numbers of erythroid precursor cells, impaired responsiveness of the erythron to proliferative signals, shortened lifespan of red blood cells, impaired iron utilization, and paraprotein-induced expansion of the plasma volume leading to dilutional anaemia.

Myeloma patients often show a blunted EPO response to their anaemic condition, which is mediated by inflammatory cytokines (IL-1, TNF-α, and interferon-γ) that suppress erythropoiesis[30,31] and EPO synthesis.[32] The inhibitory effect of these cytokines on erythropoiesis can be overcome by recombinant human erythropoietin (rhEPO).[33] Another contributing factor to patients' blunted EPO response is increased plasma viscosity, which has an adverse impact on EPO synthesis in response to anaemia.[34]

Functional iron deficiency is caused by inappropriate iron release from macrophages, even if iron stores are normal or overloaded. Activated macrophages also remove slightly damaged red blood cells from circulation, thus shortening their lifespan. Anaemia in myeloma patients may also be induced by chemotherapy or irradiation.

Table 23.5 Consequences of anaemia in myeloma

Cardiovascular system	Tachycardia Left ventricular hypertrophy Congestive heart failure Dyspnoea Pulmonary oedema Fatigue Reduced physical capacity
Central nervous system	Impairment of cognitive function Depression
Skin	Peripheral vasodilation Pallor Feeling of coldness
Sexual function	Menstrual disturbances Decreased libido Impotence
Immune system	Impaired immune defences

Anaemia associated with myeloma usually improves as the disease responds to treatment. Table 23.5 shows the various anaemia-related symptoms seen in myeloma. Almost all anaemic myeloma patients suffer from fatigue,[35] which is often associated with depression, emotional disturbances, or impaired cognitive function. Moderate to severe anaemia leads to peripheral hypoxia and vasodilation, with resultant tachycardia, left ventricular hypertrophy, and decreased physical capacity. Patients with severe anaemia may develop congestive heart failure and pulmonary oedema (Table 23.5). Because myeloma patients are usually elderly and often with other comorbid conditions, the symptoms of anaemia may be considerable even at relatively high haemoglobin levels.

Symptomatic anaemia in myeloma patients should always be treated in order to maintain an optimal quality of life. Beneficial effects of treating symptomatic mild or moderate anaemia have been clearly demonstrated in terms of significantly improved quality of life.[36,37] A number of clinical studies have shown that rhEPO treatment improves or normalizes myeloma-associated anaemia in the majority of patients.

The first pilot study, published in 1990,[38] reported increases in haemoglobin levels by at least 2 g/dl in 85% of myeloma patients who had received rhEPO at 150–300 units/kg. Symptoms of anaemia subsided, and no adverse effects occurred.[38] These results were confirmed in subsequent studies, where response rates of 78%,[39] 75%,[40] and 71%[41] were found. A lower response rate (35%) was observed in chemotherapy-refractory, poor-prognosis myeloma patients.[42] In addition to these phase II studies, several randomized trials were performed comparing the results of rhEPO treatment with those of an untreated control group (Table 23.6). Highly signifcant beneficial effects of rhEPO treatment were reported from all trials, with response rates of 60% versus 0%[43] and 75% versus 21%[44] in myeloma patients. Two trials that also included patients with non-Hodgkin's

Table 23.6 Randomized trials of recombinant human erythropoietin (rhEPO) in myeloma

Authors	Study design	No. of patients	Response rate (%)
Garton et al (1995)[43]	Placebo-controlled, two-arm[b]	20	rhEPO: 60 Control: 0
Dammacco et al (1998)[44]	Open, two-arm[c]	71	rhEPO: 75 Control: 21
Österborg et al (1995)[45,a]	Open, three-arm[d]	121	10 000 units: 60 2 000 units: 60 Control: 24
Cazzola et al (1995)[46,a]	Open, five-arm[c]	146	10 000 units: 62 5 000 units: 61 2 000 units: 31 1 000 units: 6 Control: 7
Dammacco et al (2001)[47]	Placebo-controlled, two-arm[e]	145	rhEPO: 28 Control: 47

[a] Also included patients with non-Hodgkin's lymphoma.

Response criteria:
[b] normalization of haematocrit (>38%);
[c] increase in haemoglobin by >2 g/dl;
[d] elimination of transfusion need plus increase in haemoglobin by >2 g/dl;
[e] incidence of transfusion.

lymphoma (NHL) reported response rates of 60% versus 24%[45] and 61–62% under adequate rhEPO doses versus 7%.[46] In both trials, noticably superior results were observed in myeloma patients as compared with NHL patients. A recent randomized, placebo-controlled trial confirmed the significantly decreased incidence of transfusion, regardless of the patients' transfusion history, in the rhEPO arm.[47]

The optimal initial rhEPO dose in a dose-escalation study was 5000 units/day, seven times a week,[46] which is roughly equivalent to 150 units/kg three times a week (31 500 units/week in a patient weighing 70 kg). In patients who are still unresponsive after 6 weeks, this dose may be doubled. Patients whose normal platelet counts indicate adequate bone marrow function may be treated with a low initial rhEPO dose of 5000 units, three times a week, because a response rate of 50% can be expected in such patients.[46]

Considering the effectiveness and good tolerability of rhEPO, it is obvious that the main obstacle is the treatment cost.[48] Increasing knowledge about prognostic factors at baseline or after a short treatment period may result in a considerably better cost–benefit relationship. Superior benefit may be obtained by the use of iron supplementation to meet the high iron demands of enhanced erythropoiesis. Intravenous iron supplementation has been found to reduce the weekly rhEPO requirement by 30–70% in patients with renal anaemia.[49] Individual titration of the lowest effective rhEPO maintenance dose[50] helps reduce the cost.[51] Adverse effects are negligible. They mainly consists of pain or mild erythema at the injection site in about 15% of patients.

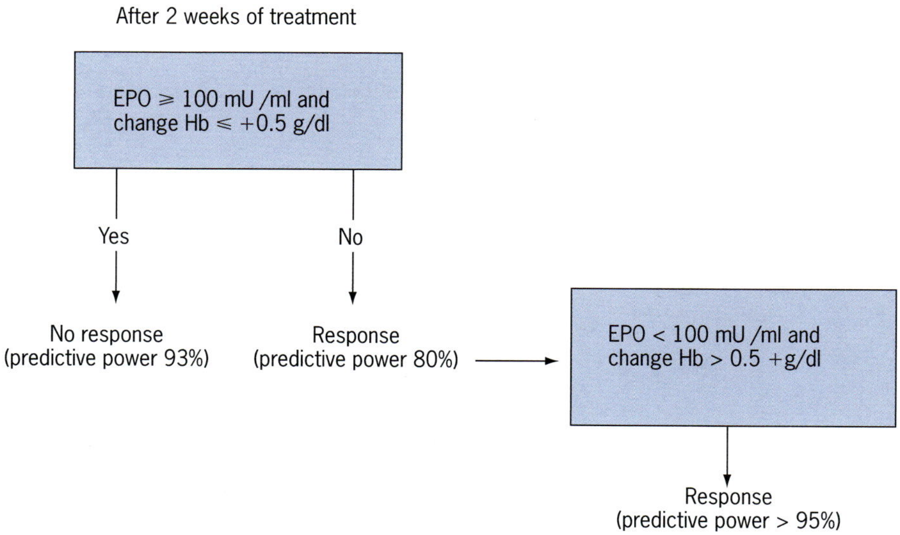

Figure 23.1 Prediction of response to recombinant human erythropoietin (rhEPO) in patients with chronic anaemia of cancer. (From Ludwig et al.[55])

Another way to economize rhEPO treatment is prediction of response in order to allow treatment to be stopped early in unresponsive patients. These predictions are based either on the patient's blunted EPO response[46] or on the first signs of therapeutic benefits during the early treatment phase.[52] The most precise predictive models combine these two criteria, and evaluate baseline EPO and the serum concentration of soluble transferrin receptor,[53] blunted EPO response and changes in haemoglobin levels,[54] or baseline EPO levels and changes in haemoglobin levels[55] (Figure 23.1).

Patients who are responsive to rhEPO therapy may benefit from this treatment for prolonged periods of time. Severe complications of the underlying disease, such as intermittent infections, or surgery may induce a transient loss of responsiveness to rhEPO, while disease progression usually results in rhEPO unresponsiveness until the disease is brought under control again.

Even though rhEPO substitution is primarily considered a supportive therapy that improves quality of life in responsive patients, recent investigations have suggested a beneficial effect of this treatment on the outcome of cancer therapy. After several large studies had demonstrated a negative influence of low haemoglobin levels on the outcome of radiotherapy,[56–58] a randomized, placebo-controlled trial, involving 375 patients with solid tumours or haematological malignancies on concurrent non-platinum-based chemotherapy, found a tendency towards increased survival in the rhEPO arm as compared with the placebo arm (median 17 months versus 11 months).[59] Several still-ongoing trials will possibly confirm the important role of prevention treatment of anaemia in the outcome of

Table 23.7 Doses of non-steroidal anti-inflammatory drugs (NSAIDs)

Drug	Oral dose (mg)	Interval (hours)
Aspirin[a]	500	4–6
Paracetamol (acetaminophen)	500	4–6
Ibuprofen[a]	400–600	4–8
Diclofenac[a,b]	25–100	6–8
Naproxen[a,b]	250–500	6–12

[a] May be contraindicated in thrombocytopenic patients; caution required if used concomitantly with corticosteroids (gastrointestinal irritation).
[b] Caution in patients with renal dysfunction.

chemotherapy in cancer patients, including those with myeloma.

The so-called 'novel erythropoiesis-stimulating protein' (NESP) stimulates erythropoiesis by the same mechanism as recombinant human erythropoietin, but has a 2–3 times longer serum half-life. Therefore, it needs to be administered only once a week. NESP has been shown to be efficient and safe in cancer patients on chemotherapy.[60] In a recent randomized, placebo-controlled trial on anaemic patients with lymphoproliferative malignancies, including myeloma, NESP induced sufficient increases in haemoglobin levels without exhibiting adverse effects.[61] Future studies will show whether the application of higher doses of NESP is still safe, and might allow even more extended treatment intervals, thus reducing the burden of injections on patients.

PAIN

Many myeloma patients suffer from moderate to severe pain, caused mainly by bone lesions. Bone lesions are painful when there is active disease or when a pathologic fracture occurs. The other causes of pain in myeloma are neurologic impairment (nerve or root compression), post-herpetic neuralgia, and unrelated causes. Although myeloma-associated pain subsides with effective chemotherapy and/or local radiation, optimal analgesia is essential in maintaining a satisfactory quality of life. The degree of pain is often estimated by patients, doctors, and nurses rather differently,[62] resulting in inadequate analgesia.[63] Pain needs to be carefully assessed, and the underlying etiology determined.

Table 23.8 Doses of opioid analgesics

Drug	Dose	Interval (hours)
Oral		
Codeine	180–200 mg	3–4
Hydrocodone	30 mg	3–4
Morphine	10–30 mg	3–4
Morphine, controlled release	90–120 mg	6–12
Levomethadone	2.5–5 mg	6–12
Buprenorphine	0.2 mg	6–8
Transdermal		
Fentanyl patch	25–100 μg/h	72

Effective pain control is possible in almost all myeloma patients using oral medications administered regularly. A three-step treatment plan, the so-called 'WHO pain treatment ladder'[64] has been widely accepted for the treatment of tumour pain.

The first step involves non-steroid anti-inflammatory drugs (NSAIDs) (Table 23.7), which may be sufficient even in patients experiencing severe pain. However, even if cyclo-oxygenase 2 (COX-2) inhibitors replace or supplement the older NSAIDs, persistent or increasing pain requires the immediate use of weak opioid drugs as step two. Strong opioids as well as specific adjuvant analgesic drugs are used in the third step, if pain still persists or increases.

Both natural and synthetic opioids exert their analgesic effect by binding to microreceptors on brain cells. Affinity for these receptors and activation of intrinsic receptor activity, the analgesic effect, are important characteristics of opioids. Substances with high intrinsic activity (morphine and pethidine) are agonists, whereas substances with high affinity that lack intrinsic activity are antagonists (naloxone and naltrexone). Agonists/antagonists (buprenorphine and pentazocine) exert relatively high intrinsic activity as well as receptor affinity, and thus can potentially replace agonists at their receptor site. Therefore, agonist and agonist/antagonist opioids must not be mixed or alternated.

Typical opioids recommended by the WHO for the second step of pain treatment are codeine, dihydrocodeine, tramadol, and tilidate. These drugs can be combined with first-line non-opioid substances.

Typical opioids for the third step of pain treatment are morphine, levomethadone, and buprenorphine (Table 23.8). Transdermal fentanyl has the advantages of long-term activity and better tolerance, with fewer gastrointestinal side-effects, but it is more expensive. Because dosing plays an important role in the extent of analgesic effect and because opioids differ widely in the duration of their activity, it is difficult to strictly differentiate between drugs belonging to the second and third steps. Table 23.8 shows recommended treatment intervals for various opioids.

Adverse effects of opioids are generally manageable by supportive measures,[65] but they may become problematic in individual patients. Nausea and emesis prevail at the start of treatment, and may require antiemetics. A number of patients complain about dryness of mouth. If impairment of vigilance and temporary confusion create problems, then treatment with antidepressants or anticonvulsants may be indicated. Major problems can evolve from impairment of visceral motor function manifested as inadequate colonic motility or bladder distension. In order to prevent constipation, a fibre-rich diet and adequate hydration should be recommended, but laxatives may also be necessary. Urinary retention because of opioid-induced bladder atony should be kept in mind if urinary retention occurs.

BONE DESTRUCTION (see also Chapter 7)

Myeloma cells interact closely with stromal cells in the bone marrow, activating osteoclasts. Because of this, skeletal lesions or osteoporosis occur in practically all myeloma patients sooner or later during their course of disease. Seventy percent of myeloma patients show osteolytic lesions, and 30% suffer from pathologic fractures, which are predominantly seen in the spine and in the ribs.

During the early stage of myeloma, increased bone resorption is still associated with increased production of bone matrix.[66] However, as the disease progresses, bone resorption increases vastly, and fails to stimulate bone growth.[67] This results in increasing osteopenia and the development of osteolytic lesions.[66]

Stimulation of osteoclasts used to be attributed to a so-called 'osteoclast-activating factor', which was discovered in supernatants of cultivated myeloma cells.[68] It is now thought that various cytokines, such as IL-1β, TNF-α and TNF-β, IL-6, macrophage colony-stimulating factor (M-CSF), and growth hormone, are responsible for the increased bone resorption in myeloma.[69] Recently, VEGF has also been indentified as an important osteoclast-activating cytokine.[70] The main source of these cytokines is the stromal cells of the bone marrow, although some (e.g. IL-6) are secreted by the myeloma cells themselves and some by osteoblasts and monocytes.

The clinical manifestations of bone resorption are bone pain, hypercalcaemia, and neurologic symptoms from spinal cord compression.

The treatment of myeloma-associated bone resorption involves optimal therapy of the underlying disease, judicious use of local irradiation, and administration of bisphosphonates. Bisphosphonates are derived from pyrophosphates by substituting a carbon atom for an oxygen atom, and modifying one or both lateral chains of the molecule. Bisphosphonates inhibit recruitment of osteoclasts from monocytes, their precursor cells, by suppressing proliferation and cellular differentiation. They also protect bones from destruction by binding to their surfaces.[71] In addition, they inhibit the production of IL-6, the most important growth factor for myeloma cells, and stimulate apoptosis of osteoclasts and myeloma cells.[72–75]

The therapeutic efficacy of the bisphosphonates clodronate and pamidronate in preventing bone lesions has been investigated in several randomized trials. Clodronate studies have yielded equivocal results. A multicentre Finnish study, using 2.4 g clodronate daily for 2 years, achieved a 50% reduction in the progression of osteolytic lesions, but no significant effects were observed on pathologic fractures, hypercalcaemia, or bone pain.[76] Contrasting results were reported from a German trial, in which significant decrease in bone pain and a trend towards reduced progression of bone lesions were observed.[77] The most extensive trial involved 536 patients randomized to receive either 1600 mg clodronate daily or placebo in addition to chemotherapy.[78] Treatment with clodronate was associated with a 50% reduction in non-vertebral fractures and a 50% decrease in the proportion of patients with severe hypercalcaemia. Significantly fewer patients in the clodronate arm suffered vertebral fractures after entry into the trial, experienced significantly less back pain and poor performance status after 24 months, and lost significantly less height over 3 years compared with patients in the placebo arm. Even patients without overt skeletal disease at enrolment benefited from clodronate. However, survival did not differ significantly between the two arms.

A multicentre Danish–Swedish randomized study of oral pamidronate (300 mg daily) showed significant reductions of bone pain and loss of height in the treatment arm, but no effect on hypercalcaemia, pathologic fractures, or progression of osteolytic lesions.[79] This was accompanied by significant reduction of circulating soluble IL-6 receptor levels, as well as a uniform tendency towards lower serum and marrow plasma levels of IL-6, IL-1β, and TNF-α in the treatment arm.[72]

The parenteral use of pamidronate (90 mg intravenously as a 4-hour infusion, monthly for 21 months) resulted in significant reductions of bone pain, number of episodes of hypercalcaemia, and skeletal complications.[80] In addition, prolonged survival times were observed in patients starting pamidronate treatment with second-line chemotherapy protocols.[81] Parenteral pamidronate treatment was safe and well tolerated by patients.[80,81] A close correlation between dose intensity and treatment effect was found in a prospective dose-escalation study on tolerability and effectiveness of repeated pamidronate infusions. Dose intensities of 25–45 mg pamidronate per week resulted in a significant palliative effect, with the best results being obtained with high doses of 60 or 90 mg pamidronate per week.[82] Pamidronate is currently used at a dose of 90 mg once a month indefinitely, because long-term treatment with this agent has been shown to be safe and efficient.[83] The infusion time can be reduced to 2 hours in the absence of hypercalcaemia.

Risedronate, a relatively new bisphosphonate, was used orally in 11 myeloma patients at a daily dose of 30 mg for 6 months, and patients were monitored for 6 additional months. The serum calcium decreased from day 4 onward. Pyridinoline and deoxypyridinoline, established markers of bone resorption, decreased to 50% of their basal values at the end of the treatment period. Significant reductions were also seen in the number of osteoclasts, their activation frequency, and their erosion depth.[84]

Intensification of bisphosphonate doses, as well as the use of newer, potentially more active, preparations such as zoledronate,[85] ibandronate,[86] or incadronate[74], may further improve treatment outcomes. Prophylactic use of bisphosphonates in patients with monoclonal gammopathy of undetermined significance (MGUS) and asymptomatic patients with early-stage myeloma might be able to prevent the development of painful bone lesions to some degree, as demonstrated for ibandronate in a murine model.[87] The inhibitory influence of bisphosphonates on myeloma-promoting cytokines[72,73] and the cytotoxic effects of bisphosphonates, particularly those of the third generation,[75,85,88] strongly suggest direct anti-myeloma activity. An in vitro study of incadronate-induced apoptosis of human myeloma cells confirmed inhibition of the mevalonate pathway as a cause of the observed antitumour effect.[74]

PSYCHOLOGICAL SUPPORT

Myeloma is an incurable disease, with a median survival of about 3–5 years. It places an enormous physical and psychological burden on patients – especially the elderly, who may lack an adequate social network of emotional support. It is essential that doctors and nurses remember the patient's emotional vulnerability in all their interactions.

Only in recent decades have physicians begun to disclose diagnoses to cancer patients. As individuals vary widely in their desire to find out details about their disease, its treatment options, and prognosis, doctors should take great care to tell the patient as much or as little as they want to know. As a general rule, younger patients prefer to be well informed, while older patients are more likely to choose a non-participatory patient role.[89] However, educational, socioeconomic, and ethnic background plays an important role in the extent of involvement that patients display or desire. Still, it has been shown that the majority of patients in all age groups prefer open communication about their disease, and express high levels of hope.

Patients who want to be involved in treatment decisions are significantly more hopeful than those who reject this involvement.[89] Participating in medical decision making returns some control over his or her fate to the patient who is utterly dependent on a medical specialist to treat the disease. This desire to take responsibility for one's own treatment might be one of the reasons for the current popularity of unproven cancer treatments. On the other hand, a sense of active mastery of the disease may explain the reported life-prolonging effect of some psychosocial therapies.[90]

One of the most serious psychological burdens on myeloma patients is uncertainty about outcome. This anxiety does not diminish during remission, because the threat of relapse remains. Patients, and sometimes also physicians, face the dilemma of approaching treatment with high hopes for cure when the natural course of myeloma eventually leads to death.

How can psychological support be provided by medical staff? The first thing is to listen to the patient. Listening relieves anxiety, and is itself therapeutic. It conveys interest in the person, and communicates the idea that problems are taken seriously. This constructive listening does have a prerequisite. Doctors and nurses of myeloma patients need to be aware of their own anxieties about incurable cancer, and must come to terms with them.

It is inappropriate to offer false hope and superficial reassurance. Fears vary among individual patients, and therefore need to be dealt with individually. Answering the wrong questions might destroy the patient's confidence.

Even though realistic information about the patient's situtation neither diminishes hope nor increases anxiety,[89] patients often need time to accept this information. It is difficult to accept news about a relapse or the necessity for chemotherapy. The patient's reaction might be denial, an important protective mechanism, or even hostility, which should never be taken personally by the doctor or the nurse.

The ability of patients to trust their physician and feel that they will never be forsaken ('given up') is essential to their emotional well-being. There is always something a doctor can do to make the patient more comfortable. Focusing on improved quality of life instead of cure will not only help the patient but also decrease frustration in doctors. It is reasonable to experience – and show – genuine sadness about a patient's poor situation. Patients will appreciate the empathy, and might subsequently become more engaged in the therapeutic alliance with their doctor.

During the course of the disease, the patient should be seen regularly by one physician or a small team of physicians, and, if possible, should be admitted to a familiar hospital ward. Continuity of care is important for the patient's sense of well-being.

Many cancer patients have an increased need for physical contact.[91] Being tenderly handled by nurses comforts the patient, and a doctor's firm handshake might also be helpful.

Myeloma and its treatment can be associated with depression, delirium, impaired cognitive function, and other psychological problems that may require psychiatric consultation[92] and specific medication. Depression also aggravates fatigue, one of the most common symptoms of myeloma. Antidepressant medication and psychotherapy are recommended for severe depression.

Even though psychological parameters such as mood and emotions do not influence response to therapy or survival,[93] mood disturbances, which are more severe in patients with myeloma than in other cancer patients,[94] objectively decrease quality of life.[94] Thus, optimal psychological support makes a vast difference to patients' emotional well-being, and may improve their quality of life.

ACKNOWLEDGEMENT

The work of the authors is supported by the Wilhelminen Cancer Research Institute of the Austrian Forum Against Cancer.

REFERENCES

1. Peest D, Coldewey R, Deicher H. Overall vs. tumor-related survival in multiple myeloma. *Eur J Cancer* 1991; **27**: 672.
2. Massaia M, Dianzani U, Bianchi A et al. Defective generation of alloreactive cytotoxic T lymphocytes (CTL) in human monoclonal gammopathies. *Clin Exp Immunol* 1988; **73**: 214–8.
3. Osterborg A, Nilsson B, Bjorkholm M et al. Natural killer cell activity in monoclonal gammopathies: relation to disease activity. *Eur J Haematol* 1990; **45**: 153–7.
4. Peest D, Holscher R, Weber R et al. Suppression of polyclonal B cell proliferation mediated by supernatants from human myeloma bone marrow cell cultures. *Clin Exp Immunol* 1989; **75**: 252–7.
5. Jacobson DR, Zolla-Pazner S. Immunosuppression and infection in multiple myeloma. *Semin Oncol* 1986; **13**: 282–90.
6. Hargreaves RM, Lea JR, Griffiths H et al. Immunological factors and risk of infection in plateau phase myeloma. *J Clin Pathol* 1995; **48**: 260–6.
7. Oken MM, Pomeroy C, Weisdorf D, Bennett JM. Prophylactic antibiotics for the prevention of early infection in multiple myeloma. *Am J Med* 1996; **100**: 624–8.
8. Salutari P, Sica S, Laurenti L et al. Incidence of sepsis after peripheral blood progenitor cells transplantation: analysis of 86 consecutive hemato oncological patients. *Leuk Lymphoma* 1998; **30**: 193–7.
9. Kolbe K, Domkin D, Derigs HG et al. Infectious complications during neutropenia subsequent to peripheral blood stem cell transplantation. *Bone Marrow Transplant* 1997; **19**: 143–7.
10. Mattsson J, Ringden O, Aschan J et al. A low incidence of grade II to IV acute GVHD, but high mortality from infection using HLA-A, -B, and -DR-identical unrelated donors and immunosuppression with ATG, cyclosporine, and methotrexate. *Transplant Proc* 1997; **29**: 735–6.
11. Chapel HM, Lee M, Hargreaves R et al. Randomised trial of intravenous immunoglobulin as prophylaxis against infection in plateau-phase multiple myeloma. The UK Group for Immunoglobulin Replacement Therapy in Multiple Myeloma. *Lancet* 1994; **343**: 1059–63.
12. Bezares R, Murro H, Diaz A et al. Prevention of infections in patients with lymphoproliferative syndromes and myeloma by nebulization of an IgA concentrate. [In Spanish.] *Sangre* 1997; **42**: 219–22.
13. Aviles A, Guzman R, Garcia EL et al. Results of a randomized trial of granulocyte colony-stimulating factor in patients with infection and severe granulocytopenia. *Anticancer Drugs* 1996; **7**: 392–7.
14. Maher DW, Lieschke GJ, Green M et al. Filgrastim in patients with chemotherapy-induced febrile neutropenia. A double-blind, placebo-controlled trial. *Ann Intern Med* 1994; **121**: 492–501.
15. Anaissie EJ, Vartivarian S, Bodey GP et al. Randomized comparison between antibiotics alone and antibiotics plus granulocyte–macrophage colony-stimulating factor (*Escherichia coli*-derived) in cancer patients with fever and neutropenia. *Am J Med* 1996; **100**: 17–23.
16. Florl C, Kofler G, Kropshofer G et al. In-vitro testing of susceptibility to amphotericin B is a reliable predictor of clinical outcome in invasive aspergillosis. *J Antimicrob Chemother* 1998; **42**: 497–502.
17. Pagano L, Girmenia C, Mele L et al. Infections caused by filamentous fungi in patients with hematologic malignancies. A report of 391 cases by GIMEMA Infection Program. *Haematologica* 2001; **86**: 862–70.
18. Bernard A, Caillot D, Couaillier JF et al. Surgical management of invasive pulmonary aspergillosis in neutropenic patients. *Ann Thorac Surg* 1997; **64**: 1441–7.
19. Klein JB, Scherzer JA, McLeish KR. IFN-gamma enhances expression of formyl peptide receptors and guanine nucleotide-binding proteins by HL-60 granulocytes. *J Immunol* 1992; **148**: 2483–8.
20. Barlogie B, Jagannath S, Dixon DO et al. High-dose melphalan and granulocyte–macrophage colony-stimulating factor for refractory multiple myeloma. *Blood* 1990; **76**: 677–80.

21. Payne RB, Carver ME, Morgan DB. Interpretation of serum total calcium: effects of adjustment for albumin concentration on frequency of abnormal values and on detection of change in the individual. *J Clin Pathol* 1979; **32**: 56–60.
22. Ralston SH, Gardner MD, Dryburgh FJ et al. Comparison of aminohydroxypropylidene diphosphonate, mithramycin and corticosteroids/calcitonin in treatment of cancer-associated hypercalcaemia. *Lancet* 1985; **ii**: 907–10.
23. Body JJ, Bartl R, Burckhardt P et al. Current use of bisphosphonates in oncology. International Bone and Cancer Study Group. *J Clin Oncol* 1998; **16**: 3890–9.
24. Carano A, Teitelbaum SI, Konsek JD et al. Bisphosphonates directly inhibit the bone resorption activity of isolated avian osteoclasts in vitro. *J Clin Invest* 1990; **85**: 456–61.
25. Pecherstorfer M, Steinhauer E-U, Pawsey SD. Ibandronic acid is more effective than pamidronate in lowering serum calcium in patients with severe hypercalcemia of malignancy (HCM), and has at least equal efficacy to pamidronate in HCM patients with lower baseline calcium levels. Results of a randomised open label comparative study. *Proc Am Soc Clin Oncol* 2001; **20**: A1535.
26. Body JJ. Dosing regimens and main adverse events of bisphosphonates. *Semin Oncol* 2001; **28** (Suppl 11): 49–53.
27. Major PP, Coleman RE. Zoledronic acid in the treatment of hypercalcemia of malignancy: results of the International Clinical Development Program. *Semin Oncol* 2001; **28** (Suppl 3): 17–24.
28. Musto P. The role of recombinant erythropoietin for the treatment of anemia in multiple myeloma. *Leuk Lymphoma* 1998; **29**: 283–91.
29. Beguin Y, Yerna M, Loo M et al. Erythropoiesis in multiple myeloma: defective red cell production due to inappropriate erythropoietin production. *Br J Haematol* 1992; **82**: 648–53.
30. Balkwill F, Osborne R, Burke F et al. Evidence for tumor necrosis factor/cachectin production in cancer. *Lancet* 1987; **ii**: 1229–32.
31. Denz H, Fuchs D, Huber H et al. Correlation between neopterin, interferon-gamma and haemoglobin in patients with haematological disorders. *Eur J Haematol* 1990; **44**: 186–9.
32. Faquin WC, Schneider TJ, Goldberg MA. Effect of inflammatory cytokines on hypoxia-induced erythropoietin production. *Blood* 1992; **79**: 1987–94.
33. Means RT, Krantz SB. Inhibition of human erythroid colony-forming units by gamma interferon can be corrected by recombinant human erythropoietin. *Blood* 1991; **78**: 2564–7.
34. Singh A, Eckardt KU, Zimmermann A et al. Increased plasma viscosity as a reason for inappropriate erythropoietin formation. *J Clin Invest* 1993; **91**: 251–6.
35. Maxwell MB. When the cancer patient becomes anemic. *Cancer Nurs* 1984; **7**: 321–6.
36. Demetri GD, Kris M, Wade J et al. Quality-of-life benefit in chemotherapy patients treated with epoetin alfa is independent of disease response or tumor type: results from a prospective community oncology study. *J Clin Oncol* 1998; **16**: 3412–25.
37. Leitgeb C, Pecherstorfer M, Fritz E, Ludwig H. Quality of life in chronic anemia of cancer during treatment with recombinant human erythropoietin. *Cancer* 1994; **73**: 2535–42.
38. Ludwig H, Fritz E, Kotzmann H et al. Erythropoietin treatment of anemia associated with multiple myeloma. *N Engl J Med* 1990; **322**: 1693–9.
39. Ludwig H, Leitgeb C, Fritz E et al. Erythropoietin treatment of chronic anemia of cancer. *Eur J Cancer* 1993; **29A**(Suppl 2): 8–12.
40. Barlogie B, Beck T. Recombinant human erythropoietin and the anemia of multiple myeloma. *Stem Cells* 1993; **11**: 88–94.
41. Mittelman M, Zeidman A, Fradin Z et al. Recombinant human erythropoietin in the treatment multiple myeloma-associated anemia. *Acta Haematol* 1997; **98**: 204–10.
42. Musto P, Falcone A, D'Arena G et al. Clinical results of recombinant erythropoietin in transfusion-dependent patients with refractory multiple myeloma; role of cytokines and monitoring of erythropoiesis. *Eur J Haematol* 1997; **58**: 314–19.
43. Garton JP, Gerz MA, Witzig TE et al. Epoetin alfa for the treatment of the anemia of multiple myeloma. A prospective, randomized, placebo-controlled, double-blind trial. *Arch Intern Med* 1995; **155**: 2069–74.
44. Dammacco F, Silvestris F, Castoldi GL et al. The effectiveness and tolerability of epoetin alfa in patients with multiple myeloma refractory to chemotherapy. *Int J Clin Lab Res* 1998; **28**: 127–34.
45. Österborg A, Boogaerts MA, Cimino R et al. Recombinant human erythropoietin in transfusion-dependent anemic patients with multiple myeloma and non-Hodgkin's lymphoma – a ran-

domized multicenter study. The European Study Group of Erythropoietin (Epoetin Beta) Treatment in Multiple Myeloma and Non-Hodgkin's Lymphoma. *Blood* 1996; **87**: 2675–82.
46. Cazzola M, Messinger D, Battistel V et al. Recombinant human erythropoietin in the anemia associated with multiple myeloma or non-Hodgkin's lymphoma: dose finding and identification of predictors of response. *Blood* 1995; **86**: 4446–53.
47. Dammacco F, Castoldi G, Rodjer S. Efficacy of epoetin alfa in the treatment of anaemia of multiple myeloma. *Br J Haematol* 2001; **113**; 172–9.
48. Beguin Y. A risk–benefit assessment of epoetin in the management of anaemia associated with cancer. *Drug Saf* 1998; **19**: 269–82.
49. Sunder-Plassmann G, Hörl WH. Importance of iron supply for erythropoietin therapy. *Nephrol Dial Transplant* 1995; **10**: 2070–6.
50. Österborg A. Recombinant human erythropoietin (rHuEPO) therapy in patients with cancer-related anaemia: What have we learned? *Med Oncol* 1998; **15**(Suppl 1): 47–9.
51. Sheffield RE, Sullivan SD, Saltiel E, Nishimura L. Cost comparison of recombinant human erythropoietin and blood transfusion in cancer chemotherapy-induced anemia. *Ann Pharmacother* 1997; **31**: 15–22.
52. Henry D, Abels R, Larholt K. Prediction of response to recombinant human erythropoietin (r-HuEPO/epoetin-alpha) therapy in cancer patients. *Blood* 1995; **85**: 1676–8.
53. Cazzola M, Ponchio L, Pedrotti C et al. Prediction of response to recombinant human erythropoietin (rHuEpo) in anemia of malignancy. *Haematologica* 1996; **81**: 434–41.
54. Henry D, Glaspy J. Predicting response to epoetin alfa in anemic cancer patients receiving chemorx. *J Clin Oncol* 1997; **16**: 49a (abst).
55. Ludwig H, Fritz E, Leitgeb C et al. Prediction of response to erythropoietin treatment in chronic anemia of cancer. *Blood* 1994; **84**: 1056–63.
56. Pedersen D, Sogaard H, Overgaard J, Bentzen SM. Prognostic value of pretreatment factors in patients with locally advanced carcinoma of the uterine cervix treated by radiotherapy alone. *Acta Oncol* 1995; **34**: 787–95.
57. Dubray B, Mosseri V, Bruin F et al. Anemia is associated with lower local-regional control and survival after radiation therapy for head and neck cancer: a prospective study. *Radiology* 1996; **201**: 553–8.
58. Lee WR, Berkey B, Marcial V et al. Anemia is associated with decreased survival and increased locoregional failure in patients with locally advanced head and neck carcinoma: a secondary analysis of RTOG 85-27. *Int J Radiat Oncol Biol Phys* 1998; **42**: 1069–75.
59. Littlewood TJ. Possible relationship of hemoglobin levels with survival in anemic cancer patients receivng chemotherapy. *Proc Am Soc Clin Oncol* 2000; **19**: 605a.
60. Glaspy J, Jadeja JS, Justice G et al. A dose-finding and safety study of novel erythropoiesis stimulating protein (NESP) for the treatment of anaemia in patients receiving multicycle chemotherapy. *Br J Cancer* 2001; **84**(Suppl 1): 17–23.
61. Hedenus M, Hansen S, Dewey C et al. A randomized, blinded, placebo-controlled, phase II, dose-finding study of novel erythropoiesis stimulating protein (NESP) in patients in lymphoproliferative malignancies. *Proc Am Soc Clin Oncol* 2001; **20**: A1569.
62. Grossman SA, Sheidler VR, Swedeen K et al. Correlation of patient and caregiver ratings of cancer pain. *J Pain Sympt Manage* 1991; **6**: 53–7.
63. Grossman SA. Undertreatment of cancer pain: barriers and remedies. *Support Care Cancer* 1993; **1**: 74–8.
64. World Health Organization. *Cancer Pain Relief and Palliative Care: Report of a WHO Expert Panel.* WHO Technical Report 804. Geneva: WHO, 1990.
65. Cherny NI, Portenoy RK. The management of cancer pain. *CA Cancer J Clin* 1994; **44**: 263–303.
66. Bataille R, Chappard D, Marcelli C et al. Recruitment of new osteoblasts and osteoclasts is the earliest critical event in the pathogenesis of multiple myeloma. *J Clin Invest* 1991; **88**: 62–6.
67. Taube T, Beneton MN, McCloskey EV et al. Abnormal bone remodelling in patients with myelomatosis and normal biochemical indices of bone resorption. *Eur J Haematol* 1992; **49**: 192–8.
68. Mundy GR, Raisz LG, Cooper RA et al. Evidence for the secretion of an osteoclast stimulating factor in myeloma. *N Engl J Med* 1974; **291**: 1041–6.
69. Bataille R, Manolagas SC, Berenson JR. Pathogenesis and management of bone lesions in multiple myeloma. *Hematol Oncol Clin North Am* 1997; **11**: 349–61.
70. Podar K, Tai YT, Davies FE et al. Vascular endothelial growth factor triggers signaling cascades mediating multiple myeloma cell growth and migration. *Blood* 2001; **98**: 428–35.

71. Siris ES. Breast cancer and osteolytic metastases: Can bisphosphonates help? *Nature Med* 1997; **3**: 151–2.
72. Abildgaard N, Rungy J, Glerup H et al. Long-term oral pamidronate treatment inhibits osteoclastic bone resorption and bone turnover without affecting osteoblastic function in multiple myeloma. *Eur J Med* 1998; **61**: 128–34.
73. Shipman CM, Rogers MJ, Apperely JF et al. Bisphosphonates induce apoptosis in human myeloma cell lines: a novel anti-tumor activity. *Br J Haematol* 1997; **98**: 665–72.
74. Shipman CM, Croucher PI, Russell RG et al. The bisphosphonate incadronate (YM175) causes apoptosis of human myeloma cells in vitro by inhibiting the mevalonate pathway. *Cancer Res* 1998; **58**: 5294–7.
75. Takahashi R, Shimazaki C, Inaba T et al. A newly developed bisphosphonate, YM529, is a potent apoptosis inducer of human myeloma cells. *Leuk Res* 2001; **25**: 77–83.
76. Lathinen R, Laakso M, Palva I et al. Randomised, placebo-controlled multicentre trial of clodronate in multiple myeloma. *Lancet* 1992; **340**: 1049–52.
77. Heim ME, Clemens MR, Queisser W et al. Prospective randomized trial of dichloromethylene bisphosphonate (clodronate) in patients with multiple myeloma requiring treatment: a multicenter study. *Onkologie* 1995; **18**: 439–48.
78. McCloskey EV, MacLennan IC, Drayson MT et al. A randomized trial of the effect of clodronate on skeletal morbidity in multiple myeloma. MRC Working Party on Leukaemia in Adults. *Br J Haematol* 1998; **100**: 317–25.
79. Brincker H, Westin J, Abildgaard N et al. Failure of oral pamidronate to reduce skeletal morbidity in multiple myeloma: a double-blind placebo-controlled trial. Danish–Swedish Co-operative Study Group. *Br J Haematol* 1998; **101**: 280–6.
80. Berenson JR, Lichtenstein A, Porter L et al. Efficacy of pamidronate in reducing skeletal events in patients with advanced multiple myeloma. *N Engl J Med* 1996; **334**: 488–93.
81. Berenson JR, Lichtenstein A, Porter L et al. Long-term pamidronate treatment of advanced multiple myeloma patients reduces skeletal events. Myeloma Aredia Study Group. *J Clin Oncol* 1998; **16**: 593–602.
82. Thürlimann B, Morant R, Jungi WF, Radziwill A. Pamidronate for pain control in patients with malignant osteolytic bone disease: a prospective dose–effect study. *Support Care Cancer* 1994; **2**: 61–5.
83. Ali SM, Esteva FJ, Hortobagyi G et al. Safety and efficacy of bisphosphonates beyond 24 months in cancer patients. *J Clin Oncol* 2001; **19**: 3434–7.
84. Roux C, Ravaud P, Cohen-Solal M et al. Biologic, histologic and densitometric effects of oral risedronate on bone in patients with multiple myeloma. *Bone* 1994; **15**: 41–9.
85. Berenson JR, Rosen LS, Howell A et al. Zoledronic acid reduces skeletal-related events in patients with osteolytic metastases. *Cancer* 2001; **91**: 1191–200.
86. Coleman RE, Purohit OP, Black C et al. Double-blind, randomised, placebo-controlled, dose-finding study of oral ibandronate in patients with metastatic bone disease. *Ann Oncol* 1999; **10**: 311–16.
87. Cruz JC, Alsina M, Craig F et al. Ibandronate decreases bone disease development and osteoclast stimulatory activity in an in vivo model of human myeloma. *Exp Hematol* 2001; **29**: 441–7.
88. Aparicio A, Gardner A, Tu Y et al. In vitro cytoreductive effects on multiple myeloma cells induced by bisphosphonates. *Leukemia* 1998; **12**: 220–9.
89. Cassileth BR, Zupkis RV, Sutton-Smith K, March V. Information and participation preferences among cancer patients. *Ann Intern Med* 1980; **92**: 832–6.
90. Spiegel D, Bloom JR, Kraemer HC, Gottheil E. Effect of psychosocial treatment on survival of patients with metastatic breast cancer. *Lancet* 1989; **2**: 888–91.
91. Leiber L, Plumb MM, Gerstenzang ML, Holland JC. The communication of affection between cancer patients and their spouses. *Psychosomatic Med* 1976; **9**: 1–17.
92. Silberfarb PM, Bates GM Jr. Psychiatric complications of multiple myeloma. *Am J Psychiatry* 1983; **140**: 788–9.
93. Silberfarb PM, Anderson KM, Rundle AC et al. Mood and clinical status in patients with multiple myeloma. *J Clin Oncol* 1991; **9**: 2219–24.
94. Poulos AR, Gertz MA, Pankratz VS, Post-White J. Pain, mood disturbance, and quality of life in patients with multiple myeloma. *Oncol Nurs Forum* 2001; **28**: 1163–71.

Part 5

Other Diseases

24

Monoclonal gammopathies of undetermined significance

Robert A Kyle, S Vincent Rajkumar

INTRODUCTION

The monoclonal gammopathies are a group of disorders characterized by the proliferation of a single clone of plasma cells that produce a homogeneous monoclonal protein (M protein or myeloma protein) that consists of two heavy polypeptide chains of the same class and subclass and two light polypeptide chains of the same type. The heavy polypeptide chains are gamma (γ) in IgG, alpha (α) in IgA, mu (μ) in IgM, delta (δ) in IgD, and epsilon (ε) in IgE. The light-chain types are kappa (κ) and lambda (λ). It is essential to differentiate between a monoclonal and a polyclonal increase in immunoglobulins, because the former is associated with a clonal process that is malignant or potentially malignant, whereas a polyclonal increase is due to a reactive or inflammatory process.

RECOGNITION OF MONOCLONAL PROTEINS

High-resolution agarose gel electrophoresis is the best method for the detection of an M protein.[1] After recognition of a localized band or spike on electrophoresis, one must determine the presence and type of M protein by performing immunofixation or immunosubtraction with capillary electrophoresis.

High-resolution agarose gel electrophoresis should be performed when myeloma, Waldenström's macroglobulinemia (WM), primary amyloidosis (AL), or a related disorder is suspected. In addition, electrophoresis is indicated in any patient with unexplained weakness or fatigue, anemia, elevation of erythrocyte sedimentation rate, unexplained back pain, osteoporosis, osteolytic lesions, fractures, hypercalcemia, Bence Jones proteinuria, renal insufficiency, or recurrent infections. Agarose gel electrophoresis should also be performed in

Portions of this chapter were first published in Kyle RA, Rajkumar SV, Monoclonal gammopathies of undetermined significance. *Hematol Oncol Clin North Am* 1999; **13:** 1181–202.

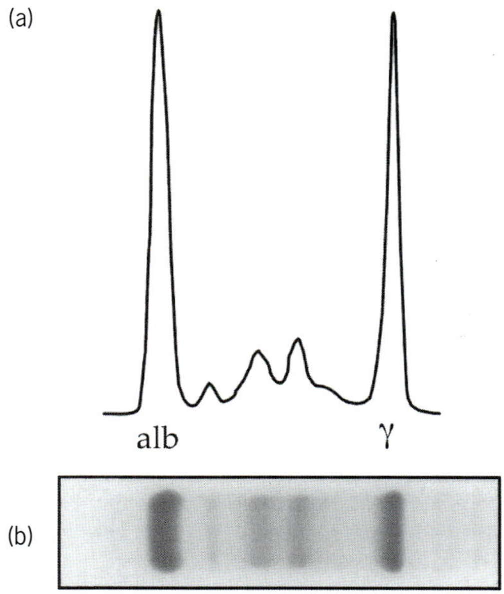

Figure 24.1 (a) Monoclonal pattern of serum protein as traced by densitometer after electrophoresis on agarose gel: tall, narrow-based peak of γ mobility. (b) Monoclonal pattern from electrophoresis of serum on agarose gel (anode on left): dense, localized band representing monoclonal protein of γ mobility. (From Kyle and Katzmann.[1] By permission of the American Society for Microbiology.)

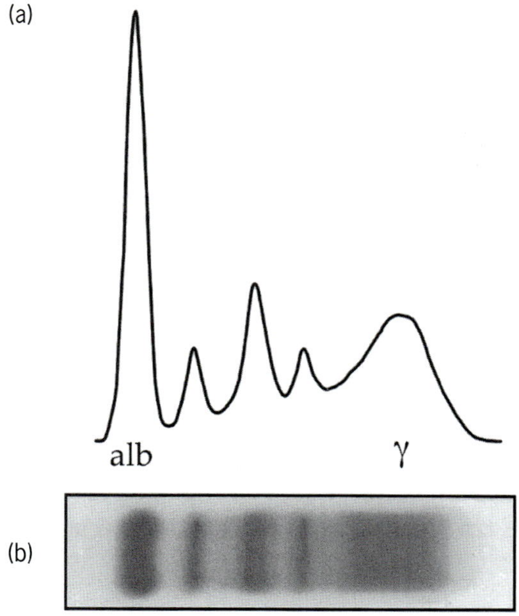

Figure 24.2 (a) Polyclonal pattern from densitometer tracing of agarose gel: broad-based peak of γ mobility. (b) Polyclonal pattern from electrophoresis in agarose gel (anode on left). The band at right is broad and extends throughout the γ area. (From Kyle and Katzmann.[1] By permission of the American Society for Microbiology.)

adults with unexplained sensory motor peripheral neuropathy, carpal tunnel syndrome, refractory congestive heart failure, cardiomyopathy, nephrotic syndrome, renal insufficiency, orthostatic hypotension, or malabsorption, because these features may result from AL.

An M protein is usually visible as a discrete band on the agarose gel electrophoretic strip or as a tall, narrow spike or peak in the γ or β region or, rarely, the α_2 area of the densitometer tracing (Figure 24.1). A polyclonal increase in immunoglobulins, which is characterized by an excess of one or more heavy-chain classes and both κ and λ light-chain types, produces a broad band or a broad-based peak, and is limited to the γ region (Figure 24.2). Two M proteins (biclonal gammopathy) occur in 3–4% of sera containing an M protein (Figure 24.3). Rarely, three M proteins are found (triclonal gammopathy).

A small M protein may be present even when the total protein, α, β, and γ components, and quantitative immunoglobulins are all within normal limits. Bence Jones proteinemia (monoclonal κ or λ light chain) is usually present in too low a concentration to be recognized as a spike. The M protein also may be small in cases with IgD myeloma. An electrophoretic pattern of the heavy-chain diseases (γ, α, and μ) is often nondiagnostic. Chronic liver disease, connective tissue disorders, or chronic infections are characterized by a large broad-based polyclonal pattern.[2] A polyclonal gammopathy may be present without evidence of an underlying inflammatory process.

The type of M protein is best determined by immunofixation. This should be performed whenever a sharp spike or band is found in the agarose gel. It is critical for the exclusion of a polyclonal increase in immunoglobulins.

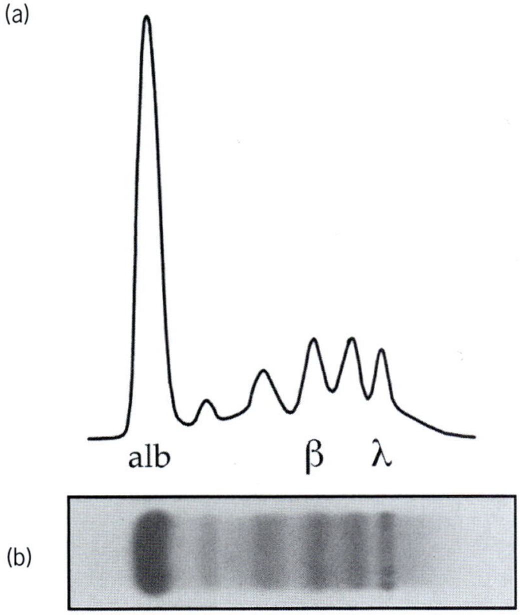

Figure 24.3 (a) Serum protein electrophoresis on agarose gel showing two γ peaks. (b) Biclonal pattern of electrophoresis of serum on agarose gel (anode on left): two discrete γ bands. (From Kyle and Katzmann.[1] By permission of the American Society for Microbiology.)

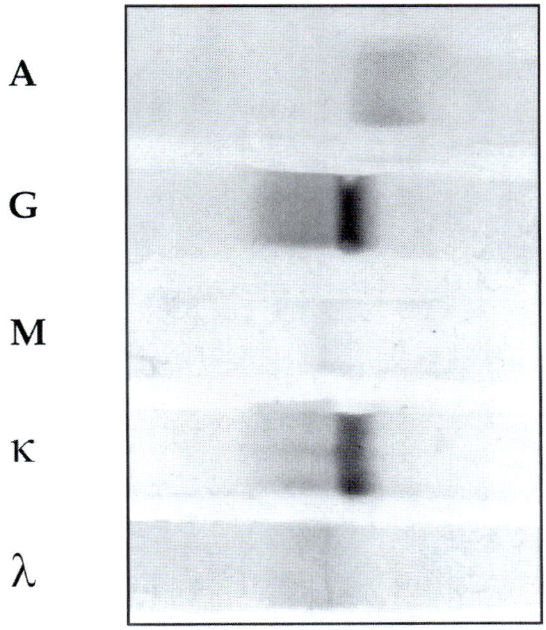

Figure 24.4 Immunofixation of serum with antisera to IgA, IgG, IgM, κ, and λ shows a localized band with IgG and κ antisera, indicating an IgGκ monoclonal protein. (From Kyle and Katzmann.[1] By permission of the American Society for Microbiology.)

Immunofixation is particularly helpful for the recognition of biclonal and triclonal gammopathies. Immunoelectrophoresis is more labor-intensive and is not as sensitive as immunofixation. Immunofixation should also be done whenever myeloma, macroglobulinemia, AL, solitary or extramedullary plasmacytoma, or a related disorder is suspected (Figure 24.4).

We use capillary zone electrophoresis for immunotyping of the M protein by immunosubtraction.[3] Capillary zone electrophoresis measures protein by absorbence; thus, protein stains are unnecessary and no point of application is seen. The immunotyping is performed by an immunosubtraction procedure in which the serum sample is incubated with sepharose beads coupled with anti-γ, -α, -μ, -κ, and -λ antisera. After incubation with each of the heavy-chain and light-chain antisera, solid-phase reagents, the sera are reanalyzed to determine which reagents have removed the electrophoretic abnormality (Figure 24.5). The immunosubtraction procedure is automated and technically less demanding, and is useful for immunotyping M proteins. If a monoclonal light chain is found in the serum (Bence Jones proteinemia), immunodiffusion or immunofixation with IgD and IgE antisera is necessary to exclude the possibility of an IgD or IgE M protein. All patients with Bence Jones proteinemia must have electrophoresis and immunofixation of a 24-hour urine specimen.

Measurement of IgG, IgA, and IgM is best performed with a rate nephelometer. Immunodiffusion for quantitation of immunoglobulins should not be done, because it is inaccurate. The levels of IgM with nephelometry may be 1000–2000 mg/dl higher than the level of the M protein in the densitometer tracing. The IgG and IgA levels also may be increased. Consequently, the clinician must measure the M protein by either or both techniques, but must not use serum protein electrophoresis and then attempt to follow the patient by comparing the M spike

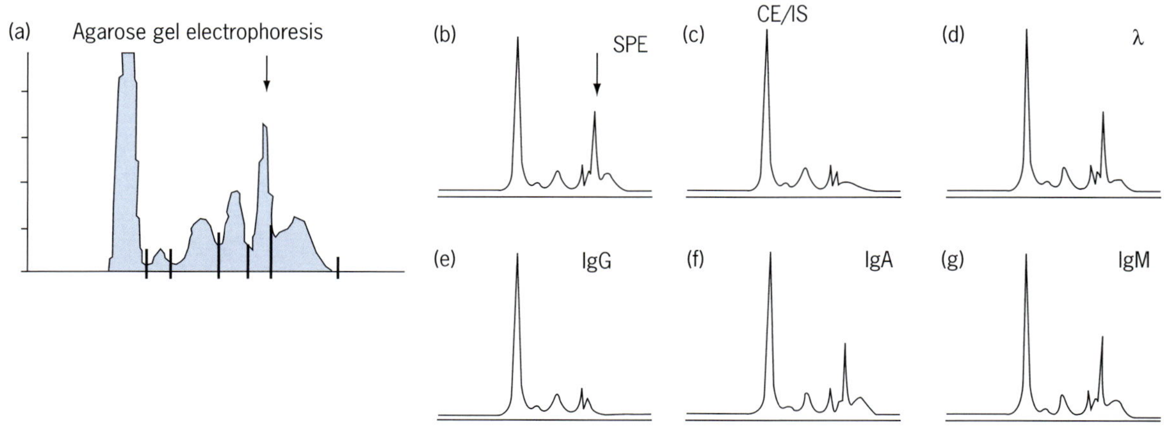

Figure 24.5 Monoclonal IgGκ: the two serum protein electrophoresis (SPE) patterns (a, b) contain a large M spike in the β–γ region (arrow). The immunosubtraction (IS) procedure using capillary electrophoresis (CE) removed the M spike with the anti-IgG and anti-κ reagents. (Note that the anti-IgG, anti-κ (c), and anti-λ (d) reagents remove all, two-thirds, and one-third of the polyclonal portion of the γ region, respectively.) The anti-IgA (f) and anti-IgM (g) reagents had little effect. (From Katzmann et al.[3] By permission of the American Society of Clinical Pathologists.)

with nephelometric measurement at the next visit. If the M protein is small, quantitation of immunoglobulins is more useful than the densitometer tracing.

The viscosity of serum should be measured if the patient has signs or symptoms of hyperviscosity syndrome, which include dilation of retinal veins, flame-shaped retinal hemorrhages, blurring or loss of vision, oronasal bleeding, headaches, vertigo, nystagmus, ataxia, paresthesias, diplopia, congestive heart failure, somnolence, stupor, or coma. The relationship of serum viscosity and the symptoms of viscosity are not precise. Therapeutic plasmapheresis is based on the clinical picture.

Patients with a serum M-protein value more than 1.5 g/dl should have electrophoresis and immunofixation of an aliquot from a 24-hour urine specimen. In addition, immunofixation of the urine should be performed initially in all patients with myeloma, WM, AL, or heavy-chain diseases, and in patients suspected to have these entities. The amount of monoclonal light chain in the urine is a direct reflection of the tumor mass.

A practical classification of monoclonal gammopathies is as given in Table 24.1.

MONOCLONAL GAMMOPATHY OF UNDETERMINED SIGNIFICANCE (MGUS)

The term 'monoclonal gammopathy of undetermined significance' denotes the presence of an M protein in persons without evidence of myeloma, WM, AL, lymphoproliferative disorders, plasmacytoma, or related disorders. The term 'benign monoclonal gammopathy' has been frequently used, but it is misleading because one does not know at the time of diagnosis whether the plasma cell proliferative process producing the M protein will remain stable and benign or will develop into symptomatic myeloma or a related disorder during long-term follow-up.

MGUS is characterized by a serum M-protein spike less than 3 g/dl, less than 5% plasma cells in the bone marrow, no or only small amounts of M protein in the urine, and no lytic bone lesions, anemia, hypercalcemia, or renal insufficiency. The proliferative rate of the plasma cells (plasma cell labeling index) is low. Most importantly, the M protein remains stable and other abnormalities do not develop during follow-up. The finding of an M protein is an unexpected event in the laboratory evaluation of an unrelated dis-

Table 24.1 Classification of monoclonal gammopathies

I. Monoclonal gammopathy of undetermined significance (MGUS)
  A. Benign (IgG, IgA, IgM, IgD)
  B. Associated with neoplasms of cell types not known to produce M proteins
  C. Biclonal gammopathies
  D. Triclonal gammopathies
  E. Idiopathic Bence Jones proteinuria

II. Malignant monoclonal gammopathies
  A. Multiple myeloma (IgG, IgA, IgD, IgE, and free κ or λ light chains)
    1. Symptomatic myeloma
    2. Smoldering myeloma
    3. Plasma cell leukemia
    4. Non-secretory myeloma
    5. Osteosclerotic myeloma (POEMS)
  B. Plasmacytoma
    1. Solitary plasmacytoma of bone
    2. Extramedullary plasmacytoma

III. Waldenström's macroglobulinemia (WM)

IV. Heavy-chain diseases (HCD)
  A. Gamma-HCD (γ-HCD)
  B. Alpha-HCD (α-HCD)
  C. Mu-HCD (μ-HCD)

V. Primary amyloidosis (AL)

order or in a general health examination. It was initially considered benign, but it is now well established that in a proportion of patients, myeloma, WM, AL, or a related disorder will evolve.

MGUS is found in approximately 3% of persons older than 70 years in Sweden,[4] the USA,[5] and France.[6] The overall rate of M protein was 1% among 6995 persons older than 25 years in the Swedish study. In a small Minnesota community with a cluster of myeloma, 15 (1.25%) of 1200 patients 50 years or older had an M protein, whereas 303 (1.7%) of 17 968 adults 50 years or older in France had an M protein. The frequency of an M protein is increased in older persons. In one study, 10% of persons older than 80 years had an M protein.[7] In another series, 23% of 439 patients aged 75–84 years had an M protein.[8]

The incidence of M proteins is higher in African-American populations than in Whites. Cohen et al[9] found a prevalence of monoclonal gammopathy of 8.4% (77 of 916 Black patients). In contrast, the incidence of the monoclonal gammopathies is less in older Japanese patients.[10] Because of the high prevalence of M proteins in many fields of clinical practice, it is important to know whether the disorder will remain stable and benign or, on the contrary, progress to a symptomatic monoclonal proliferative process requiring chemotherapy.

LONG-TERM FOLLOW-UP OF M PROTEIN

A group of 241 patients with MGUS has been followed at the Mayo Clinic for 24–38 years, and the data are updated periodically.[11–14] No patients have been lost to follow-up. The median age at diagnosis was 64 years; only 4% were younger than 40 years, and one-third were 70 years or older. There were 140 male and 101 female patients. Abnormal features on physical examination such as hepatomegaly or splenomegaly and laboratory abnormalities such as anemia, thrombocytopenia, renal insufficiency, hypoalbuminemia, or hypercalcemia were the result of unrelated disorders. The initial M-protein level ranged from 0.3 to 3.2 g/dl (median value 1.7 g/dl). The heavy-chain type was IgG in 73%, IgM in 14%, IgA in 11%, and biclonal in 2%. The light chain was κ in 62% and λ in 38%. Fifteen patients had Bence Jones proteinuria, but the amount of urinary light chain was more than 1 g/24 h in only three patients. The levels of uninvolved immunoglobulins were reduced in 29% of patients at the time of recognition of the M protein. The percentage of bone marrow cells ranged from 1% to 10% (median 3%). Unrelated disorders such as cardiovascular or cerebrovascular disease, inflammatory disorders, connective tissue diseases, and various other conditions unrelated to the M protein were found in 76%.

After follow-up of 24–38 years, the patients were categorized into four groups (Table 24.2). The number of living patients in whom the M

Table 24.2 Course of 241 patients with monoclonal gammopathy of undetermined significance[a]

Group	Description	At follow-up after 24–38 years	
		No.	%
1	No substantial increase of serum or urine monoclonal protein (benign)	25	10
2	Monoclonal protein $\geqslant$ 3.0 g/dl but no myeloma or related disease	26	11
3	Died of unrelated causes	127	53
4	Development of myeloma, macroglobulinemia, amyloidosis, or related disease	63	26
Total		241	100

[a] Modified from Kyle.[12] By permission of the American Medical Association.

protein remained stable and who are classified as having benign disease has decreased to 25 (10%). These patients are still at risk for the development of myeloma or related disorders, and continue to be followed. Twenty-six patients had an increase of the M protein to 3 g/dl or more but did not require chemotherapy for myeloma or macroglobulinemia. Three of these patients are still living. In this group, the pattern of increase was gradual in most instances. One hundred and twenty-seven patients died without myeloma or a related disorder developing. Fifty-five patients lived 10 years or more after the serum M protein was detected. The most common cause of death was cardiac (34%). Fifteen patients died of malignancy, but it was unrelated to the M protein.

In 63 patients (26%), myeloma, amyloidosis, macroglobulinemia, or a related lymphoproliferative disorder developed. The actuarial rate of development of these diseases was 16% at 10 years and 40% at 25 years (Figure 24.6). Myeloma developed in 43 (68%) of the 63 patients. The interval from recognition of the M protein to the diagnosis of myeloma ranged from 2 to 29 years (median 10 years). Myeloma was diagnosed more than 20 years after the detection of the serum M protein in nine patients. Survival after the diagnosis of myeloma was 33 months, which is similar to that in the usual patient with myeloma. Only two patients with myeloma are still alive. Development of myeloma varied from a gradual increase of the M protein to an abrupt increase. AL was found in eight patients, 6–19 years (median 9 years) after recognition of the M protein. WM developed in seven patients; the median interval from recognition of the M protein to diagnosis of WM was 8.5 years (range 4–20 years). In five patients, a malignant lymphoproliferative disorder developed 6–22 years (median 10.5 years) after recognition of the M protein. The risk of malignant transformation did not depend significantly on the type of M protein (Figure 24.7). On the basis of the proportional hazards model, the likelihood of development of myeloma or related disorders was not influenced by age, sex, class of heavy chain, IgG subclass, type of light chain, presence of hepatomegaly, values for hemoglobin, serum M-protein spike, serum creatinine, or serum albumin, or the number or appearance of bone marrow plasma cells. The living patients are still at risk for the development of myeloma or

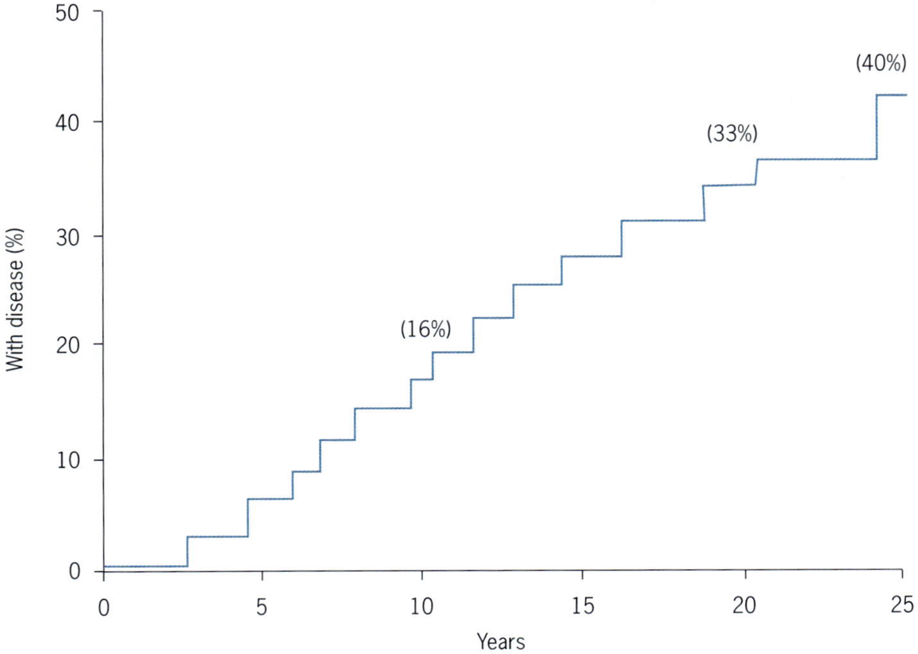

Figure 24.6 Incidence of myeloma, macroglobulinemia, amyloidosis, or lymphoproliferative disease after recognition of monoclonal protein. (From Kyle RA. Monoclonal gammopathy of undetermined significance [MGUS]. *Baillière's Clin Haematol* 1995; **8**: 761–81. By permission of Baillière Tindall.)

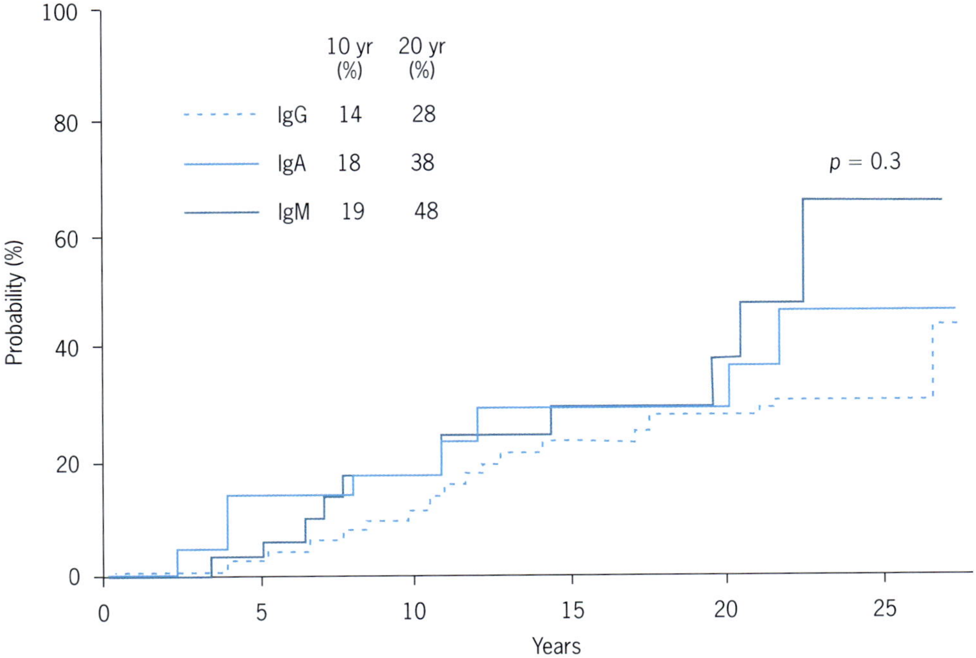

Figure 24.7 Rate of development of lymphoplasmacytic disease in 241 patients with a serum monoclonal protein, stratified by immunoglobulin class. (From Kyle.[13] By permission of the Mayo Foundation for Medical Education and Research.)

related disorders, and continue to be followed. The M protein disappeared in two patients.

In a long-term follow-up of 430 patients with an IgM M protein, 242 (56%) were considered to have MGUS. During a median follow-up of 7 years (1714 patient-years), a lymphoid malignancy developed in 40 (17%) of the 242 patients. Macroglobulinemia occurred in 22 patients, malignant lymphoproliferative disorder in 9, lymphoma in 6, primary amyloidosis in 2, and chronic lymphocytic leukemia in 1. The median duration from recognition of the IgM protein to the development of these disorders ranged from 4 to 9 years.[15]

FOLLOW-UP OF OTHER SERIES

Seven (11%) of 64 patients who had an M protein had progression of their plasma cell proliferative process during 20 years of follow-up. Three of the patients had an increase in the M protein, and one patient had a large serum IgA κ protein and light-chain proteinuria. All four were still alive and did not require chemotherapy at the time of the report.[16] Four of 20 patients had malignant transformation during a follow-up of 3–14 years.[17] In an Italian series of 313 patients with MGUS, 14% of 213 patients followed for 5–8 years and 18% of 100 patients followed for 8–13 years had a malignant transformation.[18] The average duration from recognition of the M protein until the development of serious disease was 63 months. In a series of 213 patients with MGUS, the actuarial risk for development of a malignant monoclonal gammopathy was 4.5% at 5 years, 15% at 10 years, and 26% at 15 years. For the 10 patients in whom a malignant monoclonal gammopathy developed, the median follow-up was 38 months.[19] In another series, a malignant plasma cell proliferative process developed in 13 (10.2%) of 128 patients with MGUS followed for a median of 56 months.[20] The actuarial rate of development of malignant disease was 8.5% at 5 years and 19.2% at 10 years. The median interval from recognition of the M protein to the diagnosis of the malignant process was 42 months (range 12–155 months).[20] In another report, 15 (26%) of 57 patients had development of a malignant plasma cell disorder after a median follow-up of 8.4 years.[21] In another series of 335 patients with MGUS, the frequency of progression after a median follow-up of 70 months was 6.8%.[22]

DIFFERENTIATION OF MGUS FROM MYELOMA OR MACROGLOBULINEMIA

Differentiation of a patient with MGUS from one with myeloma may be difficult. The patient with MGUS is asymptomatic, and the discovery of an M protein is unexpected during a routine medical evaluation. The size of the M protein in the serum or urine, hemoglobin value, number of bone marrow plasma cells, and the presence of hypercalcemia, renal insufficiency, and lytic lesions are helpful in the differential diagnosis.

A serum M-protein value of more than 3 g/dl usually indicates overt myeloma, but some patients may have smoldering myeloma and remain stable for long periods. Patients with smoldering myeloma have both an M-protein value of more than 3 g/dl and more than 10% bone marrow plasma cells, but they have no evidence of anemia, renal insufficiency, hypercalcemia, lytic lesions, or other clinical manifestations of myeloma.[23] Clinically and biologically, patients with smoldering myeloma actually have MGUS with a higher M-protein value and more bone marrow plasma cells. Recognition of this subset of patients is very important, because they should not be treated with chemotherapy until progression occurs. They may remain stable for many years.

Levels of uninvolved or background immunoglobulins help in differentiating benign from malignant disease. In most patients with myeloma or WM, the levels of normal, background, or uninvolved immunoglobulins are reduced. However, a reduction of uninvolved immunoglobulins may also occur in MGUS. Approximately 30% of patients with MGUS have a decrease in the uninvolved immunoglobulins.[11,22–25] Thus, reduction of uninvolved immunoglobulins is not a reliable predictor of malignant transformation. In fact, 26% of patients whose M-protein value remained stable during a median follow-up of 22 years had a decrease in normal or uninvolved immunoglobulins when the M protein was recognized.[14] In contrast, in another report, a reduction in the uninvolved immunoglobulins was significantly associated with a higher probability of malignant transformation.[22]

The presence of monoclonal light chains in the urine of a patient with a serum monoclonal gammopathy suggests a neoplastic process. However, not uncommonly, patients with newly diagnosed MGUS remain stable for many years despite the presence of a small amount of monoclonal light chain in the urine.[12] Usually the presence of more than 10% plasma cells in the bone marrow suggests myeloma, but some patients with greater plasmacytosis remain stable for long periods. Generally, the morphologic appearance of the plasma cells is of little help in differentiating malignant from benign disease. The presence of osteolytic lesions is strong evidence of myeloma, but metastatic carcinoma also may produce lytic lesions and be associated with an unrelated M protein. Magnetic resonance imaging (MRI) may be of some help in differential diagnosis. In a series of 24 patients with newly diagnosed MGUS, MRI was normal, whereas abnormalities were found in 38 (86%) of 44 patients with myeloma.[25]

Histomorphometric studies of bone biopsy specimens reveal normal bone remodeling in MGUS but increased bone resorption and increased bone formation in stage III myeloma.[26] The β_2-microglobulin levels are of little value in differentiating MGUS from myeloma, because there is considerable overlap between the two conditions. Only 1 of 35 patients with MGUS or smoldering myeloma had a serum interleukin (IL)-6 level of more than 5 U/ml. However, 41% of 85 patients with newly diagnosed myeloma also had normal levels of IL-6; thus, this measurement is of little value in differential diagnosis.[27] In another study, 14% of patients with MGUS had increased IL-6 values.[28] Thus, the serum IL-6 level does not differentiate between MGUS and myeloma. With the in situ hybridization technique, IL-1β mRNA was detectable in the plasma cells of 49 of 51 patients with myeloma, 7 of 7 with smoldering myeloma, but only 5 of 21 with MGUS. Thus, more than 95% of patients with myeloma but less than 25% of patients with MGUS are positive for IL-1β production.[29] The presence of J chains in malignant plasma cells, increased levels of plasma cell acid phosphatase, reduced numbers of $CD4^+$ lymphocytes, increased numbers of monoclonal idiotype-bearing peripheral blood lymphocytes, and an increased number of immunoglobulin-secreting cells in peripheral blood are all characteristic of myeloma, but they are not reliable for differentiation, because there is an overlap with MGUS.[30]

The plasma cell labeling index (PCLI), which measures synthesis of DNA, is useful for differentiating MGUS or smoldering myeloma from myeloma. We have developed a monoclonal antibody (BU-1) reactive with 5-bromo-2-deoxyuridine (BRD-URD) in mice. Bone marrow plasma cells are exposed to BRD-URD for 1 hour. Cells synthesizing DNA incorporate BRD-URD, which is recognized by the monoclonal antibody BU-1 (conjugated to a goat antimouse immunoglobulin–rhodamine complex). Binding with propidium iodide identifies the cells incorporating BRD-URD in S phase. The BU-1 monoclonal antibody does not require denaturation for its activity. Consequently, the use of fluorescent conjugated immunoglobulin antisera to κ and λ identifies the population of monoclonal plasma cells. The test can be done in 4–5 hours. An increased PCLI is good evidence that myeloma either is present or will soon develop. However, about 40% of patients with active myeloma have a normal PCLI. There is also a good correlation between the peripheral blood labeling index and the bone marrow labeling index.[31,32]

The presence of circulating plasma cells of the same isotype in the peripheral blood is a good marker of active disease. In a series of 57 patients with newly diagnosed smoldering myeloma, 16 had progression within 12 months. Sixty-three percent of patients who had progression had an increased number of peripheral blood plasma cells. In contrast, only 4 of 41 patients who remained stable for 1 year had an increase in peripheral blood plasma cells at diagnosis.[33,34] Billadeau et al[35] showed that clonal circulating cells are present in patients with MGUS, smoldering myeloma, and active myeloma. They used immunofluorescence microscopy with three-color flow cytometry for $CD38^{+}$, $CD45^{-}$, and $CD45^{dim}$ and the allele-specific oligonucleotide polymerase chain reaction (PCR). The PCR detected clonal cells in 13 of 16 patients with MGUS, whereas immunofluorescence and flow cytometry detected clonal plasma cells in only 4 of them. Thus, the finding of clonal cells in the peripheral blood of patients with MGUS demonstrates that the clone is present early in the disease.

Conventional cytogenetics are not useful for the differentiation of MGUS and myeloma, because the number of metaphases for study in MGUS is too low. Use of fluorescence in situ hybridization (FISH) is of interest. Zandecki et al[36] found trisomy for at least one of chromosomes 3, 7, 9, and 11 in 12–72% of bone marrow plasma cells in 12 of 14 hyperdiploid MGUS cases. Drach et al[37] found similar chromosome abnormalities in 19 (53%) of 36 patients with MGUS.

In summary, the diagnosis of MGUS is usually not difficult, and often occurs as an unexpected finding in the course of an unrelated process or a routine medical examination. No single factor can differentiate patients with MGUS from those in whom a malignant plasma cell disorder will subsequently develop.

PREDICTORS OF MALIGNANT TRANSFORMATION

There is general agreement that there are no findings at the time of diagnosis of MGUS that reliably distinguish patients who will remain stable from those in whom a malignant condition will develop. As previously mentioned, the initial hemoglobin value, the amount of serum and urine M protein, and the appearance and number of bone marrow plasma cells are helpful in differentiating MGUS from myeloma. However, they are not useful for prediction of a subsequent malignant process. Neither the increase in the initial component nor the percentage of bone marrow plasma cells added a predictive value for the malignant transformation in several series.[13,20,38]

In a report of 386 patients with a non-myelomatous gammopathy, 51 were classified as having a monoclonal gammopathy of borderline significance (MGBS) if the bone marrow plasma cell content was 10–30%. After a median follow-up of 70 months in the MGUS group and 53 months in the MGBS group, malignant disease developed in 23 of the 335 patients with MGUS and 19 of the 51 patients with MGBS. The relative risks for development of myeloma were 2.4 for each 1 g/dl increase of IgG, 3.5 for detectable light-chain proteinuria, 6.1 for age older than 70 years, and 13.1 for a reduction in two polyclonal immunoglobulins. The authors concluded that MGUS had a very low risk of evolution when the M-protein value was 1.5 g/dl or less, the bone marrow plasma cell value was less than 5%, there was no reduction in polyclonal immunoglobulins, and there was no detectable light-chain proteinuria.[22]

In a series of 263 patients with MGUS followed from 5 to 20 years, 48 (18%) had a malignant transformation. Myeloma developed in 35 patients. The actuarial risk of malignant transformation was 6% at 5 years, 15% at 10 years, and 31% at 20 years. Using the Cox proportional hazards model, the authors found that only age was a factor associated with a neoplastic event.[39]

The mode of development of myeloma is variable. In our 241 patients with MGUS, 11 had a stable M-protein value for 4–18 years (median 8 years) and gradually had an increase to myeloma during 1–4 years (median 3 years). In 7 patients, the M-protein value was stable for 2–25 years (median 8 years) and then increased rapidly in less than 1 year as myeloma developed. Seven patients had a fluctuating but gradually increasing serum M-protein value until myeloma was diagnosed 5–29 years later (median 12 years). In 7 patients, the serum M-protein value was stable for 1–16 years, followed by intervals of 2–10 years (median 4 years) before myeloma was diagnosed.

In patients whose condition evolves, myeloma usually develops after a prolonged period of stability. MGUS constitutes the premyeloma phase, which may persist for more than 20 years. A considerable number of patients with myeloma have had a previous MGUS. Of the 55 patients diagnosed with myeloma in Olmsted County, Minnesota, in recent years, 58% had a preceding MGUS, smoldering myeloma, or plasmacytoma.[40] When malignant transformation occurs, the type of M protein is always the same as it was in the MGUS state.

ASSOCIATION OF MGUS WITH OTHER DISEASES

MGUS often is associated with other diseases, such as would be expected in an older population. The association of two conditions depends on the frequency with which each occurs independently. Thus, appropriate epidemiologic and statistical studies, especially valid control populations, must be used in evaluating these associations.

Lymphoproliferative disorders

An M protein was reported in the serum of 13 patients with lymphoma or chronic lymphocytic leukemia (CLL) in 1957.[41] Three years later, Kyle et al[42] described 6 patients with lymphoma and a serum or urinary M protein in the electrophoretic pattern. Of 640 patients with non-Hodgkin's lymphoma (NHL) or CLL, 44 had an M component.[43] None of 510 patients with nodular lymphoma or Hodgkin's disease had an M protein, whereas 29 of the 640 patients with a diffuse NHL pattern had an M protein.[43]

In a series of 100 patients with CLL and M protein, IgG was found in 51, IgM in 38, IgA in 1, and light chain only in 10.[44] The presence of an IgG or an IgM protein produces no clinical differences. In another report, an M protein was found in the serum or urine in 26 (16%) of 161 cases of hairy cell leukemia.[45] Adult T-cell leukemia,[46] Sézary syndrome, and mycosis fungoides[47–49] have been reported with M proteins.

Other hematologic disorders

In one-third of patients with chronic neutrophilic leukemia, an M protein or myeloma is found.[50] M proteins have been reported in patients with refractory anemia,[51] idiopathic myelofibrosis,[52] and Gaucher's disease.[53,54] In a patient with Gaucher's disease and MGUS, myeloma developed 12 years after diagnosis of an M protein.[55]

Pernicious anemia, pure red cell aplasia, idiopathic thrombocytopenic purpura, and acute leukemia have all been reported with an M protein, but whether the incidence of an M protein is greater in patients with these conditions than in the normal population is unknown. Patients with acquired von Willebrand's disease that is due to an M protein have also been described.[56,57]

Neurologic disorders

Neuropathies may be associated with MGUS.[58,59] Of 279 patients with a sensory motor peripheral neuropathy of unknown cause, 28 (10%) had an M protein.[60] MGUS was present in 16 of the 28, AL in 7, myeloma in 3, WM in 1, and γ heavy-chain disease in 1. IgG was the most common M protein (15 cases), light chain only in 5, IgM in 4, IgA in 3, and γ heavy chain in 1.

The IgM protein binds to the myelin-associated glycoprotein (MAG) in about half of patients with an IgM protein and peripheral neuropathy.[61,62] Anti-MAG antibodies fail to distinguish a subgroup of patients with IgM sensorimotor neuropathy. Widening of the myelin lamellae may be present.[63] The neuropathy is mainly sensory, and begins in the lower extremities and extends slowly over a period of months to years. Sensory involvement is more prominent than motor. Cranial nerve and autonomic involvement is rare. Clinical and electrodiagnostic features are similar to those with chronic inflammatory demyelinating polyneuropathy. Patients with IgM MGUS have more prolonged distal latencies of the median and other motor potentials, greater slowing of the peroneal nerve conduction velocity, more often absent sensory potentials, and more severe demyelination than patients with IgG MGUS.[64]

In a Mayo Clinic study, 39 patients with peripheral neuropathy and MGUS were randomized to plasmapheresis or sham plasmapheresis in a double-blind trial.[65] Patients with IgG or IgA gammopathy had a better response to plasma exchange than those with IgM gammopathy. High-dose intravenous gammaglobulin has been reported to be of some benefit, but the results are often disappointing.[66] If there is no response to plasmapheresis, then chlorambucil in patients with an IgM protein or melphalan and prednisone in those with IgG and IgA may be useful. Other neurologic disorders such as amyotrophic lateral sclerosis, progressive muscular atrophy, and ataxia telangiectasia have been reported with M proteins, but the association may be merely coincidental.[30]

Osteosclerotic myeloma (POEMS syndrome)

POEMS syndrome is characterized by polyneuropathy (P), organomegaly (O), endocrinopathy (E), M protein (M), and skin changes (S).[67,68] Patients have a chronic inflammatory demyelinating polyneuropathy with more motor than sensory involvement. Sclerotic skeletal lesions are common and an important clue to the diagnosis. Except for papilledema, the cranial nerves are not involved. Hepatosplenomegaly and lymphadenopathy occur in some patients. Angiomatous lesions, gynecomastia, testicular atrophy, hyperpigmentation, and hypertrichosis are frequent findings. Over 90% of patients have a λ light chain. IgA is the most common heavy chain. The M component is almost always less than 3 g/dl, and the bone marrow is rarely diagnostic of myeloma. In contrast to myeloma, the hemoglobin level is normal or increased and thrombocytosis is common. Hypercalcemia, renal insufficiency, and fractures rarely occur. Diagnosis is made on the basis of monoclonal plasma cells in an osteosclerotic lesion. Radiation therapy is effective if the osteosclerotic lesion is localized.

Dermatologic diseases

Lichen myxedematosus (scleromyxedema, papular mucinosis) is characterized by papules and macules involving the skin. A cathodal IgG λ M protein is usually found.[69] Of 67 patients with pyoderma gangrenosum, 8 had an M protein.[70] IgA M protein is usually found. Necrobiotic xanthogranuloma often is associated with an IgG M protein.[71] About half of patients with plane xanthomatosis have an M protein.[72] In a report of 7 patients with subcorneal pustular dermatosis, 3 had an IgA and 1 had an IgG M protein.[73]

Immunosuppression and monoclonal gammopathies

Of 341 patients positive for human immunodeficiency virus (HIV), 11 had an M protein. In 7, the M protein disappeared during a median follow-up of 50 months. There was no apparent difference in the clinical course of those with or without an M protein.[74]

In a series of 86 patients with a liver transplant, 26 (30%) developed an M protein. In half, the M protein was transient. There was a strong correlation between the occurrence of viral infections and persistent M protein. Three of the 13 with an M protein died of a post-transplantation lymphoproliferative disorder.[75] In another report, 57 of 101 patients with a liver transplant developed an M protein. Seventy-one percent of the 7 patients with a post-transplantation lymphoproliferative disorder had an M protein.

Bone marrow transplantation also has been associated with an increased incidence of monoclonal gammopathies.[76] Twelve of 47 patients who had an allogeneic bone marrow transplantation had an M protein. All but one had a cytomegalovirus (CMV) infection.[77] In another series, 55 of 550 patients enrolled in a tandem autotransplantation trial had an abnormal protein band. These patients had a higher complete response to therapy, and thus the band was a favorable feature.[78] The presence of CMV was an important risk factor.[79] In a series of pediatric patients with a kidney transplant, 17 (57%) of 30 had an M protein, whereas only 8% of the patients without a CMV infection had an M protein.[80] In one study, an M protein developed after renal transplantation in 13% of 141 patients. Seven of the M proteins were transient.[81] In another series of 232 patients receiving immunosuppression during transplantation, 30% had an M protein. The incidence was higher in older persons.[82] In an additional group of 84 patients who had had a renal transplant, immunoelectrophoresis detected an M protein in 21%. With Western blotting, 85.5% had a monoclonal immunoglobulin. The M proteins were frequently transient.[83]

Rheumatoid arthritis and related disorders

Rheumatoid arthritis has been associated with monoclonal gammopathies.[84,85] Polymyalgia rheumatica and M proteins have been found, but both occur in an older population, and a significant relationship is questionable. Myasthenia gravis also has been reported with an M protein.[86] Angioneurotic edema caused by acquired deficiency of C1-esterase inhibitor and monoclonal gammopathy has been recognized.[72] Binding of IgG to thrombin may produce severe bleeding.[87]

Monoclonal gammopathies with antibody activity

M proteins have been reported with specificity against red blood cell polysaccharide membrane, acid polysaccharides, dextran, antistreptolysin O, antistaphylolysin, antinuclear antibody, riboflavin, von Willebrand factor, thyroglobulin, insulin, single- and double-stranded DNA, apolipoprotein, thyroxine, cephalin, lactate dehydrogenase, HIV, platelet glycoprotein III_a, transferrin, α_2-macroglobulin, cardiolipin, chondroitin sulfate, group A streptococci, CMV, and antibiotics.[30,88]

The M protein may be bound by calcium and produce a high total serum calcium level without symptoms because the ionized calcium level is normal. This possibility should be considered in asymptomatic patients with hypercalcemia.[89,90] Binding of copper by an IgG M protein has been reported.[91,92] The M protein may bind phosphate and result in a high serum phosphorus level.[93] Spurious hyperphosphatemia may also result from interference of the M protein with the phosphate chromogenic assay.[94] In a prospective study of 239 patients with hepatitis C virus (HCV), an M protein was detected in 11%, but in only 1% of the patients without HCV.[95]

VARIANTS OF MGUS

Biclonal gammopathies

Biclonal gammopathies are characterized by the production of two different M proteins. They occur in 3–4% of patients with monoclonal gammopathies. They may result from the proliferation of two different clones of plasma cells or from the production of two M proteins by a single clone of plasma cells. Two-thirds of patients have a biclonal gammopathy of undetermined significance (BGUS), and the remainder have myeloma or a malignant lymphoproliferative disorder. Thus, the clinical features of biclonal gammopathy are similar to those of monoclonal gammopathy. The second M protein is frequently not recognized until immunofixation is done, because many patients have only a single band in the agarose pattern.[96]

Triclonal gammopathies

In a report of a patient with a triclonal gammopathy (IgM κ, IgG κ, and IgA κ), the authors reviewed a group of triclonal gammopathies from the literature. Sixteen were associated with a malignant immunoproliferative disorder, five were present in non-hematologic diseases, and three were of undetermined significance.[97]

Idiopathic Bence Jones proteinuria

Although Bence Jones proteinuria is usually associated with a malignant plasma cell proliferative process, occasionally patients may excrete large amounts of Bence Jones protein and follow a benign course. One patient with a stable serum M protein and a monoclonal light chain of 0.8 g/24 h did not have myeloma or amyloidosis for almost 20 years.[98] Seven other patients with Bence Jones proteinuria ($\geq$1 g/24 h) but no serum M protein or evidence of a malignant plasma cell disorder at diagnosis have been described. During a follow-up of 7–21 years, myeloma developed in three patients, evolving myeloma in one, and asymptomatic myeloma in one. Amyloidosis developed after 12 years of follow-up in one patient, and the seventh patient has a stable level of Bence Jones proteinuria at 28 years. Consequently, myeloma or amyloidosis usually develops in patients with Bence Jones proteinuria, but they may remain stable and asymptomatic for years.[99]

IgD MGUS

The presence of an IgD M protein is almost always indicative of a malignant plasma cell disorder such as myeloma or AL. A patient with a well-documented MGUS of IgD type was followed for more than 6 years, during which no serious disease developed.[100] We have seen a patient with IgD MGUS who was followed for more than 8 years and had no evidence of malignant disease.[101]

ACKNOWLEDGEMENT

This work was supported in part by research grant CA62242 from the US National Cancer Institute.

REFERENCES

1. Kyle RA, Katzmann JA. Immunochemical characterization of immunoglobulins. In: *Manual of Clinical Laboratory Immunology*, 5th edn (Rose NR, de Macario EC, Folds JD et al, eds). Washington, DC: ASM Press, 1997: 156–76.
2. Dispenzieri A, Gertz MA, Therneau TM et al. Retrospective cohort study of 148 patients with polyclonal gammopathy. *Mayo Clin Proc* 2001; **76:** 476–87.
3. Katzmann JA, Clark R, Sanders E et al. Prospective study of serum protein capillary zone electrophoresis and immunotyping of monoclonal proteins by immunosubtraction. *Am J Clin Pathol* 1998; **110**: 503–9.
4. Axelsson U, Bachmann R, Hallen J. Frequency of pathological proteins (M-components) in 6,995 sera from an adult population. *Acta Med Scand* 1966; **179**: 235–47.
5. Kyle RA, Finkelstein S, Elveback LR, Kurland LT. Incidence of monoclonal proteins in a Minnesota community with a cluster of multiple myeloma. *Blood* 1972; **40**: 719–24.
6. Saleun JP, Vicariot M, Deroff P, Morin JF. Monoclonal gammopathies in the adult population of Finistere, France. *J Clin Pathol* 1982; **35**: 63–8.
7. Crawford J, Eye MK, Cohen HJ. Evaluation of monoclonal gammopathies in the 'well' elderly. *Am J Med* 1987; **82**: 39–45.
8. Ligthart GJ, Radl J, Corberand JX et al. Monoclonal gammopathies in human aging: Increased occurrence with age and correlation with health status. *Mech Ageing Dev* 1990; **52**: 235–43.
9. Cohen HJ, Crawford J, Rao MK et al. Racial differences in the prevalence of monoclonal gammopathy in a community-based sample of the elderly. *Am J Med* 1998; **104**: 439–44.
10. Bowden M, Crawford J, Cohen HJ, Noyama O. A comparative study of monoclonal gammopathies and immunoglobulin levels in Japanese and United States elderly. *J Am Geriatr Soc* 1993; **41**: 11–14.
11. Kyle RA. Monoclonal gammopathy of undetermined significance. Natural history in 241 cases. *Am J Med* 1978; **64**: 814–26.
12. Kyle RA. 'Benign' monoclonal gammopathy. A misnomer? *JAMA* 1984; **251**: 1849–54.
13. Kyle RA. 'Benign' monoclonal gammopathy – after 20 to 35 years of follow-up. *Mayo Clin Proc* 1993; **68**: 26–36.

14. Kyle RA. Monoclonal gammopathy of undetermined significance and solitary plasmacytoma. Implications for progression to overt multiple myeloma. *Hematol Oncol Clin North Am* 1997; **11**: 71–87.
15. Kyle RA, Garton JP. The spectrum of IgM monoclonal gammopathy in 430 cases. *Mayo Clin Proc* 1987; **62**: 719–31.
16. Axelsson U. A 20-year follow-up study of 64 subjects with M-components. *Acta Med Scand* 1986; **219**: 519–22.
17. Fine JM, Lambin P, Muller JY. The evolution of asymptomatic monoclonal gammopathies. A follow-up of 20 cases over periods of 3–14 years. *Acta Med Scand* 1979; **205**: 339–41.
18. Paladini G, Fogher M, Mazzanti G et al. Idiopathic monoclonal gammopathy. Long-term study of 313 case. [In Italian.] *Recenti Prog Med* 1989; **80**: 123–32.
19. Giraldo MP, Rubio-Félix D, Perella M et al. Monoclonal gammopathies of undetermined significance. Clinical course and biological aspects of 397 cases. [In Spanish.] *Sangre* 1991; **36**: 377–82.
20. Bladé J, Lopez-Guillermo A, Rozman C et al. Malignant transformation and life expectancy in monoclonal gammopathy of undetermined significance. *Br J Haematol* 1992; **81**: 391–4.
21. Isaksson E, Bjorkholm M, Holm G et al. Blood clonal B-cell excess in patients with monoclonal gammopathy of undetermined significance (MGUS): association with malignant transformation. *Br J Haematol* 1996; **92**: 71–6.
22. Baldini L, Guffanti A, Cesana BM et al. Role of different hematologic variables in defining the risk of malignant transformation in monoclonal gammopathy. *Blood* 1996; **87**: 912–18.
23. Kyle RA, Greipp PR. Smoldering multiple myeloma. *N Engl J Med* 1980; **302**: 1347–49.
24. Lindström FD, Dahlström U. Multiple myeloma or benign monoclonal gammopathy? A study of differential diagnostic criteria in 44 cases. *Clin Immunol Immunopathol* 1978; **10**: 168–74.
25. Bellaïche L, Laredo J-D, Lioté F et al. Magnetic resonance appearance of monoclonal gammopathies of unknown significance and multiple myeloma. *Spine* 1997; **22**: 2551–7.
26. Laroche M, Attal M, Dromer C. Bone remodelling in monoclonal gammopathies of uncertain significance, symptomatic and nonsymptomatic myeloma. *Clin Rheumatol* 1996; **15**: 347–52.
27. Bataille R, Jourdan M, Zhang XG, Klein B. Serum levels of interleukin 6, a potent myeloma cell growth factor, as a reflection of disease severity in plasma cell dyscrasias. *J Clin Invest* 1989; **84**: 2008–11.
28. Filella X, Bladé J, Guillermo AL et al. Cytokines (IL-6, TNF-α, IL-1α) and soluble interleukin-2 receptor as serum tumor markers in multiple myeloma. *Cancer Detect Prev* 1996; **20**: 52–6.
29. Lacy MQ, Donovan KA, Heimbach JK et al. Comparison of interleukin-1 beta expression by in situ hybridization in monoclonal gammopathy of undetermined significance and multiple myeloma. *Blood* 1999; **93**: 300–5.
30. Kyle RA, Lust JA. Monoclonal gammopathies of undetermined significance. In: *Neoplastic Diseases of the Blood*, 2nd edn (Wiernik PH, Canellos GP, Kyle RA, Schiffer CA, eds). New York: Churchill Livingstone, 1991: 571–94.
31. Greipp PR, Witzig TE, Gonchoroff NJ et al. Immunofluorescence labeling indices in myeloma and related monoclonal gammopathies. *Mayo Clin Proc* 1987; **62**: 969–77.
32. Witzig TE, Gonchoroff NJ, Katzmann JA et al. Peripheral blood B cell labeling indices are a measure of disease activity in patients with monoclonal gammopathies. *J Clin Oncol* 1988; **6**: 1041–6.
33. Witzig TE, Kyle RA, Greipp PR. Circulating peripheral blood plasma cells in multiple myeloma. *Curr Top Microbiol Immunol* 1992; **182**: 195–9.
34. Witzig TE, Kyle RA, O'Fallon WM, Greipp PR. Detection of peripheral blood plasma cells as a predictor of disease course in patients with smouldering multiple myeloma. *Br J Haematol* 1994; **87**: 266–72.
35. Billadeau D, Van Ness B, Kimlinger T et al. Clonal circulating cells are common in plasma cell proliferative disorders: a comparison of monoclonal gammopathy of undetermined significance, smoldering multiple myeloma, and active myeloma. *Blood* 1996; **88**: 289–96.
36. Zandecki M, Obein V, Bernardi F et al. Monoclonal gammopathy of undetermined significance: chromosome changes are a common finding within bone marrow plasma cells. *Br J Haematol* 1995; **90**: 693–6.
37. Drach J, Angerler J, Schuster J et al. Interphase fluorescence in situ hybridization identifies chromosomal abnormalities in plasma cells from patients with monoclonal gammopathy of undetermined significance. *Blood* 1995; **86**: 3915–21.

38. Carter A, Tatarsky I. The physiopathological significance of benign monoclonal gammopathy: a study of 64 cases. *Br J Haematol* 1980; **46:** 565–74.
39. Pasqualetti P, Casale R. Risk of malignant transformation in patients with monoclonal gammopathy of undetermined significance. *Biomed Pharmacother* 1997; **51**: 74–8.
40. Kyle RA, Beard CM, O'Fallon WM, Kurland LT. Incidence of multiple myeloma in Olmsted County, Minnesota: 1978 through 1990, with a review of the trend since 1945. *J Clin Oncol* 1994; **12**: 1577–83.
41. Azar HA, Hill WT, Osserman EF. Malignant lymphoma and lymphatic leukemia associated with myeloma-type serum proteins. *Am J Med* 1957; **23**: 239–49.
42. Kyle RA, Bayrd ED, McKenzie BF, Heck FJ. Diagnostic criteria for electrophoretic patterns of serum and urinary proteins in multiple myeloma: Study of one hundred and sixty-five multiple myeloma patients and of seventy-seven nonmyeloma patients with similar electrophoretic patterns. *JAMA* 1960; **174**: 245–51.
43. Alexanian R. Monoclonal gammopathy in lymphoma. *Arch Intern Med* 1975; **135**: 62–6.
44. Noel P, Kyle RA. Monoclonal proteins in chronic lymphocytic leukemia. *Am J Clin Pathol* 1987; **87**: 385–8.
45. Jansen J, Bolhuis RL, van Nieuwkoop JA et al. Paraproteinaemia plus osteolytic lesions in typical hairy-cell leukaemia. *Br J Haematol* 1983; **54**: 531–41.
46. Matsuzaki H, Yamaguchi K, Kagimoto T et al. Monoclonal gammopathies in adult T-cell leukemia. *Cancer* 1985; **56**: 1380–3.
47. Kövary PM, Suter L, Macher E et al. Monoclonal gammopathies in Sézary syndrome: a report of four new cases and a review of the literature. *Cancer* 1981; **48**: 788–92.
48. Venencie PY, Winkelmann RK, Puissant A, Kyle RA. Monoclonal gammopathy in Sézary syndrome. Report of three cases and review of the literature. *Arch Dermatol* 1984; **120**: 605–8.
49. Venencie PY, Winkelmann RK, Friedman SJ et al. Monoclonal gammopathy and mycosis fungoides. Report of four cases and review of the literature. *J Am Acad Dermatol* 1984; **11**: 576–9.
50. Rovira M, Cervantes F, Nomdedeu B, Rozman C. Chronic neutrophilic leukaemia preceding for seven years the development of multiple myeloma. *Acta Haematol* 1990; **83**: 94–5.
51. Economopoulos T, Economidou J, Giannopoulos G et al. Immune abnormalities in myelodysplastic syndromes. *J Clin Pathol* 1985; **38**: 908–11.
52. Dührsen U, Uppenkamp M, Meusers P et al. Frequent association of idiopathic myelofibrosis with plasma cell dyscrasias. *Blut* 1988; **56**: 97–102.
53. Pratt PW, Kochwa S, Estren S. Immunoglobulin abnormalities in Gaucher's disease. Report of 16 cases. *Blood* 1968; **31**: 633–40.
54. Shoenfeld Y, Berliner S, Pinkhas J, Beutler E. The association of Gaucher's disease and dysproteinemias. *Acta Haematol* 1980; **64**: 241–3.
55. Brady K, Corash L, Bhargava V. Multiple myeloma arising from monoclonal gammopathy of undetermined significance in a patient with Gaucher's disease. *Arch Pathol Lab Med* 1997; **121**: 1108–11.
56. Castaman G, Rodeghiero F, Di Bona E, Ruggeri M. Clinical effectiveness of desmopressin in a case of acquired von Willebrand's syndrome associated with benign monoclonal gammopathy. *Blut* 1989; **58**: 211–13.
57. Mant MJ, Hirsh J, Gauldie J et al. Von Willebrand's syndrome presenting as an acquired bleeding disorder in association with a monoclonal gammopathy. *Blood* 1973; **42**: 429–36.
58. Isobe T, Osserman EF. Pathologic conditions associated with plasma cell dyscrasias: a study of 806 cases. *Ann NY Acad Sci* 1971; **190**: 507–18.
59. Ropper AH, Gorson KC. Neuropathies associated with paraproteinemia. *N Engl J Med* 1998; **338**: 1601–7.
60. Kelly JJ Jr, Kyle RA, O'Brien PC, Dyck PJ. Prevalence of monoclonal protein in peripheral neuropathy. *Neurology* 1981; **31**: 1480–3.
61. Hafler DA, Johnson D, Kelly JJ et al. Monoclonal gammopathy and neuropathy: myelin-associated glycoprotein reactivity and clinical characteristics. *Neurology* 1986; **36**: 75–8.
62. Kelly JJ, Adelman LS, Berkman E, Bhan I. Polyneuropathies associated with IgM monoclonal gammopathies. *Arch Neurol* 1988; **45**: 1355–9.
63. Vital C, Vital A, Deminiere C et al. Myelin modifications in 8 cases of peripheral neuropathy with Waldenström's macroglobulinemia and anti-MAG activity. *Ultrastruct Pathol* 1997; 21: 509–16.
64. Simovic D, Gorson KC, Ropper AH. Comparison of IgM-MGUS and IgG-MGUS polyneuropathy. *Acta Neurol Scand* 1998; **97**: 194–200.

65. Dyck PJ, Low PA, Windebank AJ et al. Plasma exchange in polyneuropathy associated with monoclonal gammopathy of undetermined significance. *N Eng J Med* 1991; **325**: 1482–6.
66. Faed JM, Day B, Pollock M et al. High-dose intravenous human immunoglobulin in chronic inflammatory demyelinating polyneuropathy. *Neurology* 1989; **39**: 422–5.
67. Bardwick PA, Zvaifler NJ, Gill GN et al. Plasma cell dyscrasia with polyneuropathy, organomegaly, endocrinopathy, M-protein, and skin changes: the POEMS syndrome. Report on two cases and a review of the literature. *Medicine* 1980; **59**: 311–22.
68. Kelly JJ Jr, Kyle RA, Miles JM, Dyck PJ. Osteosclerotic myeloma and peripheral neuropathy. *Neurology* 1983; **33**: 202–10.
69. James K, Fudenberg H, Epstein WL, Shuster J. Studies on a unique diagnostic serum globulin in papular mucinosis (lichen myxedematosus). *Clin Exp Immunol* 1967; **2**: 153–66.
70. Powell FC, Schroeter AL, Su WP, Perry HO. Pyoderma gangrenosum and monoclonal gammopathy. *Arch Dermatol* 1983; **119**: 468–72.
71. Finan MC, Winkelmann RK. Necrobiotic xanthogranuloma with paraproteinemia. A review of 22 cases. *Medicine* 1986; **65**: 376–88.
72. Pascual M, Mach-Pascual S, Schifferli JA. Paraproteins and complement depletion: pathogenesis and clinical syndromes. *Semin Hematol* 1997; **34**(Suppl 1): 40–8.
73. Lutz ME, Daoud MS, McEvoy MT, Gibson LE. Subcorneal pustular dermatosis: a clinical study of ten patients. *Cutis* 1998; **61**: 203–8.
74. Lefrère JJ, Debbia M, Lambin P. Prospective follow-up of monoclonal gammopathies in HIV-infected individuals. *Br J Haematol* 1993; **84**: 151–5.
75. Pageaux GP, Bonnardet A, Picot MC et al. Prevalence of monoclonal immunoglobulins after liver transplantation: Relationship with post-transplant lymphoproliferative disorders. *Transplantation* 1998; **65**: 397–400.
76. Hammarström L, Smith CI. Frequent occurrence of monoclonal gammopathies with an imbalanced light-chain ratio following bone marrow transplantation. *Transplantation* 1987; **43**: 447–9.
77. Hebart H, Einsele H, Klein R et al. CMV infection after allogeneic bone marrow transplantation is associated with the occurrence of various autoantibodies and monoclonal gammopathies. *Br J Haematol* 1996; **95**: 138–44.
78. Zent CS, Wilson CS, Tricot G et al, Oligoclonal protein bands and Ig isotype switching in multiple myeloma treated with high-dose therapy and hematopoietic cell transplantation. *Blood* 1998; **91**: 3518–23.
79. Badley AD, Portela DF, Patel R et al. Development of monoclonal gammopathy precedes the development of Epstein–Barr virus-induced posttransplant lymphoproliferative disorder. *Liver Transplant Surg* 1996; **2**: 375–82.
80. Ginevri F, Nocera A, Bonato L et al. Cytomegalovirus infection is a trigger for monoclonal immunoglobulins in paediatric kidney transplant recipients. *Transplant Proc* 1998; **30**: 2079–82.
81. Renoult E, Bertrand F, Kessler M. Monoclonal gammopathies in HbsAg-positive patients with renal transplants. *N Engl J Med* 1988; **318**: 1205.
82. Radl J, Valentijn RM, Haaijman JJ, Paul LC. Monoclonal gammopathies in patients undergoing immunosuppressive treatment after renal transplantation. *Clin Immunol Immunopathol* 1985; **37**: 98–102.
83. Touchard G, Pasdeloup T, Parpeix J et al. High prevalence and usual persistence of serum monoclonal immunoglobulins evidenced by sensitive methods in renal transplant recipients. *Nephrol Dialysis Transplant* 1997; **12**: 1199–203.
84. Goldenberg GJ, Paraskevas F, Israels LG. The association of rheumatoid arthritis with plasma cell and lymphocytic neoplasms. *Arthritis Rheumatism* 1969; **12**: 569–79.
85. Zawadzki ZA, Benedek TG. Rheumatoid arthritis, dysproteinemic arthropathy, and paraproteinemia. *Arthritis Rheumatism* 1969; **12**: 555–68.
86. Soppi E, Eskola J, Röyttä M et al. Thymoma with immunodeficiency (Good's syndrome) associated with myasthenia gravis and benign IgG gammopathy. *Arch Intern Med* 1985; **145**: 1704–7.
87. Colwell NS, Tollefsen DM, Blinder MA. Identification of a monoclonal thrombin inhibitor associated with multiple myeloma and a severe bleeding disorder. *Br J Haematol* 1997; **97**: 219–26.
88. Merlini G, Farhangi M, Osserman EF. Monoclonal immunoglobulins with antibody activity in myeloma, macroglobulinemia and related plasma cell dyscrasias. *Semin Oncol* 1986; **13**: 350–65.
89. Annesley TM, Burritt MF, Kyle RA. Artifactual hypercalcemia in multiple myeloma. *Mayo Clin Proc* 1982; **57**: 572–5.

90. Merlini G, Fitzpatrick LA, Siris ES et al. A human myeloma immunoglobulin G binding four moles of calcium associated with asymptomatic hypercalcemia. *J Clin Immunol* 1984; **4**: 185–96.
91. Martin NF, Kincaid MC, Stark WJ et al. Ocular copper deposition associated with pulmonary carcinoma, IgG monoclonal gammopathy and hypercupremia. A clinicopathologic correlation. *Ophthalmology* 1983; **90**: 110–16.
92. Probst LE, Hoffman E, Cherian MG et al. Ocular copper deposition associated with benign monoclonal gammopathy and hypercupremia. *Cornea* 1996; **15**: 94–8.
93. Pettersson T, Hortling L, Teppo AM et al. Phosphate binding by a myeloma protein. *Acta Med Scand* 1987; **222**: 89–91.
94. Sonnenblick M, Eylath U, Brisk R et al. Paraprotein interference with colorimetry of phosphate in serum of some patients with multiple myeloma. *Clin Chem* 1986; **32**: 1537–9.
95. Andreone P, Zignego AL, Cursaro C et al. Prevalence of monoclonal gammopathies in patients with hepatitis C virus infection. *Ann Intern Med* 1998; **129**: 294–8.
96. Kyle RA, Robinson RA, Katzmann JA. The clinical aspects of biclonal gammopathies. Review of 57 cases. *Am J Med* 1981; **71**: 999–1008.
97. Grosbois B, Jégo P, de Rosa H et al. Triclonal gammopathy and malignant immunoproliferative syndrome. [In French.] *Rev Med Interne* 1997; **18**: 470–3.
98. Kyle RA, Maldonado JE, Bayrd ED. Idiopathic Bence Jones proteinuria – a distinct entity? *Am J Med* 1973; **55**: 222–6.
99. Kyle RA, Greipp PR. 'Idiopathic' Bence Jones proteinuria: long-term follow-up in seven patients. *N Engl J Med* 1982; **306**: 564–7.
100. O'Connor ML, Rice DT, Buss DH, Muss HB. Immunoglobulin D benign monoclonal gammopathy. A case report. *Cancer* 1991; **68**: 611–16.
101. Bladé J, Kyle RA. IgD monoclonal gammopathy with long-term follow-up. *Br J Haematol* 1994; **88**: 395–6.

25

Solitary plasmacytoma

Jayesh Mehta, Sundar Jagannath

INTRODUCTION

Plasmacytomas are localized tumors containing monoclonal plasma cells that arise in bones (osseous) or soft tissue (extraosseous or extramedullary). Plasmacytomas are often seen in the setting of myeloma, where the histologic appearance of the lesions is similar to that of the marrow. Plasmacytomas are sometimes seen with no marrow abnormalities, and may be single or multiple. Multiple plasmacytomas usually tend to behave clinically like myeloma.

Solitary plasmacytoma (SP), by definition, is a single tumor containing malignant plasma cells with no evidence of disease elsewhere. SP is a distinct clinical entity,[1,2] comprising less than 10% of all plasma cell dyscrasias.[2–8]

Plasmacytomas arising within a bone (solitary plasmacytoma of bone, SPB) and those arising in extraosseous locations (extramedullary plasmacytoma, EMP) differ in their natural history and prognosis. The risk of eventual progression to myeloma is considerably higher with SPB than with EMP.

The most important aspect of dealing with a patient with suspected SP is to establish the diagnosis with certainty, because the treatment approach is different for patients who do not have localized disease.

DIAGNOSIS OF SOLITARY PLASMACYTOMA

Diagnostic criteria for SPB and EMP have not been defined consistently. This may account, at least in part, for the apparent variability in the reported long-term outcome of patients with SP in terms of the risk of development of myeloma. Patients who have been diagnosed to have SP after rigorous investigations would be expected to have a lower risk of eventual progression to myeloma than those with some systemic disease (albeit minimal) that may have been overlooked.

The two important points of difference have been the extent of plasmacytosis in the bone marrow and the radiographic modality employed to look for lesions elsewhere in the body.

Some authors have included patients with up to 10% plasma cells in the marrow,[9–15] whereas others have included only patients with a 'normal' number of plasma cells (<5%).[5,7,16,17] Some authors have obtained marrow samples from two sites (iliac crest as well as sternum).[17]

Although no correlation has been described between the extent of marrow plasmacytosis and the probability of progression to myeloma, it is logical to assume that clear-cut marrow involvement with clonal cells must be considered evidence of systemic dissemination of the disease. Morphological examination is not very sensitive in identifying minimal marrow involvement, but flow cytometry for cytoplasmic immunoglobulin can identify as little as 1% light-chain-restricted plasma cells. This involvement must be considered significant (i.e. indicative of systemic involvement/spread), especially if the clone is aneuploid.[18]

The usual technique employed to look for lesions is a conventional radiographic skeletal survey, despite the fact that magnetic resonance imaging (MRI) can detect bone lesions not seen on X rays, and other newer imaging modalities (see Chapter 17) may detect other extramedullary lesions. Only two of the several published reports in the literature have reported utilising MRI to stage patients with SP.[19,20]

The MD Anderson Cancer Center group in Houston[19] performed MRI scans of the primary tumor as well as the thoracic and lumbosacral spine in 12 consecutive SPB patients. The standard skeletal survey had been negative in all of the patients. Additional lesions suggesting involvement with malignant cells were detected in 4 of 12 patients, in all of whom the abnormal protein persisted at over 50% of the baseline value following radiation treatment of the primary tumor. One of the four patients progressed to myeloma 10 months after diagnosis, and the other three were clinically stable on interferon-α at 10–31 months. At the time of disease progression, the 'occult' lesions previously visualized on MRI became detectable on conventional radiographs.

A subsequent report from the MD Anderson Cancer Center on 57 SPB patients,[20] including those reported earlier,[19] provided additional data on the usefulness of MRI scans. Amongst patients with thoracolumbar spine disease, seven of eight patients staged with plain radiographs alone developed myeloma, in comparison with one of seven patients who had MRI scans ($p = 0.08$).

We employ strict diagnostic criteria to diagnose SP (Table 25.1). These are similar to those proposed elsewhere,[2] but a normal MRI scan (*T1*, *T2*, and STIR sequences, without and with gadolinium contrast) of skull, spine, and pelvis, and flow-cytometric evaluation of the bone marrow to look for clonally restricted plasma cells and aneuploidy,[18] are essential in our criteria.

Dimopoulos et al[21] have proposed diagnostic criteria for SPB similar to those used by us for SP. They have included the absence of anemia, renal dysfunction, and hypercalcemia 'attributable to myeloma' in the criteria. The absence of these is not essential in the diagnostic criteria that we employ, because other processes could potentially account for any of these abnormalities, and the finding of myeloma as an underlying etiology, by definition, would rule out SP.

Unlike Dimopoulos et al,[21] we do not believe that the level of paraprotein or the levels of uninvolved immunoglobulins at the time of presentation make an important contribution to diagnosis, as long as all other criteria for the diagnosis of SP are satisfied, although patients with these features may merit closer follow-up for the development of systemic disease (see below).

Disappearance of paraprotein after local therapy (in patients who do have a paraprotein) within 6–12 months of completing therapy is important unless there is clear local persistence or recurrence of disease. We recognize that disappearance of the paraprotein may take longer than this in a minority of patients.[22]

Only long follow-up in a substantial number of patients will help determine the prognostic usefulness of such strict diagnostic criteria.

SOLITARY PLASMACYTOMA OF BONE

Clinical features

SPB is seen in 3–5% of patients with plasma cell disorders. As in myeloma, there is a male predominance, but, in contrast to myeloma, the median age at diagnosis is somewhat lower, and the disease may even be seen in childhood.

Over half of the tumors occur in the axial skeleton, mostly in the vertebral column,[5,9–11] and the remainder in the appendicular skeleton.

Table 25.1 Criteria for the diagnosis of solitary plasmacytoma

Solitary plasmacytoma of bone	
Single bone lesion	Complete radiographic skeletal survey MRI scan of the axial skeleton (skull, spine, and pelvis)
Clonal plasmacytosis	Biopsy of the tumor Flow cytometry or immunohistochemistry
Normal bone marrow	Morphology Lack of clonal plasma cells or aneuploidy on flow cytometry
Paraprotein	If present at diagnosis, should disappear within 6–12 months of therapy[a]
Solitary extramedullary plasmacytoma	
Single extramedullary lesion[b]	Regional CT scan
Normal skeleton	Complete radiographic skeleton survey MRI scan of the axial skeleton (skull, spine, and pelvis)
Clonal plasmacytosis	Biopsy of the tumor Flow cytometry or immunohistochemistry
Normal bone marrow	Morphology Lack of clonal plasma cells or aneuploidy on flow cytometry
Paraprotein	If present at diagnosis, should disappear within 6–12 months of therapy[a]

MRI, magnetic resonance imaging; CT, computed tomography.
[a]Assumes local eradication of plasmacytoma. If the tumor persists, paraprotein may persist too.
[b]Occasionally, more than one tumor may be present. See the discussion under 'Staging'.

Pain at the site of the lesion is a common mode of clinical presentation.[12–15] Other manifestations may include nerve root compression, spinal cord compression, other local mass effects depending upon the location of the tumor, and a palpable mass due to soft tissue extension.

Laboratory features

Blood counts, kidney function, and serum calcium levels are usually normal. Abnormalities in these, in the absence of an alternative explanation, may indicate systemic disease. A serum or urine paraprotein is seen in half of the patients.[5,7,8,10,11,16–18,20,21] Serum immunoglobulin levels (uninvolved) are usually normal. The bone marrow is normal, with no excess of plasma cells. One of the problems has been variability in the definition of a 'normal' bone marrow (see above). Flow cytometry of the peripheral blood is normal.

Biopsy of the tumor shows plasma cell infiltration that is monoclonal on flow cytometry and immunohistochemistry.

Radiologic features

Depending upon their size and the extent of bone destruction, SPB may be easily identifiable on conventional radiographs. Figure 25.1 shows

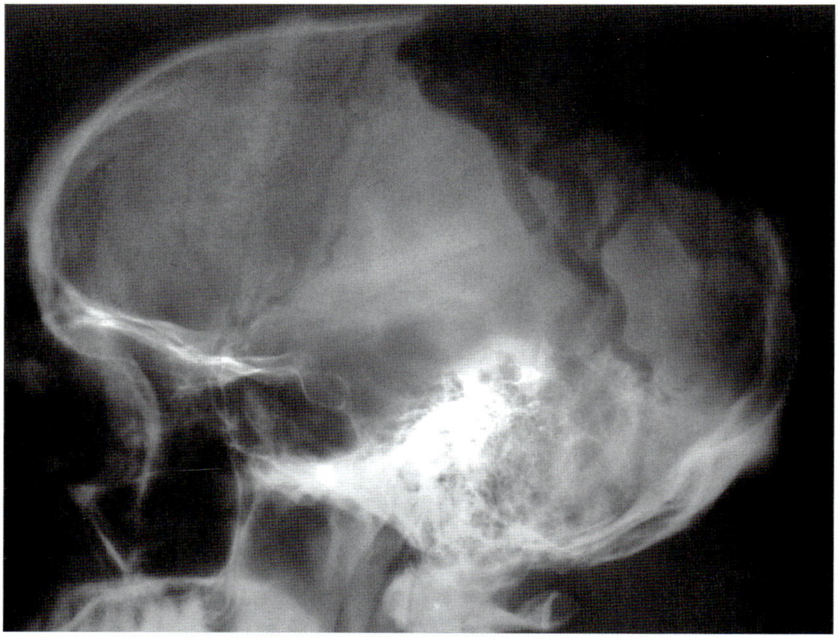

Figure 25.1 Plain radiograph of the skull of a patient with a large solitary intracranial plasmacytoma showing extensive bone destruction. All the diagnostic criteria laid down in Table 25.1 were satisfied.

extensive destruction of the skull in the parietal region in a patient with an intracranial SPB. However, computed tomography (CT) or MRI scanning is essential to delineate the exact size and extent of involvement locally, and to demonstrate the lack of involvement elsewhere. Figure 25.2 depicts the same patient's tumor on an MRI scan.

Therapy

Depending upon the mode of presentation, surgical intervention may already have occurred by the time the diagnosis is made. For example, patients presenting with a spinal SPB may have had the tumor excised and laminectomy–decompression performed. In the case of the patient depicted in Figures 25.1 and 25.2, the diagnosis was made at surgery, which was successful in resecting the entire tumor (Figure 25.3).

Additional surgical intervention required may involve spinal stabilization or internal fixation of a fractured long bone, depending upon the extent of local bone destruction.[23]

Local radiation is the treatment of choice. The field of treatment should include the entire tumor and some of the surrounding normal tissue. The dose of radiation administered, using a cobalt-60 (^{60}Co) source or a linear accelerator, is 4000–5000 cGy in 15–25 fractions over 3–5 weeks.[3,7,10,11,13–16,19,20,24–28] Lower doses

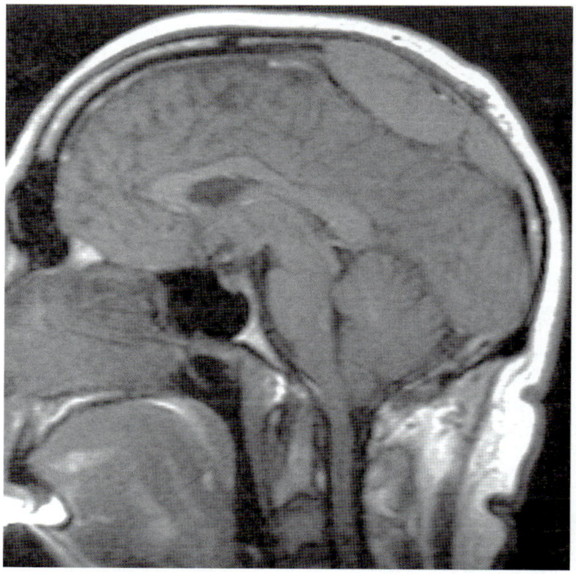

Figure 25.2 MRI scan of the patient shown in Figure 25.1.

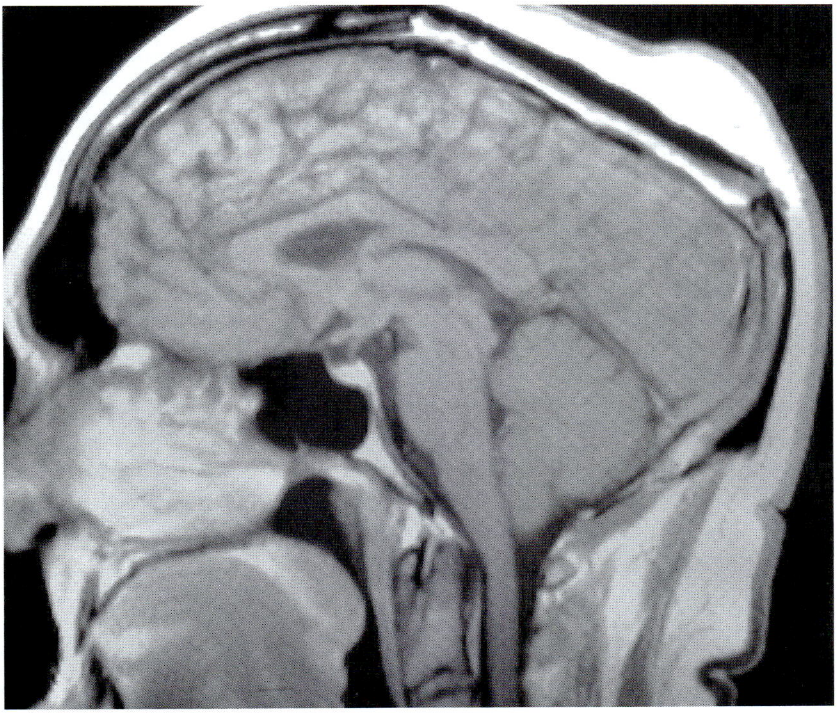

Figure 25.3 MRI scan of the patient shown in Figures 25.1 and 25.2 after surgical removal of the mass. Surgery resulted in complete removal of the mass. A prosthetic plate was placed. He received 4500 cGy local radiation subsequently.

(3500 cGy) have also been used,[29] with apparently good results, but higher rates of recurrence have been described with low doses of radiation.[30]

Reduced dose intensity (e.g. lower total dose or longer intervals between fractions) is the most common cause of treatment failure (incomplete eradication or subsequent recurrence). Some patients have tumors that are truly resistant to radiation. Radiotherapeutic management of patients with SPB is discussed in depth in Chapter 21.

Treatment approach in patients with a high likelihood of systemic disease

Patients who are detected to have disseminated disease such as plasmacytomas elsewhere or a small excess of clonal plasma cells in the marrow require systemic therapy (Chapter 18). Whether or not local radiation is used in their management depends upon the nature of the presenting lesion and the symptoms caused by it. In the absence of local problems, systemic therapy alone is reasonable. If there is significant local pain, cord compression or other local mass effects, local radiotherapy may be required in addition to systemic therapy.

Patients with a very high probability of eventually developing systemic disease,[31–33] based upon criteria such as decreased levels of uninvolved immunoglobulins or generalized osteopenia,[31,32] who otherwise have 'solitary' disease by other strictly defined criteria (Table 25.1), are treated with local therapy – similar to patients with strictly defined SP who do not exhibit these abnormalities. This is why we have not incorporated immunoparesis as an exclusion criterion in our diagnostic criteria, unlike others.[21] However, such patients must be watched much more closely for the onset of systemic disease progression. A case could be made for treating them like patients with smoldering myeloma, and they may benefit from the administration of bisphosphonates. Thalidomide[34] may also be worth investigating in this setting.

The role of adjuvant chemotherapy

Aviles et al[26] administered post-radiation adjuvant therapy with melphalan and prednisone to SPB patients in a randomized fashion in an attempt to improve disease-free survival. Between 1982 and 1989, 53 patients with SBP were randomly treated with 4000–5000 cGy local radiotherapy alone (28 patients) or similar radiation followed by melphalan–prednisone every 6 weeks for 3 years (25 patients). Disease-free and overall survival were significantly better in patients treated with combined therapy. In the experience of Mayr et al,[14] none of 5 patients receiving adjuvant chemotherapy progressed to myeloma, compared with 9 of 12 not receiving chemotherapy ($p = 0.009$). Mill et al[24] reported no progression in 4 patients treated with 'prophylactic chemotherapy', versus progression in 4 of 7 treated with radiation alone ($p = 0.1$).

On the other hand, Holland et al[15] and Bolek et al[27] could find no benefit with additional systemic chemotherapy. Delauche-Cavallier et al[17] administered adjuvant chemotherapy to 7 of 19 patients. Three of the 7 eventually developed acute leukemia.

The addition of systemic chemotherapy to radiation cannot be recommended in patients with SPB at this time. It may be an area for clinical investigation, especially in patients with features predictive for a high risk of progression to myeloma.

Follow-up after therapy

Patients with paraprotein should be monitored regularly after therapy to ensure disappearance of paraprotein. This usually occurs within a few months in the majority, but can occasionally take longer. After complete remission has been achieved, immunoglobulin levels as well as paraprotein studies should be done periodically in the long term, probably for at least 5–10 years (if not lifelong), to look for the development of immunoparesis or reappearance of paraprotein.

The utility of monitoring immunoglobulin levels and looking for paraprotein in patients who had non-secretory SPB is not defined. Certainly, in patients with myeloma, the disease does sometimes change its character (secretory to non-secretory and vice versa). This would suggest that looking for paraprotein (or decline in normal immunoglobulin levels) periodically as evidence of the onset of systemic disease may be worthwhile even in patients with non-secretory SPB.

Other investigations, depending upon the clinical situation, may include radiographic studies, bone densitometry, and even bone marrow examination. These, however, are not essential in all patients, and are only likely to be required infrequently.

Relapse

Relapse occurs in one of three different manners: local recurrence, development of additional plasmacytomas elsewhere, or development of systemic disease (myeloma).

Local recurrence may respond to additional radiation if dose-limiting radiation has not been delivered to the site already. Systemic therapy may be necessary if the tumor persists despite radiation.

The systemic treatment could be conventional chemotherapy, high-dose chemotherapy, or newer treatment approches such as thalidomide. We have treated a patient with a tumor that had not responded to 7000 cGy of local radiation cumulatively delivered elsewhere with two cycles of infusional chemotherapy (dexamethasone, cyclophosphamide, etoposide, cisplatin) and two cycles of high-dose chemotherapy (200 mg/m^2 melphalan with autologous hematopoietic stem cell transplantation). There was no apparent response to the infusional chemotherapy or the first cycle of high-dose melphalan, but complete remission was achieved with the second cycle of high-dose melphalan. When the disease recurred approximately 2 years later, the patient was started on thalidomide[34] and dexamethasone, with a partial response.

Additional plasmacytomas can be treated as an ordinary SP would be if they are single and there is no systemic disease. If they are multiple, systemic therapy is needed. The development of myeloma is an indication for treating these patients like a patient with de novo myeloma.

Prognostic factors

In patients with stringently diagnosed SPB, factors at presentation that have been identified to be predictive of a higher probability of eventual progression to myeloma include low levels of uninvolved immunoglobulins,[31–33] osteopenia,[31,32] greater age,[8,30] axial lesions,[30] presence of a paraprotein,[15,17,37] higher protein levels,[15] higher paraprotein levels,[7] and larger lesions[15] – although not in all series.[5,8,13,27,35–37]

In patients with a paraprotein at presentation, its disappearance after definitive local therapy is associated with a lower likelihood of the eventual development of myeloma.[7,20,33,38]

Natural history

With more sophisticated investigations and tighter diagnostic criteria, the number of patients with SPB will probably decrease, and the long-term survival of those diagnosed with SPB will improve.

The published series in the literature encompass patients diagnosed on the basis of heterogeneous criteria, and therefore show widely variable outcomes. The reported outcome data are summarized in Table 25.2. Overall, the prognosis of SPB is reasonably good, with overall survival exceeding 5 years in almost all patients and the median survival exceeding 10 years.

EXTRAMEDULLARY PLASMACYTOMA

Clinical features

EMPs are even more uncommon than SPB, and while they can affect soft tissues anywhere, they are most often seen in the head and neck (commonly in the nose, paranasal sinuses, nasopharynx, and tonsils; less commonly they involve other structures).[3,5,12,15,25,33,39–41] Other sites of involvement include the gastrointestinal tract, lymph nodes, spleen, skin, subcutaneous tissues, testes, and pleura.

A number of EMPs present as nasal polyps, which are common. Upon removal, nasal polyps are often not subjected to histologic examination. Therefore, it is possible that the actual incidence of EMP is higher. There is a male preponderance.[3,5,12,15,39]

Patients are either asymptomatic or present with symptoms referable to the respiratory tract, such as nasal discharge, nasal obstruction, epistaxis, dyspnea and hemoptysis. Examination reveals a smooth, fleshy, shiny tumor, which may be sessile or pedunculated. Thyroid involvement presents as a goiter, and gut involvement results in abdominal pain, weight loss, and bleeding.

Lymph nodes draining the site, especially cervical nodes, may be involved in up to one-quarter of patients.

Staging

Wiltshaw[39] and Woodruff et al[40] have utilized the following staging system for EMP:

- stage I: tumor confined to the primary site;
- stage II: involvement of drainage lymph nodes;
- stage III: evidence of metastatic spread.

The validity of this staging system may be questioned, because stage III EMP could be considered disseminated disease and perhaps classified as myeloma or 'multiple extramedullary plasmacytomas'.

Woodruff et al[40] included one patient with disease involving the antrum, cervical lymph nodes, and bone marrow in their series because of the typical nasopharyngeal plasmacytoma that the patient had. This patient died 15 months after diagnosis – presumably of systemic disease. On the other hand, Knowling et al[5]

Table 25.2 Outcome of patients with solitary plasmacytoma of bone

Authors	No. of patients	Disease progression[a]	No disease progression	Comments
Aviles et al[26]	53		66%; median 9 yr	Randomized trial of adjuvant chemotherapy. 88% disease-free in adjuvant chemotherary group and 46% in the no-chemotherapy group
Chak et al[35]	20	55%; 4–93 mo	45%; 22–218 mo	3 patients received adjuvant chemotherapy for persistent paraprotein after radiotherapy, and were progression-free at 22, 46, and 110 mo
Delauche-Cavallier et al[17]	19	68%; 9–84 mo	32%; 18–110 mo	Secondary leukemia in 4; including 3 of 7 receiving adjuvant chemotherapy
Dimopoulos et al[7]	45	51%; median 20 mo	49% (10 over 10 yr)	Only 2 of 23 relapses occurred beyond 7 yr
Frassica et al[13]	46	54%; median 18 mo	43%; 5 yr (actuarial) 25%; 10 yr (actuarial)	One-quarter of patients experiencing disease progression did so beyond 5 yr
Holland et al[15]	32	53%; 3–204 mo	45%; 16 yr (actuarial)	Four patients developing second 'solitary' plasmacytomas then had no further disease progression at 22–136 mo (median 29 mo)
Jackson and Scarffe[31]	32	63%; median 46 mo		Median survival 27 mo in patients with immunoparesis or osteopenia, and >80% survival at 10 yr with neither
Knowling et al[5]	24	54%; 7–96 mo	46%; 7–197 mo	1 of 25 reported patients excluded here (death due to unrelated causes at 6 mo)
Liebross et al[20]	57	51%; median 1.8 yr		Includes patients from Moulopoulos et al[19] and Dimopoulos et al[7]
Moulopoulos et al[19]	8	0	100%; 6–33 mo	Staged by MRI (thoracolumbar spine)
Shih et al[8]	22		58%; 5 yr (actuarial)	
Woodruff et al[16]	11	64%; 20–144 mo	36%; 12–180 mo	1 of 12 reported patients excluded here (death due to unrelated causes at 11 mo)

[a] Defined as disseminated disease, a second plasmacytoma, or local recurrence.

described a patient with skin, hand, epitrochlea, and axillary node involvement who was alive and well almost 13 years after presentation, with local therapy only.

Ganjoo and Malpas,[42] in their diagnostic criteria for EMP, require the presence of a 'solitary plasma cell tumor presenting in the head and neck', and include multiple tumors 'only in other sites of primary involvement'.

The question of whether so-called stage III EMP is SP at all or not remains unsettled on the basis of available data.

Laboratory features

These are similar to those of SPB. Blood counts, kidney function, and serum calcium levels are usually normal. A serum or urine paraprotein is seen in less than half of the patients, and the level is usually small. Serum immunoglobulin levels are usually normal, as is the bone marrow, with no excess of plasma cells.

Biopsy of the tumor shows plasma cell infiltration that is monoclonal on flow cytometry and immunohistochemistry. Demonstration of clonality of plasma cells in the tumor is particularly important in the case of nasal passage tumors, because nasal polyps often have reactive plasma cell infiltration.

Radiologic features

There are no specific characteristics of EMPs on imaging studies, which are more useful to delineate the extent of the lesion and to look for additional lesions rather than make a diagnosis.

Therapy

EMPs are exquisitely sensitive to radiation, and 4000–5000 cGy assures local control in the majority of patients. While surgical intervention has usually occurred in the majority prior to the diagnosis having been made, complete excision is not necessary. If complete local control is not achieved with radiation, then surgical excision of the remainder of the lesion may be required. This has to be done in a small proportion of patients (Table 25.3).

If more than one tumor has been detected, all involved sites should be irradiated. Involved regional nodes should be irradiated too. Whether regional nodes should be irradiated prophylactically is not known. This is routinely practiced at some centers. Details of radiation therapy are discussed in Chapter 21.

With reference to the impact of staging on therapy, the patient described by Woodruff et al[40] (see above) was treated with systemic chemotherapy in addition to local radiation. Despite good local control, the patient died 15 months later, presumably of systemic disease. On the other hand, the patient described by Knowling et al[5] (see above) remained in remission for several years, with local radiation to multiple sites.

Multiple tumors may require systemic chemotherapy, including high-dose chemotherapy and transplantation if appropriate. In fact, the first ever attempt at harnessing an immunologic graft-versus-myeloma effect[43] was made in a patient with recurrent extramedullary plasmacytomas who was allografted and subsequently given infusions of donor lymphocytes by Shimon Slavin's group in Jerusalem over a decade ago.[44]

Natural history

As Table 25.3 shows, the overall outcome of EMP is good – and is better than that of patients with SPB (Table 25.2). Local tumor eradication is achieved in a substantial proportion of patients. However, regional recurrence in draining lymph nodes is seen in up to 20% of patients.[5,12,14] Local bone invasion has also been reported, but has not always proceeded to the development of myeloma. Overall, the development of myeloma occurs in up to 40% of patients, and is less common than in patients with SPB.

Table 25.3 Outcome of patients with extramedullary plasmacytoma

Authors	No. of patients	Disease progression (myeloma)	No disease progression	Limited disease progression followed by extended period of stability[a]
Bolek et al[27]	10	11%; 10 yr (actuarial) 33%; 15 yr (actuarial)		
Corwin and Lindberg[3]	12	33%; 11–48 mo	58%; 24–320 mo	3 patient at 3 mo (5 yr)
Holland et al[15]	14	36%; 3–61 mo	65%; 10 yr (actuarial)	
Knowling et al[5]	24[b]	21%; 12–61 mo	71% 6–222 mo[c]	2 patients at 15 and 16 mo (12 and 6 yr)
Mayr et al[14]	13	23%; within 2 yr		
Meis et al[12]	13	23%; 8–52 mo	77%; 34–156 mo[d]	2 patients at 5 and 74 mo (3 and 3.5 yr)
Shih et al[8]	10		78%; 5 yr (actuarial)	
Tong et al[10]	7	0	100%; 1.5–23 yr	
Woodruff et al[16]	12[e]	25%; 3–15 mo	75%; 1.5–16 yr	

[a]The figure in parentheses is the disease-free interval after therapy of limited progression.
[b]Excludes 1 patient dying of unrelated causes at 4 mo.
[c]Includes 2 patients requiring additional therapy after failure of initial therapy to eradicate the disease completely.
[d]Includes 1 patient requiring additional therapy after failure of initial therapy to eradicate the disease completely.
[e]Excludes 1 patient dying of unrelated causes at 3 mo and 3 with short follow-up.

Why is the outcome of EMP better than that of SPB? Conceivably, the location of the tumor may have something to do with this. SPB, because of contiguity with marrow, may exhibit a greater propensity to the development of myeloma. However, there are limited data showing that the nature of the malignant cells in SPB and EMP is also different,[45] contributing to the different natural histories. Guida et al[45] studied two patients with SP: one with a mandibular SPB and one with a rhinopharyngeal EMP. Serum β_2-microglobulin, thymidine kinase, interleukin (IL)-2, IL-6, and soluble IL-2 receptor levels were higher in the patient with SPB. Flow cytometry showed 80% of the malignant cells to be aneuploid in SPB, compared with 2% of the cells in EMP, and the proportion of cells in S phase was 16% and 4%, respectively. These data suggest that plasma cells in SPB are more like myeloma plasma cells.

REFERENCES

1. Conklin R, Alexanian R. Clinical classification of plasma cell myeloma. *Arch Intern Med* 1975; **135**: 139–43.
2. Kyle RA. Monoclonal gammopathy of undetermined significance and solitary plasmacytoma. Implications for progression to overt multiple myeloma. *Hematol Oncol Clin North Am* 1997; **11**: 71–87.
3 Corwin J, Lindberg RD. Solitary plasmacytoma of bone vs. extramedullary plasmacytoma and their relationship to multiple myeloma. *Cancer* 1979; **43**: 1007–13.
4. Bartl R, Frisch B, Burkhardt R et al. Bone marrow histology in myeloma: its importance in diagnosis, prognosis, classification and staging. *Br J Haematol* 1982; **51**: 361–75.
5. Knowling MA, Harwood AR, Bergsagel DE. Comparison of extramedullary plasmacytomas with solitary and multiple plasma cell tumors of bone. *J Clin Oncol* 1983; **1**: 255–62.
6. Bataille R, Dessauw P, Sany J. Polyclonal immunoglobulins in malignant plasma cell dyscrasias. *Oncology* 1984; **41**: 314–17.
7. Dimopoulos MA, Goldstein J, Fuller L et al. Curability of solitary bone plasmacytoma. *J Clin Oncol* 1992; **10**: 587–90.
8. Shih LY, Dunn P, Leung WM et al. Localised plasmacytomas in Taiwan: comparison between extramedullary plasmacytoma and solitary plasmacytoma of bone. *Br J Cancer* 1995; **71**: 128–33.
9. Corwin J, Lindberg RD. Solitary plasmacytoma of bone vs. extramedullary plasmacytoma and their relationship to multiple myeloma. *Cancer* 1979; **43**: 1007–13.
10. Tong D, Griffin TW, Laramore GE et al. Solitary plasmacytoma of bone and soft tissues. *Radiology* 1980; **135**: 195–8.
11. Mendenhall CM, Thar TL, Million RR. Solitary plasmacytoma of bone and soft tissue. *Int J Radiat Oncol Biol Phys* 1980; **6**: 1497–501.
12. Meis JM, Butler JJ, Osborne BM, Ordonez NG. Solitary plasmacytomas of bone and extramedullary plasmacytomas. A clinicopathologic and immunohistochemical study. *Cancer* 1987; **59**: 1475–85.
13. Frassica DA, Frassica FJ, Schray MF et al. Solitary plasmacytoma of bone: Mayo Clinic experience. *Int J Radiat Oncol Biol Phys* 1989; **16**: 43–8.
14. Mayr NA, Wen BC, Hussey DH et al. The role of radiation therapy in the treatment of solitary plasmacytomas. *Radiother Oncol* 1990; **17**: 293–303.
15. Holland J, Trenkner DA, Wasserman TH, Fineberg B. Plasmacytoma. Treatment results and conversion to myeloma. *Cancer* 1992; **69**: 1513–17.
16. Woodruff RK, Malpas JS, White FE. Solitary plasmacytoma. II: Solitary plasmacytoma of bone. *Cancer* 1979; **43**: 2344–7.
17. Delauche-Cavallier MC, Laredo JD, Wybier M et al. Solitary plasmacytoma of the spine. Long-term clinical course. *Cancer* 1988; **61**: 1707–14.
18. Laso FJ, Tabernero MD, Iglesias-Osma MC. Extramedullary plasmacytoma: a localized or systemic disease? *Ann Intern Med* 1998; **128**: 156.
19. Moulopoulos LA, Dimopoulos MA, Weber D et al. Magnetic resonance imaging in the staging of solitary plasmacytoma of bone. *J Clin Oncol* 1993; **11**: 1311–15.
20. Liebross RH, Ha CS, Cox JD et al. Solitary bone plasmacytoma: outcome and prognostic factors following radiotherapy. *Int J Radiat Oncol Biol Phys* 1998; **41**: 1063–7.
21. Dimopoulos MA, Moulopulos LA, Maniatis A, Alexanian R. Solitary plasmacytoma of bone and

asymptomatic multiple myeloma. *Blood* 2000; **96**: 2037–44.
22. Alexanian R. Localized and indolent myeloma. *Blood* 1980; **56**: 521–6.
23. Durr HR, Kuhne JH, Hagena FW et al. Surgical treatment for myeloma of the bone. A retrospective analysis of 22 cases. *Arch Orth Trauma Surg* 1997; **116**: 463–9.
24. Mill WB, Griffith R. The role of radiation therapy in the management of plasma cell tumors. *Cancer* 1980; **45**: 647–52.
25. Greenberg P, Parker RG, Fu YS, Abemayor E. The treatment of solitary plasmacytoma of bone and extramedullary plasmacytoma. *Am J Clin Oncol* 1987; **10**: 199–204.
26. Aviles A, Huerta-Guzman J, Delgado S et al. Improved outcome in solitary bone plasmacytomata with combined therapy. *Hematol Oncol* 1996; **14**: 111–17.
27. Bolek TW, Marcus RB, Mendenhall NP. Solitary plasmacytoma of bone and soft tissue. *Int J Radiat Oncol Biol Phys* 1996; **36**: 329–33.
28. Jacobson RJ, Levy JI, Shulman G, De Moor NG. Solitary myeloma. A study of 10 Black patients during an 8-year period. *S Afr Med J* 1975; **49**: 1347–51.
29. Harwood AR, Knowling MA, Bergsagel DE. Radiotherapy of extramedullary plasmacytoma of the head and neck. *Clin Radiol* 1981; **32**: 31–6.
30. Bataille R, Sany J. Solitary myeloma: clinical and prognostic features of a review of 114 cases. *Cancer* 1981; **48**: 845–51.
31. Jackson A, Scarffe JH. Prognostic significance of osteopenia and immunoparesis at presentation in patients with solitary myeloma of bone. *Eur J Cancer* 1990; **26**: 363–71.
32. Jackson A, Scarffe JH. Upper humeral cortical thickness as an indicator of osteopenia: diagnostic significance in solitary myeloma of bone. *Skel Radiol* 1991; **20**: 363–7.
33. Galieni P, Cavo M, Avvisati G et al. Solitary plasmacytoma of bone and extramedullary plasmacytoma: two different entities? *Ann Oncol* 1995; **6**: 687–91.
34. Singhal S, Mehta J, Desikan R et al. Antitumor activity of thalidomide in refractory multiple myeloma. *N Engl J Med* 1999; **341**: 1565–71.
35. Chak LY, Cox RS, Bostwick DG, Hoppe RT. Solitary plasmacytoma of bone: treatment, progression, and survival. *J Clin Oncol* 1987; **5**: 1811–15.
36. Brinch L, Hannisdal E, Abrahamsen AF et al. Extramedullary plasmacytomas and solitary plasma cell tumors of bone. *Eur J Haematol* 1990; **44**: 132–5.
37. Poor MM, Hitchon PW, Riggs CE Jr. Solitary spinal plasmacytomas: management and outcome. *J Spinal Disord* 1988; **1**: 295–300.
38. Ellis PA, Colls BM. Solitary plasmacytoma of bone: clinical features, treatment and survival. *Hematol Oncol* 1992; **10**: 207–11.
39. Wiltshaw E. The natural history of extramedullary plasmacytoma and its relation to solitary myeloma of bone and myelomatosis. *Medicine (Baltimore)* 1976; **55**: 217–38.
40. Woodruff RK, Whittle JM, Malpas JS. Solitary plasmacytoma. I: Extramedullary soft tissue plasmacytoma. *Cancer* 1979; **43**: 2340–3.
41. Wollersheim HC, Holdrinet RS, Haanen C. Clinical course and survival in 16 patients with localized plasmacytoma. *Scand J Haematol* 1984; **32**: 423–8.
42. Ganjoo RK, Malpas JS. Plasmacytoma. In: *Myeloma: Biology and Management*, 2nd edn (Malpas JS, Bergsagel DE, Kyle RA, Anderson KC, eds). Oxford: Oxford University Press, 1998: 545–58.
43. Mehta J, Singhal S. Graft-versus-myeloma. *Bone Marrow Transplant* 1998; **22**: 835–43.
44. Or R, Mehta J, Naparstek E et al. Successful T cell-depleted allogeneic bone marrow transplantation in a child with recurrent multiple extramedullary plasmacytomas. *Bone Marrow Transplant* 1992; **10**: 381–2.
45. Guida M, Casamassima A, Abbate I et al. Solitary plasmacytoma of bone and extramedullary plasmacytoma: two different nosological entities? *Tumori* 1994; **80**: 370–7.

26

Amyloidosis

Morie A Gertz, Martha Q Lacy, Angela Dispenzieri

CONTENTS • **Introduction** • **When should amyloid be suspected?** • **Amyloid syndromes** • **Diagnostic confirmation of amyloidosis** • **Amyloid organ-specific syndromes** • **Therapy for amyloidosis**

INTRODUCTION

Amyloidosis is defined as deposits that bind the cotton dye Congo red and demonstrate green birefringence when viewed under polarized light. Deposits of amyloid are always seen extracellularly, and are amorphous under the light microscope. With standard hematoxylin and eosin stains, the deposits appear pink. When viewed under the electron microscope, amyloid deposits appear as rigid, non-branching fibrils of indefinite length and a width of 9.5 nm. Amyloid fibrils are insoluble but form a suspension in distilled water. Repeated homogenization with saline of tissues containing amyloid, followed by suspension in water, forms the basis for the purification of amyloid.[1]

Before much was known about the structure and sequence of amyloid, it was classified clinically on the basis of anatomic distribution.[2] Historically, three types of systemic amyloidosis were recognized. Amyloidosis seen with an autosomal dominant inheritance pattern was classified as familial.[3,4] Amyloidosis as a sequela of a long-standing infection, rheumatic disorder, or inflammatory bowel disease was classified as secondary.[5] Amyloidosis of unknown cause was considered idiopathic and designated as primary (AL). Today, amyloidosis is classified by the biochemical subunit protein constituting the amyloid fibril. A modification of the nomenclature for amyloid is given in Table 26.1. Forms other than AL are unlikely to be encountered by a hematologist or an oncologist. AL is composed of immunoglobulin light chains and is the only form of amyloid reviewed in this chapter.

It is possible to produce fibrils of AL in vitro by taking purified human Bence Jones proteins (light chains) and subjecting them to peptic digestion.[6] When the disulfide bonds between immunoglobulin light chains are reduced, amyloid can form in vitro.[7] AL is composed from the N-terminal fragment of an immunoglobulin light chain or heavy chain. The latter carries the nomenclature AH.[8] The clinical characteristics of AL and AH do not appear to be distinct. The primary structure of immunoglobulin light chains in patients who develop AL is presumed to be unique. Light chains extracted from the urine of patients with AL can produce amyloid deposits when injected into mice. The mouse amyloid deposits have been shown to be composed of human immunoglobulin light chains. The light chains from the urine of patients with myeloma who do not have AL do not produce similar deposits.[9] It is assured that certain immunoglobulin light chains have a true amyloidogenic predisposition. It is thought that

Table 26.1 Nomenclature of amyloidosis

Protein	Precursor[a]	Clinical
AL or AH	Immunoglobulin light or heavy chain	Primary or localized myeloma or macroglobulinemia association
AA	SAA	Secondary or familial Mediterranean fever
ATTR	Transthyretin	Familial and senile
$A\beta_2M$	β_2-Microglobulin	Dialysis–carpal tunnel syndrome
Aβ	ABPP	Alzheimer's disease

[a]ABPP, amyloid β protein precursor; SAA, serum amyloid A.

these light chains have a greater propensity to form a β-pleated sheet, the ultrastructure of the amyloid fibril.

In myeloma and monoclonal gammopathy of undetermined significance (MGUS), κ light chains account for two-thirds of Ig proteins. In AL patients, λ light chains represent nearly three-quarters of the deposits seen. One may infer that λ light chains are inherently more amyloidogenic. The λ_{VI} subclass of immunoglobulin light chain seems to be uniquely associated with AL, with virtually all described λ_{VI} sequences occurring in patients with AL.[10] AL patients may be classified into those with myeloma and those without myeloma.[11] The classification is usually determined by the percentage of plasma cells in the bone marrow, the presence or absence of lytic bone lesions, and whether renal insufficiency is due to deposits of amyloid in the glomerulus or to myeloma cast nephropathy. Overt myeloma is uncommon in AL, and accounts for far less than the 10% figure previously recorded. If a patient does not present with myeloma at the time when AL is diagnosed, the likelihood of myeloma developing is approximately 1 in 250.[12]

The median age of patients seen with AL at the Mayo Clinic is 62 years. The incidence of AL is 8 per million per year, a figure comparable to the incidence of agnogenic myeloid metaplasia, polycythemia rubra vera, or Hodgkin's disease.[13,14] Myeloma is fivefold more common than AL. In Olmsted County, Minnesota, the median age of patients diagnosed as having AL is 72 years, suggesting institutional referral bias.

In summary, AL is a dysproteinemia with a small number (median 5%) of monoclonal plasma cells in the bone marrow. Confusion with myeloma is common. Proteinuria is seen in both conditions. Both are treated with chemotherapy.

WHEN SHOULD AMYLOID BE SUSPECTED?

Because the symptoms and physical findings of AL are non-specific and seen in only a minority of patients, when should a clinician be alerted to the possibility of AL in a patient so that early therapy can be instituted?

Although we have seen AL in patients as young as 26 years, only 1% of patients are younger than 40 years. Males represent between 60% and 65% of patients. Only 52% of myeloma patients are males.[15] The two most common symptoms seen in AL patients are fatigue and weight loss – highly non-specific symptoms often seen in the general medical practice. In most instances, these symptoms do not help a clinician formulate a differential diagnosis that includes AL. In our experience, these presenting symptoms lead to investigation for an underlying malignancy.[16] Fatigue can often be misattributed to stress or a functional disorder. This is seen most commonly in cardiac amyloidosis, in which the objective evidence is often quite subtle. Lightheadedness, although non-specific, frequently accompanies fatigue. Its etiology is plasma volume contraction in patients with nephrotic syndrome or low stroke volume in patients who have a non-compliant left ventricle that fills poorly during diastole. Orthostatic hypotension is seen regularly in patients with renal or cardiac amyloidosis. In patients who have autonomic neuropathy associated with amyloid peripheral neuropathy, orthostatic hypotension is a consequence of autonomic failure. Syncope is seen regularly.[17]

Diagnostic physical findings are seen in the minority of patients with AL. Periorbital and facial purpura can be diagnostic of AL, but this is seen in only 10–15% of patients (Figure 26.1). The purpuric lesions are characteristic in that they occur consistently above the nipple line, typically in the webbing of the neck, eyelids, or face. Periorbital purpura is easy to overlook, because the majority represent small petechial lesions. Hepatomegaly is another important physical finding in up to 25% of patients. In the majority, the liver is enlarged only minimally, because only 10% have a liver edge palpable 5 cm below the right costal margin. Macroglossia is a specific finding for AL. Macroglossia is seen in less than 10% of patients, and can frequently be overlooked, because the enlargement tends to occur on the underside of the tongue and will be missed when the tongue is viewed in a neutral position on the floor of the mouth. Submandibular salivary gland enlargement is common, but is frequently misinterpreted as representing small submandibular lymph nodes.

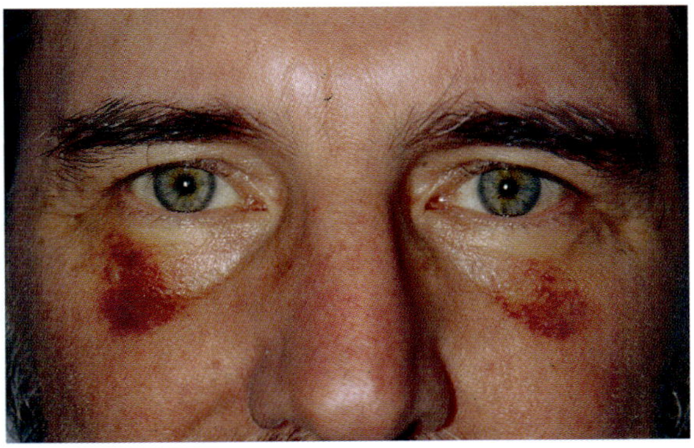

Figure 26.1 This patient demonstrates periorbital purpura classic for amyloid.

Occasionally, patients with AL present with symptoms mimicking temporal arteritis.[18–20] Patients develop amyloid occlusion of small vessels, leading to calf, buttock, shoulder, and jaw claudication. Because half of the patients with AL have a monoclonal spike in the serum, the sedimentation rate is frequently increased. This adds to the confusion and potential misdiagnosis of temporal arteritis. Empiric therapy with corticosteroids will not be helpful, and may delay the diagnosis.[21] An occasional patient is seen with skeletal muscle pseudohypertrophy and the shoulder pad sign.[22] This is a rare finding, and most patients with amyloid muscle involvement are actually profoundly weak owing to muscular atrophy from chronic reduction of blood supply to the muscles.[23] Xerostomia due to infiltration of the minor salivary glands is common.[24] In the absence of a biopsy of the minor salivary glands, Sjögren syndrome is misdiagnosed regularly.[25]

AMYLOID SYNDROMES

The clinician must be alert to the four common syndromes associated with AL and pursue appropriate screening techniques when one of these is present:

- nephrotic-range proteinuria, with or without renal insufficiency;
- heart failure secondary to restrictive cardiomyopathy;
- hepatomegaly;
- demyelinating peripheral neuropathy.

Any time an adult is seen with one of these four syndromes, amyloidosis should be included in the differential diagnosis.

Table 26.2 shows the common clinical picture with which AL presents.[26–29]

The most appropriate initial screening test is immunoelectrophoresis and immunofixation of

Table 26.2 Syndromes in primary amyloidosis (AL)

Syndrome	Patients (%)
Nephrotic syndrome (with or without renal failure)	30
Hepatomegaly	24
Congestive heart failure	22
Carpal tunnel	21
Neuropathy	17
Orthostatic hypotension	12

the serum and urine.[30] All patients with AL by definition have a light-chain-producing clone of plasma cells in their body. Detection of a free monoclonal immunoglobulin is powerful confirmation of the suspicion of amyloidosis.[31] A high proportion of patients with AL have only free light chains in the serum (Figure 26.2). Free light chains have a low molecular weight and filter through the renal glomerulus into the urine. As a consequence, they do not accumulate in the serum in sufficient quantity to produce a demonstrable M spike on serum protein electrophoresis. A visible spike will not be detected in the serum in one-third of patients with AL. Immunofixation is required to detect these small quantities of M protein. A screening protein electrophoresis is not sufficient, because the small M protein is easy to overlook on a cellulose acetate electrophoresis pattern. When intact immunoglobulin proteins are present, the peaks may be so small they can be obscured by the surrounding normal immunoglobulins.

The same concept holds true for the urine. Nearly half of patients with AL excrete 1 g or more of albumin in the urine. The urinary protein pattern is generally an ultrafiltrate of the serum, and contains all globulin fractions. The urinary protein commonly obscures the excretion of small amounts of free monoclonal light chain (Figure 26.3). Immunofixation, once again, is required to detect these small M components. If the serum and urine are both screened in patients with AL, an M component will be found in 90% of patients. Screening immunofixation of the serum and urine represents the best noninvasive screening study when a clinician is confronted with a patient with any of the four

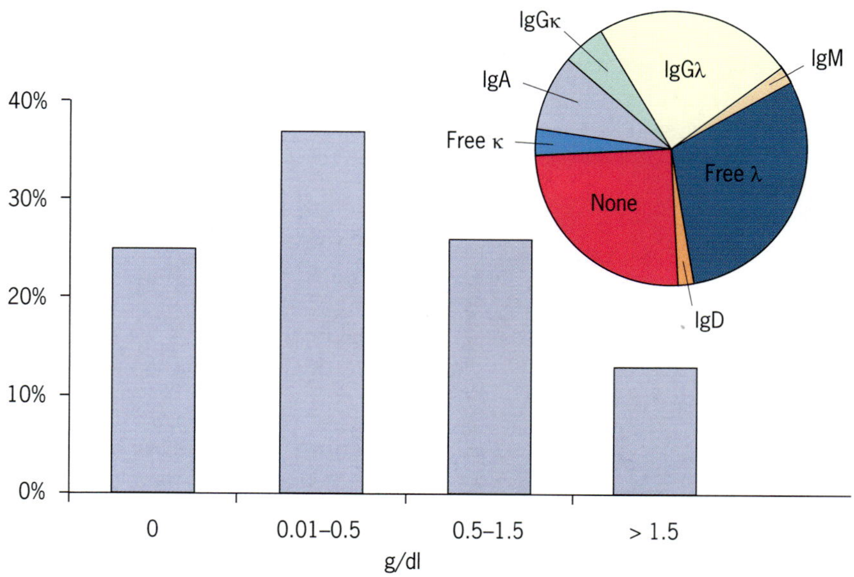

Figure 26.2 Distribution of serum M-protein findings in patients with primary amyloidosis (AL).

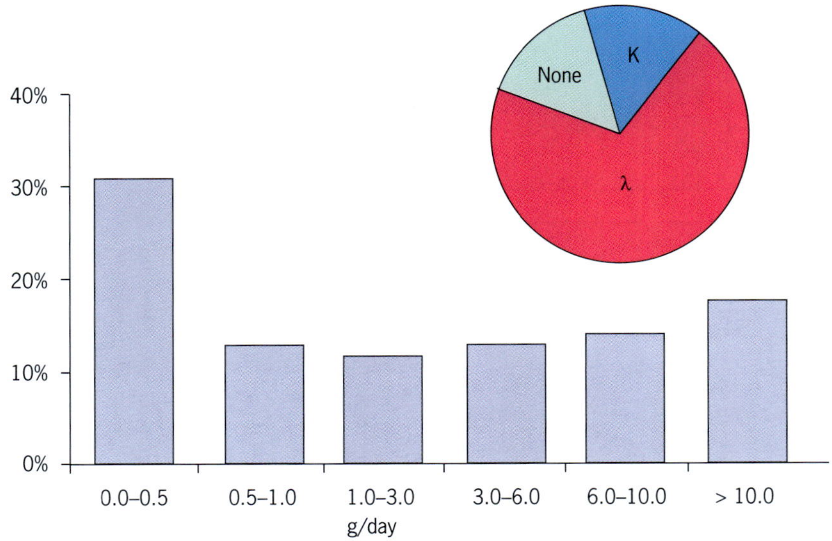

Figure 26.3 Distribution of urine M-protein findings in patients with primary amyloidosis (AL).

clinical syndromes described above (Table 26.2).[29] In the 10% of patients who do not have a detectable M component in their serum or urine, a clonal population of plasma cells in the bone marrow can virtually always be detected by immunohistochemical stains of bone marrow plasma cells or by cytoplasmic immunofluorescence or flow cytometric analysis of bone marrow plasma cells. This is the counterpart of non-secretory myeloma, and is referred to as non-secretory AL.[32,33]

DIAGNOSTIC CONFIRMATION OF AMYLOIDOSIS

Radioiodine scanning techniques can demonstrate amyloid deposits in vivo. The principle underlying the scan is the fact that amyloid deposits always contain amyloid P component, a pentagonal glycoprotein dimer that makes up approximately 10% of the amyloid fibril by weight.[34] Although these scans are highly specific for amyloid, diagnosis still requires the demonstration in biopsy tissues of deposits that bind Congo red. Patients who ultimately are shown to have renal, cardiac, hepatic, or nervous system amyloid can always have the diagnosis confirmed by direct biopsy of these organs.[34,35] In 90% of patients, however, biopsy of these organs is not required to establish a diagnosis of amyloid. Figure 26.4 shows a pathway to be followed for the diagnosis of AL.

At diagnosis, AL is generally a widespread disorder, and diffuse vascular involvement is the norm. Therefore, sampling of tissues that contain blood vessels frequently demonstrates amyloid deposits, even when there is no clinical evidence of involvement at those sites. Biopsies of minor salivary glands from the lip have been reported to demonstrate amyloid in 26 of 30 patients.[36] Biopsy of uninvolved skin regularly demonstrates deposits of amyloid in the vessels of subcutaneous tissues.[37] Rectal biopsy has been used for decades to establish the diagnosis, including those patients lacking gastrointestinal tract symptoms.[38] These acceptable techniques have the drawbacks that occasional bleeding may occur from the rectum, and biopsy samples often do not include subcutaneous tissues where blood vessels are seen.

Our current practice is simultaneous biopsy of the bone marrow and subcutaneous fat tissues, which yields the diagnosis in 80% and 50%,

Consider AL in patients with:
- Nephrotic-range proteinuria (non-diabetic)
- Cardiomyopathy (no ischemic history)
- Hepatomegaly (no filling defects by imaging)
- Peripheral neuropathy (non-diabetic)

↓

Heighten suspicion:
- Immunofixation of serum and urine

↓

Confirm diagnosis histologically:
- Fat aspirate and marrow biopsy stain with Congo red (90% sensitive)

↓

Assess prognosis:
- Echocardiography required (Doppler important)

↓

Treat:
- Melphalan and prednisone
- High-dose steroids
- Stem cell transplantation
- Organ transplantation

Figure 26.4 Diagnostic pathway for primary amyloidosis (AL).

respectively. When bone marrow and fat aspirate (Figure 26.5) are combined, amyloid deposits are detected in 90% of patients. The advantage of the subcutaneous fat aspirate is that a physician is not required to collect the sample, results can be obtained within 24 hours, and the risk is minimal. In addition, the bone marrow biopsy is required to exclude associated myeloma (Table 26.3). In the 10% of patients for whom both subcutaneous fat tissue and rectal biopsy specimen are negative, direct biopsy of the affected organ yields the diagnosis. Congo red is not a simple stain to use. False-positive results may occur because of precipitation of the dye. Overstaining may occur. Frequently,

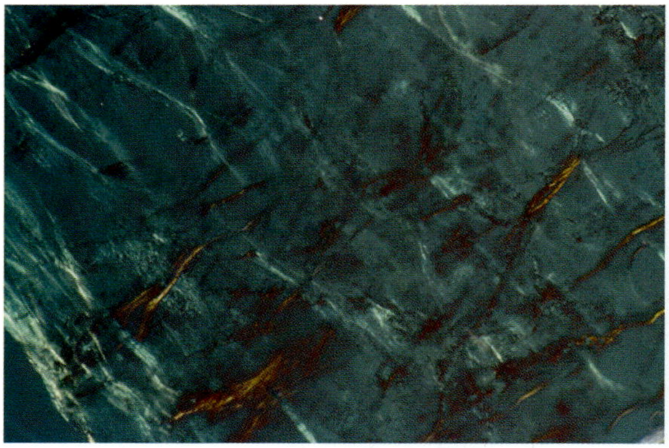

Figure 26.5 A subcutaneous fat aspirate demonstrates amyloid deposits (magnification ×100). (Slide provided by Dr C Y Li.)

collagen and elastin deposits in skin pick up Congo red. These are said to demonstrate white birefringence instead of green birefringence, but this is often a difficult distinction to make on a practical day-to-day basis.[39]

AMYLOID ORGAN-SPECIFIC SYNDROMES

Kidney

In our experience, renal involvement with amyloid is the most prevalent presentation, occurring in 33–40% of patients.[40] Amyloid is seen in approximately 2.5% of renal biopsy specimens.[26] Renal biopsy specimens obtained in adults with nephrotic syndrome who do not have diabetes contain amyloid in 10% of cases. Serum creatinine level at diagnosis is an important prognostic factor. Patients presenting with

Table 26.3 Bone marrow plasma cells in primary amyloidosis (AL)

Plasma cells (%)	Patients (%)
≤ 5	44
6–9	16
10–19	22
≥ 20	18

serum creatinine values in the normal range have a median survival of 25.6 months, compared with 14.9 months for those presenting with an abnormal creatinine value ($p < 0.01$) (Table 26.4). The 24-hour urine total protein excretion has no impact on survival in this disease. As in all other organ systems involved with amyloid, renal amyloid demonstrates a high preponderance of λ over κ light chains, with an overall ratio of 3.5 : 1. As the urinary protein excretion increases, the proportion of λ light chains also increases. With urinary protein loss in excess of 10 g, the λ : κ ratio approaches 5 : 1.

Physiologically, the nephrotic-range proteinuria results in hypoalbuminemia. The consequent reduction in serum oncotic pressure results in a marked redistribution of intravascular fluid into the extravascular space. This results in the gravitational edema characteristic of these patients. Edema can be controlled with the use of loop diuretics. Problems associated with the injudicious use of diuretics include contraction of intravascular volume, with a resultant reduction in renal blood flow and azotemia. A second consequence of the reduced intravascular volume is orthostatic hypotension associated with orthostatic syncope. The recently approved medication midodrine can decrease the symptoms of orthostatic hypotension, but its mineralocorticoid properties result in significant sodium retention and can aggravate the edema.

The greatest long-term consequence of the continuous urinary protein loss is renal tubular damage, with the ultimate development of end-stage dialysis-dependent renal disease.[41,42] One-third of patients with renal amyloidosis ultimately require dialysis support.[43] The median time from the initial diagnosis of amyloid to initiation of dialysis is 14 months. The serum creatinine concentration at presentation is the major prognostic factor in determining which patients with renal amyloid subsequently require dialysis support (Table 26.4). If patients who require emergency dialysis are considered, including those requiring dialysis after operation, the median survival of patients after initiation of dialysis is 8 months. There is no difference in survival between patients receiving hemodialysis or peritoneal dialysis.[44]

Table 26.4 Serum creatinine concentration at diagnosis in primary amyloidosis (AL)

Serum creatinine (mg/dl)	Male (%)	Female (%)
⩽ 1.2	46	68
1.3–1.9	28	14
⩾ 2.0	26	18

In most patients with renal amyloid, the most common cause of death is the development of cardiac amyloidosis with congestive heart failure, and second is hepatic failure. In patients with severe nephrotic-range proteinuria, the serum albumin value may fall below 1 g/dl. This can result in anasarca. These patients are regularly disabled as a consequence of the resultant hypotension and the massive extracellular fluid leak. Bilateral nephrectomy has been performed to eliminate the proteinuria and to restore intravascular volume to normal.[45] Early hemodialysis of patients with profound hypoalbuminemia may have the same physiologic results as nephrectomy. Dialysis in patients with a low albumin value, even with a normal creatinine value, results in a marked decrease in urine volume. The oliguria that results limits the amount of albumin lost. The serum albumin concentration increases, and the physiologic derangements associated with hypoalbuminemia are corrected.

Histologically, all patients with renal amyloid have detectable deposits, but the correlation between the extent of deposits and the degree of proteinuria is poor. Patients with small amyloid deposits can be seen with a severe nephrotic syndrome. Historically, the kidneys have been described as being enlarged in patients with AL. With the advent of routine ultrasonography of the kidney, it can be demonstrated that the overwhelming majority of patients with AL have normal-sized kidneys.[46] The urinalysis in patients with AL is consistent with other forms of nephrotic syndrome in that casts and cells are usually absent; the sediment contains protein and fat.

Heart

Restrictive cardiomyopathy is the next most frequent clinical presentation of AL patients – and the most difficult diagnosis to establish clinically.[47] Patients regularly present with profound fatigue and dyspnea on exertion; because of the restrictive nature of the process, the cardiac silhouette is normal on a chest radiograph. Echocardiography shows a preserved ejection fraction, so the diagnosis of a cardiac disorder may be overlooked. The electrocardiogram regularly demonstrates a low-voltage or a pseudoinfarction pattern, but these subtle findings are easy to overlook. Patients with a pseudoinfarction pattern have been misdiagnosed as having coronary artery disease with silent infarction.[48] A patient with this presentation can be treated incorrectly with nitrates and β-adrenergic blockers on the presumption of ischemic disease, which will lead to further depression of myocardial function and hypotension. Echocardiography regularly demonstrates infiltration of the ventricular septum and left ventricular free wall, with resultant thickening. Thickening of the left ventricle can be misinterpreted as hypertrophy. It is critical to remember that when a patient presents with cardiac symptoms and no clinical history of ischemic disease, immunofixation of the serum and urine to detect a monoclonal protein becomes an important screening test.

The physiology of cardiac amyloidosis is that of a stiff heart.[49,50] Filling of the left ventricle during diastole is impaired. The resultant reduction in left ventricular end-diastolic volume leads to a markedly reduced stroke volume, even in the presence of a completely normal ejection fraction. The myocardium frequently is hyperdynamic, and ejection fractions of 70% are not uncommon. Diastolic function abnormalities are not recognized unless specific Doppler echocardiography is performed as part of the initial examination in patients who have congestive heart failure.

The standard for assessing amyloid cardiomyopathy remains the echocardiogram. In patients with AL, the median septal wall thickness is 15 mm. The normal interventricular septal wall thickness ranges from 9 to 12 mm. Hypertension rarely causes sufficient thickening to produce a wall thickness of 15 mm. The most common echocardiographic features of amyloid are thickening of the right ventricular wall and septum and a reduced left ventricular chamber size. A granular sparkling appearance to the myocardial texture is not a reliable finding, and is highly dependent on operator proficiency.

On screening echocardiography, evidence of AL is seen in approximately 40% of patients (Table 26.5). The prevalence of congestive heart failure in patients with AL is closer to 20%. Echocardiographic evidence of amyloid does not appear to impact on the overall survival of patients with AL. The presence of clinical congestive heart failure has a powerful impact on survival (Figure 26.6), suggesting that many patients with demonstrable deposits of amyloid in the heart have little or no functional disturbance. Another important prognostic factor is the ejection fraction. An ejection fraction of less than 50% is associated with a markedly reduced survival. An occasional patient is seen whose echocardiogram does not demonstrate changes consistent with amyloid, but endomyocardial biopsy demonstrates moderate to severe deposits.[51]

Table 26.5 Echocardiographic findings in primary amyloidosis (AL)

Finding	Patients (%)
Normal	35
Abnormal non-diagnostic of AL	26
Systolic and diastolic dysfunction	16
Diastolic dysfunction only	18
Systolic dysfunction only	5

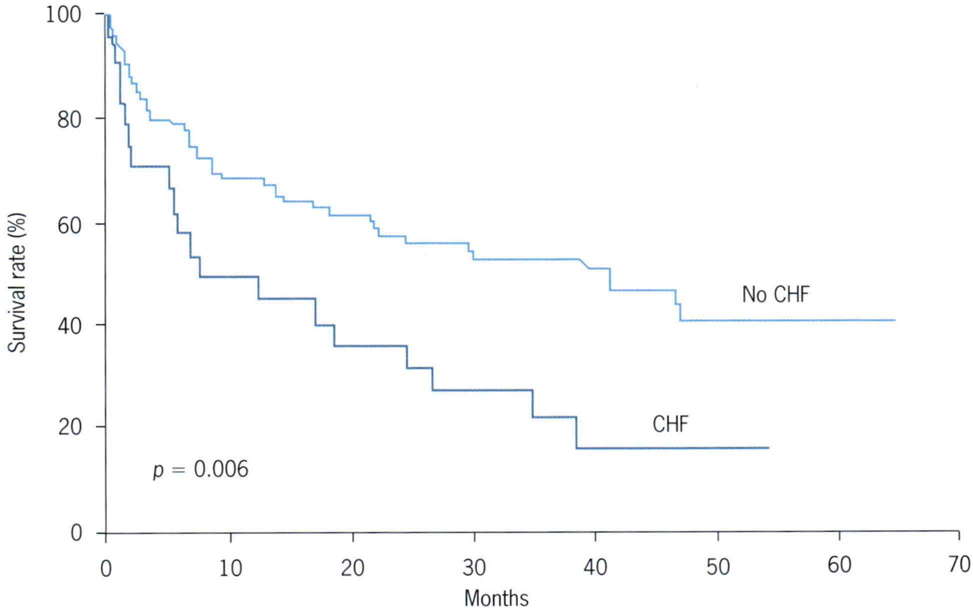

Figure 26.6 Impact of congestive heart failure (CHF) on actuarial survival in primary amyloidosis (AL).

Because infiltrative cardiomyopathy is far less common than ischemic heart disease, it would be inappropriate to consider AL in the differential diagnosis of a patient with a good history of ischemia or significant risk factors predisposing to coronary artery disease. However, a patient who presents with congestive heart failure without a good history of ischemia or obvious evidence of valvular heart disease should have AL considered in the differential diagnosis. A low-voltage echocardiogram is seen in two-thirds of patients, and is an important supportive clue.[52] The most important diagnostic test, however, would be checking immunofixation of the serum and urine for free light chains in patients presenting with heart failure of unknown etiology.

Cardiac amyloidosis can produce atrial systolic failure and dilatation of the right ventricle, and is prognostically unfavorable.[53] Physiologically, cardiac amyloidosis is characterized by abnormal relaxation. Late consequences of advanced cardiac involvement include restriction to inflow. Valvular thickening of the tricuspid and mitral valves is seen regularly, and represents an important clue. Clinically significant valvular regurgitation is rare, even though Doppler echocardiography demonstrates regurgitation in a high proportion of patients. In the past, it was easy to confuse restrictive cardiomyopathy with constrictive pericardial disease.[54,55] Patients with amyloidosis subjected to pericardial stripping rarely benefit. Right ventricular endomyocardial biopsy is virtually 100% specific for the diagnosis of amyloid. The heart is stiff, and inflow into the ventricle during diastole is impaired. The consequent stasis of blood can produce left ventricular thrombi that are potential sources of cardiac embolism and stroke.[56] A rare patient with amyloid presents because of amyloid occlusion of the small coronary vessels intramurally. This can produce classic ischemic symptoms, with exertional angina and infarction. Coronary angiography in these situations is invariably normal.[57] The diagnosis of coronary arteriolar amyloid is generally not established before death.

Prior reports have inferred that digoxin was contraindicated in amyloid heart disease, predisposing to sudden death.[58] Sudden cardiac death is seen regularly in patients with cardiac amyloidosis who do not take digoxin. It is difficult to know whether digoxin has an impact on the frequency of sudden death. We have used digoxin for control of ventricular rate when atrial fibrillation is present in patients with cardiac amyloidosis. Amyloidosis patients generally maintain normal systolic function late into the disease, and whether the inotropic benefits of digoxin produce clinical benefit is unknown. Because patients with cardiac amyloidosis have chronic heart failure, most are treated with diuretics and afterload reduction with angiotensin-converting enzyme (ACE) inhibitors.[59] Patients with amyloidosis may have difficulty tolerating diuretics and ACE inhibitors, owing to their low cardiac output and systolic hypotension.[47]

Elderly patients with heart failure can have amyloid deposits in the ventricle wall. Most of these patients have senile cardiac amyloidosis due to deposits of normal transthyretin. These patients generally do not have AL and do not have evidence of a clonal plasma cell proliferative disorder.[60] The absence of a light chain helps distinguish senile cardiac amyloid from cardiac AL. In summary, any patient who has severe fatigue, congestive heart failure without an ischemic history, or an echocardiogram that shows concentric left ventricular hypertrophy[61,62] should have immunofixation of serum and urine performed to exclude the possibility of unrecognized cardiac AL.

Liver

Enlargement of the liver is seen in 25% of patients with AL. Symptoms referable to liver dysfunction are seen in approximately 16%. The most common abnormalities are unexplained palpable hepatomegaly and an increased serum alkaline phosphatase concentration. These patients are frequently initially diagnosed as having malignant metastases to the liver. Approximately one-half of patients with amyloid in the liver have proteinuria of more than 1 g/day. This represents an important clue to the presence of a multisystem disorder. Four features that distinguish hepatic amyloidosis from other forms of liver disease include:

- the high prevalence of proteinuria;
- the presence of a monoclonal protein in serum or urine;
- the presence of Howell–Jolly bodies on a peripheral blood smear, reflecting splenic replacement by amyloid;[63]
- hepatomegaly out of proportion to the degree of abnormality on liver function test.[64]

A rare patient with liver amyloidosis presents with either hepatic or splenic rupture. Hepatic rupture is generally a fatal event.[65,66] Radioiodine serum amyloid P-component scanning demonstrates deposits of amyloid in the liver in the majority of patients with AL. Clinically important deposits are far less common. This suggests that the liver has a great capacity to accumulate amyloid without dysfunction. Jaundice in AL is a preterminal finding. Portal hypertension is rare, likely because death occurs as a consequence of extrahepatic amyloid before portal hypertension can develop. Esophageal variceal bleeding occurs in less than 1% of all patients, and is reported only rarely. Ascites is common, usually owing to the associated nephrotic-range proteinuria and not as a consequence of portal hypertension. Percutaneous liver biopsy demonstrates perisinusoidal and portal amyloid deposits. The median survival in patients with liver biopsy-proven amyloidosis is 1 year. The finding of hyposplenism is a specific sign of liver amyloid, but the converse, its absence, does not predictably reflect the absence of splenic involvement.[67] Anatomic involvement of the spleen has been seen regularly without Howell–Jolly bodies in a peripheral blood smear. Even when the anatomic involvement of the spleen is advanced, Howell–Jolly bodies may not be detected. It has been suggested that technetium-99m scanning of the spleen is a more sensitive test for the presence of amyloidosis.

Gastrointestinal tract

Virtually all patients with AL have histologic deposits of amyloid in the vessels of the gastrointestinal tract. The majority have no symptoms referable to the gastrointestinal tract. Anorexia with weight loss, which is common in AL, correlates poorly with significant deposits. Malabsorption with steatorrhea or a low serum carotene value is seen in less than 5% of patients. Amyloid in the gastrointestinal tract can cause intestinal pseudo-obstruction. Surgery in these instances is contraindicated.[68] An occasional patient requires long-term parenteral nutrition to maintain adequate muscle mass when pseudo-obstruction is present. Patients with intestinal pseudo-obstruction are nauseous and vomit, even in the fasting state. Gastric contents are generally not digested, owing to prolonged hypomotility. Abdominal distension and pain are common. Cisapride has been reported to be effective, but in our experience, the value of cisapride, cholinergic agents, and metoclopramide is limited. Pseudo-obstruction can be a direct result of deposition of amyloid in the gastrointestinal tract or can be due to autonomic dysregulation. Diarrhea, sometimes with incontinence, is also seen in patients with AL. The standard antidiarrheal agents, such as loperamide and diphenoxylate, are effective in milder cases. Cisapride and somatostatin analog have been reported to be effective for severe diarrhea.

A rare patient with AL can present with ischemic colitis.[69] Amyloid obstructs the vessels and causes mucosal ischemia. The intestinal tract lining will slough with pain and bloody diarrhea. Barium studies demonstrate luminal narrowing, thickening of mucosal folds, ulceration, and loss of colonic haustrations.[70] These radiographic changes occur most frequently in the descending and sigmoid colon. Bowel perforation as a consequence of ischemia has been reported in AL.[71] Only 8 of 769 patients with AL had symptomatic gastric amyloid.[72] The clinical symptoms were prolonged nausea, vomiting, and weight loss. Gastroparesis was recognized in three, and a gastric mass initially thought to be a neoplasm was detected in one. Six of the eight patients had concomitant small-bowel amyloid. Recovery of intestinal tract motility has not been reported.[73] Infiltration and replacement of the muscularis propria by amyloid, especially in the small intestine, are seen histopathologically. Mucosal friability and erosions are commonly seen endoscopically.

Nervous system

Patients who have amyloid in the nervous system generally present with a painful dysesthetic peripheral neuropathy involving the lower extremities. Generally, sensory symptoms precede motor symptoms, and lower-extremity dysesthesias precede upper-extremity dysesthesias. The progression of amyloid neuropathy is often indolent, and the median time between the onset of symptoms and histologic diagnosis exceeds 2 years. Muscle weakness is seen in 65% of patients. Autonomic symptoms are seen in 15% of patients. The median survival of patients with amyloid neuropathy is 36 months. Serum albumin has an important impact on overall survival, possibly reflecting the presence or absence of multisystemic disease. Carpal tunnel syndrome is associated with peripheral neuropathy in half of the patients. In patients with idiopathic peripheral neuropathy, it is important for immunofixation of serum and urine to be done as part of the initial evaluation. Peripheral neuropathy is present in 15% of AL patients. Nerve biopsy demonstrates loss of small myelinated as well as unmyelinated fibers. The predominant involvement of small unmyelinated fibers renders electromyography relatively insensitive in the early recognition of the disorder. Patients may have paresthesias of the feet with no abnormalities on electromyography. Cranial neuropathy has been reported, but is rare.[74] A high proportion of patients with amyloid neuropathy have associated proteinuria, reflecting concomitant renal involvement. Sural nerve biopsy is the most sensitive technique for the diagnosis of amyloidosis. However, there is a report in which nine patients had a sural nerve biopsy, and six demonstrated no amyloid.[75] A rare patient presents with amyloid deposits in the nerve root, leading to demyelination distally. In these instances, biopsy of the sural nerve does not demonstrate amyloid. Amyloid deposition in the peripheral nervous system is focal, and multiple sections of the sural nerve biopsy specimen must be examined to exclude the diagnosis.

Respiratory tract

Although anatomic involvement of pulmonary arteriolar blood vessels is common, clinical symptoms are rare. In most patients who have histologic pulmonary involvement, the concomitant cardiac amyloid dominates the clinical picture. Gas exchange is preserved until late into the disease. Restrictive pulmonary function studies usually reflect the presence of congestive heart failure with interstitial fluid. We reported on 35 patients with pulmonary amyloidosis presenting with radiographic evidence of an interstitial or reticulonodular infiltrate.[76] The median survival after diagnosis of pulmonary amyloid is 16 months. The chest radiograph is not specific for amyloidosis. The key to distinguishing amyloid lung disease from other interstitial processes was the presence of a monoclonal protein in the serum or urine by immunofixation.

Coagulation system

Bleeding can occur in AL. Deficiency of factor X is well recognized, but is seen in less than 5% of patients. The most common cause of bleeding is skin purpura due to fragile blood vessels. It appears that vessels infiltrated by amyloid become rigid and are easily ruptured. The coagulation test that most often has abnormal results is the thrombin time.[77] Also reported are decreased levels of α_2-plasmin inhibitor and increased levels of plasminogen.[78] Abnormal platelet aggregation has been reported. Life-threatening bleeding is rare, with the exception of patients with profound factor X deficiency or those with ischemic colitis. Melphalan and prednisone chemotherapy and splenectomy have been reported to be effective treatment for patients with severe factor X deficiency.[79]

THERAPY FOR AMYLOIDOSIS

Treatment of AL with alkylating agent-based chemotherapy has been shown in two prospective randomized studies to improve survival.[80,81] In the subset of patients who respond to melphalan and prednisone chemotherapy, the median survival can approach 90 months.[82] The majority of patients die within 1 year after diagnosis. The difficulty with alkylating agent-based chemotherapy is that the response rate for all patients is generally about 20–30%, and therefore the overall impact on survival is minimal. It is likely that part of the difficulty in treating these patients is that the organ resolution of amyloid is slow, even when the production of the precursor light-chain protein is eliminated. Many patients die of end-organ damage before sufficient time elapses for a response to occur. The body's ability to resorb amyloid deposits is limited. In our experience, the median time to recognize a response to treatment is 1 year. Many patients, particularly those with significant cardiac involvement, do not survive long enough to have an opportunity to respond.

Because the majority of patients never fulfil the response criteria for this disease, additional more effective therapies are required. For patients who are treated with alkylating agent-based chemotherapy, our standard regimen is melphalan given orally at 0.15 mg/kg per day for 7 consecutive days and prednisone at 0.8 mg/kg per day for the same 7 days, with cycles repeated every 6 weeks. We monitor the white blood cell and platelet counts every third week. The dose is generally adjusted to produce a moderate degree of leukopenia at mid-cycle. Because of the chronic myelosuppressive nature of melphalan, many patients develop chronic long-standing neutropenia, and do not recover a normal white cell count until nearly 1 year after the cessation of the medication.

When discussing treatment of AL, it is important to keep in mind the response criteria.

Responses in amyloidosis have been defined as either organ-based or responses of the M protein. Organ-based responses are generally defined as a 50% reduction in urinary protein loss in patients with renal involvement. For patients who have hepatic involvement, reduction in the serum alkaline phosphatase abnormality by 50% is considered an indication of a response. For patients with cardiac amyloidosis, the septal thickness must decrease by 2 mm without a reduction in the ejection fraction. With alkylating agent-based chemotherapy, improvement in peripheral or autonomic neuropathy is rare.

A hematologic response to chemotherapy fulfills criteria similar to those for myeloma: a 50% reduction in the serum and urine M component or, if only a free light chain is present in the serum or urine, complete eradication of the light chain. With the use of alkylating agent-based chemotherapy, a 50% reduction in the serum or urine M component does appear to correlate with improved outcome and survival. On the other hand, when we used high-dose dexamethasone to treat amyloidosis, a reduction in the M component did not appear to predict improved survival. We believe that high-dose corticosteroids prevent light-chain production, particularly in patients who have only Bence Jones proteinemia, yet this did not translate into organ resolution of amyloid. When reviewing studies on the treatment of AL, one must keep in mind the difference between a defined organ response and a defined M-protein response.

Because patients treated for AL have an improved median survival, all patients should be considered for a trial of alkylating agent-based chemotherapy. Treatment improved survival to 17 months for chemotherapy-treated patients versus 12 months for patients treated with colchicine, which represents a small although statistically significant benefit. The treatment is not without risks. As with all other alkylating agents, late myelodysplasia or acute leukemia can develop owing to chromosomal damage induced by the melphalan.[83] Characteristic cytogenetic abnormalities, such as deletion of chromosomes 5 and 7, can be seen in up to 7% of patients initially exposed. The majority are not candidates for myeloablative antileukemic therapy, and the myelodysplastic syndrome usually is the cause of death. In our experience, median survival from the onset of myelodysplasia is 8 months.

Although melphalan and prednisone may be considered standard therapy, alternatives need to be found because of the poor survival. We tested α-tocopherol[84] and interferon (IFN)-α2,[85] and found neither to be effective. High-dose dexamethasone with IFN-α has been reported to be effective in the majority of patients with AL who do not have cardiac involvement.[86] Dexamethasone has the advantage that it does not cause myelodysplasia, and the toxicity is reversible on its cessation. We have treated 44 patients with high-dose dexamethasone, both previously untreated and previously treated, and saw a response rate of less than 15%. In addition, we have seen fatal toxic responses due to bowel perforation, disseminated herpes zoster, and streptococcal sepsis as a consequence of dexamethasone therapy. We consider the utility of dexamethasone to be limited unless other alternatives do not exist.

Gianni et al[87] have reported the use of an iodinated anthracycline analog (4′-iodo-4′-deoxydoxorubicin, I-DOX). This agent appears to be able to bind and dissolve amyloid deposits. It is most effective for patients with soft tissue deposits, such as those with periarticular or tongue involvement. The response rate is less well defined for patients with visceral amyloid involving liver, kidney, and heart. This agent is not currently available in the USA. An agent that dissolves amyloid deposits may be synergistic with cytotoxic agents whose role is to destroy the light-chain-producing clone of plasma cells in the bone marrow.

I-DOX has been shown to lead to the rapid dissociation of transthyretin amyloid fibrils at physiologically achievable concentrations. After incubation with I-DOX, transthyretin amyloid becomes an amorphous material, but I-DOX does not solubilize the fibrils.[88] Transthyretin crystals soaked with I-DOX undergo rapid dissociation. It is thought that the iodine atom is buried in a pocket located between the two β-pleated sheets of the transthyretin monomer, facilitating the disruption.[89] We have treated more than 40 patients with I-DOX; our patients have had a response rate of approximately 15%. Further studies are under way. Phase II clinical trials are investigating thalidomide, an antiangiogenesis agent, and etanercept for the management of amyloid. Data have appeared in abstract form, but information is insufficient to determine whether there is benefit. These should be considered investigational agents.

An initial multicenter report suggested that the long-term outcome of cardiac transplantation for AL patients was poor.[90] Since the initial publication, there have been two papers reporting survivals of 69 and 118 months after heart transplantation,[91,92] suggesting that, with careful selection, meaningful prolongation of survival can be achieved. At the Mayo Clinic, 13 patients with amyloid heart disease were accepted for transplantation. Eight have undergone transplantation, three died on the waiting list, one was subsequently removed from the transplant list because of multiorgan failure, and one patient is waiting. The 1-year survival rate post transplant was 100% and the 2-year survival rate post transplant was 83.3%. One patient died of disseminated multiorgan amyloid 16 months after transplant. Another patient died of a post-transplant lymphoproliferative disorder 31 months after transplantation. Six patients are alive with a median follow-up of 43 months. Nephrotic syndrome developed in two of these six patients post transplant, and one received a renal transplant. Heart transplantation improved both the longevity and the quality of life. Two patients were subsequently treated with stem cell transplants in an effort to prevent recurrence of amyloid in the heart.

We have attempted more intensive chemotherapy. In a prospective randomized study of 101 patients, half received traditional therapy with melphalan and prednisone in the doses described above, and the other half received a five-drug regimen (VBMCP): vincristine, carmustine (BCNU), melphalan, cyclophosphamide, and prednisone. No survival advantage was seen for the five-drug combination compared with the standard regimen.

High-dose chemotherapy with stem cell transplantation as therapy for AL has been reported. Clinical remission has been achieved after syngeneic transplantation for AL.[93] In 25 patients with AL, 17 were alive at the time of publication. The median survival was not reached.[94] Transplantation appears to produce an unusually high prevalence of gastrointestinal tract toxicity. We have treated 19 patients with transplantation. Of these, 4 died of treatment-related causes, and 2 died within a year after transplantation of progressive AL despite the transplant. Of the remaining 13, 3 are not evaluable for response, but 9 of the remaining 10 fulfilled the criteria for organ response.

We have treated 71 AL patients with transplantation, and have follow-up data for our first 66. Of the 66 patients, 45 had renal amyloid. Forty-five patients had echocardiographic evidence of amyloid. Patients were conditioned with melphalan at 140 or 200 mg/m^2 or melphalan at 140 mg/m^2 plus 12 Gy total-body radiation. Stem cells were mobilized using granulocyte colony-stimulating factor (G-CSF) at 10 μg/kg per day or cyclophosphamide at 3 mg/m^2 followed by granulocyte–macrophage colony-stimulating factor (GM-CSF) at 5 μg/kg per day. The target goal of stem cells was 5×10^6/kg. The treatment-related mortality rate in our patient population was 14%. Five patients died of progressive cardiac amyloid – either failing to respond to transplantation or having progressive amyloid after an initial response. One patient died of myelodysplasia from oral melphalan given before transplantation. Bacteremia after transplantation was common. Coagulase-negative *Staphylococcus* was the most commonly isolated organism. Cardiac arrhythmias were seen regularly during collection and transplantation. Marked gastrointestinal tract toxic responses, including bleeding and prolonged anorexia, were also seen. Despite the high rate of toxic response, there were 32 hematologic and 31 organ responses, for an overall response rate of 62%. The responses were renal in 19, hepatic in 5, cardiac in 3, renal and cardiac in 2, renal and hepatic in 1, cardiac, renal, and neuropathic in 1, and autonomic neuropathic in 1. The median time to response was 3.6 months. The 2-year actuarial survival rate of all patients was 70%.[95,96]

Patients receiving transplants for AL are a highly selected group. It is uncertain what the survival of a comparable control group would be. A review of the Mayo Clinic's amyloid database showed that, among patients who would be eligible for stem cell transplantation, the median survival was 45.6 months. For patients younger than age 50 years, of age 51–60 years, and of age 61–70 years, the median survivals were 61, 46, and 30 months, respectively. Eligibility to receive a transplant is a favorable prognostic factor that predicts a better outcome. Patients eligible for stem cell transplantation are an inherently good-risk population, and have a superior median survival.[97]

It has been suggested that patients with significant cardiac involvement or patients with multiple organ involvement are not suitable candidates for transplant, with treatment-related mortality rates reaching 38%. We have also seen significant mortality in patients with cardiac amyloid. Moreover, we have seen excessive gastrointestinal tract toxicity that is not seen in transplantation for other malignant diseases. Following transplantation, three patients required protracted parenteral or enteral nutrition. We also saw two instances of gastrointestinal tract hemorrhage, presumably related to vascular involvement of the bowel with amyloid. Because patients who have undergone transplantation are selected by virtue of the absence of cardiac and multiorgan involvement, the selection bias that results makes it difficult to assess the overall role of transplantation in the management of AL. Nonetheless, the nine responses that we have seen are most impressive, and suggest that there is a role for transplantation in selected patients.[93] The technique of stem cell transplantation must be applied with caution, and should be limited to centers that have extensive experience in the management of patients with AL.

ACKNOWLEDGEMENT

The authors' work is supported in part by the Quade Amyloidosis Research Fund.

REFERENCES

1. Pras M, Schubert M, Zucker-Franklin D et al. The characterization of soluble amyloid prepared in water. *J Clin Invest* 1968; **47**: 924–33.
2. Cohen HJ, Minkin W. Classification of amyloidosis. *Arch Dermatol* 1971; **103**: 566–7.
3. Mahloudji M, Teasdall RD, Adamkiewicz JJ et al. The genetic amyloidoses with particular reference to hereditary neuropathic amyloidosis, type II (Indiana or Rukavina type). *Medicine (Baltimore)* 1969; **48**: 1–37.
4. Rukavina JG, Block WD, Jackson CE et al. Primary systemic amyloidosis: a review and an experimental, genetic, and clinical study of 29 cases with particular emphasis on the familial form. *Medicine (Baltimore)* 1993; **72**: 45–63.
5. Gertz MA. Secondary amyloidosis (AA). *J Intern Med* 1992; **232**: 517–18.
6. Glenner GG, Ein D, Eanes ED et al. Creation of 'amyloid' fibrils from Bence Jones proteins in vitro. *Science* 1971; **174**: 712–14.
7. Pruzanski W, Katz A, Nyburg SC, Freedman MH. In vitro production of an amyloid-like substance from gamma 3 heavy chain disease protein. *Immunol Commun* 1974; **3**: 469–76.
8. Solomon A, Weiss DT, Murphy C. Primary amyloidosis associated with a novel heavy-chain fragment (AH amyloidosis). *Am J Hematol* 1994; **45**: 171–6.
9. Solomon A, Weiss DT, Pepys MB. Induction in mice of human light-chain-associated amyloidosis. *Am J Pathol* 1992; **140**: 629–37.
10. Solomon A, Frangione B, Franklin EC. Bence Jones proteins and light chains of immunoglobulins. Preferential association of the V lambda VI subgroup of human light chains with amyloidosis AL (lambda). *J Clin Invest* 1982; **70**: 453–60.
11. Kyle RA, Bayrd ED. Amyloidosis: review of 236 cases. *Medicine (Baltimore)* 1975; **54**: 271–99.
12. Rajkumar SV, Gertz MA, Kyle RA. Primary systemic amyloidosis with delayed progression to multiple myeloma. *Cancer* 1998; **82**: 1501–5.

13. Kyle RA, Linos A, Beard CM et al. Incidence and natural history of primary systemic amyloidosis in Olmsted County, Minnesota, 1950 through 1989. *Blood* 1992; **79**: 1817–22.
14. Waterhouse D, Carman WJ, Schottenfeld D et al. Cancer incidence in the rural community of Tecumseh, Michigan: a pattern of increased lymphopoietic neoplasms. *Cancer* 1996; **77**: 763–70.
15. Kyle RA, Greipp PR. Amyloidosis (AL). Clinical and laboratory features in 229 cases. *Mayo Clin Proc* 1983; **58**: 665–83.
16. Gertz MA, Kyle RA. Primary systemic amyloidosis – a diagnostic primer. *Mayo Clin Proc* 1989; **64**: 1505–19.
17. Case Records of the Massachusetts General Hospital (Case 38-1992). *N Engl J Med* 1992; **327**: 943–50.
18. Rodon P, Friocourt P, Blanchet S, Levallois D. Temporal artery involvement revealing AL amyloidosis and IgD monoclonal gammopathy. *J Rheumatol* 1996; **23**: 189–90.
19. Salvarani C, Gabriel SE, Gertz MA et al. Primary systemic amyloidosis presenting as giant cell arteritis and polymyalgia rheumatica. *Arthritis Rheumatism* 1994; **37**: 1621–6.
20. Rao JK, Allen NB. Primary systemic amyloidosis masquerading as giant cell arteritis. Case report and review of the literature. *Arthritis Rheumatism* 1993; **36**: 422–5.
21. Gertz MA, Kyle RA, Griffing WL, Hunder GG. Jaw claudication in primary systemic amyloidosis. *Medicine (Baltimore)* 1986; **65**: 173–9.
22. Katz GA, Peter JB, Pearson CM, Adams WS. The shoulder-pad sign – a diagnostic feature of amyloid arthropathy. *N Engl J Med* 1973; **288**: 354–5.
23. Gertz MA, Kyle RA. Myopathy in primary systemic amyloidosis. *J Neurol Neurosurg Psychiatry* 1996; **60**: 655–60.
24. Schlesinger I. Multiple myeloma and AL amyloidosis mimicking Sjögren's syndrome. *South Med J* 1993; **86**: 568–9.
25. Richey TK, Bennion SD. Etiologies of the sicca syndrome: primary systemic amyloidosis and others. *Int J Dermatol* 1996; **35**: 553–7.
26. Schena FP, Pannarale G, Carbonara MC. Clinical and therapeutic aspects of renal amyloidosis. *Nephrol Dialysis Transplant* 1996; **11**(Suppl 9): 63–8.
27. Peters RA, Koukoulis G, Gimson A et al. Primary amyloidosis and severe intrahepatic cholestatic jaundice. *Gut* 1994; **35**: 1322–5.
28. Rajkumar SV, Gertz MA, Kyle RA. Prognosis of patients with primary systemic amyloidosis who present with dominant neuropathy. *Am J Med* 1998; **104**: 232–7.
29. Kyle RA, Gertz MA. Primary systemic amyloidosis: clinical and laboratory features in 474 cases. *Semin Hematol* 1995; **32**: 45–59.
30. Pascali E. Diagnosis and treatment of primary amyloidosis. *Crit Rev Oncol Hematol* 1995; **19**: 149–81.
31. Feiner HD. Pathology of dysproteinemia: light chain amyloidosis, non-amyloid immunoglobulin deposition disease, cryoglobulinemia syndromes, and macroglobulinemia of Waldenström. *Hum Pathol* 1988; **19**: 1255–72.
32. Gertz MA, Greipp PR, Kyle RA. Classification of amyloidosis by the detection of clonal excess of plasma cells in the bone marrow. *J Lab Clin Med* 1991; **118**: 33–9.
33. Wu SS, Brady K, Anderson JJ et al. The predictive value of bone marrow morphologic characteristics and immunostaining in primary (AL) amyloidosis. *Am J Clin Pathol* 1991; **96**: 95–9.
34. Gillmore JD, Hawkins PN, Pepys MB. Amyloidosis: a review of recent diagnostic and therapeutic developments. *Br J Haematol* 1997; **99**: 245–56.
35. Westermark P. Diagnosing amyloidosis. *Scand J Rheumatol* 1995; **24**: 327–9.
36. Hachulla E, Janin A, Flipo RM et al. Labial salivary gland biopsy is a reliable test for the diagnosis of primary and secondary amyloidosis. A prospective clinical and immunohistologic study in 59 patients. *Arthritis Rheumatism* 1993; **36**: 691–7.
37. Huang CY, Wang WJ, Wong CK. Skin biopsy gives the potential benefit in the diagnosis of systemic amyloidosis associated with cardiovascular involvement. *Arch Dermatol* 1998; **134**: 643–5.
38. Kyle RA, Spencer RJ, Dahlin DC. Value of rectal biopsy in the diagnosis of primary systemic amyloidosis. *Am J Med Sci* 1966; **251**: 501–6.
39. Pomerance A, Slavin G, McWatt J. Experience with the sodium sulphate–Alcian Blue stain for amyloid in cardiac pathology. *J Clin Pathol* 1976; **29**: 22–6.
40. Gertz MA, Kyle RA. Prognostic value of urinary protein in primary systemic amyloidosis (AL). *Am J Clin Pathol* 1990; **94**: 313–17.
41. Suzuki H, Konishi K, Izumi Y et al. Long-term hemodialysis in a patient with primary amyloidosis, renal failure, and a vascular necrosis of

the femoral heads. *South Med J* 1982; **75**: 1018–20.
42. Daniels JD, Hewlett JS. Renal manifestations in multiple myeloma and in primary amyloidosis. *Cleveland Clin Quart* 1970; **37**: 181–7.
43. Gertz MA, Kyle RA, O'Fallon WM. Dialysis support of patients with primary systemic amyloidosis. A study of 211 patients. *Arch Intern Med* 1992; **152**: 2245–50.
44. Stone WJ, Latos DL, Lankford PG, Baker AS. Chronic peritoneal dialysis in a patient with primary amyloidosis, renal failure, and factor X deficiency. *South Med J* 1978; **71**: 764–7.
45. Bienz N, Franklin IM, Adu D et al. Bilateral nephrectomy for uncontrollable nephrotic syndrome in primary amyloidosis, with subsequent improvement in hepatic function. *Clin Lab Haematol* 1994; **16**: 85–8.
46. Ekelund L. Radiologic findings in renal amyloidosis. *AJR* 1977; **129**: 851–3.
47. Plehn JF, Freidman BJ. Diastolic dysfunction in amyloid heart disease: restrictive cardiomyopathy or not? *J Am Coll Cardiol* 1989; **13**: 54–6.
48. Hancock EW. Low voltage, Q waves, and congestive heart failure. *Hosp Pract* 1997; **32**: 21–2.
49. Chew C, Ziady GM, Raphael MJ, Oakley CM. Functional defect in amyloid heart disease: 'the stiff heart syndrome'. *Br Heart J* 1976; **38**: 537 (abst).
50. Chew C, Ziady GM, Raphael MJ, Oakley CM. The functional defect in amyloid heart disease. The 'stiff heart' syndrome. *Am J Cardiol* 1975; **36**: 438–44.
51. Gertz MA, Grogan M, Kyle RA, Tajik AJ. Endomyocardial biopsy-proven light chain amyloidosis (AL) without echocardiographic features of infiltrative cardiomyopathy. *Am J Cardiol* 1997; **80**: 93–5.
52. Dubrey SW, Cha K, Skinner M et al. Familial and primary (AL) cardiac amyloidosis: echocardiographically similar diseases with distinctly different clinical outcomes. *Heart* 1997; **78**: 74–82.
53. Patel AR, Dubrey SW, Mendes LA et al. Right ventricular dilation in primary amyloidosis: an independent predictor of survival. *Am J Cardiol* 1997; **80**: 486–92.
54. Meaney E, Shabetai R, Bhargava V et al. Cardiac amyloidosis, constrictive pericarditis and restrictive cardiomyopathy. *Am J Cardiol* 1976; **38**: 547–56.
55. Crockett LK, Thompson M, Dekker A. A review of cardiac amyloidosis. Report of a case presenting as constrictive pericarditis. *Am J Med Sci* 1972; **264**: 149–56.
56. Browne RS, Schneiderman H, Kayani N et al. Amyloid heart disease manifested by systemic arterial thromboemboli. *Chest* 1992; **102**: 304–7.
57. Narang R, Chopra P, Wasir HS. Cardiac amyloidosis presenting as ischemic heart disease. A case report and review of literature. *Cardiology* 1993; **82**: 294–300.
58. Buja LM, Khoi NB, Roberts WC. Clinically significant cardiac amyloidosis. Clinicopathologic findings in 15 patients. *Am J Cardiol* 1970; **26**: 394–405.
59. Gertz MA, Falk RH, Skinner M et al. Worsening of congestive heart failure in amyloid heart disease treated by calcium channel-blocking agents. *Am J Cardiol* 1985; **55**: 1645.
60. Olson LJ, Gertz MA, Edwards WD et al. Senile cardiac amyloidosis with myocardial dysfunction. Diagnosis by endomyocardial biopsy and immunohistochemistry. *N Engl J Med* 1987; **317**: 738–42.
61. Presti CF, Waller BF, Armstrong WF. Cardiac amyloidosis mimicking the echocardiographic appearance of obstructive hypertrophic myopathy. *Chest* 1988; **93**: 881–3.
62. Weston LT, Raybuck BD, Robinowitz M et al. Primary amyloid heart disease presenting as hypertrophic obstructive cardiomyopathy. *Cathet Cardiovasc Diagn* 1986; **12**: 176–81.
63. Gertz MA, Kyle RA, Greipp PR. Hyposplenism in primary systemic amyloidosis. *Ann Intern Med* 1983; **98**: 475–7.
64. Gertz MA, Kyle RA. Hepatic amyloidosis: clinical appraisal in 77 patients. *Hepatology* 1997; **25**: 118–21.
65. Gastineau DA, Gertz MA, Rosen CB, Kyle RA. Computed tomography for diagnosis of hepatic rupture in primary systemic amyloidosis. *Am J Hematol* 1991; **37**: 194–6.
66. Bujanda L, Beguiristain A, Alberdi F et al. Spontaneous rupture of the liver in amyloidosis. *Am J Gastroenterol* 1997; **92**: 1385–6.
67. Seo IS, Li CY. Hyposplenic blood picture in systemic amyloidosis. Its absence is not a predictable sign for absence of splenic involvement. *Arch Pathol Lab Med* 1995; **119**: 252–4.
68. Fraser AG, Arthur JF, Hamilton I. Intestinal pseudoobstruction secondary to amyloidosis responsive to cisapride. *Dig Dis Sci* 1991; **36**: 532–5.
69. Trinh TD, Jones B, Fishman EK. Amyloidosis of the colon presenting as ischemic colitis: a case

report and review of the literature. *Gastrointest Radiol* 1991; **16**: 133–6.
70. Lee JG, Wilson JA, Gottfried MR. Gastrointestinal manifestations of amyloidosis. *South Med J* 1994; **87**: 243–7.
71. Fraser AG, Nicholson GI. Duodenal perforation in primary systemic amyloidosis. *Gut* 1992; **33**: 997–9.
72. Menke DM, Kyle RA, Fleming CR et al. Symptomatic gastric amyloidosis in patients with primary systemic amyloidosis. *Mayo Clin Proc* 1993; **68**: 763–7.
73. Tada S, Iida M, Yao T et al. Intestinal pseudo-obstruction in patients with amyloidosis: clinicopathologic differences between chemical types of amyloid protein. *Gut* 1993; **34**: 1412–17.
74. Traynor AE, Gertz MA, Kyle RA. Cranial neuropathy associated with primary amyloidosis. *Ann Neurol* 1991; **29**: 451–4.
75. Simmons Z, Blaivas M, Aguilera AJ et al. Low diagnostic yield of sural nerve biopsy in patients with peripheral neuropathy and primary amyloidosis. *J Neurol Sci* 1993; **120**: 60–3.
76. Utz JP, Swensen SJ, Gertz MA. Pulmonary amyloidosis. The Mayo Clinic experience from 1980 to 1993. *Ann Intern Med* 1996; **124**: 407–13.
77. Gastineau DA, Gertz MA, Daniels TM et al. Inhibitor of the thrombin time in systemic amyloidosis: a common coagulation abnormality. *Blood* 1991; **77**: 2637–40.
78. Mizutani AR, Ward CF. Amyloidosis associated bleeding diatheses in the surgical patient. *Can J Anaesth* 1990; **37**: 910–12.
79. Rosenstein ED, Itzkowitz SH, Penziner AS et al. Resolution of factor X deficiency in primary amyloidosis following splenectomy. *Arch Intern Med* 1983; **143**: 597–9.
80. Kyle RA, Gertz MA, Greipp PR et al. A trial of three regimens for primary amyloidosis: colchicine alone, melphalan and prednisone, and melphalan, prednisone, and colchicine. *N Engl J Med* 1997; **336**: 1202–7.
81. Skinner M, Anderson J, Simms R et al. Treatment of 100 patients with primary amyloidosis: a randomized trial of melphalan, prednisone, and colchicine versus colchicine only. *Am J Med* 1996; **100**: 290–8.
82. Gertz MA, Kyle RA, Greipp PR. Response rates and survival in primary systemic amyloidosis. *Blood* 1991; **77**: 257–62.
83. Gertz MA, Kyle RA. Acute leukemia and cytogenetic abnormalities complicating melphalan treatment of primary systemic amyloidosis. *Arch Intern Med* 1990; **150**: 629–33.
84. Gertz MA, Kyle RA. Phase II trial of alpha-tocopherol (vitamin E) in the treatment of primary systemic amyloidosis. *Am J Hematol* 1990; **34**: 55–8.
85. Gertz MA, Kyle RA. Phase II trial of recombinant interferon alfa-2 in the treatment of primary systemic amyloidosis. *Am J Hematol* 1993; **44**: 125–8.
86. Dhodapkar MV, Jagannath S, Vesole D et al. Treatment of AL-amyloidosis with dexamethasone plus alpha interferon. *Leuk Lymphoma* 1997; **27**: 351–6.
87. Gianni L, Bellotti V, Gianni AM, Merlini G. New drug therapy of amyloidoses: resorption of AL-type deposits with 4′-iodo-4′-deoxydoxorubicin. *Blood* 1995; **86**: 855–61.
88. Sebastiao MP, Merlini G, Saraiva MJ, Damas AM. The molecular interaction of 4′-iodo-4′-deoxydoxorubicin with Leu-55Pro tr 'amyloid-like' oligomer leading to disaggregation. *Biochem J* 2000; **351:** 273–9.
89. Palha JA, Ballinari D, Amboldi N et al. 4′-Iodo-4′-deoxydoxorubicin disrupts the fibrillar structure of transthyretin a. *Am J Pathol* 2000; **156:** 1919–25.
90. Hosenpud JD, DeMarco T, Frazier OH et al. Progression of systemic disease and reduced long-term survival in patients with cardiac amyloidosis undergoing heart transplantation: follow-up results of a multicenter survey. *Circulation* 1991; **84**(Suppl 3): III338–43.
91. Dubrey S, Simms RW, Skinner M, Falk RH. Recurrence of primary (AL) amyloidosis in a transplanted heart with four-year survival. *Am J Cardiol* 1995; **76**: 739–41.
92. Pelosi F Jr, Capehart J, Roberts WC. Effectiveness of cardiac transplantation for primary (AL) cardiac amyloidosis. *Am J Cardiol* 1997; **79**: 532–5.
93. van Buren M, Hene RJ, Verdonck LF et al. Clinical remission after syngeneic bone marrow transplantation in a patient with AL amyloidosis. *Ann Intern Med* 1995; **122**: 508–10.
94. Comenzo RL, Vosburgh E, Falk RH et al, Dose-intensive melphalan with blood stem-cell support for the treatment of AL (amyloid light-chain) amyloidosis: survival and responses in 25 patients. *Blood* 1998; **91**: 3662–70.
95. Gertz MA, Lacy MQ, Dispenzieri A. Myeloablative chemotherapy with stem cell rescue for the treatment of primary systemic amyloidosis: a status report. *Bone Marrow Transplant* 2000; **25:** 465–70.
96. Gertz MA, Lacy MQ, Gastineau DA et al. Blood stem cell transplantation as therapy for primary

systemic amyloidosis. *Bone Marrow Transplant* 2000; **26:** 936–9.

97. Dispenzieri A, Lacy MQ, Kyle RA et al. Eligibility for hematopoietic stem-cell transplantation for primary systemic amyloidosis is a favorable prognostic factor for survival. *J Clin Oncol* 2001; **19:** 3350–6.

98. Moreau P, Leblond V, Bourquelot P et al. Prognostic factors for survival and response after high-dose therapy and autologous stem cell transplantation in systemic AL amyloidosis: a report on 21 patients. *Br J Haematol* 1998; **101**: 766–9.

27

Waldenström's macroglobulinaemia

Meletios A Dimopoulos

INTRODUCTION

Waldenström's macroglobulinaemia (WM) is a low-grade lymphoproliferative disorder that produces monoclonal immunoglobulin M (IgM). In 1944, Jan Waldenström reported two patients with oronasal bleeding, severe anaemia, lymphadenopathy, hypofibrinogenaemia, elevated erythrocyte sedimentation rate, and the presence of large amounts of a high-molecular-weight gammaglobulin in the serum.[1] Examination of bone marrow aspirates of these patients revealed proliferation of cells with lymphocyte and plasma cell characteristics. Subsequently, the serum globulin was identified as an immunoglobulin, and was designated IgM.

According to the Revised European–American classification of lymphoid neoplasms (the REAL classification), WM represents the majority of cases that are included under the diagnosis of lymphoplasmacytoid lymphoma/immunocytoma.[2]

While all patients with Waldenström's macroglobulinaemia demonstrate a serum monoclonal IgM, the amount of the abnormal globulin and the morphology of the malignant infiltrate may vary.

Typical patients with WM present with large amounts of serum monoclonal IgM (often causing hyperviscosity), and infiltration of bone marrow, spleen, and lymph nodes by plasmacytoid lymphocytes, mast cells, and Dutcher bodies.

Some patients present with a malignant lymphoproliferative disease with moderate amounts of serum IgM. On the other hand, others present with clinical and histological features of small cell lymphocytic lymphoma or of chronic lymphocytic leukaemia (CLL) associated with an IgM paraprotein.[3]

In view of similar natural history, we believe that every patient with a low-grade malignant lymphoproliferative disease and a serum monoclonal IgM should be considered and treated as having WM.

WM affects approximately 1500 Americans each year; this disease is about 10–20% as common as myeloma. Patients' median age is about 65 years and males are more commonly affected than females. In contrast to myeloma, the disease is significantly more common among Whites than Blacks.[4,5]

ETIOLOGY

The etiology of WM is unknown. A genetic predisposition has been suggested by the identification of family clusters and by the detection of the disease in monozygotic twins.[6,7] Studies of relatives of patients with WM have shown an increased frequency of monoclonal IgM.[8]

Occupational exposure may play a role in a few cases, and exposures to leather, rubber dyes, and paints have been incriminated in some (but not all) studies.[9,10] In a case–control study, there were no differences in socioeconomic factors, past medical history, cigarette or alcohol consumption, occupational exposure, or familial cancer history between 65 patients with WM and 213 control patients.[11]

BIOLOGY

The malignant B cells in WM express monoclonal surface and cytoplasmic IgM. Several B-cell antigens such as CD19, CD20, CD21, CD22, and CD24 are present on the WM cells, while CD23 is usually absent. WM cells express CD5 at low intensity; CD5 is present on a minority of normal B cells and is strongly expressed on CLL cells.[12–14]

The immunophenotype of these cells can be used to demonstrate the presence of WM cells in the peripheral blood in patients, even if there is no absolute lymphocytosis.

Recently, DNA sequences of the Kaposi sarcoma-associated herpesvirus (KSHV; also known as human herpesvirus-8, HHV-8) have been identified in bone marrow biopsies from patients with myeloma and WM.[15,16] In other reports, however, no KSHV sequences could be amplified from patients with WM.[17] In myeloma, there is evidence that KSHV is present on bone marrow dendritic cells. Preliminary analysis of dendritic cell-enriched peripheral blood mononuclear cells from four patients with WM showed KHSV in all samples.[18] Viral interleukin (IL)-6 produced by KSHV might participate in the proliferation and/or inhibition of apoptosis of the malignant cells in myeloma or WM patients. See Chapter 3 for a detailed discussion.

Various cytogenetic abnormalities involving trisomies or deletions of chromosomes 10, 11, 12, 15, 20, and 21 have been described in up to 30% of bone marrow samples from patients with WM. Many patients had complex karyotypes.[19–21] Translocations involving the 14q32 band, where the IgH genes map, have been found, including t(14;18)(q32;q21), similar to the translocation involving the *bcl-2* gene observed in follicular lymphoma, and t(8;14)(q24;q32), similar to the translocation in Burkitt-type lymphomas involving the c-*myc* gene.[22,23]

Mutations in the tumour suppressor gene *p53* have been described, and are associated with a poor response to chemotherapy and shortened survival in some (but not all) studies.[24,25]

CLINICAL FEATURES

The clinical manifestations associated with WM can be classified into those related to direct tumour infiltration, to the amount and specific properties of circulating IgM, and to the deposition of IgM in various tissues (Table 27.1). Some aspects of this classification are arbitrary, because more than one mechanism may be responsible for a specific condition. For example, renal impairment may be due to direct infiltration of the kidney by malignant cells, to amyloid deposition, or to an immune-mediated glomerulonephritis.

Manifestations related to direct tumour infiltration

WM always involves the bone marrow. The bone marrow aspirate usually shows a diffuse proliferation of small lymphocytes, plasmacytoid lymphocytes (cells with abundant basophilic cytoplasm, but lymphocyte-like nuclei), and plasma cells.[2] Mast cells and Dutcher bodies (PAS-positive intranuclear and intracytoplasmic inclusions consisting of IgM) can also be seen.[26]

The extent of marrow infiltration is more adequately assessed with a biopsy. Bartl et al[27] distinguished three types of bone marrow involvement: lymphoplasmacytoid (47%), lymphoplasmacytic (42%), and polymorphous (11%).

Table 27.1 Waldenström's macroglobulinaemia: pathogenesis of clinical manifestations

Tumour infiltration
Bone marrow
Lymph nodes
Spleen
Liver
Miscellaneous organs
Circulating IgM
Hyperviscosity
Cryoglobulinaemia
Cold-agglutinin anaemia
Tissue IgM
Neuropathy
Glomerulopathy
Amyloidosis
Skin lesions
Malabsorption

Magnetic resonance imaging (MRI) is a non-invasive technique that complements bone marrow biopsies by sampling a large volume of bone marrow. MRI abnormalities have been demonstrated in almost all patients with WM. Most patients show a diffuse pattern of involvement, but some exhibit a variegated pattern.[28,29] The diffuse and variegated MRI patterns in WM do not differ from those observed in myeloma, and reflect a more dispersed spread of the malignant cells in the bone marrow compared with focal MRI patterns. The absence of focal MRI patterns of bone marrow involvement is in keeping with the rarity of lytic bone lesions in WM, since it is known that focal bone marrow MRI patterns are more frequently associated with destructive changes on skeletal radiographs. Lytic bone lesions have been reported in about 2% of patients with WM.[3,30] There is evidence that patients with monoclonal IgM and osteolytic lesions have a unique phenotype with characteristics of both myeloma and WM.[31]

About one-third of patients present with lymphadenopathy, splenomegaly, or hepatomegaly.[32–36] The enlarged lymph nodes are palpable or can be detected with the use of computed tomography (CT) of the abdomen and pelvis.[28]

Involvement of virtually all organs has been reported in WM. Lung involvement may manifest with diffuse pulmonary infiltrates, isolated masses, or pleural effusion.[37,38] Renal enlargement due to tumour infiltration has been reported.[39] The malignant process can involve the stomach, duodenum, and bowel.[40,41] Meningeal involvement has also been described.[42]

Manifestations related to circulating macroglobulin

Hyperviscosity syndrome

An increased concentration of monoclonal IgM may result in an increase in plasma viscosity and an expansion of plasma volume; the circulation becomes sluggish, resulting in the hyperviscosity syndrome.

Symptoms usually appear when the relative serum or plasma viscosity is above 5 (normal range 1.4–1.8). In such cases, the corresponding serum IgM is virtually always above 3 g/dl.[43,44] The symptomatic threshold, however, varies from patient to patient.

At diagnosis, the hyperviscosity syndrome is clinically evident in 10–30% of patients with WM, and is characterized by fatigue, bleeding, and ocular, neurological, and cardiovascular complications. Chronic nasal bleeding, oozing from the gums, and gastrointestinal bleeding may occur.

Ocular symptoms include blurred vision or diplopia, and fundoscopic examination reveals distended, tortuous, and 'sausage-shaped' retinal veins, haemorrhage, papilloedema, or exudates.

Neurological complaints consist of headache, tinnitus, vertigo, impaired hearing, or ataxia. In severe forms, somnolence, stupor, and coma can occur.

Occasionaly, patients with hyperviscosity syndrome can develop high-output cardiac failure, which can be aggravated by blood transfusions that further increase the already expanded plasma volume.[45]

Cryoglobulinaemia

Cryoglobulins are immunoglobulin molecules that have the unusual property of reversibly precipitating at low temperatures. When testing for cryoglobulins, specimens must be collected at body temperature, otherwise significant quantities of these proteins can be lost.

Blood is drawn into a warmed syringe and immediately allowed to clot for one to two hours at 37°C. After clotting, the serum is harvested at the warm temperature and then incubated at 0–4°C for 5–7 days. Quantitation is accomplished by direct measurement of packed volume of precipitate after centrifugation (cryocrit) or spectrophotometric determination of protein concentration. After appropriate washing the isolated cryoglobulin is redissolved at 37°C and analysed qualitatively for immunoglobulin class, light-chain type, and presence of other constituents such as complement components.

Cryoglobulins can be classified on the basis of their constituent molecules. Type I cryoglobulins consist of monoclonal IgM, and type II cryoglobulins consist of mixed immunoglobulin complexes in which the monoclonal IgM has antibody specificity for polyclonal IgG.[46]

Type I cryoglobulins are detected in 10–20% of patients with WM, but clinically evident cryoglobulinaemia occurs in less than 5% of patients.[3,35,36] The presence of cryoglobulinaemia may modify the pattern of presentation in patients with macroglobulinaemia. In some patients, the tumour load is very low, and anaemia and organomegaly may be absent. Raynaud's phenomenon, palpable purpura, arthralgias, and peripheral neuropathy may predominate. Renal involvement in the form of membranoproliferative glomerulonephritis can cause nephrotic syndrome and even irreversible renal failure.[47,48]

Cold-agglutinin disease

In approximately 10% of patients, the monoclonal IgM has cold-agglutinin activity, which may result in cold sensitivity and chronic haemolysis, with acute exacerbations related to cold exposure.

If the cold antibody is active at the temperatures of the cooler peripheral areas of circulation, it agglutinates red blood cells, leading to impaired perfusion of distal areas of the body. As a result, acrocyanosis, cold sensitivity of the Raynaud type, and livedo reticularis may develop. More severe vascular phenomena consist of chronic ulcers of the skin. Under the same circumstances, complement may become fixed, but when the red cells return to areas of the body with higher temperatures, the agglutinin dissociates and the complement remains alone on the red blood cell surface. The direct antiglobulin (Coombs) test demonstrates the presence of C3, while the IgM agglutinin is rarely detected.[49,50] In several patients, the tumour load is so low that symptoms of haemagglutination and haemolysis may occur long before any underlying tumour can be found clinically.

Manifestations related to IgM deposition

Neurological manifestations

Approximately 10% of patients with WM present with or develop symptoms and signs suggestive of polyneuropathy. Many patients with monoclonal IgM and polyneuropathy do not have evidence of lymphoma, but clonal growth may occur later. In other patients with WM and polyneuropathy, the tumour load at presentation is low, anaemia is absent, and the main discomfort is due to the neurological impairment.

We shall thus address the IgM-related polyneuropathy regardless of the presence or absence of frank WM. IgM-related polyneuropathy is composed of an immunochemically and clinically heterogeneous group of neuropathies in which the immunoglobulin appears to be an antibody to various glycoproteins or glycolipids of the peripheral nerves.

These neuropathies can be divided into the following subsets.

Demyelinating polyneuropathy with IgM anti-MAG antibodies Sera from approximately 50% of patients with IgM monoclonal gammopathy and neuropathy react with myelin-associated glycoprotein (MAG), a 100 kDa glycoprotein of the central and peripheral nerve myelin, as well as other glycoproteins or glycolipids that share antigenic determinants with MAG. Most patients with anti-MAG antibodies present with a sensory, large-fibre, demyelinating polyneuropathy. Foot numbness, paraesthesias, imbalance, and gait ataxia are the principal complaints. Some patients have aching discomfort, dysaesthesias, or lancinating pains. Weakness of the distal leg muscles with variable atrophy occurs as the illness advances. Other patients have a sensorimotor polyneuropathy with mixed features of demyelination and axonal loss.[51–54]

The CSF protein is elevated. Despite its high molecular weight, the monoclonal IgM may enter the cerebrospinal fluid (CSF) via the dorsal root ganglia that lack a blood–CSF barrier or from a disrupted root–CSF barrier.[55]

Nerve conduction studies are consistent with demyelination (slow conduction velocity and prolonged distal motor and sensory latencies). Conduction block is usually absent. The amplitude of the muscle action potential can be diminished, and the needle electromyogram often shows denervation potentials due to a concomitant axonal degeneration.

Sural nerve biopsy demonstrates a diminished number of myelinated axons. Lymphocytic infiltrates are rarely seen within the endoneurial parenchyma. On electron microscopy, there is splitting of the outer myelin lamellae, linked to the presence of IgM deposits in the same area of the split myelin sheath.[56–58]

MAG is the most extensively studied antigen recognized by the IgM paraprotein. The antigenic determinant for the anti-MAG IgM resides in the carbohydrate component of the MAG molecule, as demonstrated by the loss of reactivity following deglycosylation of purified human MAG using an immunoblotting technique.[59] The anti-MAG IgM paraproteins co-react with an acidic glycolipid in the ganglioside fraction of the human peripheral nerve.[60] This antigenic glycolipid, chromatographed between GM1 and GD1a, is a novel sulfoglucuronyl glycosphingolipid, SGPG.[61] In contrast to MAG, which is mostly present within the central nervous system, SGPG is found only in the peripheral nerve and may be the most specific antigenic target in demyelinating polyneuropathy with IgM gammopathy.

Demyelinating polyneuropathies with monoclonal IgM anti-ganglioside antibodies (but not anti-MAG) The sera of some patients with IgM monoclonal gammopathy and sensorimotor or pure sensory demyelinating polyneuropathy may not react with MAG, in spite of clinical similarities with the anti-MAG-reacting paraproteins. The IgM in several such patients reacts with various gangliosides, such as those containing a disialosyl moiety, or with GalNac-GM1b and GalNac-GD1a, two gangliosides that share epitopes with GM2, or with a combination of GM2 and GM1 or of GM1 and GM1b.[62–66]

Sensory neuropathies with monoclonal IgM anti-GD1b or anti-sulfatide antibodies Sera from a number of patients with predominantly sensory demyelinating neuropathy react with GD1b glycolipids or sulfatides.[63,66,67–68] Anti-sulfatide antibodies may bind to the surface of the dorsal root ganglionic neurones. The clinical picture is characterized by pain and paraesthesias beginning in the feet. The neuropathy associated with anti-sulphatide antibodies can be axonal or demyelinating, or can resemble dorsal root ganglioneuritis.[69]

Axonal neuropathies with monoclonal IgM anti-chondroitin sulfate antibodies A few patients with predominantly axonal neuropathy and monoclonal IgM that behaves as an anti-chondroitin sulfate antibody has been described.[70] The neuropathies are usually mixed sensorimotor in type, although some patients may have predominantly sensory or motor neuropathy.

Motor, axonal neuropathies with monoclonal IgM anti-GM1 antibodies A few patients with IgM paraprotein have a predominantly motor neuropathy that resembles a lower motor neurone syndrome. The disease is characterized by slowly progressive, painless weakness that is asymmetric or confined to one limb and by normal or reduced reflexes. An electrical conduction block in the middle or proximal regiments of the motor nerves together with normal sensory conduction in the same nerves are characteristic of this disease.[67,71,72] The IgM in some of these patients shows strong immunoreactivity with GM1 and asialoGM1 and, to a lesser degree, with GD1b.[67] Because GM1 is present on the surface of motor neurones and the nodes of Ranvier, these findings led to a search for polyclonal GM1 antibodies in patients with a variety of conditions, including patients with motor neurone diseases, patients with multifocal motor neuropathy with conduction block, and patients with Guillain–Barré syndrome.[73]

Cryoglobulinaemic neuropathy This polyneuropathy occurs most often with mixed cryoglobulinaemias, and presents as distal, sensory, symmetric polyneuropathy or as mononeuritis multiplex. The neuropathy is often axonal. The nerve biopsy shows perivascular inflammatory cuffing with axonal degeneration, which, if focal, may suggest ischaemia.[74]

Amyloid polyneuropathy In several patients with primary amyloidosis related to an IgM monoclonal protein, amyloid is deposited in the nerve or the endoneurial vessels. Such patients develop a painful sensorimotor peripheral neuropathy. Autonomic symptoms may predominate, and consist of postural hypotension, impotence, and dyfunction of bowel and bladder.[73]

Amyloidosis

Primary amyloidosis (AL) has been diagnosed in several patients with WM. In a large series of patients from the Mayo Clinic, amyloidosis developed in 2% of patients with monoclonal IgM, and 76% of cases showed a λ light chain. Cardiac, renal, hepatic, and pulmonary involvement predominated, and was the cause of death more often than the underlying macroglobulinaemia. The incidence of cardiac and pulmonary involvement appeared to be higher in patients with IgM-related amyloidosis than in the other cases of primary amyloidosis.[75]

Renal manifestations

Renal abnormalities occur infrequently in WM patients, but their spectrum and pathogenesis are different from those in myeloma. The low incidence of hypercalcaemia and the absence of significant Bence–Jones proteinuria explains the rarity of renal tubular cast formation in patients with WM.

However, glomerular abnormalities are more frequently seen in macroglobulinaemia than in myeloma. The high concentration of IgM brought about in the capillary lumen by the ultrafiltration process may lead to its local deposition. Thus, IgM can precipitate on the endothelial side of the glomerular basement membrane, occlude the capillary lumen, and cause non-selective proteinuria.[76]

A few patients have been described in whom IgM behaved as an antibody against the glomerular basement membrane and caused an immune-mediated glomerulonephritis manifested as nephritic or nephrotic syndrome.[77] In the presence of significant albuminuria, the possibility of renal amyloidosis should be considered, and the presence of rapidly progressive glomerulonephritis should raise the possibility of cryoglobulinaemia.

IgM skin deposits

Firm, translucent, flesh-coloured papules characterized by intra-epidermal deposits of IgM have occasionally been reported.[78,79] Monoclonal IgM gammopathy, and sometimes frank WM, has been also associated with urticarial skin lesions (Schniltzler syndrome).[80] Occasional patients have developed paraneoplastic pemphigus.[81]

IgM deposits in the gut

Occasional WM patients may present with or develop diarrhoea and malabsorption. Hyaline deposits, which stain positive for PAS but negative for amyloid and consist of monoclonal IgM, have been detected in some of these patients.[82,83]

LABORATORY FEATURES

Most patients with WM are anaemic – not only owing to bone marrow infiltration but also because of a dilutional effect due to plasma volume expansion.[45] Thus, the anaemia is more often apparent than real. The erythrocyte sedimentation rate is greatly increased. The leukocyte count is usually normal, but lymphocytosis is not uncommon and circulating monoclonal lymphocytes are detected with flow cytometry in virtually all patients. Significant thrombocytopenia is only occasionally present at diagnosis.[3]

All of the patients have a serum monoclonal protein, the amount of which is better evaluated from serum protein electrophoresis than by nephelometric quantitation of serum immunoglobulins. Uninvolved immunoglobulins are depressed in most patients.[3,36] Bence Jones proteinuria, usually of moderate degree, occurs in 50–80% of patients, and exceeded 1 g/day in only 3% of patients.[3,33,36] Despite the rarity of osteolytic lesions, hypercalcaemia occurred in 4% of patients.[36] Elevated levels of serum β_2-microglobulin were found in half of the patients.[36]

Abnormalities of platelet function and of clotting factors are not unusual, and predispose patients to an increased bleeding tendency. Perkins et al[84] found that several patients with WM had prolongation of bleeding time, abnormalities of platelet adhesiveness, increased prothrombin time, and decreased levels of factor VIII. Although the mechanisms are not clearly defined, it has been found that in occasional patients, the monoclonal IgM exhibited antiplatelet activity specifically against clotting factors.[85,86]

TREATMENT

Asymptomatic disease

A number of patients with WM are diagnosed by chance during routine examination and screening procedures.[3, 87] They do not have any symptoms or signs attributable to the disease. Such patients should be followed without any treatment until a complication of IgM or overt lymphoproliferative disease becomes evident. Several patients with indolent WM have survived for many years before treatment became necessary.

Treatment of IgM-induced complications

In several patients with WM, the predominant symptoms are due to the elevated serum viscosity. Because 80% of IgM is intravascular, plasmapheresis is an effective means of reducing rapidly the amount of circulating IgM.[88] Concomitant administration of systemic therapy is usually necessary in order to reduce the monoclonal protein synthesis. Nevertheless, plasma exchange has been used as the sole treatment in the occasional elderly patient with resistant disease and symptoms of hyperviscosity.[89]

In some patients with peripheral neuropathy or cryoglobulinaemia, the tumour burden at presentation is low, clinical features of WM are absent, and the main symptoms are neurological impairment or due to cryoglobulins. In such cases, an intensive series of plasma exchanges may rapidly reduce the monoclonal protein, resulting in symptomatic improvement. The observation of improvement may also provide a rationale for the subsequent administration of systemic treatment to achieve long-term disease and symptom control. In several patients with IgM demyelinating polyneuropathies, chemotherapy, plasmapheresis, and intravenous immunoglobulin (IVIG) have been associated with symptomatic improvement.[90–92] When the sensory neuropathy is axonal, treatment is, in general, disappointing. IVIG is effective in patients with motor axonal neuropathy, but repeated infusions are required.[73]

Treatment of the lymphoma

Response criteria

The response criteria utilized have not been uniform, and have usually been adapted from those used in evaluating patients with myeloma and low-grade lymphoma. In most studies, partial response is defined as a decrease in monoclonal IgM by at least 50%, with more than 50% reduction in bone marrow lymphocytosis and organomegaly. Complete response may be defined as the disappearance of the monoclonal protein by immunofixation, resolution of lymphadenopathy and splenomegaly, and less than 20% lymphocytes in the bone marrow.

Primary treatment

In view of the low incidence of macroglobulinaemia, the treatment of this disease has been adapted from established regimens used in patients with CLL, low-grade lymphoma, and myeloma. Chemotherapy with alkylating agents with or without steroids has been the standard primary therapy for patients with symptomatic macroglobulinaemia (Table 27.2). The agent most commonly used is oral chlorambucil. This agent has been administered daily at a dose of 6–8 mg and its dose has been adapted according to blood counts.[32,34,87] Intermittent chlorambucil at a dose of 8 mg/m^2 daily for 10 days and repeated at 6-week intervals with appropriate dose adjustments has also been used. Treatment with chlorambucil is usually continued until there is resolution of symptoms and stabilization of the monoclonal protein serum levels. At least 50% of patients achieve an objective response, the rate of decrease of the paraprotein is slow, and several months are usually required to determine the chemosensitivity of the disease. A randomized study has indicated that daily oral or intermittent chlorambucil were equally active, resulting in a median survival of 5.4 years.[93]

The addition of prednisone to chlorambucil did not improve patients' survival.[36] Steroids may, however, be of value in patients with immune haemolytic anemia, cold-agglutinin disease, or cryoglobulinaemia. Combinations of alkylating agents with or without a vinca alkaloid, an anthracycline or a nitrosourea have been used (Table 27.2). Although no prospective randomized trials have compared those regimens with standard chlorambucil, there is no evidence of added benefit from the combinations.[36,94,95]

The newer nucleoside analogues fludarabine and 2-chlorodeoxyadenosine (cladribine) have

Table 27.2 Primary treatment of Waldenström's macroglobulinaemia with alkylating agent-based regimens

Regimen[a]	No. of patients	Response rate (%)	Median survival (years)
Chlorambucil[93]	49	64	5.4
M2 protocol[95]	33	82	4.2
MChlP[94]	34	68	5.5
ChlP[36]	77	72	5.0
CHOP[36]	20	65	7.3

[a] M2 protocol is melphalan, cyclophosphamide, carmustine (BCNU), vincristine, and prednisone; MChlP is melphalan, chlorambucil, and prednisone; ChlP is chlorambucil and prednisone; CHOP is cyclophosphamide, doxorubicin, vincristine, and prednisone.

shown activity in patients with a variety of chronic lymphoproliferative disorders. These agents have also been administered to previously untreated patients with WM. More experience has accumulated with cladribine (Table 27.3). This agent has been administered either at a dose of 0.1 mg/kg per day for a 7-day continuous infusion or at a dose of 0.12 mg/kg by 2-hour daily intravenous infusion for 5 consecutive days at monthly intervals. Most studies have confirmed objective responses in approximately 80% of patients.[96–100] The major adverse effects of cladribine are myelosuppression and immunosuppression. Myelosuppression is usually moderate, but with repeated courses of cladribine, there is evidence of cumulative and protracted myelotoxicity. Prolonged thrombocytopenia, which can last for several months after discontinuation of cladribine, may be a significant problem. Cladribine therapy causes significant reduction of monocytes and lymphocytes, which results in an increased risk for opportunistic infections.[96]

In order to avoid significant myelosuppression and immunosuppression, the treatment strategy at the MD Anderson Cancer Center in Houston has been to administer only two courses of cladribine at a dose of 0.1 mg/kg per day as a 7-day continuous infusion using a portable pump through a central venous catheter. Responding patients are followed without further therapy, and receive two additional courses of cladribine at the time of progression. This resulted in responses in 80% of patients. The median time to 50% reduction in IgM was 1.2 months, and gradual reduction of abnormal protein continued in all responding patients even after cladribine therapy was stopped. The median duration of unmaintained remission was approximately 18 months, and the disease responded in most patients when cladribine treatment was resumed at the time of relapse.[96]

Although primary treatment of WM with cladribine has not been prospectively compared with the use of chlorambucil, because of its rapid cytoreduction, cladribine may be the treatment of choice when rapid disease control is desirable because of hyperviscosity, pancytopenia, or severe peripheral neuropathy. Preliminary data suggest that the combination of subcutaneous cladribine and oral cyclophosphamide is very active.[101] In the same series, it was found that cladribine-containing regimens, administered to 58 previously untreated patients, induced a significantly higher response rate (75%) than that observed previously in 115 patients treated with alkylating agent-based therapy (55%; $p = 0.01$).

Fludarabine has also been studied as first-line treatment of WM. A preliminary report suggested that only 33% of previously untreated patients achieved an objective response.[102] This figure is lower than that seen with cladribine.

Table 27.3 Primary treatment of Waldenström's macroglobulinaemia with cladribine

Series	No. of patients	Response	
		No.	%
Dimopoulos et al[96]	26	22	85
Delannoy[97]	11	8	73
Fridrik et al[98]	10	9	90
Lui et al[99]	7	4	57
Hellmann et al[100]	7	5	71
Total	61	48	79

The final analysis of this important study will help determine the role of fludarabine as primary treatment for WM.

Treatment of disease previously treated with alkylating agents

Several patients with WM do not respond to the initial alkylating agent-based treatment, and virtually all responding patients eventually experience disease progression. Until recently, few effective treatments were available for patients whose disease was resistant to alkylating agents.

There have been limited trials of second-line treatments, including doxorubicin, high-dose steroids, interferon (IFN)-γ, and splenectomy, with some benefit.[103–107] IFN-α has also been administered to several previously treated WM patients. Using different doses and response criteria, an antitumour effect was seen in 20–50% of patients.[108–110] These data indicate that IFN-α may have a role to play in the treatment of WM. Studies are required to assess its effect as maintenance therapy in responding patients and in previously untreated patients with low tumour burden.

Fludarabine and cladribine afford an opportunity for effective salvage therapy in many patients with resistant macroglobulinaemia. Fludarabine was the first nucleoside analogue to induce responses in about one-third of patients who had been resistant to previous treatments.[111] These results were subsequently confirmed by other studies.[112–114] The recommended dose of fludarabine is 25 mg/m^2 intravenously daily for 5 days every 4 weeks. Cladribine has also shown activity in previously treated WM patients.[104,105,115–117] As shown in Table 27.4, approximately half of the patients achieve an objective response.

Table 27.4 Treatment of resistant Waldenström's macroglobulinaemia with nucleoside analogues[97, 99, 112–114, 116, 117]

	Fludarabine	Cladribine
No. of patients	109	114
Response rate (%)	31	46

The status of the disease at the time of salvage treatment with a nucleoside analogue is an important predictor of the likelihood and durability of the response.[116] Patients relapsing from an unmaintained remission (relapse off treatment) and those who had never responded to previous treatments (primary resistant) are more likely to benefit. The response rates for these two groups of patients were 78% and 44%, respectively. The duration of primary resistance is also an important parameter: 57% of patients with primary resistance duration of less than 1 year responded to cladribine, compared with 17% of patients with a longer duration of primary resistance. Patients who were treated while their disease was relapsing despite salvage therapy (refractory relapse) had a significantly lower response rate (21%) and a median survival of 13 months. The median progression-free survival of all responding patients is about 12 months.[116]

Nucleoside analogues are the treatment of choice in patients who do not respond to primary treatment with alkylating agents. The much lower response rate among patients with a longer duration of primary resistance or during refractory relapse may be due to the evolution, over time, of resistant clones. Prior resistance to fludarabine is associated with cross-resistance to cladribine. While three of four patients who had previously responded to fludarabine and had relapsed from an unmaintained remission achieved a partial response with cladribine, only one of ten patients with disease resistant to fludarabine responded to cladribine.[118] Thus, patient groups unlikely to respond to a nucleoside analogue are candidates for new agents or for more intensive chemotherapy.

Paclitaxel was inactive in six previously untreated patients with WM.[119] Preliminary evidence suggests that rituximab (an anti-CD20 monoclonal antibody) and high-dose therapy with autologous stem cell support may have a role to play in the management of WM.[120,121]

PROGNOSIS

The median survival of patients with WM is 5 years, but at least 20% of patients survive for more than 10 years, and up to one-fifth of patients die of unrelated causes.[3,34,35,36,122] Because WM is an uncommon disorder, relatively few studies have defined prognostic factors for this disease.

Parameters associated with inferior survival are shown in Table 27.5. In most series, patients older than 60 or 70 years have a worse prognosis. Bartl et al[27] distinguished three types of bone marrow involvement, which had significantly different median survival times. Anaemia, which is usually due to marrow infiltration, is also associated with worse prognosis. Morel et al[123] recently indicated that the combination of age, albumin level, and blood cell counts provided a simple prognostic model for survival in WM. Using these readily available parameters, patients were stratified into three groups with low, intermediate, and high risk, and with probabilities of 5-year survival of 86%, 61%, and 26%, respectively.[123]

Patients with WM who respond to treatment live longer than non-responders. Mackenzie and Fudenberg[32] reported a mean survival of 49 months for patients responding to chemotherapy and 24 months for the non-responders. In the MD Anderson series,[36] patients achieving an objective response lived a median of 7.7 years, in comparison with a median of 2.5 years for unresponsive patients; 10% of patients achieved a complete response and survived for a median of 11 years.

Table 27.5 Adverse prognostic factors in Waldenström's macroglobulinaemia

- Advanced age[34–36,123]
- Male gender[34]
- Weight loss[35]
- Anaemia[25,34,35,123]
- Neutropenia[25,34,123]
- Hypoalbuminaemia[33, 123]
- Cryoglobulinaemia[35]
- Pattern of bone marrow involvement[27]

Most patients with WM die of progressive disease that has become refractory to treatment. The use of alkylating agents has been associated with the development of myelodysplastic syndrome and secondary acute leukaemia.[124,125] In some patients, the disease may transform into a diffuse large cell lymphoma (Richter syndrome) characterized by the development of fever, weight loss, rapidly enlarging lymph nodes, extranodal involvement, and reduction of monoclonal protein synthesis. Despite treatment with combinations of agents with activity in high-grade lymphomas, the outcome of these patients is poor.[126,127]

CONCLUSIONS AND FUTURE DIRECTIONS

WM is an uncommon low-grade lymphoid malignancy that may involve several organs through a variety of pathogenetic mechanisms. This disease has unique clinical and laboratory features that rarely occur in other lymphoproliferative disorders. There is no evidence that treatment of asymptomatic patients is of benefit. Therapy consists of treatment of IgM-induced complications and treatment of the lymphoma. Although standard primary chemotherapy consists of oral chlorambucil, we believe that limited therapy with cladribine may provide the best opportunity for rapid disease control in symptomatic patients with WM. Further studies are needed in order to elucidate the optimal dose and duration of cladribine treatment and the activity of cladribine combined with other agents such as cyclophosphamide or mitoxantrone. For disease resistant to alkylating agents, either fludarabine or cladribine can induce responses in about one-third of patients. These agents are more effective when administered soon after resistance has been documented. Patients in resistant relapse are candidates for treatment with investigational agents. There is preliminary evidence that high-dose therapy with peripheral blood stem cell support and treatment with IFN-α or with monoclonal anti-CD20 antibody (rituximab) may have a role to play in the treatment of WM. More data are required to assess the value of these approaches for outcome.

ACKNOWLEDGEMENT

The excellent editorial and secretarial assistance of Dimitra Gika is greatly appreciated.

REFERENCES

1. Waldenström J. Incipient myelomatosis or 'essential' hyperglobulinemia with fibrinogenopenia – a new syndrome? *Acta Med Scand* 1944; **216**: 433–4.
2. Harris NL, Jaffe ES, Stein H et al. A Revised European–American classification of lymphoid neoplasms: a proposal from the International Lymphoma Study Group. *Blood* 1994; **84**: 1361–92.
3. Kyle RA, Garton JP. The spectrum of IgM monoclonal gammopathy in 430 cases. *Mayo Clin Proc* 1987; **62**: 719–31.
4. Herrinton LJ, Weiss NS. Incidence of Waldenström's macroglobulinemia. *Blood* 1993; **82**: 3148–50.
5. Groves FD, Travis LB, Devesa SS et al. Waldenström's macroglobulinemia: incidence patterns in the United States, 1988–1994. *Cancer* 1998; **82**: 1078–81.
6. Fine JM, Mullier JY, Rochu D. Waldenström's macroglobulinemia in monozygotic twins. *Acta Med Scand* 1989; **220**: 369–73.
7. Renier G, Ifrah N, Chevalier A et al. Four brothers with Waldenström's macroglobulinemia. *Cancer* 1989; **64**: 1554–9.
8. Seligmann M, Danon F, Mihaesco C et al. Immunoglobulin abnormalities in families of patients with Waldenstrom's macroglobulinemia. *Am J Med* 1967; **43**: 66–83.
9. Williamson LM, Greaves M, Waters JR et al. Waldenström's macroglobulinaemia: three cases in shoe repairers. *BMJ* 1989; **298**: 498–9.
10. Tepper A, Moss CE. Waldenström's macroglobulinemia: search for occupational exposure. *J Occup Med* 1989; **36**: 133–6.
11. Linet MS, Humphrey RL, Mehl ES et al. A case–control and family study of Waldenström's macroglobulinemia. *Leukemia* 1993; **7**: 1363–9.
12. Kucharska-Pulczynska M, Ellegard J, Hokland P. Analysis of leucocyte differentiation antigens in blood and bone marrow from patients with Waldenström's macroglobulinaemia. *Br J Haematol* 1987; **65**: 395–9.
13. Feiner HD, Rizk CC, Finfer MD et al. IgM monoclonal gammopathy/Waldenström's macroglobulinemia: a morphological and immunophenotypic study of the bone marrow. *Mod Pathol* 1990; **3**: 348–56.
14. Jensen GS, Andrews EJ, Mant MJ et al. Transitions in CD45 isoform expression indicate continuous differentiation of a monoclonal CD5+CD11b+B lineage in Waldenström's macroglobulinemia. *Am J Hematol* 1991; **37**: 20–30.
15. Said JW, Retting MR, Heppner K et al. Localization of Kaposi's sarcoma-associated herpesvirus in bone marrow samples from patients with multiple myeloma. *Blood* 1997; **90**: 4278–83.
16. Agbalika F, Mariette X, Pierre Matolleau JP et al. Detection of human herpesvirus-8 DNA in bone marrow biopsies from patients with multiple myeloma and Waldenström's macroglobunemia. *Blood* 1998; **91**: 4393–4.
17. Brouset P, Theriault C, Roda D et al. Kaposi's sarcoma-associated herpesvirus (KSHV) in bone marrow biopsies of patients with Waldenström's macroglobulinaemia. *Br J Haematol* 1998; **102**: 795–7.
18. Rettig M, Vescio R, Ma H et al. Detection of Kaposi's sarcoma associated herpesvirus in the dendritic cells of Waldenström's macroglobulinemia and primary amyloidosis patients. *Blood* 1997; **90**(Suppl 1): 86a (Abst 374).
19. Palka G, Spadano A, Geraci L et al. Chromosome changes in 19 patients with Waldenström's macroglobulinemia. *Cancer Genet Cytogenet* 1987; **29**: 261–9.
20. Calasanz MJ, Cigudosa JC, Odero MD et al. Cytogenetic analysis of 280 patients with multiple myeloma and related disorders: primary break points and clinical correlations. *Genes Chromosomes Cancer* 1997; **18**: 84–93.
21. Louviaux I, Michaux L, Hagemeijer A et al. Cytogenetic abnormalities in Waldenström's disease: a single center study on 45 cases. *Blood* 1998; **92**(Suppl 1): 184b (Abst 3776).
22. Nishida K, Taniwaki M, Misawa S et al. Nonrandom rearrangement of chromosome 14 at band q32,33 in human lymphoid malignancies with mature B-cell phenotype. *Cancer Res* 1989; **49**: 1275–81.

23. Chong YY, Lau LC, Lui WO et al. A case of t(8;14) with total and partial trisomy 3 in Waldenström macroglobulinemia. *Cancer Genet Cytogenet* 1998; **103**: 65–7.
24. Dohner H, Fischer K, Bentz M et al. p3 gene delection predicts for poor survival and non-response to therapy with purine analogs in chronic B-cell leukemias. *Blood* 1995; **85**: 1580–9.
25. Andriko JA, Aguilea NS, Chu WS et al. Waldenström's macroglobulinemia: a clinicopathologic study of 22 cases. *Cancer* 1997; **80**: 1926–35.
26. Dutcher TF, Fahey JL The histopathology of macroglobulinemia of Waldenström. *J Nat Cancer Inst* 1959; **22**: 887–917.
27. Bartl R, Frisch B, Mahl G et al. Bone marrow histology in Waldenström's macroglobulinemia. Clinical relevance of subtype recognition. *Scand J Haematol* 1983; **31**: 359–75.
28. Moulopoulos LA, Dimopoulos MA, Varma DG et al. Waldenström macroglobulinemia: MR imaging of the spine and computed tomography of the abdomen and pelvis. *Radiology*, 1993; **188**: 669–73.
29. Duhem, Ries F, Dicato M. Accuracy of magnetic resonance imaging (MRI) of bone marrow in Waldenström's macroglobulinemia. *Blood* 1994; **84**(Suppl 1): 653a (Abst 2598).
30. Leb L, Grimes ET, Balogh K et al. Monoclonal macroglobulinemia with osteolysic lesions. *Cancer* 1997; **39**: 227–31.
31. Haghighi B, Yanagihara R, Cornbleet PJ. IgM myeloma: case report with immunophenotypic profile. *Am J Hematol* 1998; **59**: 302–8.
32. Mackenzie MR, Fudenberg HH. Macroglobulinemia: an analysis of forty patients. *Blood* 1972; **39**: 874–89.
33. Krajny M, Pruzanski W. Waldenström's macroglobulinemia: review of 45 cases. *Can Med Assoc J* 1976; **114**: 899–905.
34. Facon T, Brouillard M, Duhamel A et al. Prognostic factors in Waldenström's macroglobulinemia: a report of 167 cases. *J Clin Oncol* 1993; **11**: 1553–8.
35. Gobbi P, Bettini R, Montecucco C et al. Study of prognosis in Waldenström's macroglobulinemia: a proposal for a simple binary classification with clinical and investigational utility. *Blood* 1994; **83**: 2939–45.
36. Dimopoulos MA, Alexanian R. Waldenström's macroglobulinemia. *Blood* 1994; **83**: 1452–9.
37. Rausch RG, Herion JC. Pulmonary manifestations of Waldenström's macroglobulinemia. *Am J Hematol* 1980; **9**: 201–9.
38. Fadil A, Taylor DE. The lung and Waldenström's macroglobulinemia. *South Med J* 1998; **91**: 681–5.
39. Moore DF, Moulopoulos LA, Dimopoulos MA. Waldenström's macroglobulinemia presenting as renal or perirenal mass: clinical and radiographic features. *Leuk Lymphoma* 1995; **14**: 331–4.
40. Rosenthal JA, Curran WJ, Schuster SJ. Waldenström's macroglobulinemia resulting from localized gastric lymphoplasmacytoid lymphoma. *Am J Hematol* 1998; **58**: 244–5.
41. Yasui O, Tukamoto F, Sasaki N et al. Malignant lymphoma of the transverse colon associated with macroglobulinemia. *Am J Gastroenterol* 1997; **92**: 2299–301.
42. Torrey JJ, Katakkar SB. Treatable meningeal involvement in Waldenström's macroglobulinemia. *Ann Intern Med* 1984; **101**: 345–7.
43. MacKenzie MR, Lee TK. Blood viscosity in Waldenström macroglobulinemia. *Blood* 1977; **49**: 507–10.
44. Crawford J, Cox EB, Cohen HJ. Evaluation of hypervisosity in monoclonal gammopathies. *Am J Med* 1985; **79**: 13–22.
45. Alexanian R. Blood volume in monoclonal gammopathy. *Blood* 1977; **49**: 301–4.
46. Brouet JC, Clauvel JP, Danon F et al. Biologic and clinical significance of cryoglobulins. *Am J Med* 1974; **57**: 775–88.
47. Goveric PD, Kassad HJ, Levo Y et al. Mixed cryoglobulinemia: clinical aspects and long-term follow up of 40 patients. *Am J Med* 1980; **69**: 287–308.
48. Invernizzi F, Galli M, Serino G et al. Secondary and essential cryoglobulinemias. *Acta Haematol* 1983; **70**: 73–82.
49. Pruzanski W, Shumak H. Biologic activity of cold reactive autoantibodies. *N Engl J Med* 1977; **297**: 538–44.
50. Rose WF, Adams J, Logue G. Hemolysis by complement and cold reaction antibody. *Am J Hematol* 1977; **2**: 259–70.
51. Dalakas MC, Engle WK. Polyneuropathy with monoclonal gammopathy. *Ann Neurol* 1981; **10**: 45–52.
52. Latov N, Braun PE, Gross RB et al. Plasma cell dyscrasia and peripheral neuropathy: Identification of the myelin antigens that react with human paraproteins. *Proc Natl Acad Sci USA* 1981; **78**: 7139–42.

53. Dellagi K, Dupouey P, Brouet JC et al. Waldenström's macroglobulinemia and peripheral neuropathy: a clinical and immunologic study of 25 patients. *Blood* 1983; **62**: 280–5.
54. Nobile-Orazio E, Marmireli P, Baldini L et al. Peripheral neuropathy in macroglobulinemia. *Neurology* 1987; **37**: 1506–14.
55. Dalakas MC, Papadopoulos NM. Paraproteins in the spinal fluid of patients with paraproteinemic polyneuropathies. *Ann Neurol* 1984; **15**: 590–3.
56. Meier C. Polyneuropathy in paraprotenemia. *J Neurol* 1985; **48:** 204–14.
57. Mendell JR, Sahhenk Z, Whitaker JN et al. Polyneuropathy and monoclonal gammopathy: studies on the pathogenetic role of anti-myelin-associated glycoprotein antibody. *Ann Neurol* 1985; **17**: 243–54.
58. Vital A, Vital C, Julien J et al. Polyneuropathy associated with IgM monoclonal gemmopathy. Immunological and pathological study in 31 patients. *Acta Neuropathol* 1989; **79**: 160–7.
59. Ilyas AA, Quarles RH, Mclntosh TD et al. IgM in a human neuropathy related to paraproteinemia binds to a carbohydrate determinant in the myelin-associated glycoprotein and to a ganglioside. *Proc Natl Acad Sci USA* 1984; **81**: 1225–9.
60. Ilyas AA, Quaries RH, Dalakas MC et al. Polyneuropathy with monoclonal gammopathy glycolipids are frequently antigens for IgM paraproteins. *Proc Natl Acad Sci USA* 1985; **82**: 6697–700.
61. Ilyas AA, Dalakas MC, Brady RO et al. Sulfated glucuronyl glycolipids reacting with anti-myelin associated glycoproterin monoclonal antibodies including IgM paraproteins in neuropathy species distribution and partial characterization of epitopes. *Brain* 1986; **385**: 1–9.
62. O'Shannessy DJ, Ilyas AA, Dalakas MC et al. Specificity of human IgM monoclonal antibodies from patients with peripheral neuropathy. *J Neuroimmunol* 1986; **11**: 131–6.
63. Ilyas AA, Quarles RH, Dalakas MC et al. Monoclonal IgM in a patient with paraproteinemic neuropathy binds to gangliosides containing disialossyl groups. *Ann Neurol* 1985; **15**: 655–9.
64. Ilyas A, Willison HJ, Dalakas MC et al. Identification and characterization of gangliosides reacting with IgM paraproteins in three patients with neuropathy associated with biclonal gammopathy. *J Neurochem* 1988; **51**: 851–8.
65. Freddo L, Yu RK, Latov N et al. Gangliosides GM1 and GD1b are antigens for IgM M-proteins in a patient with motor neuron disease. *Neurology* 1986; **36**: 454–8.
66. Duane GC, Farrer RG, Dalakas MC et al. Sensory neuropathy associated with monoclonal IgM to GD 1b ganglioside. *Ann Neurol* 1992; **31**: 683–5.
67. Latov N. Antibodies to glycoconjugates in neuropathy and motor neuron disease. *Prog Brain Res* 1993; **101**: 295–303.
68. Ilyas AA, Cook SD, Dalakas MC et al. Anti-MAG IgM paraproteins from some patients with polyneuropathy associated with IgM paraprotenemic neuropathy also react with sulfatide. *J Neuroimmunol* 1992; **37**: 85–92.
69. Quatrinni A, Corbo M, Dhaliwal SK et al. Anti-sulfatide antibodies in neurological disease, binding to rat dorsal root ganglia neurons. *J Neurol* 1992; **112**: 152–9.
70. Nobile-Orazio E, Manfredini E, Carpo M et al. Frequency and clinical correlates of anti-neuronal IgM antibodies in neuropathy associated with IgM monoclonal gammopathy. *Ann Neurol* 1994; **36**: 416–24.
71. Latov N, Hays AP, Donofrio PD et al. Monoclonal IgM with unique specificity to gangliosides GM1 and GD1b, and to lacto-N-tetraose, associated with human motor neuron disease. *Neurology* 1988; **38**: 763–8.
72. Sadiq SA, Thomas FP, Kilidireas K et al. The spectrum of neurologic disease associated with anti-GM1 antibodies. *Neurology* 1990; **40**: 1067–72.
73. Ropper AH, Gorson KC. Neuropathies associated with paraproteinemia. *N Engl J Med* 1998; **338**: 1601–7.
74. Garsia-Bragado F, Fermandez JM, Navarro C et al. Peripheral neuropathy in essential mixed cryoglobulinemia. *Arch Neurol* 1988; **45**: 1210–14.
75. Gertz MA, Kyle RA, Noel P. Primary systemic amyloidosis: a rare complication of immnoglobulin M monoclonal gammopathies and Waldenström's macroglobulinemia. *J Clin Oncol* 1993; **11**: 914–20.
76. Morel L, Basch A, Danon F et al. Pathology of the kidney in Waldenström's macroglobulinemia. *N Engl J Med* 1970; **283**: 123–9.
77. Meyrier A, Simon P, Mignon F et al. Rapidly progressive glomerulonephritis and monoclonal gammopathies. *Nephron* 1984; **38**: 156–62.
78. Lowe L, Fitzpatrick JE, Huff JC et al. Cutaneous macroglobulinosis. *Arch Dermatol* 1992; **128**: 377–80.

79. Whittaker SJ, Bhogla BS, Black MM. Acquired immunobullous disease: a cutaneous manifestation of IgM macroglobulinaemia. *Br J Dermatol* 1996; **35**: 283–6.
80. Schnitzler L, Schubert B, Boasson M et al. Urticaire chronique, lésions osseuses, macroglobulinémié IgM: maladie de Waldenström? *Bull Soc Fr Dermatol* 1974; **81**: 363.
81. Becker LR, Bastian BC, Wesselmann U et al. Paraneoplastic pemphigus treated with dexamethasone/cyclophosphamide pulse therapy. *Eur J Dermatol* 1998; **8**: 551–3.
82. Pruzanski W, Warren RE, Goldie JH et al. Malabsorption syndrome with infiltration of the intestinal wall by extracellular monoclonal macroglobulin. *Am J Med* 1973; **58**: 811–18.
83. Tait RC, Oagarah PK, Houghton JB et al. Waldenström's macroglobulinemia secreting a paraprotein with lupus anticoagulant activity: possible association with gastrointestinal tract disease and malabsorption. *Clin Pathol* 1993; **46**: 678–80.
84. Perkins HA, Mackenzie MR, Fudenberg HH. Hemostatic defects in dysproteinemias. *Blood* 1970; **35**: 694–707.
85. Varticovski L, Pick AI, Schattner A et al. Antiplatelet and anti-DNA IgM in Waldenström's macroglobulinemia and ITP. *Am J Hematol* 1987; **24**: 351–5.
86. Castaldi PA, Penney R. A macroglobulin with inhibitory activity against coagulation factor VIII. *Blood* 1970; **35**: 370–6.
87. McCallister BD, Bayrd ED, Harrison EG et al. Primary macroglobulinemia. *Am J Med* 1967; **43**: 394–404.
88. Schwab PJ, Fahey JL. Treatment of Waldenström's macroglobulinemia by plasmapheresis. *N Engl J Med* 1960; **263**: 574–9.
89. Buskard NA, Galton DAG, Goldman JM et al. Plasma exchange in the long-term treatment of Waldenström's macroglobulinemia. *Can Med Assoc J* 1977; **117**: 135–7.
90. Dyck PJ, Low PA, Windebank AJ. Plasma exchange in polyneuropathy associated with monoclonal gammopathy of undetermined significance. *N Engl J Med* 1991; **325**: 1482–6.
91. Nobile-Orazio E, Baldini L, Barbieri A et al. Treatment of patients with neuropathy and anti-MAG IgM M-proteins. *Ann Neurol* 1988; **24**: 93–7.
92. Cook D, Dalakas M, Galdi A et al. High-dose intravenous immunoglobulin in the treatment of demyelinating neuropathy associated with monoclonal gammopathy. *Neurology* 1990; **40**: 212–14.
93. Kyle RA, Greipp P, Gertz M et al. Waldenström's macroglobulinemia: a prospective study comparing daily versus intermittent oral chlorambucil. *Blood* 1998; **92**(Suppl 1): 279b (Abst 4204).
94. Petrucci MT, Avvisati G, Tribalto M et al. Waldenström's macroglobulinemia: results of a combined oral treatment in 34 newly diagnosed patients. *J Intern Med* 1989; **226**: 443–7.
95. Case DC, Ervin TJ, Boyd MA. Long term results and disease characteristics of patients with Waldenström's macroglobulinemia treated with the M-2 protocol. *Blood* 1993; **82**(Suppl 1): 561a (Abst 2230).
96. Dimopoulos MA, Kantarjian H, Weber D et al. Primary therapy of Waldenström's macroglobulinemia with 2-chlorodeoxyadenosine. *J Clin Oncol* 1994; **12**: 2694–8.
97. Delannoy A. 2-Chlorodeoxyadenosine: clinical applications in hematology. *Blood Rev* 1996; **10**: 148–60.
98. Fridrik MA, Jager G, Baldinger C et al. First-line treatment of Waldenström's disease with cladribine. *Ann Hematol* 1997; **74**: 7–10.
99. Liu F, Burian C, Miller W et al. Bolus administration of cladribine in the treatment of Waldenström's macroglobulinaemia. *Br J Haematol* 1998; **103**: 690–5.
100. Hellmann A, Lewandowski K, Zancha JM et al. Treatment of Waldenström's macroglobulinemia with 2–chlorodeoxyadenosine. *Br J Haematol* 1998; **102**: 244 (Abst 0973).
101. Weber D, Delasalle K, Gavino M et al. Primary treatment of Waldenström's macroglobulinemia with subcutaneous 2-chlorodeoxyadenosine and oral cyclophosphamide. *Blood* 1997; **90**(Suppl 1): 357a (Abst 1592).
102. Dhodapkar M, Jacobson J, Gertz M et al. Phase II intergroup trial of fludarabine in Waldenström's macroglobulinemia: results of Southwest Oncology Group trial in 220 patients. *Blood* 1997; **90**(Suppl 1): 577a (Abst 2571).
103. Claman GH, Corder MP, Burus CP. Successful doxorubicin therapy of primary macroglobulinemia resistant to alkylating agents. *Am J Hematol* 1980; **9**: 221–3.
104. Jane SM, Salem HH. Treatment of resistant Waldenström's macroglobulinemia with high dose glucocorticoids. *Aust NZ J Med* 1988; **18**: 77–8.

105. Quesada JR, Alexanian R, Kurzrock R et al. Recombinant interferon gamma in hairy cell leukemia, multiple myeloma, and Waldenström's macroglobulinemia. *Am J Hematol* 1988; **29**: 1–4.
106. Humphrey JS, Lockard C. Durable complete remission of macroglobulinemia after splenectomy. *Am J Hematol* 1995; **48**: 262–6.
107. Takemori N, Hirai k, Onodera R et al. Durable remission after splenectomy for Waldenström's macroglobulinemia with massive splenomegaly in leukemic phase. *Leuk Lymphoma* 1997; **26**: 387–93.
108. Ohno R, Kodera Y, Ogura M et al. Treatment of plasma cell neoplasm with recombinant leukocyte α-interferon and human lymphoblastoid interferon. *Cancer Chemother Pharmacol* 1985; **14**: 34–7.
109. Rotoli B, De Renzo A, Frigeri F et al. A phase II trial on alpha-interferon effect in patients with monoclonal IgM gammopathy. *Leuk Lymphoma* 1994; **13**: 463–9.
110. Legouffe E, Rossi JF, Laporte JP et al. Treatment of Waldenström's macroglobulinemia with very low doses of alpha interferon. *Leuk Lymphoma* 1995; **19**: 337–42.
111. Kantarjian HM, Alexanian R, Koller CA et al. Fludarabine therapy in macroglobulinemic lymphoma. *Blood* 1990; **75**: 1928–31.
112. Dimopoulos MA, O'Brien S, Kantarjian H et al. Fludarabine therapy in Waldenström's macroglobulinemia. *Am J Med* 1993; **95**: 49–52.
113. Zinzani PL, Gherlinzoni F, Blendandi M et al. Fludarabine treatment in resistant Waldenström's macroglobulinemia. *Eur J Hematol* 1995; **54**: 120–3.
114. Leblond V, Ben-Othman T, Deconinck E et al. Activity of fludarabine in previously treated Waldenström's macroglobulinemia: a report of 71 cases. Group Cooperatif Macroglobulinémié. *J Clin Oncol* 1998; **16**: 2060–4.
115. Dimopoulos MA, Kantarjian HM, Estey EH et al. Treatment of Waldenström's macroglobulinemia with 2-chlorodeoxyadenosine. *Ann Intern Med* 1993; **118**: 195–8.
116. Dimopoulos MA, Weber D, Delasalle KB et al. Treatment of Waldenström's macroglobulinemia resistant to standard therapy with 2-chlorodeoxyadenosine: identification of prognostic factors. *Ann Oncol* 1995; **6**: 49–52.
117. Betticher DC, Hsu Schmitz SF, Ratschiller D et al. Cladribine (2-CDA) given as subcutaneous bolus injection is active in pretreated Waldenström's macroglobulinaemia. Swiss Group for Clinical Cancer Research. *Br J Haematol* 1997; **99**: 358–63.
118. Dimopoulos MA, Weber DM, Kantarjian H et al. 2-Chlorodeoxyadenosine therapy of patients with Waldenström macroglobulinemia previously treated with fludarabine. *Ann Oncol* 1994; **5**: 288–9.
119. Dimopoulos MA, Luckett R, Alexanian R. Primary therapy of Waldenström's macroglobulinemia with paclitaxel. *J Clin Oncol* 1994; **12**: 1998.
120. Byrd JC, White CA, Link B et al. Rituximab therapy in previously treated Waldenström's macroglobulinemia: preliminary evidence of activity. *Blood* 1998; **92**(Suppl 1): 106a (Abst 433).
121. Desikan R, Dhodapkar M, Siegel D et al. High dose therapy with autologous peripheral blood stem cell support for Waldenström's macroglobulinemia: a pilot study. *Blood* 1998; **92** (Suppl 1): 660a (Abst 2271).
122. Frase LL, Stone MJ. Long-term survival in Waldenström's macroglobulinemia. *Am J Med* 1998; **104**: 507–8.
123. Morel P, Monconduit M, Jacomy D et al. A new scoring system in Waldenström's macroglobulinemia; description on 232 patients with validation on 167 other patients. *Blood* 1997; **90**(Suppl 1): 243a (Abst 1069).
124. Rosner F, Grunwald HW. Multiple myeloma and Waldenström's macroglobulinemia terminating in acute leukemia. *NY State J Med* 1980; **80**: 558–70.
125. Rodriguez JN, Fernandez-Jurado A, Martino ML et al. Waldenström's macroglobulinemia complicated with acute myeloid leukemia. Report of a case and review of the literature. *Hematologica* 1998; **83**: 91–2.
126. Leonhard SA, Muhleman AF, Hurtubise PF et al. Emergence of immunoblastic sarcoma in Waldenström's macroglobulinemia. *Cancer* 1980; **45**: 3102–7.
127. Garcia R, Hernandez JM, Caballero MD et al. Immunoblastic lymphoma and associated non-lymphoid malignancies following two cases of Waldenström's macroglobulinemia. *Eur J Hematol* 1993; **50**; 299–301.

28

Multicentric Castleman's disease

Glauco Frizzera, Amy Chadburn

INTRODUCTION

The clinicopathologic entity known as Castleman's disease (CD; also referred to as giant lymph node hyperplasia and angiofollicular lymph node hyperplasia) has evolved over time to include three different disorders.

- CD as originally described by Castleman et al[1] consisted of localized lymph node hyperplasia characterized by abnormal follicles with small germinal centers simulating Hassal's corpuscles, and by marked capillary proliferation.
- A second localized form of the disease, described 13 years later, was characterized morphologically by hyperplastic germinal centers, abundant plasma cells in the interfollicular area, and persistence of sinuses, and clinically by systemic symptoms and laboratory abnormalities.[2–4] These two forms of CD were subsequently termed 'hyaline–vascular' (HV) and 'plasma cell' (PC) variants, respectively.[4]
- A third form, with histologic features similar to those of the other two, but with more extensive lymphadenopathy and systemic clinical manifestations (B symptoms, increased levels of acute-phase reactants, hypergammaglobulinemia, autoimmune manifestations) was described by Leibetseder and Thurner in 1973[5] and by Gaba and associates in 1978.[6] It has subsequently appeared in the literature under a variety of terms, including multicentric angiofollicular lymphoid hyperplasia,[7] angiofollicular and plasmacytic polyadenopathy,[8] systemic lymphoproliferative disorder with morphologic features of CD,[9,10] idiopathic plasmacytic lymphadenopathy with polyclonal hypergammaglobulinemia,[11] plasma cell dyscrasia,[12,13] lymphogranulomatosis X with excessive plasmacytosis,[14] and, most commonly, multicentric CD (MCD).

MCD has been reported both as an autonomous disease process and in association with a number of disease entities, making it one of the most ubiquitous associations in medicine[15] (Table 28.1). This is because its characteristic manifestations are the clinicopathologic endpoint of a cytokine-overloaded environment – increased levels of interleukin (IL)-6 and possibly other cytokines – that is common to all these different entities. Thus, it may be argued that the clinicopathologic entity usually referred to as 'MCD' should more correctly be indicated as 'IL-6 syndrome' and its histopathologic changes in lymphoid tissue as 'IL-6 lymphadenopathy.'

Table 28.1 Disorders associated with the histology or the clinicopathologic complex of 'MCD' (IL-6 syndrome)

- Autoimmune diseases:
  Rheumatoid arthritis[225]
  Sjögren syndrome[226]
  Systemic lupus erythematosus (SLE)[228]
  Mixed connective tissue disease[205]
- Human immunodeficiency virus (HIV) infection[108, 166–173]
- Human herpesvirus (HHV)-8/Kaposi sarcoma-associated herpesvirus (KSHV) infection[29, 71, 99–104]
- Kaposi sarcoma[7, 10, 29, 67, 102, 112, 141, 178–180, 182, 183, 185]
- Plasma cell dyscrasias, especially the POEMS syndrome[13, 48, 68, 189, 191–194, 196, 199–203]
- Other neoplasms, especially Hodgkin's disease[70,91, 209–217]
- Others:[15]
  Primary immunodeficiencies
  Glomerulopathy
  Skin diseases

A role for IL-6 in CD was first suggested in 1989 by Yoshizaki et al,[16] who reported increased serum IL-6 levels in two cases – one localized and one multicentric – and the disappearance of all symptoms and all laboratory abnormalities after the excision of a lymph node in the former but not in the latter. This finding has been confirmed several times.[17–28] Other pathologic and clinical evidence suggests an essential role for IL-6 in the pathogenesis of MCD. Cultured cells from the involved tissues produce human (hu)IL-6,[16,19] and IL-6-positive cells have been detected by immunohistochemistry and/or mRNA in situ hybridization in involved lymphoid tissue, although their identification is somewhat disputed.[16,18–20,24,29, 30] The positive cells have been found in germinal centers, and considered to be either B cells[16,18,24] or follicular dendritic cells.[29,30] They have also been found scattered in the interfollicular area of the node (lymphoid and non-lymphoid cells).[18–20,24,29,30] Peripheral blood B cells from patients with MCD have been shown to express a higher density of the IL-6 receptor (IL-6R, CD126) and to be hyper-responsive to IL-6.[31] Treatment with an anti-IL-6 antibody in a patient with localized CD[24] and another with MCD[32] led to normalization of IL-6 serum levels and resolution of symptoms and laboratory abnormalities.

Finally, there is experimental evidence to support the importance of IL-6 in the pathogenesis of MCD. In congenitally anemic mice, reconstitution with marrow cells transduced with a retroviral vector carrying IL-6 coding sequences produced clinical and pathologic changes similar to those of CD.[33] Mice lacking a negative transcriptional regulator of IL-6, C/EBPβ, developed a lymphoproliferative disorder similar to MCD, including high serum levels of IL-6, and the simultaneous inactivation of both the *IL-6* and *C/EBPβ* genes, in a $IL\text{-}6^{-/-}$, $C/EBP\beta^{-/-}$ double-knockout mouse, prevented the development of such a disorder.[34,35] Local overexpression of *IL-6* and *IL-6R* genes, by introducing expression vectors in Wistar rats via the trachea, resulted in lymphocytic interstitial pneumonia,[36] as observed in some patients with MCD.[37]

IL-6 is a pleiotropic lymphokine produced by various types of normal cells: B and T lymphocytes, monocytes/macrophages, fibroblasts, endothelial cells, epidermal keratinocytes, mesangial cells, and syncytiotrophoblasts.[38,39]

IL-6 is important for the terminal differentiation of activated B cells to plasma cells,[31] the growth of plasma cells and myeloma cells in vitro, possibly through an anti-apoptotic mechanism,[40] and the regulation of T-cell activation.[38] It stimulates hematopoiesis, and is a potent inducer of platelet and macrophage differentiation. It is an endogenous pyrogen, and stimulates the production of acute-phase reactants (such as C-reactive protein, fibrinogen, and haptoglobin) from hepatocytes, but inhibits the secretion of albumin.[33,41]

The production of IL-6 explains many of the clinicopathologic manifestations of MCD: B-cell hyper-reactivity, plasmacytosis in the lymphoid tissues, B symptoms, elevated erythrocyte sedimentation rate (ESR) and acute-phase reactants, hypergammaglobulinemia, and hypoalbuminemia. It does not, however, explain all the manifestations: thrombocytopenia (rather than thrombocytosis, as one would expect), skin manifestations, or neurologic changes.

Other factors are also produced in excess in patients with MCD:[16,17,21,25–27,38] tumor necrosis factor (TNF)-α,[17,21] TNF-β,[25] interferon (IFN)-γ,[25] macrophage colony-stimulating factor (M-CSF),[21] IL-1,[17] and vascular endothelial growth factor (VEGF).[42,43]

These cytokines may act synergistically to induce the systemic manifestations seen in MCD,[17,25] or may have a pathogenetic role in other facets of the disease. For example, elevated VEGF levels may induce angiogenesis, as evidenced by the increased vascularity in the lymph nodes,[42,43] and may also drive the development of glomeruloid hemangiomas.[44]

IL-6 is thought to play a pathogenetic role in several disorders (see Chapter 4) – the same ones in which an association with MCD is so often described: autoimmune diseases,[27,38,39] human immunodeficiency virus (HIV) and other infections,[27,45–47] plasma cell dyscrasias[39] (including POEMS syndrome[48]), Kaposi sarcoma (KS),[49] and lymphomas.[50–56] IL-6 is both produced by and has an autocrine effect on the spindle cells of KS.[49] While production of IL-6 in culture was not detected in a series of low-grade B-cell lymphomas,[50] it was detected by in situ hybridization (ISH) and immunohistochemistry in 24 patients, mostly HIV-positive, with high-grade B-cell lymphomas.[51] Reed–Sternberg cells have been shown to produce IL-6,[52–56] and elevated serum IL-6 levels are present in patients with Hodgkin's disease.[52]

In this chapter, we attempt to develop a framework that, within this vast and heterogenous 'IL-6 syndrome', distinguishes categories of possibly different clinical significance and – as very recent evidence indicates – different etiology (Table 28.2).

We look first at those cases of 'MCD' that are not associated with any other well-defined disease process and thus might be referred to as 'primary'. These fit a combined clinicopathologic definition, which we have previously used[10,57] and includes the following criteria:

- histopathology of CD, most usually of the PC type;
- predominantly lymphadenopathic disease, involving multiple sites;
- manifestations of multisystem involvement (especially bone marrow, liver, or kidney);
- 'idiopathic' nature.

Table 28.2 Forms of multicentric Castleman's disease (MCD; IL-6 syndrome)

Primary

- Not related to HHV-8/KSHV
- Related to HHV-8/KSHV

Secondary[a]

- In HIV infection (with or without KS)
- In KS
- In plasma cell dyscrasias
- In malignant lymphomas
- In autoimmune diseases
- In other clinical situations

IL-6, interleukin-6; HHV-8/KSHV, human herpesvirus-8/Kaposi sarcoma-associated herpesvirus; HIV, human immunodeficiency virus; KS, Kaposi sarcoma.
[a]May or may not be related to HHV-8/KSHV.

The pathologic and clinical features of this primary disorder, as described below and listed in Tables 28.3 and 28.4, are summarized from evaluation of the six published series of such cases (for a total of 44),[7,10,58–61] as well as of single case reports. Recent evidence suggests that, in some patients with 'MCD', the clinicopathologic manifestations of the IL-6 syndrome may be secondary to lymphoid tissue infection by human herpesvirus (HHV)-8 (also known as Kaposi sarcoma-associated herpesvirus, KSHV), with expression of the viral homologue of IL-6 (vIL-6). Cases of HHV-8-related 'MCD' may occur in the absence of associated diseases, and, for this reason and convenience of presentation, we

Table 28.3 Main clinical findings in 44 patients with primary multicentric Castleman's disease (MCD)[7,10,58–61]

Finding	%
Symptoms	98
Lymphadenopathy	100
Peripheral	100
Abdominal	33
Mediastinal	9.5
Splenomegaly	69
Hepatomegaly	54
Edema or effusions	23
Skin rash	20
Neurologic changes	11

Table 28.4 Main laboratory findings in 44 patients with primary multicentric Castleman's disease (MCD)[7,10,58–61]

Finding	%
Elevated erythrocyte sedimentation rate	90
Anemia	88
Hypergammaglobulinemia	82
Hypoalbuminemia	67
Thrombocytopenia	62.5
Proteinuria	16

discuss them as a subset of primary MCD, although not idiopathic in nature.

We shall then evaluate separately, as 'secondary', the diverse categories of MCD reported in association with HIV infection and/or KS, plasma cell dyscrasias, other neoplasms, and, finally, autoimmune diseases. Some of these secondary MCDs also appear to be related to an HHV-8 infection (with vIL-6 production) superimposed on the original disease. Others are not, and result from huIL-6 overproduction due to various etiologies. Whether the HHV-8-positive cases of MCD, be they primary or secondary, are clinically distinct from the HHV-8-negative cases is not clear at the present time, but this may become a very relevant issue in the future.

'PRIMARY' MULTICENTRIC CASTLEMAN'S DISEASE

Histopathologic features

The histopathologic features of primary MCD in the nodes are similar to those described in localized CD, PC type, and include relative preservation of the architecture, frequent dilatation of the sinuses, abundance and prominent alterations of the germinal centers, and marked plasmacytic infiltration of the interfollicular regions (Figures 28.1 and 28.2).[8,9,13,62,63]

The germinal centers may show the usual hyperplastic features; however, most are markedly abnormal, owing to an increase in vessels (which are frequently hyalinized), a decrease in lymphocytes, and a prominence of follicular dendritic cells and histiocytes. Occasionally, they appear similar to those of the HV variant of CD.[4] These basic histologic features in the lymph node, however, can vary in different cases. In some, there is an abundance of

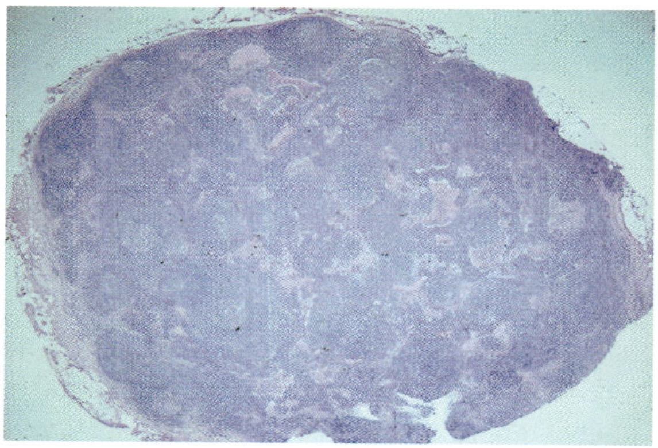

Figure 28.1 Primary multicentric Castleman's disease (MCD): large lymph node with hyperplastic, abnormal germinal centers, dilated sinuses, and prominent plasmacytosis.

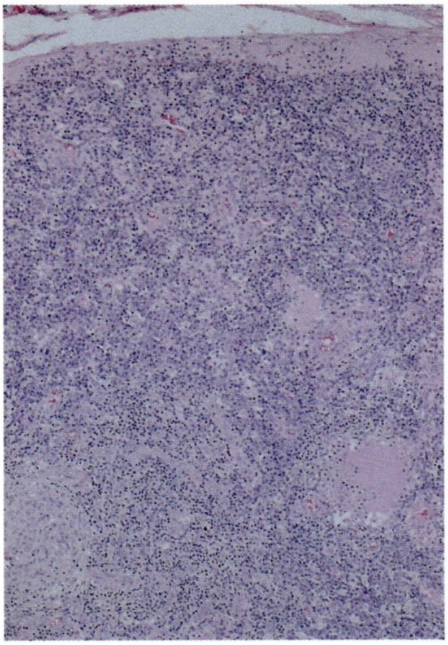

Figure 28.2 Primary multicentric Castleman's disease (MCD): higher power of the same lymph node seen in Figure 28.1, showing a hyaline–vascular germinal center (left lower corner), prominent plasmacytosis, and sinuses filled with hyperchromatic lymph.

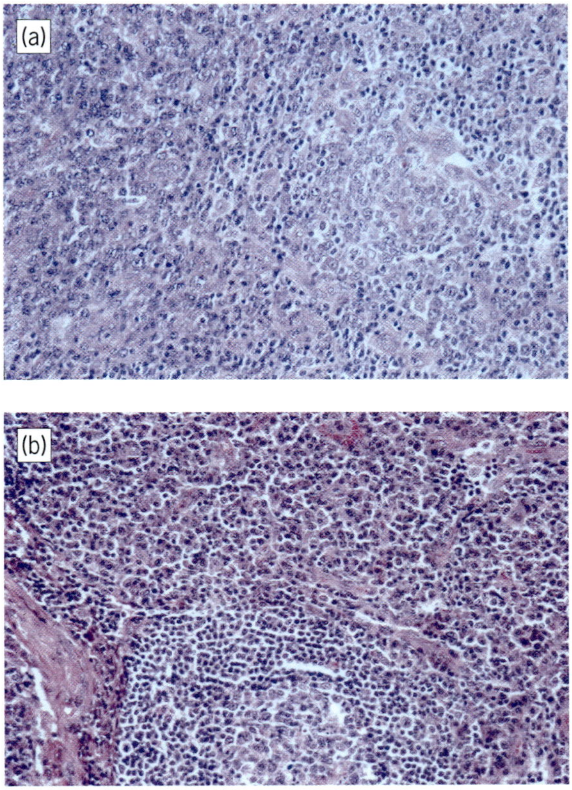

Figure 28.3 Primary multicentric Castleman's disease (MCD). (a) A small germinal center, with attenuated mantle zone, is surrounded by abundant blood vessels and a mixture of mature plasma cells and large transformed cells ('proliferative' pattern). (b) In another case, around a germinal center with well-developed mantle zone, mature plasma cells predominate and vascularity is normal ('accumulative' pattern).

high endothelial venules and immunoblasts, as well as many mitoses in the interfollicular area (Figure 28.3a). In other instances, blood vessels are not increased in the interfollicular area, and immunoblasts and mitoses are few (Figure 28.3b). Examination of multiple, sequential biopsies from the same patient have shown that these two latter patterns represent successive phases in the evolution of this disease process, termed 'proliferative' and 'accumulative'.[9] An additional histologic pattern observed in some patients is a burned-out stage, with abundant HV germinal centers, sclerotic interfollicular blood vessels, and few plasma cells. This last pattern most likely accounts for cases reported in the literature as MCD of the HV or mixed type.[7,62,64–71] Finally, in the subset of patients with HHV-8-related MCD, there is a distinct component of medium-sized plasmacytoid cells that are localized in the mantle zone of the follicles: this variant has been referred to as the 'plasmablastic' type of MCD.[72]

The extranodal pathology of MCD is non-specific, and does not, in our opinion, permit a definitive diagnosis of this disorder, because similar changes can be seen in other inflammatory conditions and atypical lymphoproliferative disorders.[9] In the spleen, there can be variable abnormalities of germinal centers – fibrosis, hemosiderin deposits, and lymphoid depletion of the periarteriolar lymphoid sheaths – and plasmacytosis in the red pulp.[9,73] Bone marrow biopsies may show focal infiltrates of plasma cells; and, in the lung, thickening of the alveolar walls with a diffuse infiltrate of immunoblasts, plasma cells and fibroblasts, was seen in one of our cases[9] and reported by

Japanese groups as lymphocytic interstitial pneumonia.[37,74,75]

There are occasional reports in the literature of a disorder characterized by multiple reddish-brown skin nodules with[76–78] or without[79,80] CD-like adenopathy and laboratory abnormalities. These cases, too, have been interpreted as MCD or idiopathic plasmacytic lymphadenopathy with polyclonal hypergammaglobulinemia.[11]

Immunophenotypic, genotypic, and cytogenetic features

The immunohistochemical findings in the lymph node lesions of MCD are similar to those described in the localized form of CD. The central regions of the abnormal follicles display an irregular network of follicular dendritic cells associated with sparse T cells.[81,82] The mantle zones are composed of small B cells that, in contrast to normal mantle cells, have been shown to be $CD5^{+}$[81] and $CD45RA^{-}$ (with the Ki-B3 antibody) and to preferentially express λ light chain;[69] thus, they are thought to correspond to a normal murine lymphocyte subset referred to as Ly-1 sister B lymphocytes.[69]

The interfollicular tissue contains T-cell subsets in normal proportions[81,83,84] and a prominent population of plasma cells, which, in the majority of cases, is polyclonal. Within this background, a monoclonal plasma cell component may develop[13,69,70,81,85–89] – a phenomenon particularly common (29%) in cases of MCD associated with the POEMS (polyneuropathy, organomegaly, endocrinopathy, M proteins, skin lesions) syndrome.[13] These focal proliferations are mostly of IgGλ or IgAλ isotype, and are often associated with a serum paraprotein. It has been shown in several studies that the presence of a monoclonal plasma cell population is not associated with a shortened survival.[69,87,89]

Molecular genetic analysis of antigen receptor genes in primary MCD has been performed in a small number of cases.[70,81,84,88–90] However, a monoclonal rearrangement of the immunoglobulin heavy-chain gene was detected in 33% of cases studied by Southern blotting and in 7% of those studied by polymerase chain reaction (PCR). A minor T-cell clone, mostly on a polyclonal background, was reported in 25% of specimens studied by Southern blotting and, in one of our cases, it was associated with clonal rearrangements of both the Ig heavy- and light-chain genes.[84]

Finally, molecular techniques have only occasionally detected Epstein–Barr virus (EBV) in the tissues of MCD,[29,84,88,91] suggesting that this virus is not involved in the pathogenesis of the disease. Two reports have described cytogenetic abnormalities in MCD: ins(1)(1pter→1cen::?::1cen→1qter) in one case[88] and a t(7;14)(p22;q22) in another.[92] The latter case is particularly interesting, because the patient had high IL-6 serum levels – a phenomenon possibly related to the involvement of the *IL-6* gene, located at 7p21–22.[92]

HHV-8 studies

HHV-8 is a gamma-herpesvirus implicated in the pathogenesis of KS and primary effusion lymphoma. The viral genome contains several homologues of human genes,[93,94] including the *IL-6* gene.[95,96] The HHV-8 *IL-6* gene product (vIL-6) has many functional similarities to human IL-6;[97,98] however, it differs somewhat in its structural and receptor binding properties.[98]

Genomic sequences of HHV-8 have been detected in MCD by several groups.[29,71,99–104] Excluding cases associated with KS and other diseases, HHV-8 sequences were detected by PCR in 16 of 34 (47%) cases of MCD in the nodal tissue,[28,29,71,72,99–103] peripheral blood mononuclear cells,[105] or lung[75] (Figure 28.4). This is in contrast with the finding of HHV-8 by PCR in over 95% of 'MCD' occurring in HIV-positive patients,[71,72,99,103,106–109] 90% of those associated with the POEMS syndrome,[29,71,110] and 7% of reactive lymph nodes.[100–102,111–113] HHV-8 has also been detected by PCR in peripheral blood mononuclear cells of both HIV-negative/KS-negative[105] and HIV-positive (with or without KS) MCD patients.[106,107] In some of these cases, the viral DNA load was shown to vary in paral-

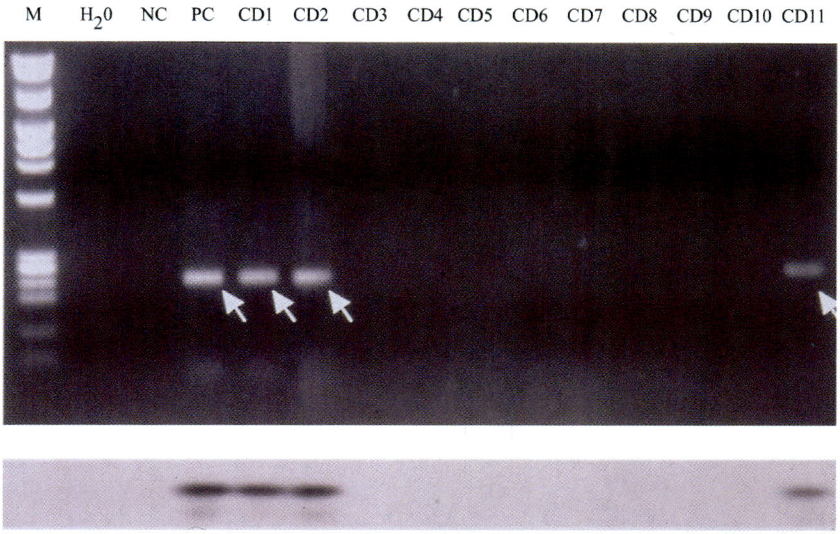

Figure 28.4 Results of PCR amplification of 11 cases of Castleman's disease for the presence of human herpesvirus-8/Kaposi sarcoma-associated herpesvirus (HHV-8/KSHV) using primers to the ORF75 region of the virus. Electrophoresis of the PCR amplification products as visualized in an ethidium bromide-stained agarose gel. Hybridization of the PCR products to an internal oligonucleotide probe after transfer to a nitrocellulose filter. Cases CD1, CD2, CD4, CD8, and CD11 are cases of multicentric Castleman's disease (MCD); the remaining cases are localized Castleman's disease. Cases CD1, CD2 and CD11, (all MCD) are positive for HHV-8. M, molecular-weight marker; H_2O, water; NC, negative control; PC, positive control.

lel with the clinical activity of the disease.[106] The HHV-8-infected cells, identified in HIV-positive 'MCD' using a monoclonal antibody to a latent nuclear antigen of the virus, had immunoblastic features and were found in small numbers in the mantle zone of follicles.[103] In another study,[114] using mRNA-ISH for the latent/lytic gene *TO.7* and the lytic gene *nut-1*, the signal for these viral antigens co-localized in the same few cells that contained high copy levels of vIL-6 and corresponded primarily to λ-bearing plasma cells.

vIL-6-producing cells have been identified by immunohistochemistry,[29,72,109,112] mRNA-ISH,[114] or reverse-transcriptase PCR (RT-PCR)[104] in cases of MCD associated with HHV-8. These cells, very much like the cells containing the viral latent nuclear antigen mentioned above,[103] are located in the mantle zone, where they represent a minority of the resident cells.[29,72,109,112,114] They have the appearance of large plasmacytoid cells,[72,109,112] and express λ light-chain immunoglobulin[72,114] (Figure 28.5).

It is apparent from these studies that, in a proportion of cases of MCD, mantle zone B cells latently infected by HHV-8 may produce vIL-6. Importantly, however, other HHV-8 genes, homologous to human *cyclin D*, *bcl-2*, and *IL-8R* genes, were also found to be expressed in one case of MCD by RT-PCR.[115]

See Chapter 3 for a detailed discussion of the role of viruses in plasma cell disorders.

Clinical findings

MCD is primarily a disease of older individuals (range 19–85 years, median 55.5 years), more often male (M : F =1.4 : 1). Only rare cases have been reported in children,[20,116,117] (reviewed in reference 118); however, it is possible that some of these are cases of primary immunodeficiency with 'MCD-like' manifestations.

MCD presents with systemic symptoms and with multiple peripheral lymphadenopathies. Involvement of deeper nodal regions is

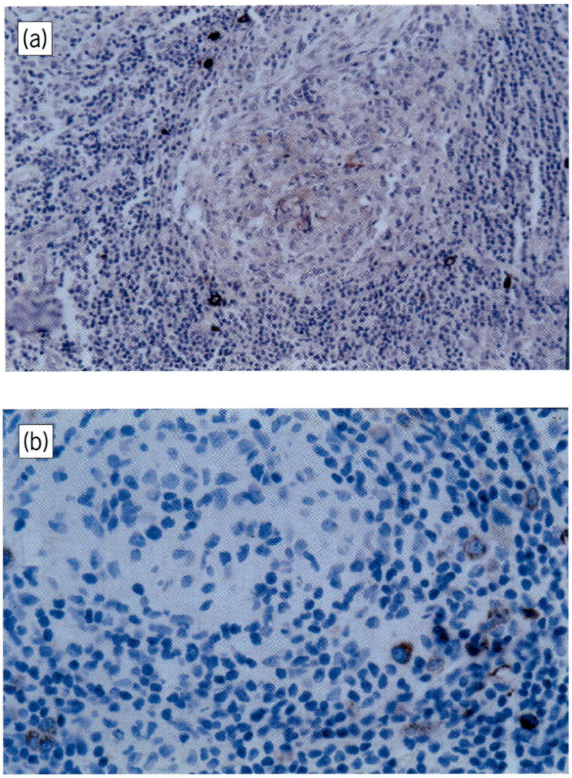

Figure 28.5 Multicentric Castleman's disease (MCD) in an HIV-positive patient. In two adjacent sections, medium-sized plasmacytoid cells around the same abnormal germinal center express vIL-6 (a), detected with a polyclonal antibody, and immunoglobulin λ light chains (b).

uncommon at presentation, although it occurs with increasing frequency with disease progression.[10] Splenomegaly, with or without hepatomegaly, is quite common. Skin manifestations include non-specific rashes, as well as a host of other changes:[119,120]

- pemphigus;
- lichenoid, nodular, or miscellaneous maculopapular eruptions;
- cutaneous necrotizing vasculitis;
- generalized plane xanthomas;
- vitiligo.

A unique skin manifestation of the disease, described only in the Far East, consists of multiple violaceous nodules that histologically show infiltration of the dermis by plasma cells.[76–78] In addition, skin lesions with an unusual histology ('glomeruloid hemangioma') have been described in a few patients.[44,121]

Neurologic manifestations are relatively uncommon in primary MCD (described in 5 of 44 cases), and include poorly defined central nervous system (CNS) changes,[10,58] persistent seizures,[7] and peripheral neuropathy.[7,61] In addition, isolated cases of peripheral neuropathy, usually sensorimotor, have been reported.[6,86,122] Furthermore, an interesting small study described the association of nodal MCD with a distinct syndrome of peripheral neuropathy, pseudotumor cerebri, IgA dysproteinemia (monoclonal in one patient only), and thrombocytosis in four women.[123] These cases raise the issue of the overlap of MCD and POEMS syndrome[124] (see below). In one case of MCD, the CNS symptoms were associated with the presence of plasma cells in the cerebrospinal fluid without evidence of lesions in the brain by computed tomography or magnetic resonance imaging scan.[125]

A wide variety of rheumatologic symptoms and signs can accompany MCD, including arthralgia, myalgia, joint effusions, keratoconjunctivitis sicca, xerostomia, and Raynaud's phenomenon.[7,8,10,126] It may, in fact, be difficult in some cases to distinguish MCD from an autoimmune disease.[127]

Gastrointestinal manifestations, such as antral ulcers and neutropenic enterocolitis, are rarely reported.[128,129]

The most common laboratory findings in patients with MCD have been listed in Table 28.4, and reflect the involvement of multiple systems in this disorder. Anemia is found in the majority of patients, and is often autoimmune in origin.[7,8,10,120,130–133] Thrombocytopenia is common, and may also be autoimmune.[130] In one patient, the simultaneous occurrence of autoimmune hemolytic anemia and immune thrombocytopenia (Evan's syndrome) has been reported.[120] Anti-erythropoietin antibodies, with an accompanying hyperviscosity syndrome, have been described in another patient.[134] The bone marrow often shows mild plasmacytosis.

The ESR is frequently elevated, as is the

level of γ-globulins in the serum. These γ-globulins are usually polyclonal, but monoclonal gammopathy, either at presentation[86] or developing on a polyclonal background,[58] has also been described. Antinuclear antibodies, rheumatoid factor, inhibitors of factors VII and VIII, cryoglobulins, cold agglutinins,[6,135] and anti-smooth-muscle, anti-gastric, anti-salivary-gland and anti-phospholipid antibodies[8,64,131] have also been found occasionally.

Lymphocyte function studies have demonstrated various abnormalities, such as a decrease in the number of T cells, inversion of the $CD4^+ : CD8^+$ ratio, and T-cell unresponsiveness to mitogens,[60,77,136,137] as well as cell-mediated immunodeficiency[137,138] and reduced natural killer (NK)-cell activity.[136] In addition, in four HIV-negative patients with MCD, abnormalities in T-cell and NK-cell function similar to those occurring in AIDS patients have been reported.[19] As already mentioned, increased serum levels of IL-6 and other cytokines seem to be a consistent feature of patients with MCD.

Renal dysfunction is relatively uncommon: proteinuria in 16% and hematuria in 7% of our reviewed cases. These changes and/or evidence of renal insufficiency are also described in many single case reports.[22,131,139,140,141] The histopathology, where available, was heterogeneous, and included: (a) no specific abnormalities; (b) membranous, mesangioproliferative, or membranoproliferative glomerulonephritic patterns; (c) interstitial nephritis;[22,131,141] and (d) amyloidosis.[142,143] In addition, there are rare reports of renal thrombotic microangiopathy, which was thought to be due to autoantibodies.[131] In two patients, a unique combination of mesangial proliferation and interstitial plasma cell infiltration with negative immunofluorescence study was reported. These findings were thought to be related to overproduction of IL-6, a known growth factor for mesangial cells.[22]

MCD has been associated with a variety of syndromes. Amyloidosis is one, although it is less common than in localized CD. In localized CD, it involves the lymphoid mass or single organs, or is systemic in distribution; it is characteristically of AA type,[144–147] and is thought to be related to an excess of the acute-phase reactant serum amyloid A secondary to IL-6 overproduction;[144,145,147] excision of the lymphoid mass results in improvement of the clinical signs of amyloidosis.[144,145,147] The amyloidosis reported in MCD is systemic,[148] renal,[142,143] and intestinal,[149] and is also of AA type.[143,148,149] Amyloidosis in primary MCD appears to be different from that described in 'MCD' associated with myeloma, in which the amyloid is of the AL (λ) type.[150]

Other reported associations in MCD include thrombotic thrombocytopenic purpura,[135] myelofibrosis,[140] pure red cell aplasia,[143] γ heavy-chain disease,[151] vasculitis,[7] pulmonary hyalinizing granuloma,[152] and myasthenia gravis.[153] In one case, MCD (with elevated serum IL-6) was diagnosed after a long history of Behçet's disease, and, interestingly, the two diseases responded to various therapies and recurred together after discontinuation of therapy.[28] Peliosis hepatis, a feature also seen in association with monoclonal lymphoproliferative disorders, such as myeloma and Waldeström's macroglobulinemia, has been reported in two cases of MCD.[119,154]

MCD follows three patterns of clinical evolution: an aggressive, rapidly fatal course, a chronic course with sustained clinical symptoms, or a course characterized by recurrent exacerbations and remissions. These were seen in 19%, 37%, and 44%, respectively, of a total of 27 patients.[7,10,60] Of the 44 patients evaluated, 45% died, with infection being the most common cause of death (60%) and lymphoproliferative disorder being mentioned as the sole cause in 20% of patients. The overall median survival time in this group (excluding the patients who had neoplastic complications) was 34 months. However, the median survival was 14 months for the patients who died, and over 46 months for those who survived. In our series,[10] we found that male gender, presence of enlarged mediastinal lymph nodes, and an episodic pattern of disease were the three clinical features that together best predicted a fatal outcome ($p = 0.002$). The only morphologic feature significantly associated with a fatal outcome was a persistent proliferative pattern in multiple biopsies ($p = 0.005$).

The clinical course of the subset of patients with HHV-8-related 'primary' MCD is poorly defined, since there are only eight evaluable patients in the literature,[28,29,72,75,102,105] but appears to be heterogenous. These patients ranged in age from 21 to 79 years (median 70.5 years). Four of seven patients were alive at the time of the report (including one with associated Behçet's disease, who has been followed for 6 years,[28] and three died within 3 months of their diagnosis.

Therapy

It is difficult to draw conclusions on the management of MCD from our data or those presented in the literature, given the multiplicity of treatments used, the variability of the clinical situations, and the difficulty of exactly defining treatment response retrospectively.[10,155] It appears that all treatment modalities have been able to produce at least some transient improvement in some of the patients.

The treatments used have included steroids alone, chemotherapy (single or multiagent) and – in unique cases – surgery alone (splenectomy or excision of the main nodal mass)[10,133] and radiation therapy alone.[60] Overall, however, steroids appear to be associated with a better survival rate (69%) compared with chemotherapy (36%). Death by infectious complications was equally frequent in patients treated with either approach.

New treatments reported to produce favorable responses in MCD in the more recent literature include interferon-γ (IFN-γ),[28,156] 2-chlorodeoxyadenosine (cladribine),[157] thalidomide (J Mehta, personal communication), cimetidine (which, as a downregulator of T cells that express histamine H_2 receptors, is thought to act by dampening autoimmune phenomena),[158] and even autologous bone marrow transplantation in a refractory case.[159] In addition, the systemic symptoms may be alleviated by the administration of monoclonal anti-huIL-6 antibody.[24, 32]

From accrued experience, a stepwise management strategy has been devised to treat patients with MCD.[155] Some patients may experience a spontaneous remission or may not require therapeutic intervention. Other patients might initially be treated with corticosteroids, which appear to have less toxicity and can result in long-term remissions. Chemotherapy may need to be used in steroid-refractory cases.

Pathogenesis

IL-6 overproduction plays a central role in producing most of the pathologic and clinical manifestations of MCD. However, other factors are probably also involved in the pathogenesis of this disorder.

Autoimmune manifestations are frequently present, at times making it difficult to distinguish MCD from a *bona fide* autoimmune disease. One explanation for the autoimmune phenomena centers around the anti-apoptotic role of IL-6 and proposes that increased IL-6 production in the germinal centers affects the normal elimination of B cells that have undergone 'inappropriate Ig gene mutations', resulting in the emergence of autoreactive clones.[27] A somewhat different explanation emerges from the evidence, discussed above, that the lymphocytes of the abnormal lymphoid follicles of CD may correspond to the long-lived memory B-cell subset Ly-1 in the mouse and to the human $CD5^+$ subset, which naturally produces autoantibodies.[160] This same B-cell population has also been shown to account for a case of neuropathy associated with IgM monoclonal gammopathy.[161] These data complement the IL-6 data already discussed, and suggest a general pathogenetic picture of MCD as a lymphoproliferation of a specific autoantibody-producing B-cell subset, driven by IL-6 and resulting in the sustained production and accumulation of plasma cells.

A final pathogenetic factor in MCD may be the existence of underlying defects of immune regulation.[10,15] The evidence for this includes: (a) the occurrence of the disease in older age groups ('senescent' immune system); (b) the high frequency of intercurrent infections; and (c) the previously discussed abnormalities in the number and functions of lymphoid subsets identified in some patients.[19,60,77,136–138,162]

The distinct subset of cases of MCD related to HHV-8 fits well in this pathogenetic scenario. HHV-8 infection of the lymphoid tissue by itself does not appear to lead to the histologic or clinical manifestations of MCD, since this virus has been found in lymph nodes with other (specific and non-specific) reactive features.[71,101,102,111] However, in the lymphoid tissue of MCD, HHV-8 infection has been found to be associated with the expression of vIL-6,[29,104,114] and HHV-8 mRNA[114] by ISH and vIL-6 protein by immunohistochemistry are both localized in sparse mantle zone B cells.[29,72,109,112,114] Since vIL-6 mimics in vitro[32] and in athymic mice[97] the effects of huIL-6, it may serve as an autocrine growth factor in MCD, as it does in cases of primary effusion lymphoma,[97,163,164] and may account for the characteristic clinical and laboratory manifestations of MCD. This pathogenetic scenario, however, may not yet be complete.

First, the different expression of viral genes reported in different cases raises the question as to whether other HHV-8 genes, in addition to v*IL-6*, are necessary to produce the manifestations of MCD. v*IL-6*, v*cyclin D*, v*bcl-2*, and v*IL-8R* genes were all found to be expressed in one case of MCD, while only the first two were expressed in cases of florid follicular hyperplasia.[115] Similarly, 'several HHV-8 genes' were expressed in another MCD case;[32] but v*IL-6* alone (and not other viral RT-PCR transcripts) was detected in one case of MCD associated with primary effusion lymphoma.[104] Secondly, in an HIV-positive patient with MCD, it was shown that huIL-6, not vIL-6, was responsible for the systemic manifestations of the disease, since these were alleviated by neutralizing anti-huIL-6 monoclonal antibodies.[32] Thus, HHV-8 may not necessarily act via viral homologues of human proteins, but by deregulating in vivo the production of human cytokines;[32] alternatively, HHV-8-infected cells may also produce human cytokines, as observed in vitro with primary effusion lymphoma cell lines, which released not only vIL-6, but also huIL-6 and huIL-10.[164]

One last unresolved issue in MCD is its relationship to localized CD, a point that has been discussed elsewhere in detail.[10] Striking histological and clinical similarities exist between these two forms of disease. The reports of elevated serum levels of IL-6 and IL-6 production in lymphoid tissue in cases of localized CD[16,30] explain some of the similarities. In these cases, IL-6 may act locally in a paracrine fashion, rather than systemically as in MCD. However, there are obvious clinical differences between the localized and multicentric cases:[57] MCD patients are older and have peripheral, rather than central, nodal disease and a more aggressive clinical course, often associated with infection. Some of these differences 'may be due to . . . the more profound immunologic deficit'[7] of the patients with multicentric compared with those with localized disease. It is also possible that the etiology is different: HHV-8, in fact, has been detected in only one[105] of 26 cases of localized CD.[29,99–102] Whatever the answer to this question, it is clear from experience that the management of these disorders is different: the localized lesion is surgically treatable, whereas the multicentric form requires systemic therapy.[10,59,61,155]

'SECONDARY' MULTICENTRIC CASTLEMAN'S DISEASE

As already mentioned, this term is useful to distinguish the instances of 'MCD' (IL-6 syndrome) that occur in association with other diseases. Like 'primary' MCD, these cases appear to have different etiologies (Table 28.5). A large proportion of MCD developing in patients with HIV infection and/or KS[71,72,99,103] and with the POEMS syndrome[29,71,110,165] have been shown to be related to HHV-8. For others, however – especially those developing with autoimmune diseases or adjacent to Hodgkin's disease – such a relationship has not been established, and the IL-6 syndrome may have another explanation. It may, in fact, become important in the future to determine

Table 28.5 Etiology of various forms of multicentric Castleman's disease (MCD)

	HHV-8-positive (%)	HHV-8-negative (%)
'Primary' MCD	47	53
'Secondary' MCD, associated with:		
Kaposi sarcoma	87.5	12.5
HIV infection and Kaposi sarcoma	100	
HIV infection only	95.6	4.4 (?)
POEMS syndrome	90	10 (?)
Non-Hodgkin's lymphoma	'Plasmablastic'	'Late' lymphomas
Hodgkin's disease	—	Paracrine IL-6 disease
Autoimmune disease	?	Most cases?

which 'MCDs' are HHV-8/vIL-6-related and which are HHV-8-negative/huIL-6-related, as well as to determine whether these two groups are clinically and prognostically different.

MCD associated with HIV infection and/or Kaposi sarcoma

One of the various histologic forms of HIV-related lymphadenopathy manifests the 'angio-follicular changes' considered characteristic of CD.[108,166–173] When separated from the mixed (follicular hyperplasia and follicular involution) and the follicular involution histologic stages,[174] this form accounted for 2% or less of the HIV-associated lymph nodes evaluated in three large series.[169,171,173] It has recently been proposed that this association (MCD and HIV infection) represents 'a distinct clinicopathological entity that can be differentiated from other types of HIV-associated systemic lymphoproliferative disorders'.[171] The clinical presentation and laboratory findings in this group of patients were very similar to those of MCD in general: fever and splenomegaly (100%), peripheral lymphadenopathy (90%), severe weight loss (70%), edema (55%), anemia (100%), high level of C-reactive protein (90%), hypergammaglobulinemia (89%), and hypoalbuminemia (56%). This syndrome (which was associated with HHV-8 in all cases) differed from MCD observed in HIV-negative patients because of the younger age at presentation (median 39 years), predominance of men (M : F = 19 : 1), a higher prevalence of pulmonary symptoms (cough, dyspnea, interstitial infiltrates: 65%), more frequent pancytopenia (35%), and a higher incidence of KS (75%). Remission was obtained in most patients with low-dose and usually single-agent chemotherapy, but the mortality rate was high (70%), with a median survival of 9.5 months in the entire series and 12.5 months among those who survived.

The outcome in these HIV-positive MCD patients, however, may be dependent on the added burden of KS (Table 28.6). If one considers (in this[171] and other reports[72,107,108]) only the patients without KS, then only half of them died – a mortality figure similar to that of primary MCD. However, if one separates those with KS,[32,72,107,114,167,168,171,172,175,176] then the mortality rate increases to 75%, with survivals varying from a few weeks to 39 months (median 7 months): in these patients, death was due to infection, organ failure, or KS, in similar proportions. A cluster of three patients with this combination (HIV infection, MCD, and KS) and rapidly progressive course (fatal in two) has been reported during highly active antiretroviral therapy for AIDS: it was concluded that this combination should be considered as a medical emergency.[177] Therefore, it is possible that it is the concurrence of KS, sug-

Table 28.6 Clinical comparison of primary multicentric Castleman's disease (MCD) and MCD associated with other diseases

	Primary MCD[a]	HIV-positive MCD[b]	MCD with KS	
			HIV-positive[c]	HIV-negative[d]
No. of patients	44	10	29	26
Age (years):				
Range	19–85	28–62	21–67	26–87
Median	55.5	40.5	36	67
Males (%)	59	90	93	62
Alive (%)	55	50	25	19
Dead (%)	45	50	75	81
Range (months)	3–72	1–19	Weeks–39	1–42
Median (months)	14	7	7	6

[a]References 7, 10, 58–61. [b]References 72, 107, 108, 171. [c]References 32, 72, 107, 114, 167, 168, 171, 172, 175, 176. [d]References 7, 10, 29, 67, 102, 112, 141, 178–183.

gesting a more disseminated HHV-8 infection, that accounts for the poor prognosis of these MCD patients, not the HIV infection per se.

The association of KS and MCD is also reported in the absence of HIV infection, in a total of 26 patients.[7,10,29,67,102,112,141,178–183] These patients, who manifested the characteristic clinical features of MCD, had a mortality rate (81%) and median survival (6 months) quite similar to those of the HIV-positive MCD patients with KS, but were much older (69% were 60 years or more) and almost equally male and female (Table 28.6). This, however, does not appear be a homogeneous group, since it includes: (a) patients who manifested an acute disease, with both MCD and KS diagnosed in their lymph nodes, and died within a few months of various causes;[29,67,178,179,184] (b) patients with long-standing KS, who later (16–156 months) developed 'MCD' and died of a lymphoproliferative disease or KS after a longer period of time from the diagnosis of MCD (median 23 months);[7,10,183] and (c) patients initially diagnosed with MCD who later (weeks to 24 months) developed cutaneous KS, and most of whom died, of various causes, 8–19 months after the diagnosis of MCD.[10,141,180–182,185] It is quite possible that the first two subgroups represent instances of primary HHV-8 infection and vIL-6 production, resulting in KS and, simultaneously or later, lymphoid tissue disease (MCD), while the third is composed of patients with MCD, possibly autoimmune in origin and driven by huIL-6, who later acquired a secondary HHV-8 infection (and KS) on the basis of their immunocompromised status. In one of the patients from this third group, in fact, HHV-8 was detected in the KS, but not in the MCD nodal lesion.[181]

MCD and POEMS syndrome

A multisystem disorder combining peripheral polyneuropathy, organomegaly, endocrine abnormalities, various forms of plasma cell dyscrasia, and skin lesions, as well as a host of less consistent manifestations, was first reported by Crow[186] in Britain and later by several groups in Japan.[187,188] This syndrome has been referred to as 'Crow-Fukase',[189] 'Takatsuki',[190] or, more frequently, POEMS.[191] The polyneuropathy syndrome, which is sensory–motor in type, is characteristically bilateral, distal, with progressive proximal spread. Organomegaly includes lymphadenopathy and hepatosplenomegaly. The endocrine disorders are variable; however, the most common is diabetes mellitus, followed by hypogonadism and hypothyroidism. The most frequent skin changes are hyperpigmentation, thickening, hyperthrichosis, and angiomas. The plasma cell dyscrasia is most usually manifested by a serum monoclonal IgGλ or IgAλ spike, and spans the spectrum from classic myeloma, osteosclerotic myeloma, Waldenström's macroglobulinemia, monoclonal gammopathy of undetermined significance (MGUS), to polyclonal hypergammaglobulinemia.[48,189,191–195]

In fact, the definition of POEMS syndrome and the clinical findings in the different series have varied, largely owing to the criteria used for 'plasma cell dyscrasia': some studies accept all types of plasma cell disorders (including myeloma and polyclonal hypergammaglobulinemia),[189] others include only cases with serum monoclonal proteins (with or without bone lesions),[48,194] while others equate POEMS syndrome with osteosclerotic myeloma.[193] Osteosclerotic myeloma, however, is the most common form of plasma cell dyscrasia in all series.[194] A unifying pathogenetic hypothesis for such varied manifestations is not yet available, although it is generally accepted that the anti-tissue effects of immunoglobulins,[196] especially anti-nerve antibodies,[197,198] and one or more soluble factors produced by the plasma cells are responsible for most of the clinical symptoms and laboratory abnormalities seen in this syndrome.[194]

Lymphadenopathy is a feature of 42–73% of patients with the POEMS syndrome, depending on the definition of the latter.[48,189,192–194] However, the histologic findings in the lymph nodes are variable, and include Castleman's-like changes, plasmacytoma, non-specific abnormalities, and normal histology. Overall, these various histologic forms account for 63%, 7%, 30%, and 0%, respectively, in Japan[189] and 63%, 13%, 13%, and 11%, respectively, in a compilation of 68 non-Asian patients.[194] Japanese pathologists were the first to recognize that some patients presenting with the combination of clinical findings later referred to as POEMS syndrome showed lymph node lesions closely resembling those of CD.[13] They also noted that 29% of these lymph nodes contained sheet-like or nodular accumulations of monoclonal plasma cells within a background of polyclonal plasma cells, blurring somewhat the distinction between MCD with a monoclonal component and nodal plasmacytoma.[13] These observations have since been confirmed in the West.[68,85,191,196,199–203]

Along with the histologic nodal lesions of CD, patients with POEMS syndrome may present with clinical and laboratory features characteristic of MCD: weight loss, splenomegaly, edema, effusions, nephropathy, autoimmune manifestations (such as systemic lupus erythematosus (SLE) or mixed connective tissue disease),[204,205] and cutaneous glomeruloid hemangiomas.[202] In recent large series of POEMS patients, the incidence of the MCD clinicopathologic complex is 38–50%.[48,110,165]

In addition, in many, but not all,[194] POEMS patients, there are increased serum levels of the same cytokines that are elevated in MCD.[48,203,205,206] More specifically, elevated serum levels of IL-6, TNF-α, and IL-1β are found in 67–93% of patients with POEMS.[48] Although it has been suggested that the activation of these proinflammatory cytokines, coupled with decreased levels of the antagonist, transforming growth factor (TGF)-β1, accounts for the manifestations of POEMS syndrome, it is most likely that IL-6 overproduction accounts instead for the MCD-like manifestations, since IL-6 levels have not been found to be increased in POEMS patients without MCD.[207]

There is, therefore, overlap between the POEMS syndrome and MCD, which is best explained by overproduction of IL-6 in a subset of POEMS patients. More recently, it has been shown by PCR analysis of lymphoid (and hematopoietic) tissues that 90% of POEMS patients with MCD,[29,71,110] but only 17% of those without MCD,[110] were HHV-8-positive. In one study, which evaluated the ORF26 region of the virus, only subgroup B was detected, rather than subgroup A, which is found in KS and MCD.[110] By serologic means, HHV-8 was identified in 75–78%,[110,208] or 20%[165] of POEMS patients with MCD, versus 13–22% of POEMS patients without MCD.[110,208] This evidence is strong enough to support the concept that a subset of patients with the POEMS syndrome (most of them with osteosclerotic myeloma) is associated with HHV-8-driven MCD.[110] As HHV-8 is a lymphotropic virus and the lymphoid tissues are sites of virus latency, it has been suggested that the course of this subset of POEMS patients might be complicated by an immunodeficiency state or an unknown cofactor. This may induce reactivation of HHV-8, possibly of a specific subtype, resulting in an increased systemic viral load, production of lymphokines, and, ultimately, the development of MCD.[110] The pathogenesis of MCD in the remaining HHV-8-negative POEMS patients is unclear, but may involve production of human, rather than viral, IL-6 by the plasma cells.

The above explanation of the overlap between POEMS syndrome and MCD allows for the various clonal plasma cell patterns described in POEMS patients. In the usual case, a bone marrow plasma cell dyscrasia is complicated by IL-6 overproduction (or HHV-8 infection), which results in the classic polyclonal CD lymph node lesion. In other patients, the polyclonal CD nodal lesion might be associated with a monoclonal plasma cell component – either a metastasis from the marrow clone or a local clonal evolution of the polyclonal nodal plasma cell proliferation. Alternatively, a de novo nodal plasmacytoma (without bone marrow involvement) may be responsible for the serum gammopathy and its effects. And, finally, a primary (HHV-8-positive or HHV-8-negative) MCD (polyclonal) could be the underlying cause of the unusual cases of POEMS syndrome – in its complete or incomplete[123] form – without plasma cell dyscrasia.[189]

CD and other neoplasms

The sparse reports of patients with both 'CD', of either localized or multicentric type, and neoplasms other than KS or plasma cell dyscrasia fall into two categories: those describing synchronous occurrence of CD and a neoplasm, and others describing the even more uncommon, subsequent development of a neoplasm in patients with CD.

Most commonly (a total of 30 cases), CD has been described in association with Hodgkin's disease (HD).[70,91,209–217] In all cases, except one,[216] the histologic lesions of CD and HD were intermixed in the same tissue specimen. In several reports,[91,211,213] HD was initially diagnosed on a second biopsy, but review of the previous specimen, diagnosed as CD, revealed the presence of occult HD. Thus, the only reported case of CD followed six years later by HD[216] might be an example of HD unrecognized the first time.

The unanimous interpretation of the association of HD and CD is that 'CD' is a non-specific pathologic finding,[53,210–215] thought to occur (a) as a local manifestation of the abnormal immune status of patients with HD[210,212,214,215] or (b) as the result of cytokine production by HD. The role of IL-6 is suggested by the increased serum levels of IL-6 in over half of the patients with HD[52] and by the detection of IL-6 in supernatants of HD cell lines.[52] Furthermore, IL-6 has been detected by immunohistochemistry and molecular techniques in Reed–Sternberg cells and/or the background inflammatory cells.[52,53,55,56] Finally, IL-6R is also found to be expressed by Reed–Sternberg cells, suggesting that IL-6 may be involved in the pathogenesis of HL via an autocrine or paracrine mechanism.[52]

Non-Hodgkin's lymphomas have similarly been reported to occur in association with CD, of either localized or multicentric type.[7,71,72,104,171,172,180,218–220] In some patients, the lymphoma presents simultaneously with the 'MCD' clinicopathologic syndrome[7,172,180] or develops rapidly (within 2–9 months) during the course of the syndrome.[7,58,70,72] These 'early' lymphomas include various types: diffuse large cell,[7] diffuse mixed peripheral T-cell,[7] immunoblastic,[171] and the recently described 'plasmablastic lymphomas', composed of medium-sized cells, with amphophilic cytoplasm and prominent nucleolus(i).[72] This latter type of lymphoma is unique in that it is reported to occur in patients with the HHV-8-positive 'plasmablastic variant' of MCD, the lymphoma cells often contain HHV-8, and the tumor cells only express the λ light chain. Thus, plasmablastic lymphoma may be a new disease entity associated with HHV-8, *au pair* with KS, primary effusion lymphoma, and some cases of MCD.[72] Therefore, in some patients with MCD who develop 'early' lymphomas, both diseases might be etiologically related to HHV-8. In others, such as those with lymphoma of peripheral T-cell type,[7,218] other explanations might apply, such as a coincidental occurrence, the development of both diseases on the basis of an immunodeficient status, or development of a MCD driven by the huIL-6 produced by the lymphoma.

A second group of lymphomas were reported to develop much later (3–14 years) after the diagnosis of MCD[7,10,59,62,69,79,104,138,221] ('late' lymphomas). In our review of 44 primary cases of MCD, lymphoma developed in 5 patients (11%) – a figure similar to that arrived at in a series of MCD without neuropathy (15%).[62,69] These late lymphomas were classified as of diffuse mixed or large cell type according to the Working Formulation; in only a rare case is there any immunophenotypic[79] and in none a genotypic documentation of clonality and/or cell lineage. The pathogenesis of these lymphomas is unclear, but may be different from that of early lymphomas. However, HHV-8 has been detected in one case.[104]

Finally, there are very rare reports of non-lymphoid tumors associated with 'CD'. Some were diagnosed simultaneously with CD, and include rectal carcinoma,[128] neurofibromatosis and pheochromocytoma,[222] and renal cell carcinoma;[223] one patient had both thyroid and kidney carcinoma.[224] In these cases, the 'CD' was of the PC type (either localized or multicentric), and was probably due to IL-6 production by the tumor,[222,223] as in the cases of CD associated with Hodgkin's disease discussed above. Other neoplasms occurred as late complications of MCD. These include colon carcinoma,[10] carcinoma of the prostate,[221] renal cell carcinoma,[21] myeloproliferative disorder, and thymoma.[7]

MCD associated with autoimmune diseases

It has already been mentioned that clinical and laboratory manifestations of autoimmunity are occasionally reported in MCD. In fact, in some cases, the distinction of MCD from an autoimmune disease is a moot point, the lymph node pathology being of no help because of its lack of specificity. The overlap between MCD and autoimmune disease in individual cases has been explained in a variety of ways: (a) as a concurrence of MCD with an autoimmune disease, such as rheumatoid arthritis,[225] Sjögren syndrome,[226] or mixed connective tissue disease;[205] (b) as MCD presenting with aspects of an autoimmune disease;[126,127,227] or (c) as an autoimmune disease (SLE) manifesting with the histopathologic features of MCD.[228] A similar issue arises in the rare patients with MCD who present with lung infiltrates composed of lymphoid cells and plasma cells,[9,37,74,75] since these findings of 'diffuse lymphoid hyperplasia' or lymphocytic interstitial pneumonitis are also common in patients with connective tissue diseases.[37]

This clinicopathologic overlap may be explained by pathologic data suggesting that primary MCD might be a lymphoproliferative disorder of a specific autoantibody-producing B-cell subset. Thus, at least in the cases in which this proliferation produces clinical and laboratory autoimmune manifestations, MCD may indeed be seen as a specific form of autoimmune disease, characterized, as it has been suggested, by 'unremitting or progressive lymphadenopathy'.[227] Thus, whether these overlap cases are best classified as autoimmune disorders or as MCD is a matter of opinion. From a practical point of view, if the lymphoproliferation predominates over autoimmune phenomena,[9] and the pattern of clinical and serologic findings is insufficient for a definitive diagnosis of a specific rheumatologic entity,[155] then the diagnosis is most likely MCD.

REFERENCES

1. Castleman B, Iverson L, Menendez VP. Localized mediastinal lymph node hyperplasia resembling thymoma. *Cancer* 1956; **9**: 822–30.
2. Flendrig JA. Benign giant lymphoma: clinicopathologic correlation study. Chicago: Year Book Medical 1970: 296–9.
3. Flendrig JA, Schillings PHM. Benign giant lymphoma: the clinical signs and symptoms. *Folia Med Neerl* 1969; **12**: 119–20.
4. Keller AR, Hochholzer L, Castleman B. Hyaline–vascular and plasma-cell types of giant lymph node hyperplasia of the mediastinum and other locations. *Cancer* 1972; **29**: 670–83.
5. Leibetseder F, Thurner J. Angiofollikulare Lymphknotenhyperplasie (Zwiebelschalenlymphom). *Med Klin* 1973; **68**: 817–20.
6. Gaba AR, Stein RS, Sweet DL, Variakojis D. Multicentric giant lymph node hyperplasia. *Am J Clin Pathol* 1978; **69**: 86–90.
7. Weisenburger DD, Nathwani BN, Winberg CD, Rappaport H. Multicentric angiofollicular lymph node hyperplasia: a clinicopathologic study of 16 cases. *Hum Pathol* 1985; **16**: 162–72.
8. Diebold J, Tulliez M, Bernadou A et al. Angiofollicular and plasmacytic polyadenopathy: a pseudotumourous syndrome with dysimmunity. *J Clin Pathol* 1980; **33**: 1068–76.
9. Frizzera G, Banks PM, Massarelli G, Rosai J. A systemic lymphoproliferative disorder with morphologic features of Castleman's disease. Pathological findings in 15 patients. *Am J Surg Pathol* 1983; **7**: 211–31.
10. Frizzera G, Peterson BA, Bayrd ED, Goldman A. A systemic lymphoproliferative disorder with morphologic features of Castleman's disease: clinical findings and clinicopathologic correlations in 15 patients. *J Clin Oncol* 1985; **3**: 1202–16.
11. Mori S, Mohri N, Uchida T, Shimamine T. Idiopathic plasmacytic lymphadenopathy with polyclonal hyperimmunoglobulinemia. A syndrome related to giant lymph node hyperlasia of plasma cell type. *J Jpn Soc Res* 1981; **20**(Suppl): 85–94.
12. Mori N, Tsunoda R, Kojima K. Multicentric lymphadenopathy histologically simulating Castleman's disease. *J Jpn Soc Res* 1981; **20**(Suppl): 55–66.
13. Kojima M, Sakuma H, Mori N. Histopathological features of plasma cell dyscrasia with polyneuropathy and endocrine disturbances, with special reference to germinal center lesions. *Jpn J Clin Oncol* 1983; **13**: 557–75.
14. Knecht H, Schwarze EW, Lennert K. Histological, immunohistological and autopsy findings in lymphogranulomatosis X (including angioimmunoblastic lymphadenopathy). *Virchows Arch A Pathol Anat Histopathol* 1985; **406**: 105–24.
15. Frizzera G. Castleman's disease: more questions than answers. *Hum Pathol* 1985; **16**: 202–5.
16. Yoshizaki K, Matsuda T, Nishimoto N et al. Pathogenic significance of interleukin-6 (IL-6/BSF-2) in Castleman's disease. *Blood* 1989; **74**: 1360–7.
17. Herbelin C, Roux-Lombard P, Herbelin A et al. Inflammation: 'a natural experiment' for the systemic pathogenicity of cytokines. *Eur Cytokine Netw* 1998; **9**: 57–60.
18. Hsu SM, Waldron JA, Xie SS, Barlogie B. Expression of interleukin-6 in Castleman's disease. *Hum Pathol* 1993; **24**: 833–9.
19. Ishiyama T, Nakamura S, Akimoto Y et al. Immunodeficiency and IL-6 production by peripheral blood monocytes in multicentric Castleman's disease. *Br J Haematol* 1994; **86**: 483–9.
20. Kinney MC, Hummell DS, Villiger PM et al. Increased interleukin-6 (IL-6) production in a young child with clinical and pathologic features of multicentric Castleman's disease. *J Clin Immunol* 1994; **14**: 382–90.
21. Lee M, Hirokawa M, Matuoka S et al. Multicentric Castleman's disease with an increased serum level of macrophage colony-stimulating factor. *Am J Hematol* 1997; **54**: 321–3.
22. Lui SL, Chan KW, Li FK et al. Castleman's disease and mesangial proliferative glomerulonephritis: the role of interleukin-6. *Nephron* 1998; **78**: 323–7.
23. Mandler RN, Kerrigan DP, Smart J et al. Castleman's disease in POEMS syndrome with elevated interleukin-6. *Cancer* 1992; **69**: 2697–703.
24. Beck JT, Hsu SM, Wijdenes J et al. Alleviation of systemic manifestations of Castleman's disease by monoclonal anti-interleukin-6 antibody. *N Engl J Med* 1994; **330**: 602–5.
25. Winter SS, Howard TA, Ritchey AK et al. Elevated levels of tumor necrosis factor-beta, gamma-interferon, and IL-6 mRNA in Castleman's disease. *Med Pediatr Oncol* 1996; **26**: 48–53.
26. Veldhuis GJ, van der Leest AH, de Wolf JT et al. A case of localized Castleman's disease with sys-

temic involvement: treatment and pathogenetic aspects. *Ann Hematol* 1996; **73**: 47–50.
27. Emilie D, Zou W, Fior R et al. Production and roles of IL-6, IL-10, and IL-13 in B-lymphocyte malignancies and in B-lymphocyte hyperactivity of HIV infection and autoimmunity. *Methods* 1997; **11**: 133–42.
28. Strohal R, Tschachler E, Breyer S et al. Reactivation of Behçet's disease in the course of multicentric HHV8-positive Castleman's disease: long-term complete remission by a combined chemo/radiation and interferon-alpha therapy regimen. *Br J Haematol* 1998; **103**: 788–90.
29. Parravicini C, Corbellino M, Paulli M et al. Expression of a virus-derived cytokine, KSHV vIL-6, in HIV-seronegative Castleman's disease. *Am J Pathol* 1997; **151**: 1517–22.
30. Leger-Ravet MB, Peuchmaur M, Devergne O et al. Interleukin-6 gene expression in Castleman's disease. *Blood* 1991; **78**: 2923–30.
31. Ishiyama T, Koike M, Nakamura S et al. Interleukin-6 receptor expression in the peripheral B cells of patients with multicentric Castleman's disease. *Ann Hematol* 1996; **73**: 179–82.
32. Foussat A, Fior R, Girard T et al. Involvement of human interleukin-6 in systemic manifestations of human herpesvirus type 8-associated multicentric Castleman's disease. *AIDS* 1999; **13**: 150–2.
33. Brandt SJ, Bodine DM, Dunbar CE, Nienhuis AW. Dysregulated interleukin 6 expression produces a syndrome resembling Castleman's disease in mice. *J Clin Invest* 1990; **86**: 592–9.
34. Screpanti I, Romani L, Musiani P et al. Lymphoproliferative disorder and imbalanced T-helper response in C/EBP beta-deficient mice. *EMBO J* 1995; **14**: 1932–41.
35. Screpanti I, Musiani P, Bellavia D et al. Inactivation of the IL-6 gene prevents development of multicentric Castleman's disease in C/EBP beta-deficient mice. *J Exp Med* 1996; **184**: 1561–6.
36. Yoshida M, Sakuma J, Hayashi S, et al. A histologically distinctive interstitial pneumonia induced by overexpression of the interleukin 6, transforming growth factor beta 1, or platelet-derived growth factor B gene. *Proc Natl Acad Sci USA* 1995; **92**: 9570–4.
37. Johkoh T, Muller NL, Ichikado K et al. Intrathoracic multicentric Castleman disease: CT findings in 12 patients. *Radiology* 1998; **209**: 477–81.
38. Yoshizaki K, Kuritani T, Kishimoto T. Interleukin-6 in autoimmune disorders. *Semin Immunol* 1992; **4**: 155–66.
39. Akira S, Taga T, Kishimoto T. Interleukin-6 in biology and medicine. *Adv Immunol* 1993; **54**: 1–78.
40. Kawano MM, Mihara K, Huang N et al. Differentiation of early plasma cells on bone marrow stromal cells requires interleukin-6 for escaping from apoptosis. *Blood* 1995; **85**: 487–94.
41. Ramadori G, Christ B. Cytokines and the hepatic acute-phase response. *Semin Liver Dis* 1999; **19**: 141–55.
42. Foss HD, Araujo I, Demel G et al. Expression of vascular endothelial growth factor in lymphomas and Castleman's disease. *J Pathol* 1997; **183**: 44–50.
43. Nishi J, Arimura K, Utsunomiya A et al. Expression of vascular endothelial growth factor in sera and lymph nodes of the plasma cell type of Castleman's disease. *Br J Haematol* 1999; **104**: 482–5.
44. Chan JK, Fletcher CD, Hicklin GA, Rosai J. Glomeruloid hemangioma. A distinctive cutaneous lesion of multicentric Castleman's disease associated with POEMS syndrome. *Am J Surg Pathol* 1990; **14**: 1036–46.
45. Marfaing-Koka A, Aubin JT, Grangeot-Keros L et al. In vivo role of IL-6 on the viral load and on immunological abnormalities of HIV-infected patients. *J Acquir Immune Defic Syndr Hum Retrovirol* 1996; **11**: 59–68.
46. Suffredini AF, Fantuzzi G, Badolato R et al. New insights into the biology of the acute phase response. *J Clin Immunol* 1999; **19**: 203–14.
47. Presterl E, Lassnigg A, Mueller-Uri P et al. Cytokines in sepsis due to *Candida albicans* and in bacterial sepsis. *Eur Cytokine Netw* 1999; **10**: 423–30.
48. Gherardi RK, Belec L, Soubrier M, et al. Overproduction of proinflammatory cytokines imbalanced by their antagonists in POEMS syndrome. *Blood* 1996; **87**: 1458–65.
49. Miles SA, Rezai AR, Salazar-Gonzalez JF et al. AIDS Kaposi sarcoma-derived cells produce and respond to interleukin 6. *Proc Natl Acad Sci USA* 1990; **87**: 4068–72.
50. Burger R, Wendler J, Antoni K et al. Interleukin-6 production in B-cell neoplasias and Castleman's disease: evidence for an additional paracrine loop. *Ann Hematol* 1994; **69**: 25–31.
51. Emilie D, Coumbaras J, Raphael M et al. Interleukin-6 production in high-grade B

lymphomas: correlation with the presence of malignant immunoblasts in acquired immunodeficiency syndrome and in human immunodeficiency virus-seronegative patients. *Blood* 1992; **80**: 498–504.
52. Tesch H, Jucker M, Klein S et al. Hodgkin and Reed–Sternberg cells express interleukin 6 and interleukin 6 receptors. *Leuk Lymphoma* 1992; **7**: 297–303.
53. Hsu SM, Xie SS, Hsu PL, Waldron JA Jr. Interleukin-6, but not interleukin-4, is expressed by Reed–Sternberg cells in Hodgkin's disease with or without histologic features of Castleman's disease. *Am J Pathol* 1992; **141**: 129–38.
54. Hsu SM, Hsu PL. Autocrine and paracrine functions of cytokines in malignant lymphomas. *Biomed Pharmacother* 1994; **48**: 433–44.
55. Foss HD, Herbst H, Oelmann E et al. Lymphotoxin, tumour necrosis factor and interleukin-6 gene transcripts are present in Hodgkin and Reed–Sternberg cells of most Hodgkin's disease cases. *Br J Haematol* 1993; **84**: 627–35.
56. Jucker M, Abts H, Li W et al. Expression of interleukin-6 and interleukin-6 receptor in Hodgkin's disease. *Blood* 1991; **77**: 2413–8.
57. Frizzera G. Castleman's disease and related disorders. *Semin Diagn Pathol* 1988; **5**: 346–64.
58. Kessler E. Multicentric giant lymph node hyperplasia. A report of seven cases. *Cancer* 1985; **56**: 2446–51.
59. Herrada J, Cabanillas F, Rice L et al, The clinical behavior of localized and multicentric Castleman disease. *Ann Intern Med* 1998; **128**: 657–62.
60. Artusi T, Bonacorsi G, Saragoni A et al. Castleman's lymphoadenopathy: twenty years of observation. II. Generalized form. *Haematologica* 1982; **67**: 124–42.
61. Bowne WB, Lewis JJ, Filippa DA et al. The management of unicentric and multicentric Castleman's disease: a report of 16 cases and a review of the literature. *Cancer* 1999; **85**: 706–17.
62. Menke DM, Camoriano JK, Banks PM. Angiofollicular lymph node hyperplasia: a comparison of unicentric, multicentric, hyaline vascular, and plasma cell types of disease by morphometric and clinical analysis. *Mod Pathol* 1992; **5**: 525–30.
63. Nguyen DT, Diamond LW, Hansmann ML et al. Castleman's disease. Differences in follicular dendritic network in the hyaline vascular and plasma cell variants. *Histopathology* 1994; **24**: 437–43.
64. Summerfield GP, Taylor W, Bellingham AJ, Goldsmith HJ. Hyaline–vascular variant of angiofollicular lymph node hyperplasia with systemic manifestations and response to corticosteroids. *J Clin Pathol* 1983; **36**: 1005–11.
65. Rosen LB, Robinson MJ, Rywlin AM. Familial multicentric angiofollicular lymphoid hyperplasia. *South Med J* 1983; **76**: 1183–4.
66. Cousineau S, Beauchamp G, Boileau J. Extramedullary plasmacytoma associated with angiofollicular lymph node hyperplasia. *Arch Pathol Lab Med* 1986; **110**: 157–8.
67. Leoncini L, del Vecchio MT, Minacci C et al. Kaposi's sarcoma of lymph nodes associated with multicentric angiofollicular hyperplasia. *Appl Pathol* 1989; **7**: 329–32.
68. Gould SJ, Diss T, Isaacson PG. Multicentric Castleman's disease in association with a solitary plasmacytoma: a case report. *Histopathology* 1990; **17**: 135–40.
69. Menke DM, Tiemann M, Camoriano JK et al. Diagnosis of Castleman's disease by identification of an immunophenotypically aberrant population of mantle zone B lymphocytes in paraffin-embedded lymph node biopsies. *Am J Clin Pathol* 1996; **105**: 268–76.
70. Soulier J, Grollet L, Oksenhendler E et al. Molecular analysis of clonality in Castleman's disease. *Blood* 1995; **86**: 1131–8.
71. Soulier J, Grollet L, Oksenhendler E et al. Kaposi's sarcoma-associated herpesvirus-like DNA sequences in multicentric Castleman's disease. *Blood* 1995; **86**: 1276–80.
72. Dupin N, Diss T, Kellam P et al. HHV-8 is associated with a plasmablastic variant of Castleman's disease that is linked to HHV-8 positive plasmablastic lymphoma. *Blood* 2000; **95**: 1406–12.
73. Weisenburger DD. Multicentric angiofollicular lymph node hyperplasia. Pathology of the spleen. *Am J Surg Pathol* 1988; **12**: 176–81.
74. Torii K, Ogawa K, Kawabata Y et al. Lymphoid interstitial pneumonia as a pulmonary lesion of idiopathic plasmacytic lymphadenopathy with hyperimmunoglobulinemia. *Intern Med* 1994; **33**: 237–41.
75. Hayashi M, Aoshiba K, Shimada M et al. Kaposi's sarcoma-associated herpesvirus infection in the lung in multicentric Castleman's disease. *Intern Med* 1999; **38**: 279–82.
76. Watanabe S, Ohara K, Kukita A, Mori S. Systemic plasmacytosis. A syndrome of peculiar multiple skin eruptions, generalized lymphadenopathy,

and polyclonal hypergammaglobulinemia. *Arch Dermatol* 1986; **122**: 1314–20.

77. Kitamura K, Tamura N, Hatano H et al. A case of plasmacytosis with multiple peculiar eruptions. *J Dermatol* 1980; **7**: 341–9.
78. Kubota Y, Noto S, Takakuwa T et al. Skin involvement in giant lymph node hyperplasia (Castleman's disease). *J Am Acad Dermatol* 1993; **29**: 778–80.
79. Nitta Y. Case of malignant lymphoma associated with primary systemic plasmacytosis with polyclonal hypergammaglobulinemia. *Am J Dermatopathol* 1997; **19**: 289–93.
80. Skelton HG, Smith KJ. Extranodal multicentric Castleman's disease with cutaneous involvement. *Mod Pathol* 1998; **11**: 93–8.
81. Hall PA, Donaghy M, Cotter FE et al. An immunohistological and genotypic study of the plasma cell form of Castleman's disease. *Histopathology* 1989; **14**: 333–46.
82. Weisenburger DD, Lipscomb Grierson H, Purtilo D. Immunologic studies of multicentric (M) and unicentric (U) angiofollicular lymphoid hyperplasia (AFH). *Lab Invest* 1986; **54**: 68A.
83. Martin JM, Bell B, Ruether BA. Giant lymph node hyperplasia (Castleman's disease) of hyaline vascular type. Clinical heterogeneity with immunohistologic uniformity. *Am J Clin Pathol* 1985; **84**: 439–46.
84. Hanson CA, Frizzera G, Patton DF et al. Clonal rearrangement for immunoglobulin and T-cell receptor genes in systemic Castleman's disease. Association with Epstein–Barr virus. *Am J Pathol* 1988; **131**: 84–91.
85. Case records of the Massachusetts General Hospital. Weekly clinicopathological exercises. Case 10-1987. A 59-year-old woman with progressive polyneuropathy and monoclonal gammopathy. *N Engl J Med* 1987; **316**: 606–18.
86. Hineman VL, Phyliky RL, Banks PM. Angiofollicular lymph node hyperplasia and peripheral neuropathy: association with monoclonal gammopathy. *Mayo Clin Proc* 1982; **57**: 379–82.
87. Radaszkiewicz T, Hansmann ML, Lennert K. Monoclonality and polyclonality of plasma cells in Castleman's disease of the plasma cell variant. *Histopathology* 1989; **14**: 11–24.
88. Ohyashiki JH, Ohyashiki K, Kawakubo K et al. Molecular genetic, cytogenetic, and immunophenotypic analyses in Castleman's disease of the plasma cell type. *Am J Clin Pathol* 1994; **101**: 290–5.
89. Liu K, Liu J, Mann KP et al. B-cell clonality in Castleman's disease, plasma cell type. *Mod Pathol* 1997; **10**: 129a (abst).
90. Nagai M, Irino S, Uda H et al. Molecular genetic and immunohistochemical analyses of a case of multicentric Castleman's disease. *Jpn J Clin Oncol* 1988; **18**: 149–57.
91. Murray PG, Deacon E, Young LS et al. Localization of Epstein–Barr virus in Castleman's disease by in situ hybridization and immunohistochemistry. *Hematol Pathol* 1995; **9**: 17–26.
92. Nakamura H, Nakaseko C, Ishii A et al. Chromosomal abnormalities in Castleman's disease with high levels of serum interleukin-6. [In Japanese.] *Rinsho Ketsueki* 1993; **34**: 212–7.
93. Brooks LA, Wilson AJ, Crook T. Kaposi's sarcoma-associated herpesvirus (KSHV)/human herpesvirus 8 (HHV8) – a new human tumour virus. *J Pathol* 1997; **182**: 262–5.
94. Cesarman E, Mesri EA. Virus-associated lymphomas. *Curr Opin Oncol* 1999; **11**: 322–32.
95. Nicholas J, Ruvolo VR, Burns WH et al. Kaposi's sarcoma-associated human herpesvirus-8 encodes homologues of macrophage inflammatory protein-1 and interleukin-6. *Nature Med* 1997; **3**: 287–92.
96. Neipel F, Albrecht JC, Ensser A et al. Human herpesvirus 8 encodes a homolog of interleukin-6. *J Virol* 1997; **71**: 839–42.
97. Aoki Y, Jaffe ES, Chang Y et al. Angiogenesis and hematopoiesis induced by Kaposi's sarcoma-associated herpesvirus-encoded interleukin-6. *Blood* 1999; **93**: 4034–43.
98. Wan X, Wang H, Nicholas J. Human herpesvirus 8 interleukin-6 (vIL-6) signals through gp130 but has structural and receptor-binding properties distinct from those of human IL-6. *J Virol* 1999; **73**: 8268–78.
99. Gessain A, Sudaka A, Briere J et al. Kaposi sarcoma-associated herpes-like virus (human herpesvirus type 8) DNA sequences in multicentric Castleman's disease: Is there any relevant association in non-human immunodeficiency virus-infected patients? *Blood* 1996; **87**: 414–6.
100. Corbellino M, Poirel L, Aubin JT et al. The role of human herpesvirus 8 and Epstein–Barr virus in the pathogenesis of giant lymph node hyperplasia (Castleman's disease). *Clin Infect Dis* 1996; **22**: 1120–1.
101. Luppi M, Barozzi P, Maiorana A et al. Human herpesvirus-8 DNA sequences in human immunodeficiency virus-negative angioimmunoblastic

lymphadenopathy and benign lymphadenopathy with giant germinal center hyperplasia and increased vascularity. *Blood* 1996; **87**: 3903–9.

102. Chadburn A, Cesarman E, Nador RG et al. Kaposi's sarcoma-associated herpesvirus sequences in benign lymphoid proliferations not associated with human immunodeficiency virus. *Cancer* 1997; **80**: 788–97.
103. Dupin N, Fisher C, Kellam P et al. Distribution of human herpesvirus-8 latently infected cells in Kaposi's sarcoma, multicentric Castleman's disease, and primary effusion lymphoma. *Proc Natl Acad Sci USA* 1999; **96**: 4546–51.
104. Teruya-Feldstein J, Zauber P, Setsuda JE et al. Expression of human herpesvirus-8 oncogene and cytokine homologues in an HIV-seronegative patient with multicentric Castleman's disease and primary effusion lymphoma. *Lab Invest* 1998; **78**: 1637–42.
105. Kikuta H, Itakura O, Taneichi K, Kohno M. Tropism of human herpesvirus 8 for peripheral blood lymphocytes in patients with Castleman's disease. *Br J Haematol* 1997; **99**: 790–3.
106. Grandadam M, Dupin N, Calvez V et al. Exacerbations of clinical symptoms in human immunodeficiency virus type 1-infected patients with multicentric Castleman's disease are associated with a high increase in Kaposi's sarcoma herpesvirus DNA load in peripheral blood mononuclear cells. *J Infect Dis* 1997; **175**: 1198–201.
107. Dupin N, Gorin I, Deleuze J et al. Herpes-like DNA sequences, AIDS-related tumors, and Castleman's disease. *N Engl J Med* 1995; **333**: 798.
108. Revuelta MP, Nord JA. Successful treatment of multicentric Castleman's disease in a patient with human immunodeficiency virus infection. *Clin Infect Dis* 1998; **26**: 527.
109. Cannon JS, Nicholas J, Orenstein JM et al. Heterogeneity of viral IL-6 expression in HHV-8-associated diseases. *J Infect Dis* 1999; **180**: 824–8.
110. Belec L, Mohamed AS, Authier FJ et al. Human herpesvirus 8 infection in patients with POEMS syndrome-associated multicentric Castleman's disease. *Blood* 1999; **93**: 3643–53.
111. Huh J, Kang GH, Gong G et al. Kaposi's sarcoma-associated herpesvirus in Kikuchi's disease. *Hum Pathol* 1998; **29**: 1091–6.
112. Matsushima AY, Strauchen JA, Lee G et al. Posttransplantation plasmacytic proliferations related to Kaposi's sarcoma-associated herpesvirus. *Am J Surg Pathol* 1999; **23**: 1393–400.
113. Chang Y, Cesarman E, Pessin MS et al. Identification of herpesvirus-like DNA sequences in AIDS-associated Kaposi's sarcoma. *Science* 1994; **266**: 1865–9.
114. Staskus KA, Sun R, Miller G et al. Cellular tropism and viral interleukin-6 expression distinguish human herpesvirus 8 involvement in Kaposi's sarcoma, primary effusion lymphoma, and multicentric Castleman's disease. *J Virol* 1999; **73**: 4181–7.
115. Luppi M, Barozzi P, Maiorana A et al. Expression of cell-homologous genes of human herpesvirus-8 in human immunodeficiency virus-negative lymphoproliferative diseases. *Blood* 1999; **94**: 2931–3.
116. O'Reilly PE Jr. Joshi VV, Holbrook CT, Weisenburger DD. Multicentric Castleman's disease in a child with prominent thymic involvement: a case report and brief review of the literature. *Mod Pathol* 1993; **6**: 776–80.
117. Smir BN, Greiner TC, Weisenburger DD. Multicentric angiofollicular lymph node hyperplasia in children: a clinicopathologic study of eight patients. *Mod Pathol* 1996; **9**: 1135–42.
118. Parez N, Bader-Meunier B, Roy CC, Dommergues JP. Paediatric Castleman disease: report of seven cases and review of the literature. *Eur J Pediatr* 1999; **158**: 631–7.
119. Sherman D, Ramsay B, Theodorou NA et al. Reversible plane xanthoma, vasculitis, and peliosis hepatis in giant lymph node hyperplasia (Castleman's disease): a case report and review of the cutaneous manifestations of giant lymph node hyperplasia. *J Am Acad Dermatol* 1992; **26**: 105–9.
120. Marsh JH, Colbourn DS, Donovan V, Staszewski H. Systemic Castleman's disease in association with Evan's syndrome and vitiligo. *Med Pediatr Oncol* 1990; **18**: 169–72.
121. Yang SG, Cho KH, Bang YJ, Kim CW. A case of glomeruloid hemangioma associated with multicentric Castleman's disease. *Am J Dermatopathol* 1998; **20**: 266–70.
122. Scherokman B, Vukelja SJ, May E. Angiofollicular lymph node hyperplasia and peripheral neuropathy. Case report and literature review. *Arch Intern Med* 1991; **151**: 789–90.
123. Feigert JM, Sweet DL, Coleman M et al. Multicentric angiofollicular lymph node hyperplasia with peripheral neuropathy, pseudotumor cerebri, IgA dysproteinemia, and thrombocytosis

in women. A distinct syndrome. *Ann Intern Med* 1990; **113**: 362–7.

124. Gherardi RK, Malapert D, Degos JD. Castleman disease–POEMS syndrome overlap. *Ann Intern Med* 1991; **114**: 520–1.
125. Stanley MW, Frizzera G, Dehner LP. Castleman's disease, plasma-cell type. Diagnosis of central nervous system involvement by cerebrospinal fluid cytology. *Acta Cytol* 1986; **30**: 481–6.
126. Kingsmore SF, Silva OE, Hall BD et al. Presentation of multicentric Castleman's disease with sicca syndrome, cardiomyopathy, palmar and plantar rash. *J Rheumatol* 1993; **20**: 1588–91.
127. Gohlke F, Marker-Hermann E, Kanzler S et al. Autoimmune findings resembling connective tissue disease in a patient with Castleman's disease. *Clin Rheumatol* 1997; **16**: 87–92.
128. Wengrower D, Libson E, Okon E, Goldin E. Gastrointestinal manifestations in Castleman's disease. *Am J Gastroenterol* 1990; **85**: 1179–81.
129. Burak KW, Bridges RJ, Blahey WB. Castleman's disease and neutropenic enterocolitis presenting as Crohn's disease. *Can J Gastroenterol* 1998; **12**: 270–2.
130. Carrington PA, Anderson H, Harris M et al. Autoimmune cytopenias in Castleman's disease. *Am J Clin Pathol* 1990; **94**: 101–4.
131. Lajoie G, Kumar S, Min KW, Silva FG. Renal thrombotic microangiopathy associated with multicentric Castleman's disease. Report of two cases. *Am J Surg Pathol* 1995; **19**: 1021–8.
132. Liberato NL, Bollati P, Chiofalo F et al. Autoimmune hemolytic anemia in multicentric Castleman's disease. *Haematologica* 1996; **81**: 40–3.
133. Lerza R, Castello G, Truini M et al. Splenectomy induced complete remission in a patient with multicentric Castleman's disease and autoimmune hemolytic anemia. *Ann Hematol* 1999; **78**: 193–6.
134. Steinberg JJ, Huang PL, Ljubich P, Lee-Huang S. Anti-erythropoietin antibodies in hyperviscosity syndrome associated with giant lymph node hyperplasia (GLNH; Castleman's disease). *Br J Haematol* 1990; **74**: 543–4.
135. Couch WD. Giant lymph node hyperplasia associated with thrombotic thrombocytopenic purpura. *Am J Clin Pathol* 1980; **74**: 340–4.
136. Massey GV, Kornstein MJ, Wahl D et al. Angiofollicular lymph node hyperplasia (Castleman's disease) in an adolescent female. Clinical and immunologic findings. *Cancer* 1991; **68**: 1365–72.
137. Shohat B, Cohen I, Fogel R, Zaizov R. Suppressor mononuclear cells in giant lymph node hyperplasia and thymoma. *Cancer* 1981; **48**: 923–6.
138. Perez Peña F, Tejero Lamarca J, Martin Rodilla C et al. Castleman's disease: Is diffuse histiocytic lymphoma in the evolution of hyalinovascular lymphonodular hyperplasia a benign entity? [In Spanish.] *Rev Clin Esp* 1980; **158**: 83–6.
139. Said R, Tarawneh M. Membranoproliferative glomerulonephritis associated with multicentric angiofollicular lymph node hyperplasia. Case report and review of the literature. *Am J Nephrol* 1992; **12**: 466–70.
140. Karcher DS, Pearson CE, Butler WM et al. Giant lymph node hyperplasia involving the thymus with associated nephrotic syndrome and myelofibrosis. *Am J Clin Pathol* 1982; **77**: 100–4.
141. Chim CS, Lam KY, Chan KW. Castleman's disease with Kaposi's sarcoma and glomerulonephritis. *Am J Med* 1999; **107**: 186–8.
142. Moon WK, Kim SH, Im JG et al. Castleman disease with renal amyloidosis: imaging findings and clinical significance. *Abdom Imaging* 1995; **20**: 376–8.
143. Hattori K, Irie S, Isobe Y et al. Multicentric Castleman's disease associated with renal amyloidosis and pure red cell aplasia. *Ann Hematol* 1998; **77**: 179–81.
144. Ordi J, Grau JM, Junque A et al. Secondary (AA) amyloidosis associated with Castleman's disease. Report of two cases and review of the literature. *Am J Clin Pathol* 1993; **100**: 394–7.
145. Ikeda S, Chisuwa H, Kawasaki S et al. Systemic reactive amyloidosis associated with Castleman's disease: serial changes of the concentrations of acute phase serum amyloid A and interleukin 6 in serum. *J Clin Pathol* 1997; **50**: 965–7.
146. Tanaka K, Horita M, Shibayama H et al. Secondary amyloidosis associated with Castleman's disease. *Intern Med* 1995; **34**: 122–6.
147. Perfetti V, Bellotti V, Maggi A et al. Reversal of nephrotic syndrome due to reactive amyloidosis (AA-type) after excision of localized Castleman's disease. *Am J Hematol* 1994; **46**: 189–93.
148. Kanoh T, Shimada H, Uchino H, Matsumura K. Amyloid goiter with hypothyroidism. *Arch Pathol Lab Med* 1989; **113**: 542–4.
149. Miura A, Sato I, Suzuki C. Fatal diarrhea in a patient with Castleman's disease associated with

intestinal amyloidosis. *Intern Med* 1995; **34**: 1106–9.
150. West KP, Morgan DR, Lauder I. Angiofollicular lymph node hyperplasia with amyloidosis. *Postgrad Med J* 1989; **65**: 108–11.
151. Okuda K, Himeno Y, Toyama T et al. Gamma heavy chain disease and giant lymph node hyperplasia in a patient with impaired T cell function. *Jpn J Med* 1982; **21**: 109–14.
152. Atagi S, Sakatani M, Akira M et al. Pulmonary hyalinizing granuloma with Castleman's disease. *Intern Med* 1994; **33**: 689–91.
153. Pasaoglu I, Dogan R, Topcu M, Gungen Y. Multicentric angiofollicular lymph-node hyperplasia associated with myasthenia gravis. *Thorac Cardiovasc Surg* 1994; **42**: 253–6.
154. Molina T, Delmer A, Le Tourneau A et al. Hepatic lesions of vascular origin in multicentric Castleman's disease, plasma cell type: report of one case with peliosis hepatis and another with perisinusoidal fibrosis and nodular regenerative hyperplasia. *Pathol Res Pract* 1995; **191**: 1159–64.
155. Peterson BA, Frizzera G. Multicentric Castleman's disease. *Semin Oncol* 1993; **20**: 636–47.
156. Pavlidis NA, Briassoulis E, Klouvas G, Bai M. Is interferon-α an active agent in Castleman's disease? *Ann Oncol* 1992; **3**: 85–6.
157. Bordeleau L, Bredeson C, Markman S. 2-Chlorodeoxyadenosine therapy for giant lymph node hyperplasia. *Br J Haematol* 1995; **91**: 668–70.
158. Barbounis V, Efremidis A. A plasma cell variant of Castleman's disease treated successfully with cimetidine. Case report and review of the literature. *Anticancer Res* 1996; **16**: 545–7.
159. Repetto L, Jaiprakash MP, Selby PJ et al. Aggressive angiofollicular lymph node hyperplasia (Castleman's disease) treated with high dose melphalan and autologous bone marrow transplantation. *Hematol Oncol* 1986; **4**: 213–7.
160. Kasaian MT, Casali P. Autoimmunity-prone B-1 (CD5 B) cells, natural antibodies and self recognition. *Autoimmunity* 1993; **15**: 315–29.
161. Lee KW, Inghirami G, Spatz L et al. The B-cells that express anti-MAG antibodies in neuropathy and non- malignant IgM monoclonal gammopathy belong to the CD5 subpopulation. *J Neuroimmunol* 1991; **31**: 83–8.
162. Ishiyama T, Koike M, Kakimoto T et al. The presence of CD28-negative T cells in a patient with multicentric Castleman's disease. *Ann Hematol* 1996; **73**: 199–200.
163. Gillison ML, Ambinder RF. Human herpesvirus-8. *Curr Opin Oncol* 1997; **9**: 440–9.
164. Jones KD, Aoki Y, Chang Y et al. Involvement of interleukin-10 (IL-10) and viral IL-6 in the spontaneous growth of Kaposi's sarcoma herpesvirus-associated infected primary effusion lymphoma cells. *Blood* 1999; **94**: 2871–9.
165. Papo T, Soubrier M, Marcelin AG et al. Human herpesvirus 8 infection, Castleman's disease and POEMS syndrome. *Br J Haematol* 1999; **104**: 932–3.
166. Harris NL. Hypervascular follicular hyperplasia and Kaposi's sarcoma in patients at risk for AIDS. *N Engl J Med* 1984; **310**: 462–3.
167. Lachant NA, Sun NC, Leong LA et al. Multicentric angiofollicular lymph node hyperplasia (Castleman's disease) followed by Kaposi's sarcoma in two homosexual males with the acquired immunodeficiency syndrome (AIDS). *Am J Clin Pathol* 1985; **83**: 27–33.
168. Lowenthal DA, Filippa DA, Richardson ME et al. Generalized lymphadenopathy with morphologic features of Castleman's disease in an HIV-positive man. *Cancer* 1987; **60**: 2454–8.
169. Ost A, Baroni CD, Biberfeld P et al. Lymphadenopathy in HIV infection: histological classification and staging. *APMIS Suppl* 1989; **8**: 7–15.
170. Racz P, Tenner-Racz K, van Vloten F et al. Classification of histopathological changes of lymph nodes in HIV-1 infection. Significance of Castleman's disease-like lymph node lesion concerning the diagnosis of HIV-1-related Kaposi's sarcoma. *Antibiot Chemother* 1991; **43**: 201–13.
171. Oksenhendler E, Duarte M, Soulier J et al. Multicentric Castleman's disease in HIV infection: a clinical and pathological study of 20 patients. *AIDS* 1996; **10**: 61–7.
172. Perlow LS, Taff ML, Orsini JM et al. Kaposi's sarcoma in a young homosexual man. Association with angiofollicular lymphoid hyperplasia and a malignant lymphoproliferative disorder. *Arch Pathol Lab Med* 1983; **107**: 510–3.
173. Diebold J, Audouin J, Le Tourneau A et al. Lymph node reaction patterns in patients with AIDS or AIDS-related complex. *Curr Top Pathol* 1991; **84**: 189–221.
174. Chadburn A, Metroka C, Mouradian J. Progressive lymph node histology and its prognostic value in patients with acquired immunodeficiency syndrome and AIDS-related complex. *Hum Pathol* 1989; **20**: 579–87.

175. Dominguez F, Riera JR, Junco P et al. Generalized lymphadenopathy with morphologic findings of multicentric angiofollicular ganglionic hyperplasia in a patient with AIDS. [In Spanish.] *Rev Clin Esp* 1993; **193**: 299–302.
176. Wynia MK, Shapiro B, Kuvin JT, Skolnik PR. Fatal Castleman's disease and pulmonary Kaposi's sarcoma in an HIV-seropositive woman. *AIDS* 1995; **9**: 814–6.
177. Zietz C, Bogner JR, Goebel FD, Lohrs U. An unusual cluster of cases of Castleman's disease during highly active antiretroviral therapy for AIDS. *N Engl J Med* 1999; **340**: 1923–4.
178. Rywlin AM, Recher L, Hoffman EP. Lymphoma-like presentation of Kaposi's sarcoma. Three cases without characteristic skin lesions. *Arch Dermatol* 1966; **93**: 554–61.
179. Chen KT. Multicentric Castleman's disease and Kaposi's sarcoma. *Am J Surg Pathol* 1984; **8**: 287–93.
180. Dickson D, Ben-Ezra JM, Reed J et al. Multicentric giant lymph node hyperplasia, Kaposi's sarcoma, and lymphoma. *Arch Pathol Lab Med* 1985; **109**: 1013–8.
181. Kwong YL, Chan AC. Absence of Kaposi's sarcoma associated herpesvirus-like DNA sequences (KSHV) in HIV-negative multicentric Castleman's disease complicated by KSHV-positive Kaposi's sarcoma. *Br J Haematol* 1997; **96**: 881–2.
182. Zeidman A, Fradin Z, Cohen AM, Mittelman M. Kaposi's sarcoma associated with Castleman's disease. *Eur J Haematol* 1999; **63**: 67–70.
183. Kessler E, Beer R. Multicentric giant lymph node hyperplasia clinically simulating angioimmunoblastic lymphadenopathy. Associated Kaposi's sarcoma in two of three cases. *Isr J Med Sci* 1983; **19**: 230–4.
184. Lubin J, Rywlin AM. Lymphoma-like lymph node changes in Kaposi's sarcoma. Two additional cases. *Arch Pathol* 1971; **92**: 338–41.
185. De Rosa G, Barra E, Guarino M, Gentile R. Multicentric Castleman's disease in association with Kaposi's sarcoma. *Appl Pathol* 1989; **7**: 105–10.
186. Crow RS. Peripheral neuritis in myelomatosis. *BMJ* 1956; **2**: 802–4.
187. Shimpo S, Nishitani H, Tsunematsu T, Fukase M. Solitary plasmacytoma with polyneuritis and endocrine disturbances. *Nippon Rinsho* 1968; **26**: 2444–56.
188. Takatsuki K, Uchiyama T, Sagawa K, Yodoi J. Plasma cell dyscrasia with polyneuropathy and endocrine disorder; review of 32 patients. In: *Proceedings of 16th International Congress of Hematology, 1977, Kyoto*. Amsterdam: Excerpta Medica, 1977: 454.
189. Nakanishi T, Sobue I, Toyokura Y et al. The Crow–Fukase syndrome: a study of 102 cases in Japan. *Neurology* 1984; **34**: 712–20.
190. Pruzanski W. Takatsuki syndrome: a reversible multisystem plasma cell dyscrasia. *Arthritis Rheum* 1986; **29**: 1534–5.
191. Bardwick PA, Zvaifler NJ, Gill GN et al. Plasma cell dyscrasia with polyneuropathy, organomegaly, endocrinopathy, M protein, and skin changes: the POEMS syndrome. Report on two cases and a review of the literature. *Medicine (Baltimore)* 1980; **59**: 311–22.
192. Takatsuki K, Sanada I. Plasma cell dyscrasia with polyneuropathy and endocrine disorder: clinical and laboratory features of 109 reported cases. *Jpn J Clin Oncol* 1983; **13**: 543–55.
193. Miralles GD, O'Fallon JR, Talley NJ. Plasma-cell dyscrasia with polyneuropathy. The spectrum of POEMS syndrome. *N Engl J Med* 1992; **327**: 1919–23.
194. Soubrier MJ, Dubost JJ, Sauvezie BJ. POEMS syndrome: a study of 25 cases and a review of the literature. French Study Group on POEMS Syndrome. *Am J Med* 1994; **97**: 543–53.
195. Pavord SR, Murphy PT, Mitchell VE. POEMS syndrome and Waldenström's macroglobulinaemia. *J Clin Pathol* 1996; **49**: 181–2.
196. Farhangi M, Merlini G. The clinical implications of monoclonal immunoglobulins. *Semin Oncol* 1986; **13**: 366–79.
197. Adams D, Said G. Ultrastructural characterisation of the M protein in nerve biopsy of patients with POEMS syndrome. *J Neurol Neurosurg Psychiatry* 1998; **64**: 809–12.
198. Ropper AH, Gorson KC. Neuropathies associated with paraproteinemia. *N Engl J Med* 1998; **338**: 1601–7.
199. Bitter MA, Komaiko W, Franklin WA. Giant lymph node hyperplasia with osteoblastic bone lesions and the POEMS (Takatsuki's) syndrome. *Cancer* 1985; **56**: 188–94.
200. Rolon PG, Audouin J, Diebold J et al. Multicentric angiofollicular lymph node hyperplasia associated with a solitary osteolytic costal IgG lambda myeloma. POEMS syndrome in a South American (Paraguayan) patient. *Pathol Res Pract* 1989; **185**: 468–75; discussion 76–9.

201. Muñoz G, Geijo P, Moldenhauer F et al. Plasmacellular Castleman's disease and POEMS syndrome. *Histopathology* 1990; **17**: 172–4.
202. Judge MR, McGibbon DH, Thompson RP. Angioendotheliomatosis associated with Castleman's lymphoma and POEMS syndrome. *Clin Exp Dermatol* 1993; **18**: 360–2.
203. Rose C, Zandecki M, Copin MC et al. POEMS syndrome: report on six patients with unusual clinical signs, elevated levels of cytokines, macrophage involvement and chromosomal aberrations of bone marrow plasma cells. *Leukemia* 1997; **11**: 1318–23.
204. Murphy N, Schumacher HR Jr. POEMS syndrome in systemic lupus erythematosus. *J Rheumatol* 1992; **19**: 796–9.
205. Nanki T, Tomiyama J, Arai S. Mixed connective tissue disease associated with multicentric Castleman's disease. *Scand J Rheumatol* 1994; **23**: 215–7.
206. Pasqui AL, Bova G, Saletti M et al. POEMS syndrome with vascular lesions and renal carcinoma – possible role of cytokines. *Eur J Med Res* 1998; **3**: 304–6.
207. Emile C, Danon F, Fermand JP, Clauvel JP. Castleman disease in POEMS syndrome with elevated interleukin-6. *Cancer* 1993; **71**: 874.
208. Belec L, Authier FJ, Mohamed AS, Soubrier M, Gherardi RK. Antibodies to human herpesvirus 8 in POEMS (polyneuropathy, organomegaly, endocrinopathy, M protein, skin changes) syndrome with multicentric Castleman's disease. *Clin Infect Dis* 1999; **28**: 678–9.
209. Brice P, Marolleau JP, D'Agay MF et al. Autoimmune hemolytic anemia disclosing Hodgkin's disease associated with Castleman's disease. *Nouv Rev Fr Hematol* 1991; **33**: 273–4.
210. Drut R, Larregina A. Angiofollicular lymph node transformation in Hodgkin's lymphoma. *Pediatr Pathol* 1991; **11**: 903–8.
211. Maheswaran PR, Ramsay AD, Norton AJ, Roche WR. Hodgkin's disease presenting with the histological features of Castleman's disease. *Histopathology* 1991; **18**: 249–53.
212. Pettit C, Ferry JA, Harris NL. Simultaneous occurrence of Hodgkin's disease and angiofollicular hyperplasia (Castleman's disease): report of 3 cases. *Mod Pathol* 1990; **4**: 81A.
213. Molinie V, Perie G, Melo I et al. Association of Castleman's disease and Hodgkin's disease. Eight cases and review of the literature. [In French.] *Ann Pathol* 1994; **14**: 384–91.
214. Zarate-Osorno A, Medeiros LJ, Danon AD, Neiman RS. Hodgkin's disease with coexistent Castleman-like histologic features. A report of three cases. *Arch Pathol Lab Med* 1994; **118**: 270–4.
215. Abdel-Reheim FA, Koss W, Rappaport ES, Arber DA. Coexistence of Hodgkin's disease and giant lymph node hyperplasia of the plasma-cell type (Castleman's disease). *Arch Pathol Lab Med* 1996; **120**: 91–6.
216. McAloon EJ. Hodgkin's disease in a patient with Castleman's disease. *N Engl J Med* 1985; **313**: 758.
217. Doggett RS, Colby TV, Dorfman RF. Interfollicular Hodgkin's disease. *Am J Surg Pathol* 1983; **7**: 145–9.
218. Hanchard B, Williams N, Green M. Concurrent multicentric angiofollicular lymph node hyperplasia and peripheral T-cell lymphoma. *West Indian Med J* 1987; **36**: 104–7.
219. Buijs L, Wijermans PW, van Groningen K et al. Hyaline–vascular type Castleman's disease with concomitant malignant B-cell lymphoma. *Acta Haematol* 1992; **87**: 160–2.
220. Orcioni GF, Mambelli V, Ascani S et al. Concurrence of localized Castleman's disease and peripheral small B-lymphocytic lymphoma within the same lymph node. *Gen Diagn Pathol* 1998; **143**: 327–30.
221. Baker WJ, Vukelja SJ, Weiss RB, Dich N. Multicentric angiofollicular lymph node hyperplasia and associated carcinoma. *Med Pediatr Oncol* 1994; **22**: 384–8.
222. Stelfox HT, Stewart AK, Bailey D, Harrison D. Castleman's disease in a 44-year-old male with neurofibromatosis and pheochromocytoma. *Leuk Lymphoma* 1997; **27**: 551–6.
223. Tissier F, de Pinieux G, Thiounn N et al. Castleman's disease and chromophobe carcinoma of the kidney. An incidental association? [In French.] *Ann Pathol* 1998; **18**: 429–31.
224. Mizutani N, Okada S, Tanaka J et al. Multicentric giant lymph node hyperplasia with ascites and double cancers, an autopsy case. *Tohoku J Exp Med* 1989; **158**: 1–7.
225. Ben-Chetrit E, Flusser D, Okon E et al. Multicentric Castleman's disease associated with rheumatoid arthritis: a possible role of hepatitis B antigen. *Ann Rheum Dis* 1989; **48**: 326–30.
226. Tavoni A, Vitali C, Baglioni P et al. Multicentric Castleman's disease in a patient with primary Sjögren's syndrome. *Rheumatol Int* 1993; **12**: 251–3.

227. Suwannaroj S, Elkins SL, McMurray RW. Systemic lupus erythematosus and Castleman's disease. *J Rheumatol* 1999; **26**: 1400–3.
228. Kojima M, Nakamura S, Itoh H et al. Systemic lupus erythematosus (SLE) lymphadenopathy presenting with histopathologic features of Castleman' disease: a clinicopathologic study of five cases. *Pathol Res Pract* 1997; **193**: 565–71.

29

Light-chain deposition disease

Alan Solomon, Deborah T Weiss, Guillermo A Herrera

CONTENTS • **Introduction** • **clinical features** • **Pathogenesis** • **Pathophysiologic manifestations** • **Experimental systems** • **Diagnosis** • **Treatment**

INTRODUCTION

Light-chain deposition disease (LCDD) represents a monoclonal plasma cell dyscrasia that is characterized by the presence of punctate or granular, electron-dense, homogeneous light-chain immunoglobulin (Ig) molecules in basement membranes of the kidney and other vital organs.[1–7] The relentless progression of this deposition eventually leads to renal, cardiac, or hepatic failure, and accounts for the poor prognosis of patients with this illness.[8]

The distinctive nature and anatomic distribution of the pathologic deposits found in the organs of patients with LCDD distinguish it from other monoclonal plasma cell dyscrasias such as myeloma, primary (AL) amyloidosis, or adult Fanconi syndrome, in which monotypic Ig molecules are deposited as amorphous casts, fibrils, or crystals, respectively.[5] In LCDD, as well as these other disorders, monoclonal free light chains, (i.e. Bence Jones proteins) are responsible for the observed pathology. Although it is now known that heavy chains (or even complete Ig molecules) can also form morphologically similar types of tissue deposits,[2,3] this chapter will focus primarily on the role of the light chain as the major causative factor in the pathologic ramifications of LCDD.

CLINICAL FEATURES

It is only within the past two decades or so that LCDD has been recognized as a distinct clinicopathologic entity. Following the first detailed description of this illness by Randall et al[9] in 1976, numerous reports on the subject have appeared in the medical literature. A comprehensive review of the salient clinical features, immunopathology, and molecular biology of LCDD and related disorders was provided in 1992 by Buxbaum[3] and updated by Gallo et al.[7]

The incidence of LCDD is unknown. Although it is seemingly one of the least common of the monoclonal plasma cell dyscrasias, its clinical importance is underlined by the invariable renal dysfunction that occurs in patients with this disorder. The disease is often not diagnosed owing to the subtle nature of the morphologic alterations that are found, and because many of the changes mimic those seen in other types of renal disease such as nodular diabetic glomerulosclerosis.

LCDD is now recognized with increasing frequency as the cause of 'unexplained' proteinuria, renal failure, hematuria, or hypertension.[4] Similarly, because LCDD is not limited to the kidney and can affect organs throughout the body, other medical specialists should consider this entity when making a differential diagnosis of disease associated with cardiac, hepatic, or pulmonary insufficiency (Table 29.1).

LCDD lacks many of the clinical characteristics of myeloma, and occurs in younger (30–50 years), predominantly female, patients. Osteolytic skeletal lesions are absent and, usually, bone marrow plasmacytosis and monoclonal gammopathy are not striking. Individuals with this disorder invariably have varying degrees of renal dysfunction that results from the pathologic deposition of light chains in the glomeruli and in tubular and vascular basement membranes. Most commonly, LCDD presents initially in the form of acute renal failure or a more chronic process that is manifested by non-selective proteinuria, nephrotic syndrome, or hematuria. In 7–10% of cases, the disease progresses to exhibit features typical of myeloma; conversely, LCDD-like lesions have been found in a comparable percentage of individuals with myeloma.[5]

At some point in their illness, virtually all patients require dialysis. Renal transplants have obviated the need for this procedure, but continued production of the abnormal protein eventually results in its deposition in the transplanted kidney or other organs. The heart also can be a target organ in LCDD, and light-chain deposits in the myocardial basement membranes or vasculature result in irreversible cardiomyopathy.[10–13] Therefore, efforts have been directed towards suppressing monoclonal Ig production through the use of chemotherapeutic agents. Although such treatment has extended survival, the overall prognosis remains poor, and death eventually results from infection and failure of vital organs targeted by the disease process.

Table 29.1 Organs affected in patients with light-chain deposition disease[a]

Organ	Occurrence (%)
Kidney	94
Heart	79
Liver	77
GI tract	33
Nerves	22
Lung	?

[a]Data from reference 3 include patients with light- and heavy-chain deposition disease (LHCDD).

PATHOGENESIS

Light-chain structure

The two types of light chains, kappa (κ) and lambda (λ), are characterized by a common structure consisting of two domains that include a ~107- to 111-residue amino-terminal variable (V_L) portion and a 107-residue carboxyl-terminal constant (C_L) portion. The V_L is the product of two genes, *V* and *J*, that encode the first ~95–99 and remaining ~12 amino acids, respectively. Variation in V_L primary structure results from (a) the presence of ~30 V_κ and V_λ germline genes that, on the basis of sequence homology, are divided into four major V_κ (*κ1, κ2, κ3, κ4*) and five V_λ (*λ1, λ2, λ3, λ6, λ8*) subgroups or families; (b) somatic mutation; and (c) differences that result from recombination of the *V*- and *J*-gene encoded segments.[14–16] As will be discussed subsequently, this inherent variability in primary structure accounts for the fact that certain light chains are pathologic while others are apparently benign.

Light-chain synthesis and catabolism

Circulating Igs are products of terminally differentiated B cells (plasma cells). Light chains, both κ and λ, are typically synthesized in excess of heavy chains, and are secreted from the cell in the 'free' state.[17] κ molecules occur predominately as monomers or non-covalent dimers (~22 kDa and 44 kDa, respectively), whereas λ proteins usually exist as covalent dimers[18]

Approximately 0.3 mg/kg per hour of these components are synthesized daily and rapidly catabolized within the kidney (with a half-life of about 2 hours).[19,20] Owing to their relatively low molecular weights, they are readily filtered through the glomeruli. However, certain physiochemical properties determined by the V_L portion of the molecule (e.g. isoelectric point and hydrophobicity) may adversely affect glomerular clearance.[21–23] After filtration, about 90% of light chains are reabsorbed by endocytosis in the proximal tubules.[20] Initially, these proteins bind to a low-affinity, high-capacity light-chain-specific receptor located on the tubular brush border,[24] or to another glycoprotein receptor, cubilin (Gp280), that is also involved in endocytosis and cell trafficking of other low-molecular-weight proteins such as lysozyme, insulin, cytochrome *c*, myoglobin, and β_2-microglobulin.[25] Although light chains may undergo proteolysis at the brush border, the major site of degradation is intracellular. After endocytosis, these components are entrapped in vesicles that fuse with lysosomes, and are then degraded enzymatically. Once the endocytic receptor(s) is saturated, light chains pass into the distal nephron and are eventually excreted in the urine.

These physiologic processes are altered in LCDD, where there is an increased synthesis of free monoclonal light chains. Although there is increased proteinuria, the catabolism of light chains by the kidneys decreases, resulting in an increase in their serum concentration.[20,21] Additionally, certain Bence Jones proteins may be inherently pathologic.[26,27]

Under normal circumstances, free heavy chains are not found in the circulation. In patients who have heavy-chain-related disease, the excess production of these molecules may be associated with basement membrane precipitates.[2,3,7] However, there is no information currently available on how such proteins are processed by the kidney.

Molecular features of pathologic light chains

There is no obvious relationship between the amount of Bence Jones protein excreted daily and the presence or absence of light-chain-related pathology.[28] This is because certain primary and tertiary structural features of light chains influence their pathologic potential.

It has been reported that LCDD-associated Bence Jones proteins, in contrast to those found in AL amyloidosis and myeloma (cast) nephropathy, tend to have higher isoelectric points (>8.2)[13,23] and that the cationic nature of these molecules may facilitate their interaction with anionic basement membrane constituents.[13] Further, LCDD-associated monoclonal Igs are predominantly κ-type, whereas a predominance of λ light chains is found in AL amyloidosis.[5,16] This discordance may be related to the different quaternary structural properties of κ and λ light chains mentioned above. These differences could affect their rate of glomerular filtration as well as renal catabolism, and account for the finding that the ratio of κ to λ chains in urine is 2 : 1, while it is the opposite in serum.[29]

Additionally, κ Bence Jones proteins may possess structural features that render them more prone to form punctate deposits, as evidenced by the discovery that light chains of two particular V_κ subgroups – $V_\kappa1$ and $V_\kappa4$ – are seemingly overrepresented in LCDD.[13,30–34] In the case of $V_\kappa1$, although seven gene families have been identified, the pathologic proteins are predominantly products of only two: L12A and 018-08[13,32] ($V_\kappa4$ is a single gene family[14]). In contrast to the hemoglobinopathies, there is no single, site-specific residue that differentiates between pathologic and non-pathologic κ and λ components.[29] Rather, it has become apparent that certain substitutions located at particular positions within the V_L domain affect the stability of these molecules, result in partial unfolding, and lead to their propensity to aggregate.[13,35] Despite the fact that light chains are rarely glycosylated, there is a prevalence of such proteins among LCDD- and AL-associated components.[36] However, in contrast to amyloid, LCDD-related deposits are not congophilic and do not contain

P component or other 'accessory' molecules, such as glycosaminoglycans and apolipoprotein E.[12]

PATHOPHYSIOLOGIC MANIFESTATIONS

Glomerular pathology

Nodular glomerulosclerosis resulting from the co-deposition of light chains with extracellular matrix proteins is the pathologic hallmark of LCDD (Figure 29.1).

Well-defined mesangial nodules can be seen throughout the glomeruli, and the peripheral capillary walls appear thickened. Light-chain deposits, most often κ-type, are evidenced immunohistochemically in subendothelial and mesangial areas. Ultrastructurally, this material appears punctate and electron-dense, and may extend into the lamina densa of glomerular basement membranes or even into subepithelial zones, resulting eventually in obliteration of the glomerulus. As a result of the progressive damage to the glomeruli, the kidney loses its ability to retain serum proteins, including albumin, and nephrotic syndrome develops. Other manifestations of glomerular injury can be noted, especially in the initial phase of the disease process. These alterations mimic 'minimal change' or mesangial, membranoproliferative, and crescentic glomerulopathies.

Although, by definition, LCDD is associated with the pathologic deposition of light chains, a similar disease process can result from the precipitation of monoclonal heavy chains or both heavy and light chains in the basement membranes of the kidney and other organs.[2,3,7] Accordingly, the illnesses resulting from this process have been designated HCDD (heavy-chain deposition disease) or LHCDD (light- and heavy-chain deposition disease), respectively; they are seemingly rare.

Tubular pathology

Tubular interstitial disease[37,38] is also a pathologic feature of LCDD, and is manifested by thickened basement membranes that sometimes acquire a ribbon-like refractile appearance (Figure 29.2).

The observed abnormalities are similar to those found in acute tubular necrosis, and include vacuolation, fragmentation, desquamation, and, ultimately, total loss of the brush border. The lumens may be filled with cell nuclei and cytoplasmic fragments, and, by immunoelectron microscopy, monotypic light chains can be visualized within lysosomal compartments and outer aspects of the basement membranes.[39–43] Tubular interstitial disease adversely affects renal function, as evidenced by the failure of the kidney to concentrate or acidify urine.

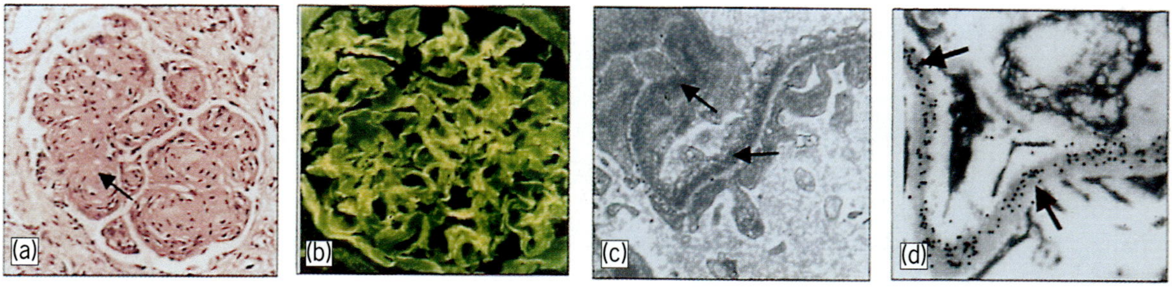

Figure 29.1 Glomerular pathology in LCDD: nodular glomerulosclerosis. (a) Glomerulus with mesangial nodules (arrow); hematoxylin–eosin stain; original magnification ×750. (b) Linear κ-chain deposits in capillary walls of glomerulus; immunofluorescence technique, anti-κ antibody; original magnification × 750. (c) Punctate, electron-dense deposits (arrows) along peripheral capillary wall; Electron–photomicrograph, uranyl acetate and lead citrate stain; original magnification × 8500. (d) κ-chain deposits (arrows) in peripheral capillary wall; immunoelectron–photomicrograph; immunogold (10 nm)-labeled anti-κ antibody; original magnification × 9500.

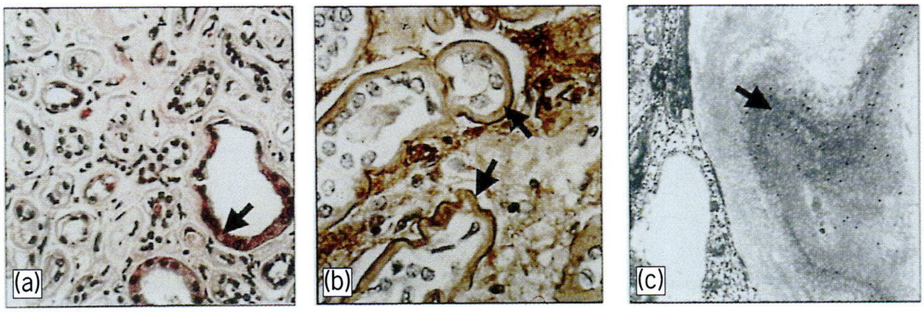

Figure 29.2 Tubular pathology in LCDD. (a) Thickened distal tubular wall (arrow); hematoxylin–eosin stain; original magnification x350. (b) κ-chain deposits in tubular basement membranes (arrows); immunoperoxidase technique, anti-κ antibody; original magnification x500. (c) Punctate electron-dense κ-chain deposits (arrow); immunoelectron–photomicrograph; immunogold (10 nm)-labeled anti-κ antibody; original magnification x13 300.

A less commonly recognized pattern of monoclonal light-chain-mediated tubular injury is associated with an inflammatory process that imitates acute interstitial nephritis. Cellular infiltrates consisting primarily of lymphocytes or plasma cells can be an early manifestation of LCDD.[4,41]

The coexistence in individual patients of LCDD and AL amyloid fibrillar deposits has been reported.[44–46] In such cases, the light chains that constitute the two types of pathologic deposits appear to be identical.[46] We have also noted the presence of tubular proteinaceous casts with an adjacent giant cell reaction analogous in appearance to myeloma (cast) nephropathy. However, whether this material is composed of Bence Jones proteins or, more likely, represents polyclonal Ig (or other serum protein) remains to be seen.

Vascular pathology

In LCDD, the characteristic punctate light-chain deposits are also present in renal blood vessel walls (Figure 29.3).[4,37] In some cases, this deposition leads to a proliferative vasculopathy that may result in renal hypoperfusion and contributes to loss of renal function.[4]

Extrarenal pathology

The characteristic morphologic lesions associated with LCDD – punctate Ig-containing basement membrane deposits – are not limited to the kidney. The involvement of other organs by this process has been demonstrated through immunohistochemical and electron-microscopic analyses of tissue obtained from patients with

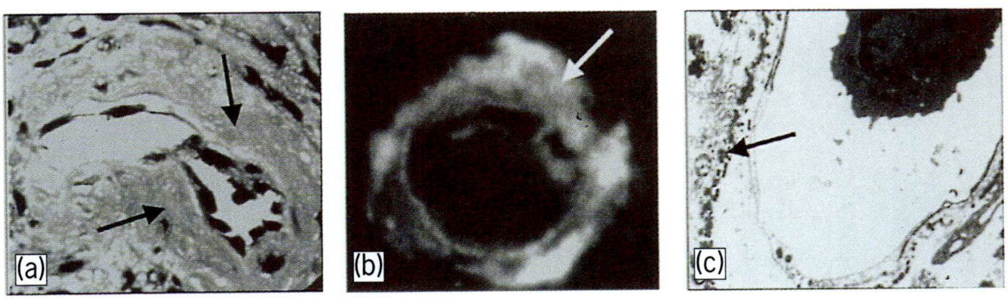

Figure 29.3 Vascular pathology in LCDD. (a) Thickened arterial tubular wall (arrows); hematoxylin–eosin stain; original magnification x750. (b) κ-chain deposits in vascular wall (arrow); immunofluorescence technique, anti-κ antibody; original magnification x750. (c) Punctate electron-dense deposits (arrow) along the wall of a peritubular capillary; electron–photomicrograph; uranyl acetate and lead citrate stain; original magnification x7500.

this disorder. The sites most commonly affected include the liver (Figure 29.4), heart, and lungs, and such deposits eventually lead to organ failure.[3] We hypothesize that the widespread nature of this process results from the affinity of certain light chains for one or more constituents of the basement membrane. In support of this, examination of skin biopsies obtained from patients with LCDD has revealed the presence of pathologic deposits at the dermal–epidermal junction.[47]

EXPERIMENTAL SYSTEMS

Protein (light-chain) factors

The pre-eminent role of monoclonal light chains in the pathogenesis of LCDD has been demonstrated experimentally. For example, it has been shown in vitro that perfusion of rat tubules with human 'tubulopathic' Bence Jones proteins induces the typical morphologic changes associated with cellular injury (e.g. vacuolation, fragmentation, and desquamation), as well as physiologic abnormalities such as impairment of water, glucose, and chloride absorption.[26,27,48–50] Further, through size-exclusion chromatography, it is possible to distinguish 'toxic' from 'non-toxic' light chains on the basis of polymer formation.[51]

Conclusive evidence that the protein itself is primarily responsible for LCDD has come from an in vivo experimental model where mice were injected with Bence Jones proteins obtained from patients with LCDD and other monoclonal plasma cell disorders.[28,52,53] The presence or absence of light-chain-related nephropathology found in the animals correlated with that seen in the patients from whom the proteins were derived. Thus, light chains that were associated with basement membrane precipitates, as well as tubular casts or crystals in patient kidneys, were deposited in similar fashion in the mouse.[28,53] No pathology occurred using non-nephrotoxic components.

That the primary structure of light chains can render certain molecules pathologic has also been evidenced in other studies where recombinant V_L fragments were utilized.[54–56] These experiments have revealed that particular amino acid substitutions so alter the tertiary conformation of the protein that it becomes partially or completely unfolded, and, owing to reduced stability, the molecule is more prone to aggregate.[57] Computer modeling offers a powerful new tool for predicting the three-dimensional impact imparted on a protein by modification of and interactions between amino acids. Such information can have both prognostic and therapeutic relevance in the identification of LCDD-associated proteins and the

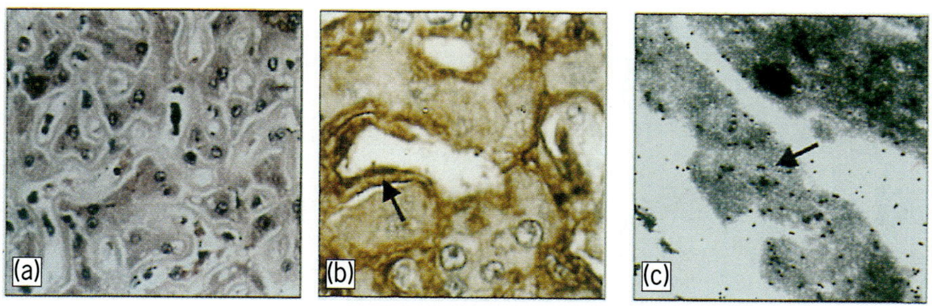

Figure 29.4 Extrarenal pathology in LCDD: liver sinusoids. (a) Hematoxylin–eosin stain; original magnification x350. (b) κ-chain deposits (arrow); immunoperoxidase, anti-κ antibody; original magnification x500. (c) Punctate, electron-dense κ-chain deposits (arrow); immunoelectron–photomicrograph; immunogold (10 nm)-labeled anti-κ antibody; original magnification x7500.

development of drugs designed to stabilize these molecules.

Ancillary (host) factors

In addition to specific structural features that may render light chains toxic, other factors, such as accessory molecules, are seemingly important in disease pathogenesis. Indeed, it has been shown experimentally that the precipitation of Bence Jones proteins as casts requires interaction with Tamm–Horsfall protein, a low-molecular-weight glycoprotein synthesized by the thick ascending limb of Henle's loop.[58] In the case of LCDD, co-culture of 'glomerulopathic' Bence Jones proteins with human mesangial cells has shown that pathologic deposition is initiated by an interaction between light chains and putative, as yet uncharacterized, mesangial cell surface receptors.[59,60]

Initially, cellular proliferation occurs concomitantly with alteration in calcium homeostasis,[61] as well as activation of platelet-derived growth factor β (PDGF-β).[60] This cytokine has been localized to arterial walls, and may play a role in the hyperplastic vasculopathy seen in some patients with LCDD. Subsequently, transforming growth factor β (TGF-β) activity also increases, while that of collagenase IV decreases.[59,60]

These effects are associated with enhanced production of extracellular matrix proteins (e.g. tenascin, collagen IV, laminin, and fibronectin), as found in the glomerular mesangial nodules of patients with LCDD and other disorders.[59,60,62,63] The alterations induced by LCDD-derived proteins do not occur when non-pathologic light chains are incubated with the mesangial cells.

DIAGNOSIS

In order to diagnose LCDD definitively, a kidney biopsy is essential.[64] Because pathologic deposition is often subtle and not easily recognized, particularly in the earliest stages of disease, it is most important that the specimen be examined by a nephropathologist who has a special interest and expertise in this disorder. The procedure can be safely performed under computed tomography guidance. A sufficient amount of tissue should be obtained for light- and electron-microscopic examination and for immunohistochemical studies. Two specimens are required. One is fixed in Carson Millonig's solution for routine staining (hematoxylin–eosin, periodic acid Schiff (PAS), trichrome, Jones silver–methenamine, and Congo red or Thioflavin T), immunoperoxidase analyses (if needed), and electron microscopy. The second is placed in Michel's or Zeus' transport medium for immunofluorescence studies.

There are pitfalls in diagnosing LCDD: the lesion most often seen in renal biopsies – nodular glomerulosclerosis – may also be found in diabetic nephropathy and, in some instances, in other nodular glomerulopathies such as type I or type II membranoproliferative glomerulonephritis (dense deposit disease) and in amyloidosis.[37,64] Through the use of electron microscopy and immunoelectron microscopy, LCDD can be differentiated from these other entities by demonstration that the pathognomonic punctate protein deposits are present and are monoclonal (κ or λ). However, the monotypic nature of this material can be obscured by the presence of entrapped normal Ig. This problem can be obviated through the use of serially diluted anti-light-chain antisera, where the reactivity of such reagents with confounding proteins becomes diminished while that of the pathologically deposited Ig is maintained. We have found that the use of the immunofluorescence versus the immunoperoxidase technique to establish light-chain monoclonality often results in less 'background' staining. Further, structural modifications of the deposited protein may render the molecule undetectable by commercial antisera. In this situation, the diagnosis of LCDD must be made solely on the basis of morphologic criteria. In those instances where nodular glomerulosclerosis is not a prominent feature, monoclonal light-chain deposits can be visualized in the tubular interstitial and vascular compartments. Recognition of this form of pathologic light-chain deposition may require detailed analyses such as immunoelectron microscopy that can only be performed in specialized laboratories.

The diagnosis of LCDD can also be inferred from detection in skin biopsies of the characteristic electron-dense, punctate monoclonal light-chain deposits in the dermal–epidermal junction.[47]

Often, pathologic light-chain renal deposits typical of LCDD are detected unexpectedly in kidney biopsies performed on patients with unexplained proteinuria or renal insufficiency. In these situations, the diagnosis of this monoclonal Ig plasma cell dyscrasia is made retrospectively through examination of bone marrow, blood, and urine specimens.

The presence in the bone marrow of monoclonal plasma cells is a characteristic feature of LCDD as well as myeloma, AL amyloidosis, and adult Fanconi syndrome. In myeloma, the percentage of plasma cells is usually high (> 20%), and therefore it is not difficult to document their monoclonal nature. In contrast, this percentage is usually low (<5%) in LCDD, and consequently the bone marrow is reported as 'normal'. To establish monoclonality in such cases, immunophenotyping analyses should be performed on cytospin preparations where the number of plasma cells has been enriched by sedimentation through polysucrose/sodium diatrizoate (Histopaque-1077, Sigma Diagnostics, St Louis, MO). For these studies, highly specific anti-light-chain reagents or those that have V_L subgroup reactivity are required (Figure 29.5).[65]

Another typical diagnostic feature of LCDD and other monoclonal plasma cell disorders is the finding of homogeneous serum and/or urinary Ig-related M proteins. These can be identified using analytical methods, such as agarose gel and immunofixation electrophoresis, that are readily available in clinical laboratories. It should be noted that Bence Jones proteinuria is frequently unrecognized in cases where the amount excreted is low (<0.3 mg/ml) or is obscured by transferrin or other 'serum' proteins, as occurs in nephrosis. In this situation, the urine sample must be concentrated at least 10- to 20-fold prior to analysis (Figure 29.6). However, because of the extreme sensitivity of immunofixation, free polyclonal light chains can also be detected. They appear not as a single but as multiple, closely spaced bands, most commonly κ-type, and should not be misconstrued as Bence Jones proteins. This pattern has been referred to as a 'ladder' configuration, and can be found in specimens obtained from apparently normal individuals.[66]

The concentration of serum or urinary M components can be determined by densitometric

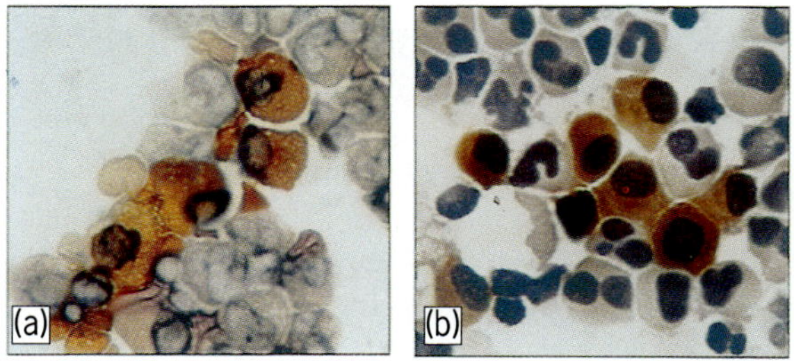

Figure 29.5 Immunophenotyping analysis of LCDD-associated bone marrow specimen: plasma cells containing monoclonal κ light chains. Reactivity with anti-free-κ (a) and anti-$V_\kappa 4$ (b) subgroup-specific monoclonal antibodies; immunoperoxidase technique, original magnification x400.

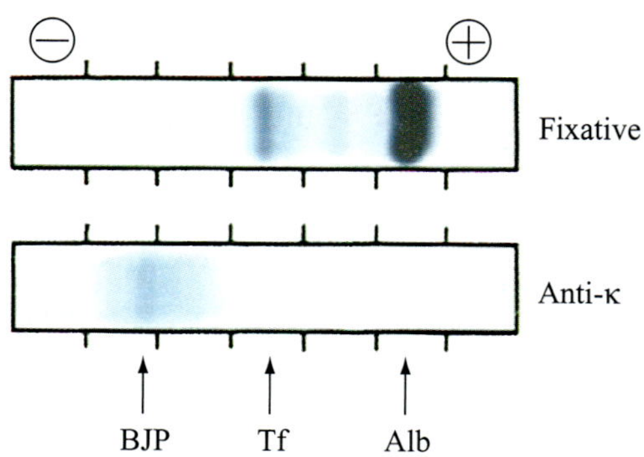

Figure 29.6 Bence Jones proteinuria in LCDD: immunofixation analyses of a reconstituted (50 mg/ml) lyophilized urine specimen obtained from a patient with LCDD. The locations of the κ Bence Jones protein (BJP), transferrin (Tf), and albumin (Alb) are as indicated.

analyses of proteins separated by agarose gel electrophoresis, or, alternatively, through nephelometry or serologic techniques utilizing specific anti-heavy-chain or anti-light-chain antibodies. Such measurements are necessary to document response to therapy or relapse.

TREATMENT

Owing to the pre-eminent role of monoclonal Igs in the pathogenesis of LCDD, major therapeutic efforts have been directed towards reducing or eliminating the synthesis of these components.[67] This can best be achieved by chemotherapeutic regimens that are effective in myeloma, such as melphalan–prednisone (MP), vincristine–doxorubicin–dexamethasone (VAD), and high-dose dexamethasone.[68] A more complete and sustained suppression of monoclonal Ig synthesis has been achieved with even larger doses of chemotherapy in conjunction with autologous/allogeneic hematopoietic stem cell transplantation.[69,70] Plasmapheresis could be an effective, albeit temporary, measure for patients in whom rapid reduction in the concentration of circulating Bence Jones proteins is deemed essential, such as those with acute renal failure.[71] Because factors in addition to pathologic M-component deposits can adversely affect kidney function in patients with LCDD, hypercalcemia, electrolyte imbalance, anemia, and infection should be treated appropriately.

Although certain forms of pathologic Ig deposits, such as cast nephropathy, may be reversible, the nephropathology found in patients with LCDD rarely regresses.[3,7] Invariably, there is a progressive worsening of renal (and other organ) function that leads to oliguric kidney failure requiring dialysis. Such patients should be considered candidates for renal transplantation if, after a year, they meet acceptable medical criteria, including disease stability and no evidence of clinically significant extrarenal deposition.[72] Recurrence of pathologic deposits in the transplanted kidney is less likely if monoclonal Ig production has been suppressed by chemotherapy. After transplantation, it is important to test urine specimens periodically for the reappearance of monoclonal protein and to reinstitute chemotherapy if necessary.

Other treatment strategies currently under study are those directed towards suppression of plasma cell proliferation by immune- or gene-mediated therapy.[73] New approaches will include the development of compounds that can inhibit the binding of monoclonal Igs to basement membranes. For example, TGF-β, which plays a role in mediating glomerulosclerosis in LCDD,[74] could be a potential target.[75] The identification of compounds that can inhibit the formation or effect resolution of pathologic protein aggregates may also prove beneficial.

ACKNOWLEDGEMENTS

We thank Valerie Brestel and Lolita Davis for manuscript preparation. This work was supported in part by USPS Research Grant CA10056 from the US National Cancer Institute (AS) and Grant 6198–98 from the Leukemia Society of America (GAH). AS is an American Cancer Society Clinical Research Professor.

REFERENCES

1. Gallo G, Picken M, Buxbaum J, Frangione B. The spectrum of monoclonal immunoglobulin deposition disease associated with immunocytic dyscrasias. *Semin Hematol* 1989; **26**: 234–45.
2. Buxbaum JN, Chuba JV, Hellman GC et al. Monoclonal immunoglobulin deposition disease: light chain and light and heavy chain deposition diseases and their relation to light chain amyloidosis. Clinical features, immunopathology, and molecular analysis. *Ann Intern Med* 1990; **112**: 455–64.
3. Buxbaum J. Mechanisms of disease: monoclonal immunoglobulin deposition. Amyloidosis, light chain deposition disease, and light and heavy chain deposition disease. *Hematol Oncol Clin North Am* 1992; **6**: 323–46.

4. Sanders PW, Herrera GA. Monoclonal immunoglobulin light chain-related renal diseases. *Semin Nephrol* 1993; **13**: 324–41.
5. Dhodapkar MV, Merlini G, Solomon A. Biology and therapy of immunoglobulin deposition diseases. *Hematol Oncol Clin North Am* 1997; **11**: 89–110.
6. Cohen AH. The kidney in plasma cell dyscrasias: Bence-Jones cast nephropathy and light chain deposit disease. *Am J Kidney Dis* 1998; **32**: 529–32.
7. Gallo GR, Lazowski P, Kumar A et al. Renal and cardiac manifestations of B-cell dyscrasias with nonamyloidotic monoclonal light chain and light and heavy chain deposition diseases. *Adv Nephrol Necker Hosp* 1998; **28**: 355–82.
8. Pozzi C, Fogazzi GB, Banfi G et al. Renal disease and patient survival in light chain deposition disease. *Clin Nephrol* 1995; **43**: 281–7.
9. Randall RE, Williamson WC Jr, Mullinax F et al. Manifestations of systemic light chain deposition. *Am J Med* 1976; **60**: 293–9.
10. Staros E, Katz SM. Myocardial necrosis in light chain deposition. *Am Heart J* 1985; **110**: 1295–6.
11. Peng SK, French WJ, Cohen AH, Fausel RE. Light chain cardiomyopathy associated with small-vessel disease. *Arch Pathol Lab Med* 1988; **112**: 844–6.
12. McAllister HA Jr, Seger J, Bossart M, Ferrans VJ. Restrictive cardiomyopathy with κ light chain deposits in myocardium as a complication of multiple myeloma. Histochemical and electron microscopic observations. *Arch Pathol Lab Med* 1988; **112**: 1151–4.
13. Gallo G, Goñi F, Boctor F et al. Light chain cardiomyopathy. Structural analysis of the light chain tissue deposits. *Am J Pathol* 1996; **148**: 1397–1406.
14. Klein R, Jaenichen R, Zachau HG. Expressed human immunoglobulin κ genes and their hypermutation. *Eur J Immunol* 1993; **23**: 3248–62.
15. Kawasaki K, Minoshima S, Nakato E et al, One-megabase sequence analysis of the human immunoglobulin λ gene locus. *Genome Res* 1997; **7**: 250–61.
16. Solomon A, Weiss DT. Protein and host factors implicated in the pathogenesis of light chain amyloidosis (AL amyloidosis). *Int J Exp Clin Invest* 1995; **2**: 269–79.
17. Buxbaum J. Aberrant immunoglobulin synthesis in light chain amyloidosis. Free light chain and light chain fragment production by human bone marrow cells in short-term tissue culture. *J Clin Invest* 1986; **78**: 798–806.
18. Stevens FJ, Solomon A, Schiffer M. Bence Jones proteins: a powerful tool for the fundamental study of protein chemistry and pathophysiology. *Biochemistry* 1991; **30:** 6803–5.
19. Solomon A, Waldmann TA, Fahey JL, McFarlane AS. Metabolism of Bence Jones proteins. *J Clin Invest* 1964; **43**: 103–17.
20. Waldmann TA, Strober W, Mogielnicki RP. The renal handling of low molecular weight proteins. II. Disorders of serum protein catabolism in patients with tubular proteinuria, the nephrotic syndrome, or uremia. *J Clin Invest* 1972; **51**: 2162–74.
21. Coward RA, Delamore IW, Mallick NP, Robinson EL. The importance of urinary immunoglobulin light chain isoelectric point (p*I*) in nephrotoxicity in multiple myeloma. *Clin Sci* 1984; **66**: 229–32.
22. Bellotti V, Merlini G, Bucciarelli E et al. Relevance of class, molecular weight and isoelectric point in predicting human light chain amyloidogenicity. *Br J Haematol* 1990; **74**: 65–69.
23. Herrera GA. Low molecular weight proteins and the kidney: physiological and pathologic considerations. *Ultrastruct Pathol* 1994; **18**: 89–98.
24. Batuman V, Guan S. Receptor-mediated endocytosis of immunoglobulin light chains by renal proximal tubule cells. *Am J Physiol* 1997; **272**: F521–30.
25. Batuman V, Verroust PJ, Navar GL et al. Myeloma light chains are ligands for cubilin (gp 280). *Am J Physiol* 1998; **275**: F246–54.
26. Sanders PW, Herrera GA, Galla JH. Human Bence Jones protein toxicity in rat proximal tubule epithelium in vivo. *Kidney Int* 1987; *32*: 851–61.
27. Sanders PW, Herrera GA, Chen A et al. Differential nephrotoxicity of low molecular weight proteins including Bence Jones proteins in the perfused rat nephron in vivo. *J Clin Invest* 1988; **82**: 2086–96.
28. Solomon A, Weiss DT, Kattine AA. Nephrotoxic potential of Bence Jones proteins. *N Engl J Med* 1991; **324**: 1845–51.
29. Abe M, Goto T, Kosaka M et al. Differences in kappa to lambda (κ : λ) ratios of serum and urinary free light chains. *Clin Exp Immunol* 1998; **111**: 457–62.
30. Denoroy L, Deret S, Aucouturier P. Over-representation of the VκIV subgroup in light chain deposition disease. *Immunol Lett* 1994; **42**: 63–6.

31. Rocca A, Khamlichi AA, Touchard G et al. Sequences of VκI subgroup light chains in Fanconi's syndrome. Light chain V region gene usage restriction and peculiarities in myeloma-associated Fanconi's syndrome. *J Immunol* 1995; **155**: 3245–52.
32. Stevens FJ, Weiss DT, Solomon A. Structural basis of light chain-related pathology. In: *Antibodies*, Vol 5 (Capra JD, Zanetti M, eds). Langhorne, PA: Gordon & Breach, 1999: 175–208.
33. Cogne M, Preud'homme JL, Bauwens M et al. Structure of a monoclonal kappa chain of the VκIV subgroup in the kidney and plasma cells in light chain deposition disease. *J Clin Invest* 1991; **87**: 2186–90.
34. Khamlichi AA, Aucouturier P, Silvain C et al. Primary structure of a monoclonal κ chain in myeloma with light chain deposition disease. *Clin Exp Immunol* 1992; **87**: 122–6.
35. Stevens FJ, Myatt EA, Chang CH et al. A molecular model for self-assembly of amyloid fibrils: immunoglobulin light chains. *Biochemistry* 1995; **34**: 10697–702.
36. Preud'homme JL, Aucouturier P, Touchard G et al. Monoclonal immunoglobulin deposition disease (Randall type). Relationship with structural abnormalities of immunoglobulin chains. *Kidney Int* 1994; **46**: 965–72.
37. Sanders PW, Herrera GA, Kirk KA et al. Spectrum of glomerular and tubulointerstitial renal lesions associated with monotypical immunoglobulin light chain deposition. *Lab Invest* 1991; **64**: 527–37.
38. Picken MM, Shen S. Immunoglobulin light chains and the kidney: an overview. *Ultrastruct Pathol* 1994; **18**: 105–12.
39. Herrera GA, Paul R, Turbat-Herrera EA et al. Ultrastructural immunolabeling in the diagnosis of light chain-related renal disease. *Pathol Immunopathol Res* 1986; **5**: 170–87.
40. Silver MM, Hearn SA, Walton JC et al. Immunogold quantitation of immunoglobulin light chains in renal amyloidosis and κ light chain nephropathy. *Am J Pathol* 1990; **136**: 997–1007.
41. Herrera GA, Sanders PW, Reddy BV et al. Ultrastructural immunolabeling: a unique diagnostic tool in monoclonal light chain-related renal diseases. *Ultrastruct Pathol* 1994; **18**: 401–16.
42. Sanders PW, Herrera GA, Lott RL, Galla JH. Morphologic alterations of the proximal tubules in light chain-related renal disease. *Kidney Int* 1988; **33**: 881–9.
43. Strom EH, Fogazzi GB, Banfi G et al. Light chain deposition disease of the kidney. Morphological aspects in 24 patients. *Virchows Arch* 1994; **425**: 271–80.
44. Ganeval D, Noël LH, Preud'homme JL et al. Light-chain deposition disease: its relation with AL-type amyloidosis. *Kidney Int* 1984; **26**: 1–9.
45. Jacquot C, Saint-Andre JP, Touchard G et al. Association of systemic light-chain deposition disease and amyloidosis: a report of three patients with renal involvement. *Clin Nephrol* 1985; **24**: 93–8.
46. Kaplan B, Vidal R, Kumar A et al. Amino-terminal identity of co-existant amyloid and non-amyloid immunoglobulin kappa light chain deposits. A human disease to study alterations of protein conformation. *Clin Exp Immunol* 1997; **110**: 472–8.
47. Picken MM, Gallo GR. Non-invasive diagnosis of light chain depostion disease. In: *Amyloid and Amyloidosis* (Kisilevesky R, Benson MD, Frangione B et al, eds). London: Parthenon, 1993: 226–8.
48. Clyne DH, Pollak VE. Renal handling and pathophysiology of Bence Jones proteins. *Contrib Nephrol* 1981; **24**: 78–87.
49. Smolens P, Venkatachalam M, Stein JH. Myeloma kidney cast nephropathy in a rat model of multiple myeloma. *Kidney Int* 1983; **24**: 192–204.
50. Smolens P, Barnes JL, Stein JH. Effect of chronic administration of different Bence Jones proteins on rat kidney. *Kidney Int* 1986; **30**: 874–82.
51. Myatt EA, Westholm FA, Weiss DT et al. Pathogenic potential of human monoclonal immunoglobulin light chains: relationship of in vitro aggregation to in vivo organ deposition. *Proc Natl Acad Sci USA* 1994; **91**: 3034–8.
52. Khamlichi AA, Rocca A, Touchard G et al. Role of light chain variable region in myeloma with light chain deposition disease: Evidence from an experimental model. *Blood* 1995; **86**: 3655–9.
53. Solomon A, Weiss DT, Williams TK. Experimental model of human light-chain-associated disease. *Curr Top Microbiol Immunol* 1992; **182**: 261–7.
54. Hurle MR, Helms LR, Li L et al. A role for destabilizing amino acid replacements in light-chain amyloidosis. *Proc Natl Acad Sci USA* 1994; **91**: 5446–50.
55. Stevens PW, Raffen R, Hanson DK et al. Recombinant immunoglobulin variable domains generated from synthetic genes provide a system for in vitro characterization of light-chain amyloid proteins. *Protein Sci* 1995; **4**: 421–32.

56. Helms LR, Wetzel R. Specificity of abnormal assembly in immunoglobulin light chain deposition disease and amyloidosis. *J Mol Biol* 1996; **257**: 77–86.
57. Wetzel R. Domain stability in immunoglobulin light chain deposition disorders. *Adv Protein Chem* 1997; **50**: 183–242.
58. Huang ZQ, Sanders PW. Biochemical interaction between Tamm–Horsfall glycoprotein and Ig light chains in the pathogenesis of cast nephropathy. *Lab Invest* 1995; **73**: 810–17.
59. Zhu L, Herrera GA, Murphy-Ullrich JE et al. Pathogenesis of glomerulosclerosis in light chain deposition disease. Role for transforming growth factor-β. *Am J Pathol* 1995; **147**: 375–85.
60. Herrera GA, Russell WJ, Isaac J et al. Glomerulopathic light chain–mesangial cell interactions modulate in vitro extracellular matrix remodeling and reproduce mesangiopathic findings documented in vivo. *Ulstruct Pathol* 1999; **23**: 107–26.
61. Zhu L, Herrera GA, White CR, Sanders PW. Immunoglobulin light chain alters mesangial cell calcium homeostasis. *Am J Physiol* 1997; **272**: F319–F24.
62. Turbat-Herrera EA, Isaac J, Sanders PW et al. Integrated expression of glomerular extracellular matrix proteins and beta 1 integrins in monoclonal light-chain related renal diseases. *Mod Pathol* 1997; **10**: 485–95.
63. Bruneval P, Foidart JM, Nochy D et al. Glomerular matrix proteins in nodular glomerulosclerosis in association with light chain deposition disease and diabetes mellitus. *Hum Pathol* 1985; **16**: 477–84.
64. Isaac J, Herrera GA. Renal biopsy as a primary diagnostic tool in plasma cell dyscrasias. *Pathol Case Rev* 1998; **3**: 183–9.
65. Abe M, Goto T, Kennel SJ et al. Production and immunodiagnostic applications of anti human light chain monoclonal antibodies. *Am J Clin Pathol* 1993; **100**: 67–74.
66. Harrison HH. The 'ladder light chain' or 'pseudo-oligoclonal' protein in urinary immunofixation electrophoresis (IFE) studies: a distinctive IFE pattern and an exploratory hypothesis relating it to free polyclonal light chains. *Clin Chem* 1991; **37**: 1559–64.
67. Heilman RL, Velosa JA, Holley KE et al. Long-term follow-up and response to chemotherapy in patients with light-chain deposition disease. *Am J Kidney Dis* 1992; **20**: 34–41.
68. Alexanian R, Dimopoulos MA. Management of multiple myeloma. *Semin Hematol* 1995; **32**: 20–30.
69. Jagannath S, Vesole DH, Glenn L et al. Low-risk intensive therapy for multiple myeloma with combined autologous bone marrow and blood stem cell support. *Blood* 1992; **80**: 1666–72.
70. Attal M, Harousseau JL. Standard therapy versus autologous transplantation in multiple myeloma. *Hematol Oncol Clin North Am* 1997; **11**: 133–46.
71. Blade J, Fernandez-Llama P, Bosch F et al. Renal failure in multiple myeloma: presenting features and predictors of outcome in 94 patients from a single institution. *Arch Intern Med* 1998; **158**: 1889–93.
72. Gerlag PG, Koene RA, Berden JH. Renal transplantation in light chain nephropathy: case report and review of the literature. *Clin Nephrol* 1986; **25**: 101–4.
73. Teoh G, Chen L, Urashima M et al. Adenovirus vector-based purging of multiple myeloma cells. *Blood* 1998; **92**: 4591–601.
74. Border WA, Nobel NA. TGF-β in kidney fibrosis: a target for gene therapy. *Kidney Int* 1997; **51**: 1388–96.
75. Lipkowitz MS, Klotman ME, Bruggeman LA et al. Molecular therapy for renal diseases. *Am J Kidney Dis* 1996; **28**: 475–92.

Index

Notes: Page references in bold refer to topics which appear only in figures or captions. Page references in italics refer to topics in tables only. Abbreviations used in subheadings are: FISH = fluorescence in situ hybridization; HIV = human immunodeficiency virus; IFN = interferon; IL-6 = interleukin-6; KSHV = Kaposi sarcoma-associated herpesvirus; MAPK = mitogen-activated protein kinase; MGUS = monoclonal gammopathy of undetermined significance; MP = melphalan–prednisone; M protein = monoclonal protein; MRI = magnetic resonance imaging; PCD = plasma cell disorder; PCLI = plasma cell labeling index; SKY = spectral karyotyping; SPB = solitary plasmacytoma of bone; TBI = total-body irradiation; vFLIP = viral FLICE-inhibitory protein.